3D Diagnosis and Treatment Planning in Orthodontics

Jean-Marc Retrouvey • Mohamed-Nur Abdallah
Editors

3D Diagnosis and Treatment Planning in Orthodontics

An Atlas for the Clinician

Springer

Editors
Jean-Marc Retrouvey
Leo Rogers Endowed Chair and Professor
Department of Orthodontics
University Missouri Kansas City
Kansas City, MO
USA

Mohamed-Nur Abdallah
Department of Orthodontics
School of Dentistry
University of Detroit Mercy
Detroit, MI
USA

ISBN 978-3-030-57222-8 ISBN 978-3-030-57223-5 (eBook)
https://doi.org/10.1007/978-3-030-57223-5

This Springer imprint is published by the registered company Springer Nature Switzerland AG
The registered company address is: Gewerbestrasse 11, 6330 Cham, Switzerland

Introduction

Diagnostic and treatment planning are very important tools in orthodontic treatment and are used prior to initiating any type of comprehensive treatment by the majority of orthodontists. New advent in digital technology and increased needs for more accurate diagnostic tools in orthodontically related issues such as complex adult treatment, TMJ dysfunctions, or sleep disturbances have shown that our conventional 2D diagnostic may not be sufficient to correctly diagnose and treatment plan these problems.

This book will present the most up-to-date diagnostic tools to better identify and treatment plan malocclusions with cone beam CT, intraoral scans, and MRI as well as present software that allow for combining these technologies to obtain the most accurate diagnostic and guide the busy practitioner in designing the most appropriate biomechanical approach to address these malocclusions.

Contents

Contributors

Reinaldo Abdala-Junior, DDS, MSc Department of Radiology, UniFSP, Avaré, SP, Brazil

School of Dentistry, University of São Paulo, São Paulo, Brazil

Mohamed-Nur Abdallah, BDS, MSc, PhD Department of Orthodontics, School of Dentistry, University of Detroit Mercy, Detroit, MI, USA

Asta Abunevičiūtė, DDS, MDS Private Practice, Vilnius, Lithuania

BIOMEDE (International Association for Development and Spread of Orthodontic Biomechanics Knowledge), Lugano, Switzerland

Walaa Magdy Ahmed, BDS, MSc, Dip Pros, PhD, FRCD(C) Department of Restorative Dentistry, Faculty of Dentistry, King Abdulaziz University, Jeddah, Saudi Arabia

Faculty of Dentistry, University of British Columbia, Vancouver, BC, Canada

Bassam Alalola, BDS, MSc, FRCD(C), ABO College of Dentistry, King Saud bin Abdulaziz University for Health Sciences, Riyadh, Saudi Arabia

King Abdullah International Medical Research Center, Riyadh, Saudi Arabia

Mohammed Alsaloum, BDS, MSc, Dip (Pros), FRCD(C) College of Dentistry, King Saud bin Abdulaziz University for Health Sciences, Riyadh, Saudi Arabia

King Abdullah International Medical Research Center, Riyadh, Saudi Arabia

Emad Eddin Alzoubi, BDS, MOrth RCS, MOrth RCPS, MFDS Department of Child Dental Health and Orthodontics, Faculty of Dental Surgery, University of Malta, Msida, Malta

Department of Restorative Dentistry, Faculty of Dental Surgery, University of Malta, Msida, Malta

James Andrew Faculty of Dentistry, University of British Columbia, Vancouver, BC, Canada

Normand Boucher, DDS Department of Orthodontics, University of Pennsylvania, Philadelphia, PA, USA

Marco Caminiti, DDS, Med, FRCDC (OMFS) Oral and Maxillofacial Surgery, Faculty of Dentistry, University of Toronto, Toronto, ON, Canada

Oral and Maxillofaical Surgery, Humber River Hospital, Toronto, ON, Canada

Jaw Deformity Clinic, Holland Bloorview Kids Rehabilitation Hospital, Toronto, ON, Canada

Arthur Rodriguez Gonzalez Cortes, DDS, MSc, PhD Department of Dental Surgery, Faculty of Dental Surgery, University of Malta, Msida, Malta

Hakan El, DDS, PhD School of Dental Medicine—Department of Orthodontics, Hacettepe University, Ankara, Turkey

Manhal Eliliwi, DDS School of Dental Medicine—Department of Orthodontics, Case Western Reserve University, Cleveland, OH, USA

Tarek Elshebiny, BDS, MSD School of Dental Medicine—Department of Orthodontics, Case Western Reserve University, Cleveland, OH, USA

Giorgio Fiorelli, MD, DMD Orthodontic Department, University of Siena, Siena, Italy

BIOMEDE (International Association for Development and Spread of Orthodontic Biomechanics Knowledge), Lugano, Switzerland

Marius Hack, BSc, PhD Hack Dental, Răzvad, Romania

John Kaku, DDS, MSD Private Practice, Tokyo, Japan

Suzanne Lacombe Department of Orthodontics, University of Missouri Kansas City, Kansas City, MO, USA

Luca Lombardo, DDS, MDS Ferrara University, Ferrara, Italy

Tiantong Lou, DMD, MSc, FRCDC (Ortho) Private Practice, Toronto, ON, Canada

Giuliano Bortolo Maino, DDS, MDS Ferrara University, Ferrara, Italy

Kensuke Matsumoto, DMD, MSc Department of Periodontics and Orthodontics, University of Pennsylvania, Philadelphia, PA, USA

Muralidhar Mupparapu, DMD, MDS, Dip.ABOMR Division of Oral and Maxillofacial Radiology Department of oral Medicine, University of Pennsylvania, Philadelphia, PA, USA

Juliana No-Cortes, DDS, MSc Department of Restorative Dentistry, Faculty of Dental Surgery, University of Malta, Msida, Malta

Juan Martin Palomo, DDS, MSD School of Dental Medicine—Department of Orthodontics, Case Western Reserve University, Cleveland, OH, USA

Mario Palone, DDS, MDS Ferrara University, Ferrara, Italy

Nearchos Panayi, DDS, MSc, PhD Medical School of Athens, National and Kapodistrian University of Athens, Athens, Greece

Emanuele Paoletto Ferrara University, Ferrara, Italy

Fernando Pugliese School of Dental Medicine—Department of Orthodontics, Case Western Reserve University, Cleveland, OH, USA

Jean-Marc Retrouvey, DMD, MSc Leo Rogers Endowed Chair and Professor, Department of Orthodontics, University Missouri Kansas City, Kansas City, MO, USA

Shadi Samawi, BDS, MMedSci(Orth), MOrth RCSED Samawi Dental and Orthodontic Center—SDOC, Amman, Jordan

Franklin She Tsang Tsang, BDS, MOrth, MOrthRCS, FHKAM Orthodontics, Faculty of Dentistry, The University of Hong Kong, Hong Kong, China

BIOMEDE (International Association for Development and Spread of Orthodontic Biomechanics Knowledge), Lugano, Switzerland

Giuseppe Siciliani, DMD, MDS Ferrara University, Ferrara, Italy

Neda Stefanovic, DDS, MSc, PhD Faculty of Dental Medicine—Department of Orthodontics, University of Belgrade, Belgrade, Serbia

Apostolos Tsolakis, DDS, MSD, PhD Department of Orthodontics, Faculty of Dentistry, National and Kapodistrian University of Athens, Athens, Greece

Yona R. Vandersluis, BSc, DDS, MSc (Ortho), FRCD(C) Discipline of Orthodontics, Faculty of Dentistry, University of Toronto, Toronto, ON, Canada

Sivabalan Vasudavan, BDSc, MDSc, MPH, MOrth RCS Private Practice, Perth, WA, Australia

Tyler Verhaeghe, DDS, MEd Faculty of Dentistry, University of British Columbia, Vancouver, BC, Canada

Reviewers

Mohamed-Nur Abdallah, BDS, MSc, PhD Department of Orthodontics, School of Dentistry, University of Detroit Mercy, Detroit, MI, USA

Walaa Magdy Ahmed, BDS, MSc, Dip Pros, PhD, FRCD(C) Department of Restorative Dentistry, Faculty of Dentistry, King Abdulaziz University, Jeddah, Saudi Arabia

Faculty of Dentistry, University of British Columbia, Vancouver, BC, Canada

Arthur Rodriguez Gonzalez Cortes, DDS, MSc, PhD Department of Dental Surgery, Faculty of Dental Surgery, University of Malta, Msida, Malta

Tiantong Lou, DMD, MSc, FRCDC (Ortho) Private Practice, Toronto, ON, Canada

Jean-Marc Retrouvey, DMD, MSc Leo Rogers Endowed Chair and Professor, Department of Orthodontics, University Missouri Kansas City, Kansas City, MO, USA

Shadi Samawi, BDS, MMedSci(Orth), MOrth RCSED Samawi Dental and Orthodontic Center—SDOC, Amman, Jordan

Yona R. Vandersluis, BSc, DDS, MSc (Ortho), FRCD(C) Discipline of Orthodontics, Faculty of Dentistry, University of Toronto, Toronto, ON, Canada

About the Editors

Jean-Marc Retrouvey, DMD, MSc, FRCD (C), is the Leo Rogers Endowed Chair of the Orthodontic Department at the University of Missouri Kansas City.

He is a RCDC (Royal College of Dentists of Canada) examiner, an NDEB advisor, member of the AAO, the American College of Dentists, The Angle East Society of Orthodontist, a Fellow in the Académie Dentaire du Quebec, and the past president of the Canadian Association of Orthodontists.

As a teacher, he has received the McGill Dental Society and the Wood, Katz and Silverstone awards for excellence in teaching. Dr. Retrouvey also received the Bravo award for his implication in teaching and research at McGill University. Dr. Retrouvey is also involved with HVO (Health Volunteer Overseas) in the development of blended teaching program for emerging countries and is president of the International Foundation for Dental Education, a nonprofit organization offering orthodontic course in developing countries.

He is the principal investigator (PI) for the NIH-supported research project dental aspect of the Longitudinal Study of Osteogenesis Imperfecta and was the PI for the "Dental Malocclusion and Craniofacial Development in OI." These research projects are conducted by the Brittle Bone Disease Consortium from the RDCRN network of the NIH and have been renewed for a second phase. He is now PI for the NIH-supported project: Use of clear aligner for the treatment of dental malocclusion in individuals with osteogenesis imperfecta types III and IV.

Mohamed-Nur Abdallah is a dental clinician and a biomaterial scientist. In addition to working in private practice, he is an Adjunct Associate Professor at the Division of Graduate Orthodontics at the University of Detroit Mercy and an Instructor at the Faculty of Dentistry/University of Toronto.

Dr. Abdallah obtained his dental degree from the University of Jordan and then worked as a general dentist for 3 years. He completed his first MSc degree focused on Biomaterials and his PhD in Craniofacial Health Sciences at McGill University in Canada. He then pursued an MSc/Orthodontic specialty program at the University of Toronto and worked as a graduate researcher at the Mt. Sinai Hospital (Lunenfeld-Tanenbaum Research Institute) in Toronto.

Dr. Abdallah received numerous academic scholarships and awards, including the Orthodontic & Craniofacial Clinical and Translational Research Award from International Association for Dental Research (IADR) as well as several Graduate Excellence Awards in Dentistry and the Southern Ontario Surgical Orthodontic Study Club Award for the best clinical presentation. So far, he has authored and coauthored more than 35 articles published in peer-reviewed journals and six book chapters as well as filed three patents.

Part I

Techniques Used in Orthodontic Diagnosis

1 Evolution of the Orthodontic Diagnosis in the Age of Artificial Intelligence

Jean-Marc Retrouvey, Nearchos Panayi, and Apostolos Tsolakis

1.1 The Objectives of an Orthodontic Diagnosis

Capturing diagnostic information to analyze the craniofacial complex is a demanding process in modern orthodontics. The craniofacial structures are highly organized with many vital functions and dynamic interactions. Breathing, mastication, swallowing, speech, and facial expressions are controlled by complex neuromuscular functions that must be in balance [1]. These interactions play a large role in the development of malocclusions but are still not well understood. They are also difficult to correlate with our current diagnostic methods [2, 3]. The temporomandibular joints are the most complex joints in our body. They are potentially associated with craniofacial dysfunctions but their imaging is currently not a routine part of a conventional orthodontic diagnosis [4], although dental models are sometimes mounted on a semi-adjustable articulator to give better 3D orientation of the dentition in relation to condylar position. All clinical information needed to obtain an accurate orthodontic diagnosis are not readily available with conventional records since malocclusions develop in three planes of space and may involve the entire craniofacial complex [5]. 3D imaging and advances in digital technologies have significantly increased the potential for integrating different formats of orthodontic records to enhance the accuracy of the orthodontic diagnosis process [6] (Fig. 1.1).

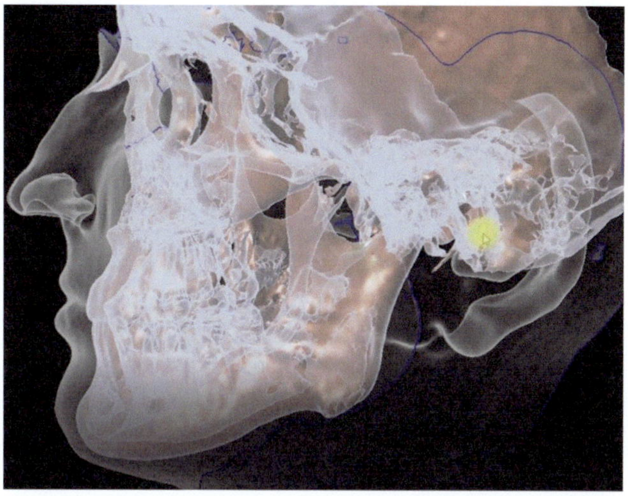

Fig. 1.1 Relationship between the dentition and the craniofacial complex

The goals for accurate orthodontic diagnoses are to record and analyze interactions between the dentition and surrounding craniofacial structures, and to obtain a problem list to formulate a treatment plan [7]. A large quantity of information is gathered from an orthodontic clinical examination, analyses of 2D radiographs and orthodontic study models, as well as other relevant records of a patient. These orthodontic records are usually taken in a static state [8, 9]. Consequently, these records only partially reflect the intricacies of craniofacial and dentoalveolar structures, and therefore limit their diagnostic power [10]. As traditional diagnosis and treatment planning procedures are usually performed without a patient being present, orthodontic records are aimed to faithfully replicate clinical presentations of a patient in order to facilitate these procedures [11]. To obtain an orthodontic diagnosis, most orthodontists still rely mainly on 2D radiographs such as a cephalogram [12] and a panoramic radiograph [13, 14],

J.-M. Retrouvey (✉)
Leo Rogers Endowed Chair and Professor, Department of Orthodontics, University Missouri Kansas City, Kansas City, MO, USA
e-mail: jean-marc.retrouvey@umkc.edu

N. Panayi
Medical School of Athens, National and Kapodistrian University of Athens, Athens, Greece

Private Orthodontist, Limassol, Cyprus
e-mail: dr.panayi@cytanet.com.cy

A. Tsolakis
Department of Orthodontics, Faculty of Dentistry, National and Kapodistrian University of Athens, Athens, Greece
e-mail: apostso@otenet.gr

J.-M. Retrouvey, M.-N. Abdallah (eds.), *3D Diagnosis and Treatment Planning in Orthodontics*,
https://doi.org/10.1007/978-3-030-57223-5_1

in addition to plaster dental casts which have been in use since the eighteenth century. Each element of these records provides orthodontists with a different type of information. Orthodontists combine all these data from clinical experiences and derive a differential diagnosis of the observed malocclusions. The process of recording a 3D structure on 2D radiograph causes a significant loss of data [15]. This is due to the fact that a conventional 2D radiograph is a mere "shadow" of a 3D object and provide only a partial or incomplete detail of projected structures. As a result, clinicians must always use their considerable skill and experience to "interpret" radiographs in a "forward propagation" method [16] in an attempt to arrive at an accurate diagnosis as each element of these conventional orthodontic records is variably formatted. They cannot be digitally integrated to recreate a virtual patient for the purpose of diagnosis and treatment planning. The inability of these conventional diagnostic tools to accurately portray malocclusion and its associated craniofacial structures in three dimensions may result in an incomplete diagnosis or a misdiagnosis [17, 18]. An integrable set of 3D orthodontic records recreating a real patient's anatomy and function is therefore desirable to increase diagnostic accuracy, and to ensure that a treatment option selected can be effectively implemented [19, 20] (Fig. 1.2).

For the past 15 years, significant changes have taken place in the field of orthodontic diagnosis. These changes include uses of digital photography, digital examination forms, cone beam radiography [21], digital dental models [22], and intraoral scanning. They have allowed for a large amount of clinical information to be gathered. The additional diagnostic information has opened new possibilities for orthodontists. Sequential records easily obtained with intraoral scanning, digital photography and radiography facilitate various treatment simulations and may further customize orthodontic treatment approaches, and even perform in-house 3D printing [23]. Despite these advances, there is still a significant paucity of knowledge required to optimize the use of 3D digital technologies for orthodontic records [24]. A recent data mining technology offers new possibilities to improve on orthodontic diagnostic process [25]. The goals of gathering and computing digital orthodontic data are:

1. To obtain the most accurate depiction of the patient's unique occlusal and craniofacial structures
2. To store the data efficiently
3. To simulate different treatment options
4. To formulate a final treatment plan
5. To compare the findings to other types of malocclusions
6. To facilitate an analysis of treatment progress
7. To plan for orthognathic surgery
8. To produce individualized and customized appliances
9. To communicate with other specialties (Figs. 1.3 and 1.4)

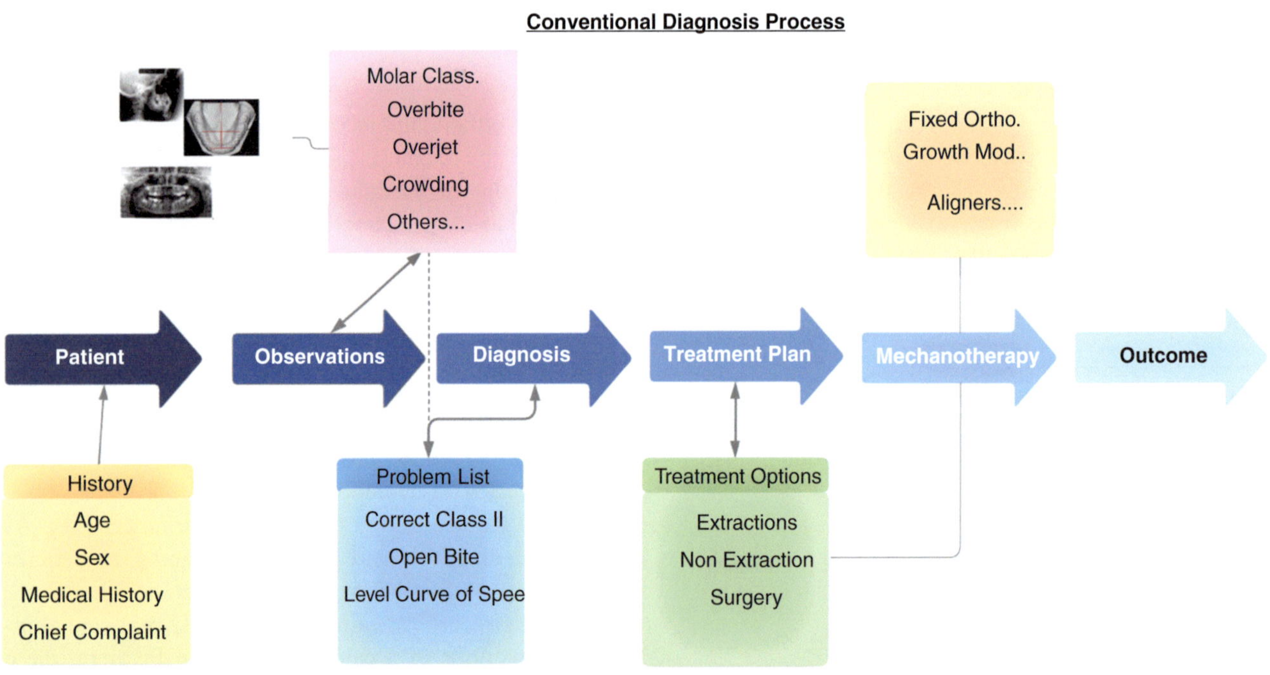

Fig. 1.2 A conventional "going forward" workflow to plan an orthodontic case. The process starts from a patient and stops at an outcome. No feedback loop is present

1.2 Evolution of the Orthodontic Record Overtime

1.2.1 Examination Form

Paper-based forms have been widely used to gather relevant patient information. They include a questionnaire, a medical history, recording of extra- and intraoral examination, and patient's chief complaints. These collected data are rarely reviewed during treatment and almost never incorporated into any database.

1.2.1.1 Dental Photographs

Dental photographs were introduced several decades ago [26]. Extraoral photographs provide valuable information on a patient's facial features while intraoral photographs record conditions and positions of teeth in relation to each other and to surrounding soft tissues [27]. Dental photographs are not quantifiable, unless properly calibrated. They mostly provide qualitative data used by most clinicians to validate their physical observation of patients [28] (Fig. 1.5).

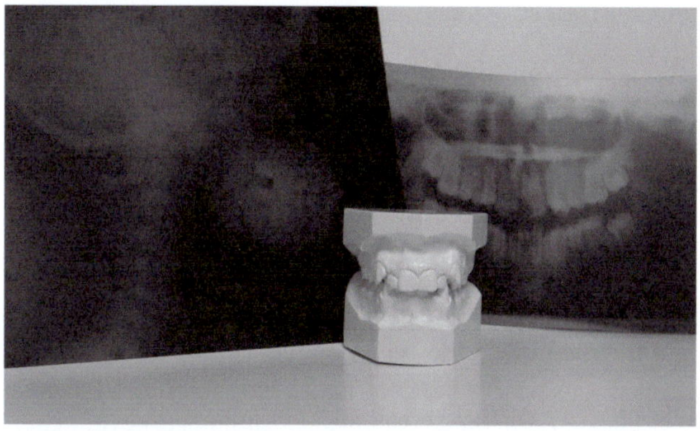

Fig. 1.3 Montage of diagnostic tools consisting of a panoramic radiograph, a cephalometric radiograph, and dental casts

1.2.1.2 Panoramic Radiographs

A panoramic radiograph is based on the concept of focal plane tomography as described by Pickens et al. [29]. Widely used in orthodontics, it enables clinicians to visualize all teeth present, temporomandibular joints, the alveolus, and other orofacial structures in a single radiograph [14]. For a routine diagnostic process, a panoramic radiograph offers several advantages including low costs and easy access. It dispenses low amount of radiation. It is considered more like a screening radiograph and does not allow for consistent and reliable measurements. Despite its benefits, the radiograph provides an incomplete rendering of the anatomy or pathology presented by a patient. Both false positive and negative interpretations occur frequently [30]. As an example, the following panoramic radiograph (Fig. 1.6) shows impacted canines but does not provide any spatial information or their relationship to the rest of the dentition [31]. The condition of the lateral incisor roots is also very challenging to assess. The use of Cone Beam Computed Tomography (CBCT) allows clinicians to accurately assess the condition of the lateral incisor roots (Fig. 1.7).

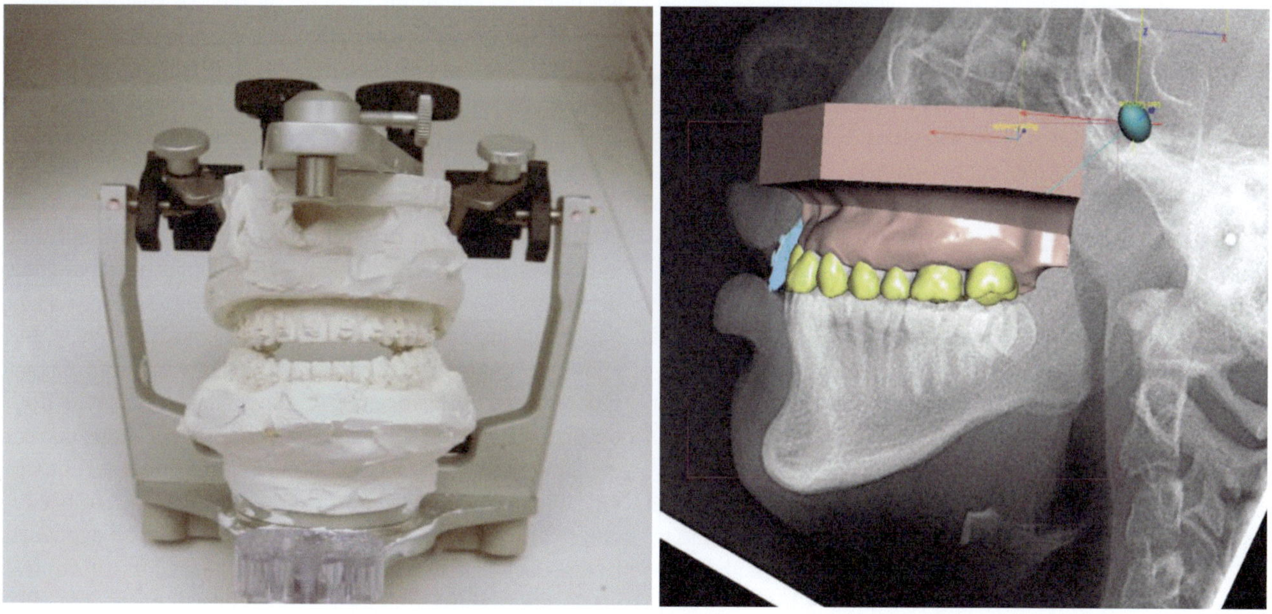

Fig. 1.4 Semi-adjustable articulator and virtual 3D articulator that allows an orientation of dental casts in space more accurately

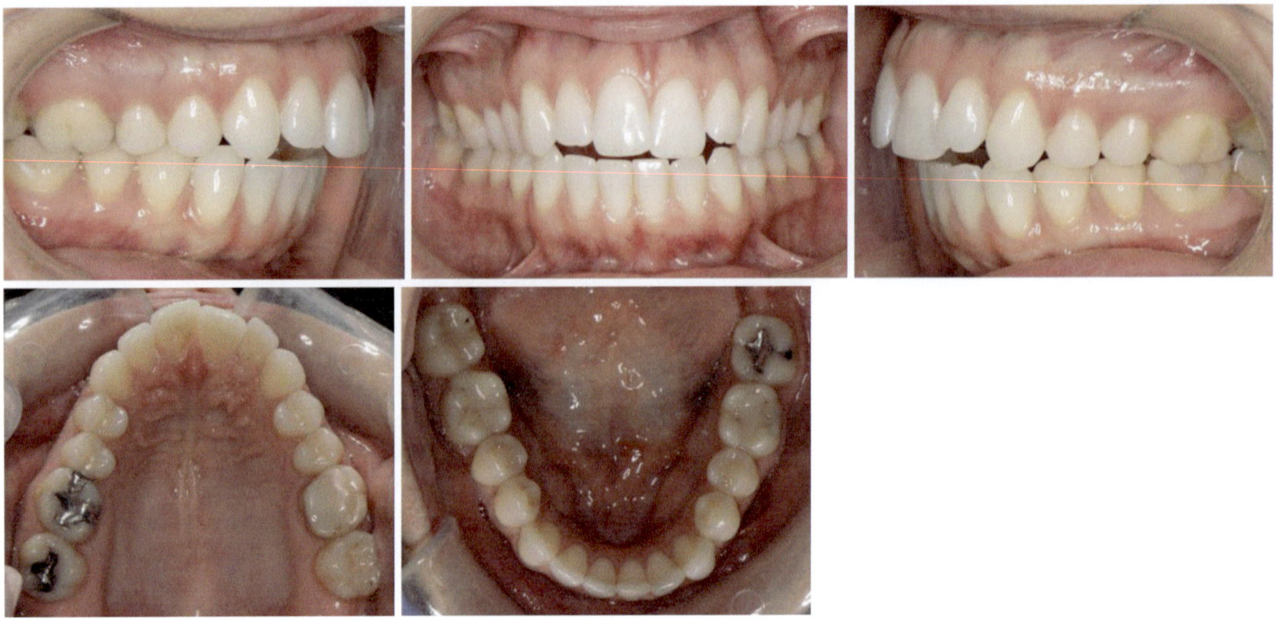

Fig. 1.5 Digital intraoral photographs

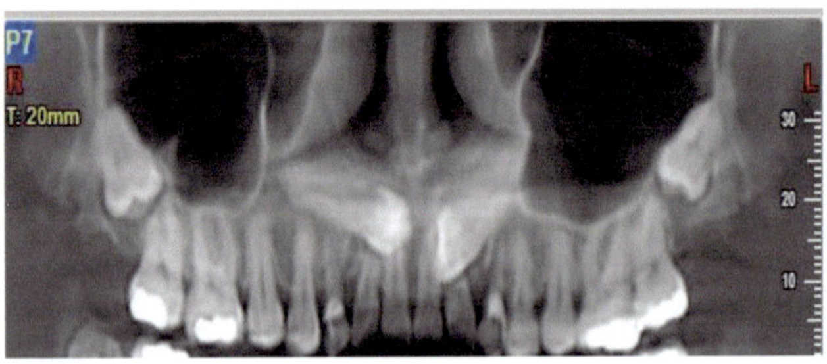

Fig. 1.6 Panoramic radiograph showing impacted canines

1.2.1.3 Cephalometric Radiograph

The lateral cephalogram depicts a projection of the entire craniofacial structures onto a sagittal 2D plane [32]. It is mainly used to perform cephalometric analyses to compare a patient's measurements to standard norms [33]. Cephalometric radiographs are very valuable in orthodontics as they provide a measurable assessment of maxilla, mandible, dentition, and their spatial relationships in the anteroposterior and vertical dimensions [34]. Anatomical structures such as the condyles, temporal fossa, and auditory meatus are sometimes more challenging to identify as they are not located on the mid-sagittal plane [35]. The 2D posteroanterior cephalogram is not commonly employed as a part of routine orthodontic records despite its usefulness in transverse analyses. This could be due to the fact that landmarks used in the aforementioned analyses are difficult to identify and reproduce [36] (Fig. 1.8).

1.2.1.4 Orthodontic Study Models

Orthodontic study models are usually composed of free-posteriorly standing maxillary and mandibular dental casts trimmed in a trimmed in centric occlusion relationship. They are traditionally made of plaster of Paris. They provide invaluable information on multiple parameters that influences orthodontic diagnosis and treatment planning [37]. The models are not three-dimensionally oriented to the surrounding craniofacial complex, particularly regarding the condylar position. They are useful to obtain information on relative spatial relationship of the dentition and allow for measurements of teeth and dentoalveolar structures. However, it is impossible using orthodontic study models to determine accurate root positions and their relations to surrounding dentoalveolar bones using orthodontic study models. It is also very tedious to perform a simulation of an orthodontic treatment plan on plaster models. Each simulation requires a considerable effort and time to achieve. In general, they have less diagnostic capabilities when compared to their digital counterparts [38] (Fig. 1.9).

In conclusion, the conventional diagnostic process has allowed orthodontists to obtain a reasonably accurate diagnosis in the past [39]. However, validity of the process with fragmented 2D records has often been challenged in this current digital era. The conventional orthodontic records do not significantly improve a diagnostic power despite a carefully conducted clinical examination [16, 39]. This could be explained by the fact that there may be a significant loss of clinical information from these disintegrated formats of records [40].

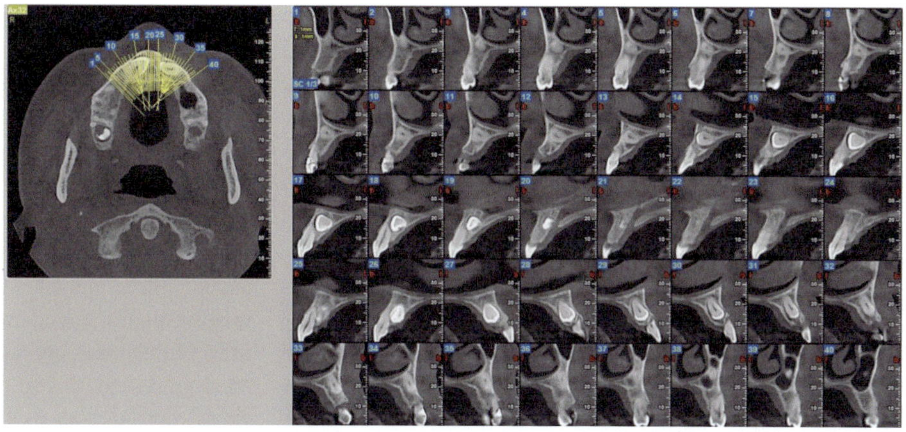

Fig. 1.7 Cone beam radiograph of same patient showing lateral incisor root resorption

	Value	Norm	Std Dev
SNA (°)	78.7	81.0	3.0
SNB (°)	71.9	78.0	3.0
ANB (°)	6.8	3.0	2.0
Facial Angle (FH-NPo) (°)	85.5	88.0	4.0
Wits Appraisal [Glupker]	-3.2	2.0	2.0
MP - SN (°)	47.3	33.0	3.0
Y-Axis (SGn-SN) (°)	75.6	60.0	4.0
U1 - NA (°)	23.2	23.0	6.0
L1 - NB (°)	32.4	27.5	5.0
Interincisal Angle (U1-L1	117.6	130.0	7.0
IMPA (L1-MP) (°)	693.3	91.4	4.0
Mandibular length (Co-G	109.8	122.3	4.0
Maxillary length (Co-A)	79.3	90.0	5.0

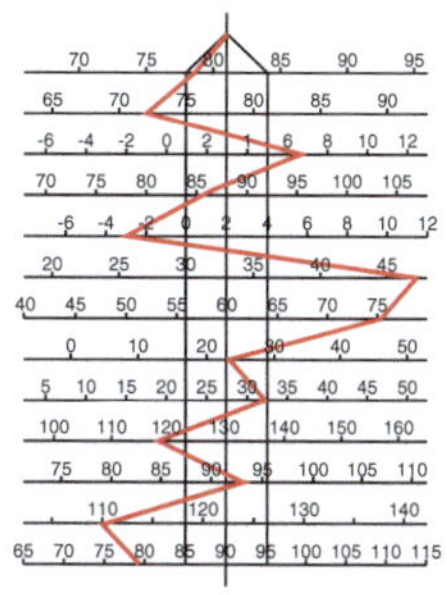

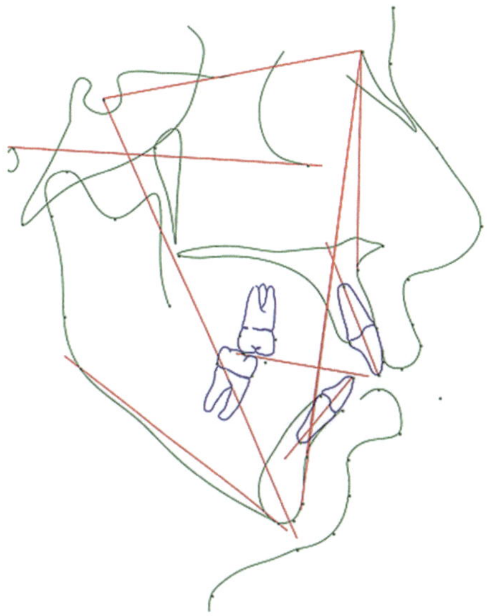

Fig. 1.8 Cephalometric tracing with a cephalometric analysis

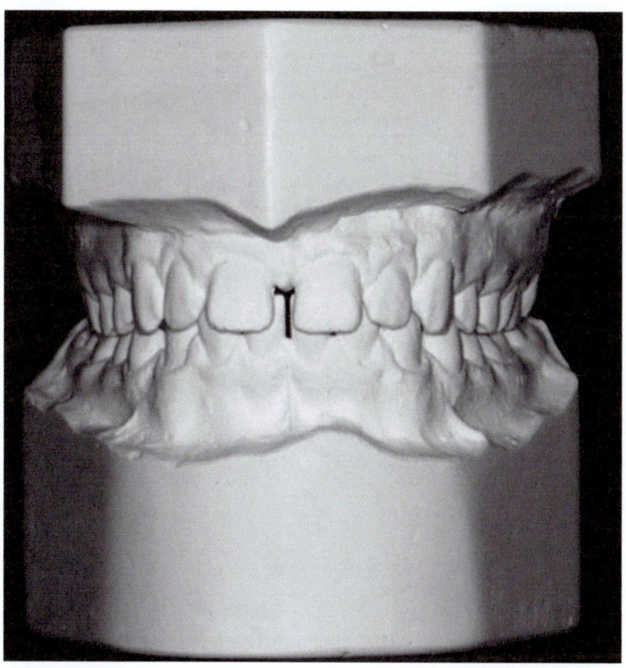

Fig. 1.9 Dental casts trimmed to orthodontic standards. No spatial relationship to the cranial structures is present

1.3 The Rationale for 3D Digital Orthodontic Records: A More Accurate Method to Analyze the Craniofacial Complex

The digital technology with its inherent characteristics of accuracy, speed, and reproducibility is fast gaining acceptance by the orthodontic community [41]. In a digital orthodontic office, a patient file is created by a practice management software prior to patient's initial visit. During the diagnostic phase of an orthodontic treatment, an electronic orthodontic screening form, 3D radiographic records (e.g., CBCT in DICOM file format), intraoral photographs, and intraoral dental scan (in STL file format) can all be merged into a single digital patient dataset [42]. This dataset is then transferred to a Computer-Assisted Design (CAD) software to create an individualized and interactive 3D rendering of an orthodontic patient. One of the most promising application of this digitally integrated patient data is the ability to analyze multiple variables of a malocclusion and its surrounding craniofacial structures.

This also allows orthodontists to fully customize a treatment plan to address the specific needs of a patient [43, 44]. With this technology, 3D analyses of craniofacial structures, occlusion, and dentoalveolar support measurements can be simultaneously performed to formulate the most appropriate treatment plan and alternatives. After patients agree and consent to a treatment plan, this integrated digital data set can also be used to create individualized appliances with Computer-Aided-Design (CAD) software and Computer-Assisted Manufacturing (CAM) technology. Customization and individualization of the entire treatment process are some of the major advantages of digital technology [45]. Currently both clear aligners and orthodontic fixed appliances can be fabricated in-house as a result of these technologies [46].

Once an electronic patient's file is created, any forms, charts, communications, and digital records can be digitally added. These files can be kept in local servers or by using cloud storage. The stored data may be used for treatment planning and communication with the patient and other clinicians in any location with a secure internet connection [47]. Data backups can also be performed automatically on a regular basis. The digital charts are patient-centered and other clinicians can add their entries to a shared file while maintaining their original data sets [10]. Major advantages of these digital files include shareability, retrievability, and storability. The main disadvantage of these cloud- or server-based files is that the files can be hacked [48]. Companies usually charge annual fees for storage and/or security for the files. And these fees can amount to significant expenses for orthodontic offices (Fig. 1.10).

1.3.1 Digital Photography

Digital photography became popular around the early 2000s [28]. The digital format allows clinicians to store and use images from multiple locations. Photographic software such as Photoshop™ (San Jose, California, USA) and DigitalSmileDesign™ (Madrid, Spain), if specifically designed for orthodontic purpose, can enhance the quality and edit these images. They allow for the digital photographs to be easily integrated into a digital data set [49]. Even though most of the commercially available software use 2D images, the digital rendering of these clinical photographs still offers significant advantages over their analog counterparts especially when combined with CBCT and intraoral dental scans [50]. Chapter 2 will cover in detail the role of photography as a contributing diagnostic tool when combined with intraoral scans and CBCT (Fig. 1.11).

3D photograph technology such as the one developed by 3DMD™ (Atlanta, Georgia, USA) uses a special setup consisting of two cameras placed at a strategic angle to each other to create a 3D image. They use complex algorithms capable of digitally reconstructing a patient's facial features from 3D data captured from both cameras. This technology is more commonly used in research and not widely adopted in clinical orthodontics due to its high cost and fairly narrow range of application [51] (Fig. 1.12 and Table 1.1).

1.3.1.1 Cone Beam Radiography

As 2D radiography proved to have limited accuracy in depicting craniofacial structures, the development of a 3D radiographic imaging system became highly desirable in

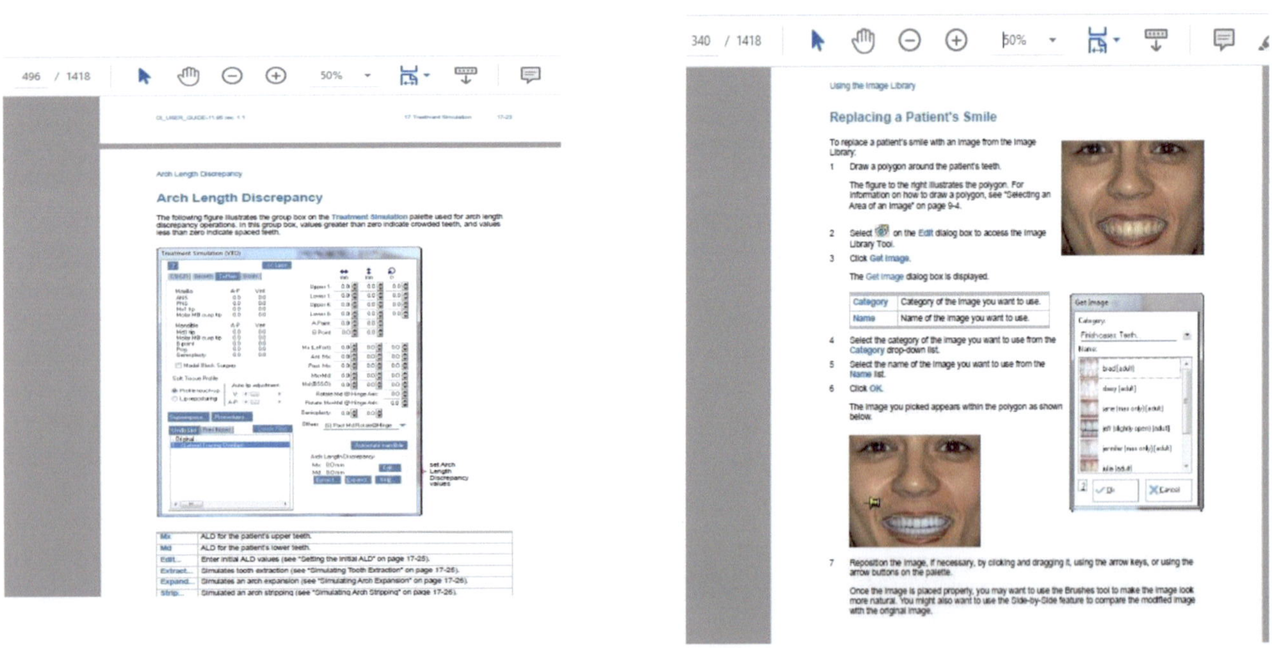

Fig. 1.10 Examples of electronic forms with data entry capability

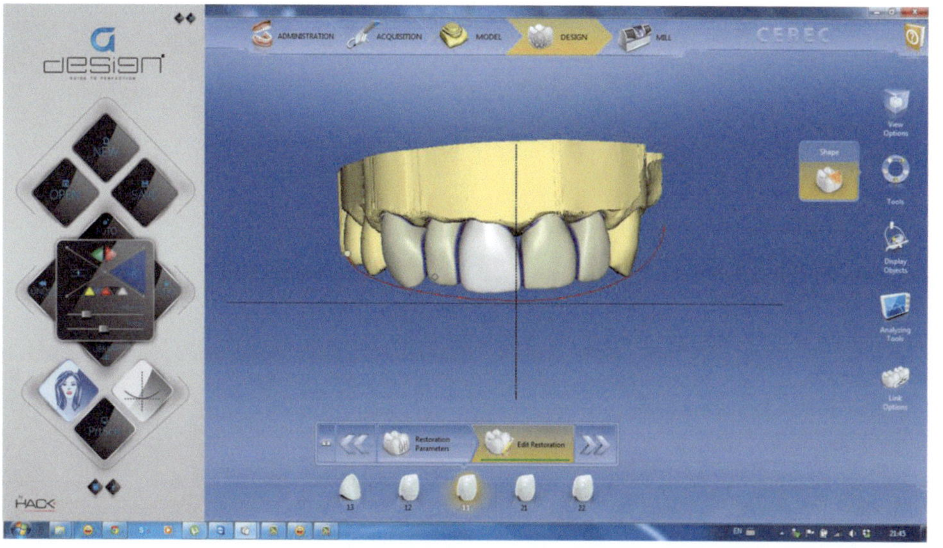

Fig. 1.11 Smile design software using scanned models

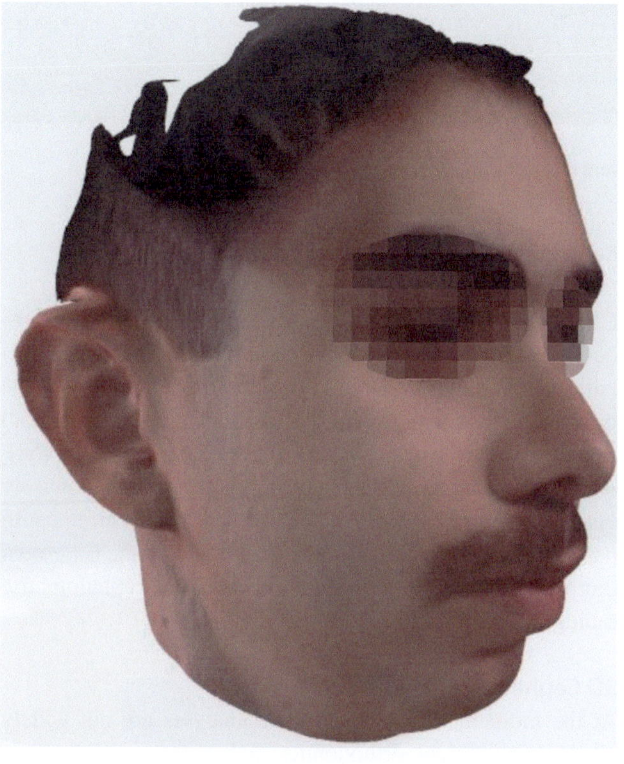

Fig. 1.12 3D photograph of a patient in pre-surgical stage

Table 1.1 Comparison between 2D and 3D photographs in various parameters

Comparison	2D photos	3D photos
Shots	Multiple shots—angle	Single shot
Combine with CBCT	No	Yes
Capture	Static	Static
Orthognathic surgery planning	Satisfactory	Excellent
Prediction of surgical outcome	Satisfactory	Excellent
Craniofacial deformities (syndromes, clefts)	Satisfactory	Excellent

orthodontic diagnosis [52]. The cone beam computerized tomography (CBCT) was first introduced by Sir Godfrey N. Hounsfield in 1967. It was initially used for general medical imaging [53]. The first successful craniofacial cone beam machine was introduced in 1996 by QR s.r.l™ (NewTom 9000). The 3D rendering gives orthodontists an ability to visualize the craniofacial complex from different angles focusing on different structures (teeth, bone, and soft tissue) just by changing filters provided in a software. The tomography in different planes provides significantly more details in comparison to traditional 2D radiographs. A CBCT may replace the need for most other radiographic images commonly used in orthodontics including a panoramic x-ray, and a lateral cephalogram. Significant technological progress has decreased the amount of radiation and the exposure time required for obtaining a diagnostically valid CBCT, while the image quality has considerably increased. CBCT technology and its indications will be further discussed in subsequent chapters (Fig. 1.13).

Bone density can only be approximated as a Hounsfield scale which is not reliable in CBCT radiography [54]. A CBCT offers orthodontists the following advantages over a conventional 2D radiograph [55, 56].

1. More accurate representation of the craniofacial structures.
2. More precise radiographic data.
3. Structures are visible in their exact positions with their exact shapes.
4. No radiographic projection errors.
5. No enlargement or distortion of structures.
6. Ease of landmark identification.
7. Superimposition with 3D facial photograph.
8. Ability of accurately comparing several CBCTs of the same patient [57] (Figs. 1.14 and 1.15).

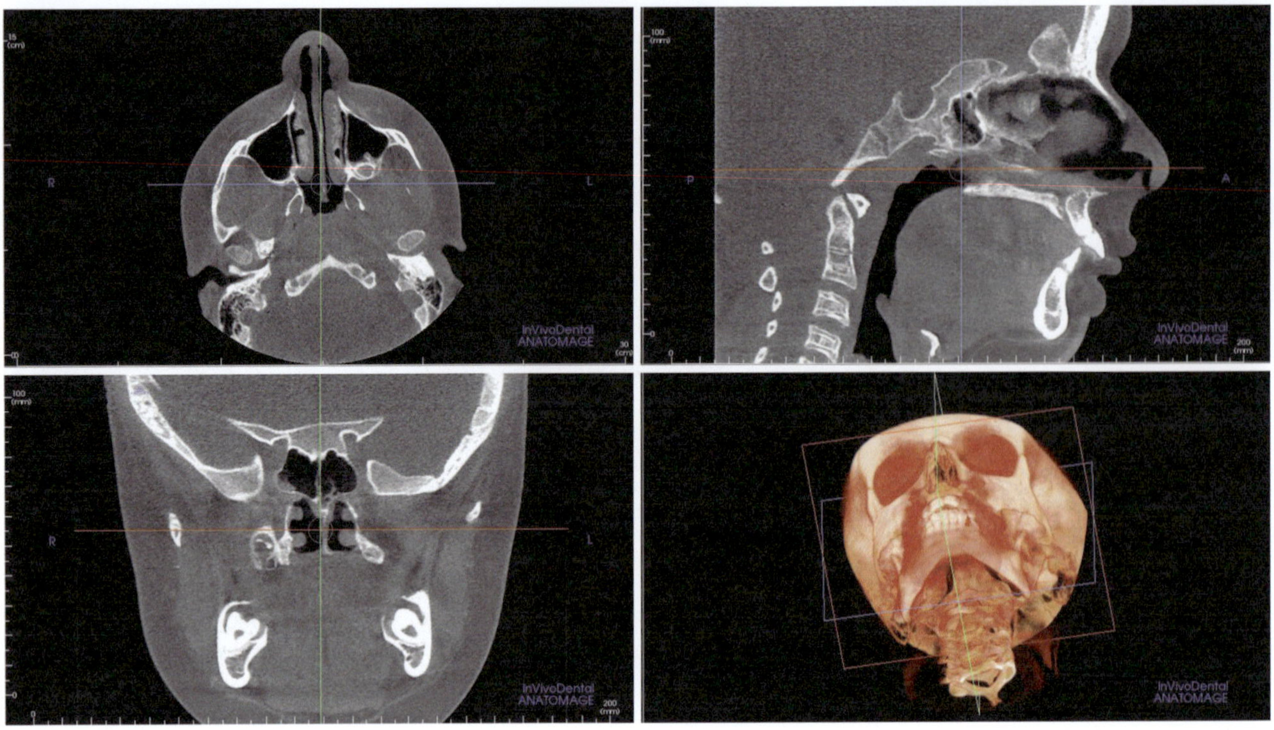

Fig. 1.13 CBCT images of a 12-year-old patient who presented with a severe maloccusion

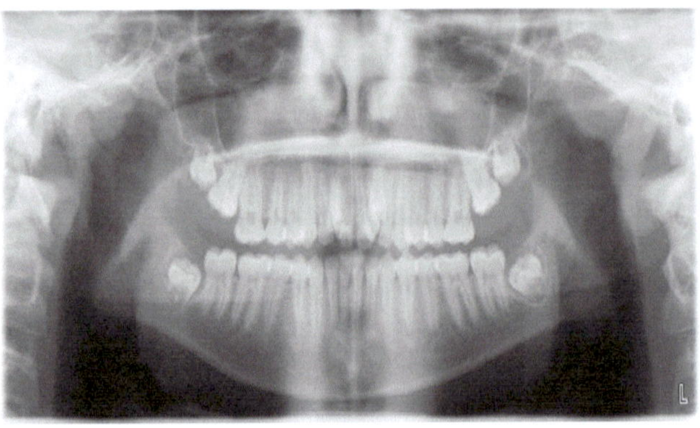

Fig. 1.14 A 2D panoramic radiograph showing a patient without any observable condylar change

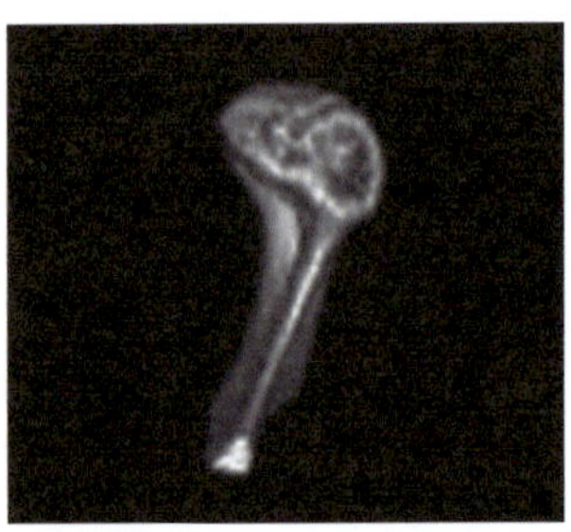

Fig. 1.15 A 3D radiograph showing the same patient with a significant condylar resorption

Reformatted Panoramic and Cephalometric Radiographs

CBCT software presents many useful functions for orthodontic diagnosis procedures including an ability to digitally reconstruct a panoramic (not totally containing all the informations that a traditional panoramic x-ray contains) and a cephalometric radiograph from a CBCT data set [58]. A central cut of the CBCT allows practitioners to precisely visualize the cranial base angle, an essential measurement in patients affected by craniofacial disorders, a measurement more difficult to obtain with a conventional cephalometric radiograph [59] (Fig. 1.16).

3D Cephalometric Analysis

At the moment, 3D cephalometric analyses are not widely adopted in clinical orthodontics and orthognathic surgery as their advantages over the 2D analyses are not yet evident to the clinician [60, 61]. Artificial intelligence may have a potential to easily integrate the CBCT data into 3D cephalometric analyses using automatic voxel recognition [62]. This will allow 3D cephalometric analyses to become a routine part of an orthodontic diagnosis, and increase the accuracy of superimpositions. It will also provide invaluable assistance to clinicians to recognize and quantify craniofacial asymmetries as well as growth deficiencies [63] (Fig. 1.17 and Table 1.2).

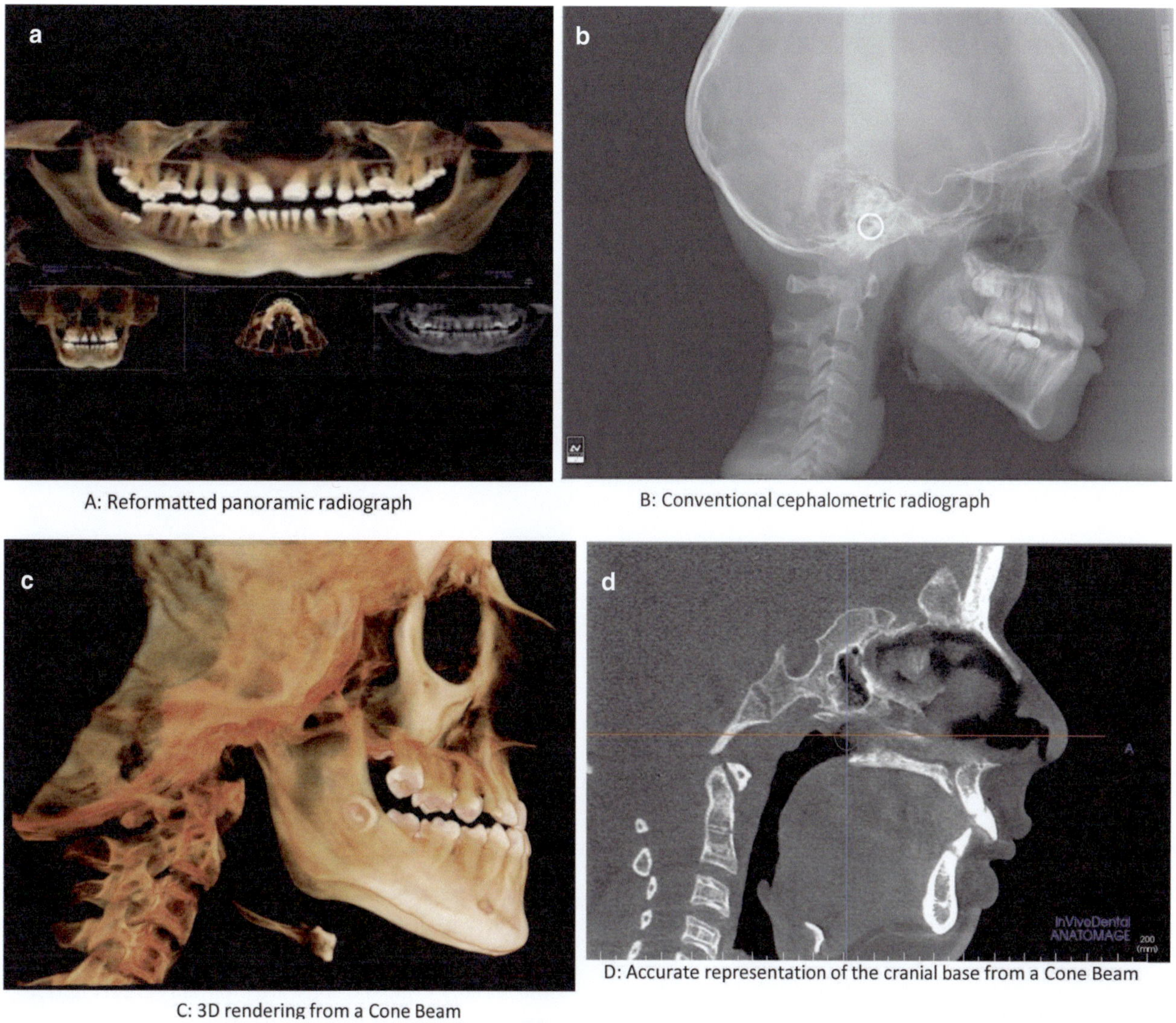

Fig. 1.16 (**a**) A panoramic radiograph reconstructed from CBCT data. (**b**) A conventional 2D cephalometric radiograph showing superimposition of different craniofacial structures. (**c**) A 3D rendering of a CBCT illustrating the 3D relationship of craniofacial structures. (**d**) A mid-sagittal cut of a CBCT showing the cranial base clearly

1.3.1.2 Intraoral Scanner and Digital Model

Prior to the advent of intraoral scanners, digital dental models were made either by tabletop scanners or by a CT scan. A digital stereolithographic file (also known as Standard Tessellation Language or STL) was produced [64]. Cerec™ introduced the first intraoral scanner in the 1980s for restorative dentistry [65]. Itero™ followed with the introduction of full-arch intraoral scanners in the 1990s. Multiple intraoral scanners are now commercially available. All employ STL or PLY files to reproduce dental anatomy and related structures. The digital orthodontic models were shown to be as reliable as plaster casts in orthodontic diagnosis and treatment planning [66].

STL 3D Digital Orthodontic Models and Software Programs to Analyze the Dentition

3D digital orthodontic models have replaced plaster models in many orthodontic practices. Currently these digital models are stored as STL files. Importing these files into a software to analyze the dentition is the next step in the diagnostic process. These software programs provide a visualization of occlusal contacts, overjet, overbite, molar and canine relationships. One major advantage of an STL virtual model is its versatility. A single STL file can be used for record keeping, simulations, superimpositions, and comparisons of different treatment options [67]. The software also allows common orthodontic analyses such as tooth/arch size analysis, Bolton analysis, intercanine, and intermolar measurements to be performed with more efficiency and accuracy [68] (Fig. 1.18).

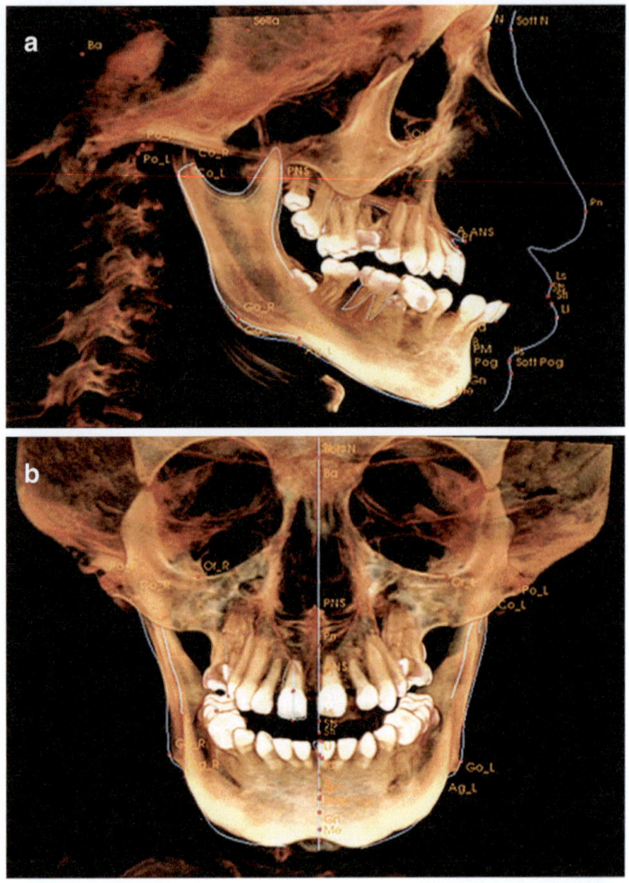

Fig. 1.17 (**a**) Lateral 3D cephalometric analysis. (**b**) Anteroposterior 3D analysis. (**c**) A reformatted image for 3D cephalometric interpretation

Table 1.2 Comparison of panoramic radiograph vs CBCT

Problem	Panoramic	CBCT
Dental fusion	++	+++
Clefts	+	+++
Supernumerary position	+	+++
Bone density	–	++
TMJ evaluation	+	+++
Bone pathology	++	+++
Root resorption	+	+++
TAD placement	–	+++
Roots proximity to sinus, assessment	++	+++
Root length (hypoplastic)	+	+++

– Not available, + Limited diagnostic value, ++ Moderate diagnostic value, +++ Reliable diagnostic value

In an STL virtual file, the upper and lower digital models are individual "solid" entities. Segmentation of the dentition is required for treatment simulation or virtual orthodontic movements. The process of segmentation is carried out by a tooth recognition in some softwares artificial intelligence is used as an segmentation-assistant [69]. Following segmentation, each tooth becomes disconnected from the adjacent teeth and gingival base. It becomes movable in three planes of space [70]. These software programs create realistic and accurate movements of the dentition. They allow for orthodontic simulations and planning of tooth movements [71]. 3 Shape™ (Copenhagen, Denmark), Onyxceph™ (Chemnitz, Germany), Maestro™ (New Age, Piza, Italy), Suresmile™ (Orametrix,Richardson, USA), Deltaface (Limoges, France) and Align™ (San Jose, California, USA) are some of the commercially available software programs [72] (Fig. 1.19).

For clear aligners fabrication, orthodontists now have the ability to simulate an orthodontic treatment plan using a CAD software once the teeth are segmented [73]. The clinical crowns of teeth are moved by different algorithms into the desired position. The amount and direction of these movements are recorded in three planes of space [74]. However, an STL orthodontic model file does not contain data on root positioning. Therefore, the software calculates an approximate position of the roots. Once these orthodontic movements are accepted, the software will then analyze these movements, apply proprietary biomechanical manipulations to the movements prescribed, add interproximal reduction, attachments and other relevant auxiliaries. The sequence will then be divided into multiple stages and transferred to a CAM software for the fabrication of programmed STL files. The staging of aligners being established, the production of individualized aligners can be initiated [75, 76]. It is noteworthy that STL files allow for segmentation of dental arches and make treatment simulation possible but this is done without relating the dentition to surrounding craniofacial structures. These software do not have the capacity to accurately predict the biological response to conduct totally accurate tooth movement [77] (Figs. 1.20 and 1.21).

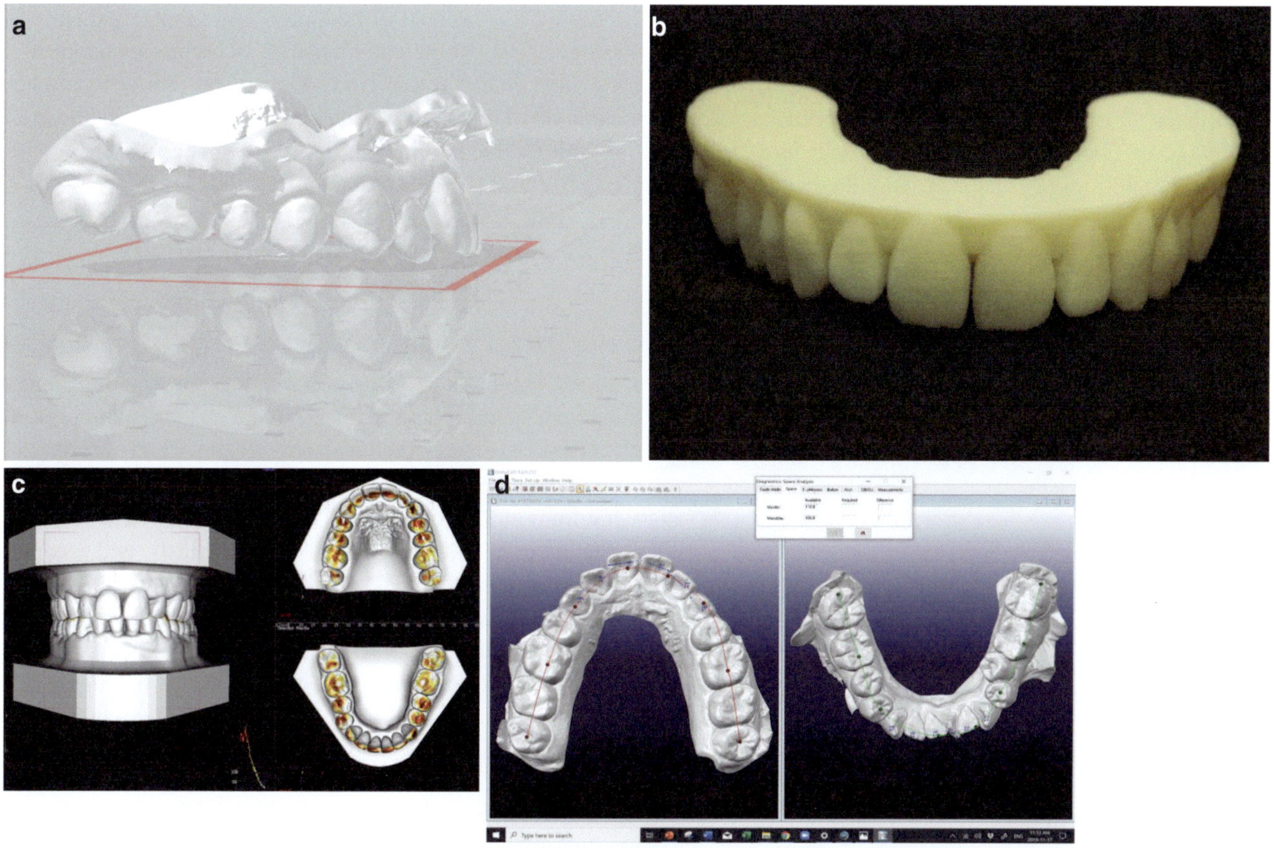

Fig. 1.18 (**a**) Stereolithographic file. (**b**) 3D model using fused deposition modeling. (**c**) Occlusal mapping using DDP™ software. (**d**) Dental arch measurements using OrthoCAD™

Fig. 1.19 Automatic segmentation of teeth using OrthoAnalyzer Software 3Shape™

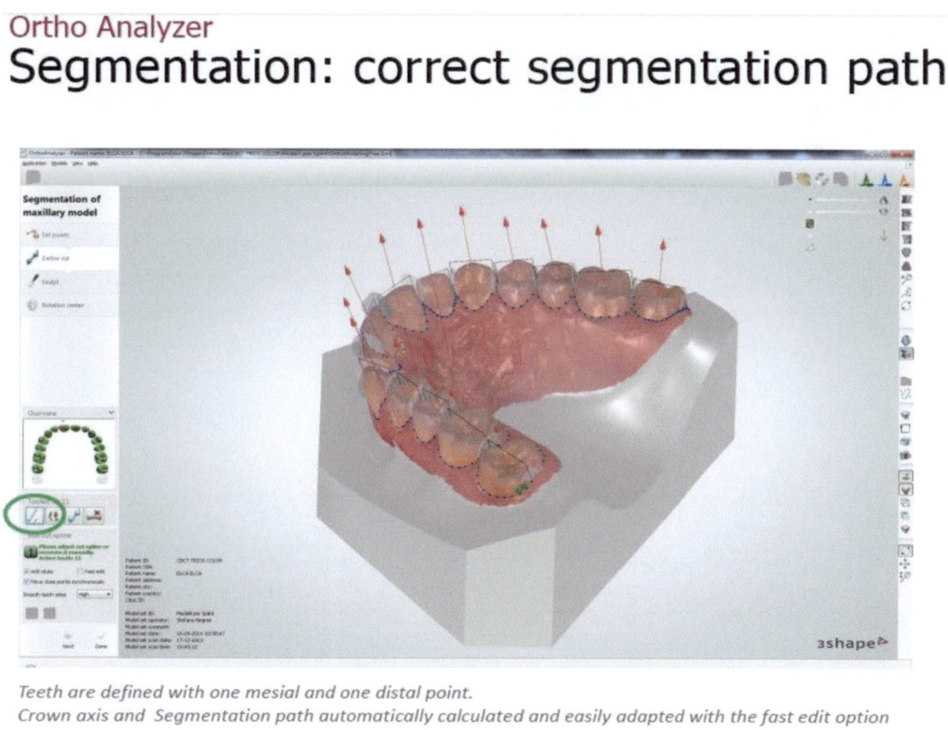

Currently, the most popular appliances produced by CAD/CAM technologies are clear aligners and programmed indirect bonding trays. Recently, CAD-CAM customized brackets have been introduced to take an advantage of this unique interaction between a treatment simulation and production of an individualized bracketing system [78]. Lingual orthodontics has adopted part of this system [79]. Robotically created archwires as advocated by Suresmile™ (Orametrix, Richardson, USA) is another example of a technology that employs an individualization of orthodontic treatment approach [80] (Fig. 1.22).

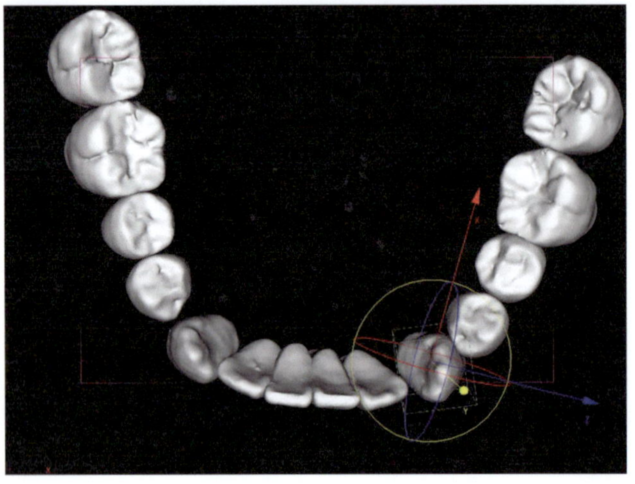

Fig. 1.20 Teeth are repositioned three-dimensionally with DDP software

1.3.2 Integration of 3D Files: A Fusion of STL-DICOM

The ultimate goal of obtaining CBCT, intraoral scans, and digital photographs is to accurately reproduce a patient's dentofacial morphology by accurate 3D orientation [81]. Software such as Anatomage(TM) (Santa Clara, USA) can now integrate a DICOM data set from CBCT with an STL file from an intraoral scan. The software may also incorporate 2D or 3D photographs to create a realistic and accurate virtual patient [82]. This combination of different files help to position the dentition in its exact spatial relationship with the surrounding craniofacial structures. This process is a significant improvement over a conventional set of fragmented 2D diagnostic records [83]. An addition of accurate root positioning data to the spatial positions of clinical crowns

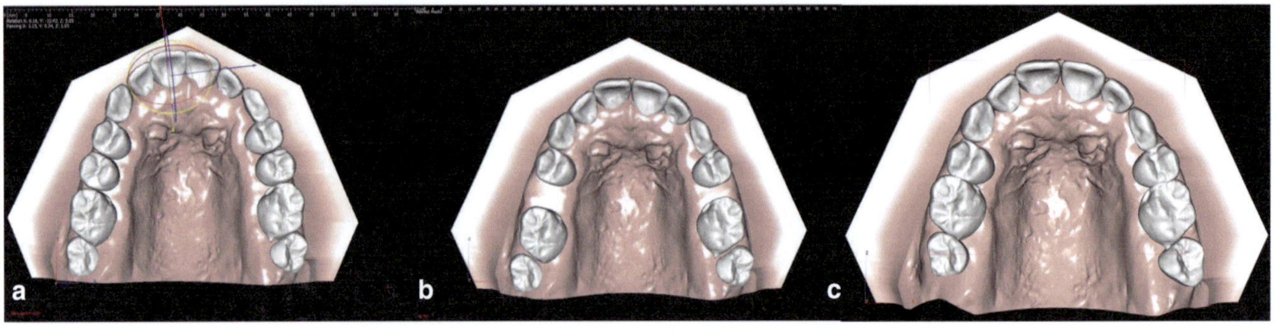

Fig. 1.21 3D tooth movement (**a**): Prior to orthodontic tooth movement, (**b**): Mid treatment, (**c**): End of treatment

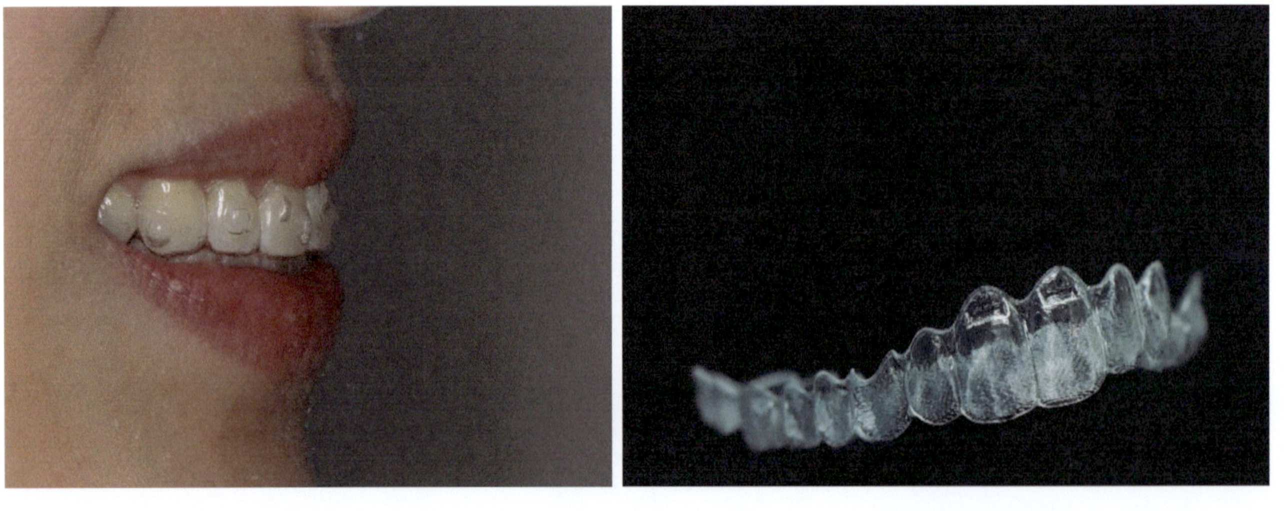

Fig. 1.22 Aligners from Invisalign™

further enhances the predictability of clinical outcomes [42]. A new fully integrated 3D spatial relationship between an entire dentoalveolar complex and its surrounding craniofacial structures is obtained and can be reliably studied and evaluated. Eventually with artificial intelligence and the judicious use of big data, these simulation software will be able to reasonably predict how clinical crowns and roots can be moved in relation to their alveolar bone housing as well as predict clinical changes of their surrounding craniofacial structures [84] (Fig. 1.23).

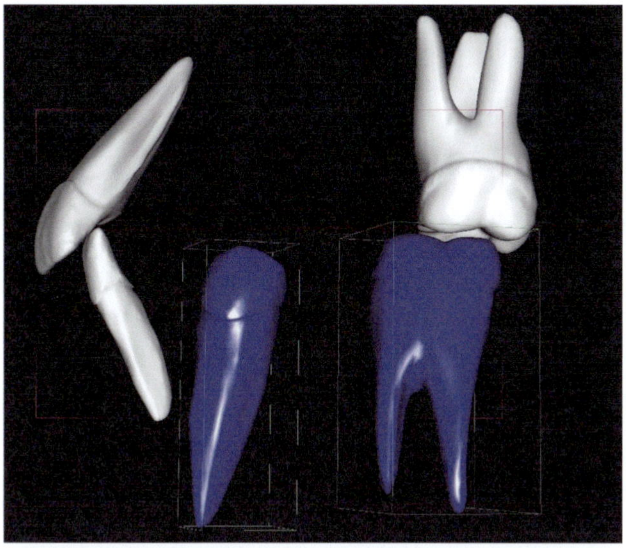

Fig. 1.23 Teeth have been segmented and incorporated into the cone beam for biomechanical simulations using DDP™ software

At the moment, seamless STL-DICOM integration capability is not readily present in commercially available orthodontic simulation software. To circumvent this, several companies are offering new versions of their software with an ability to segment each tooth and root from a DICOM file and then reassemble them as an STL orthodontic model file. Figure 1.24. demonstrates an example of total integration of STL, CBCT, and DPP simulation software to move clinical crowns and roots at the same time [83] (Fig. 1.25).

1.4 Introduction of Data Mining, Artificial Intelligence, and Machine Learning

An integration of DICOM and STL files provides clinicians a potential to relate clinical crowns and roots of the dentition to their surrounding craniofacial structures in a static state. As all magnitude and direction of each orthodontic movement can be constantly recorded by the software, the next logical step is to input all these collected data into statistical models to improve our understandings of potential correlations that may exist between all diagnostic variables and the resulting movements [85]. This will allow orthodontists to correlate entirely measurable diagnostic findings, with treat-

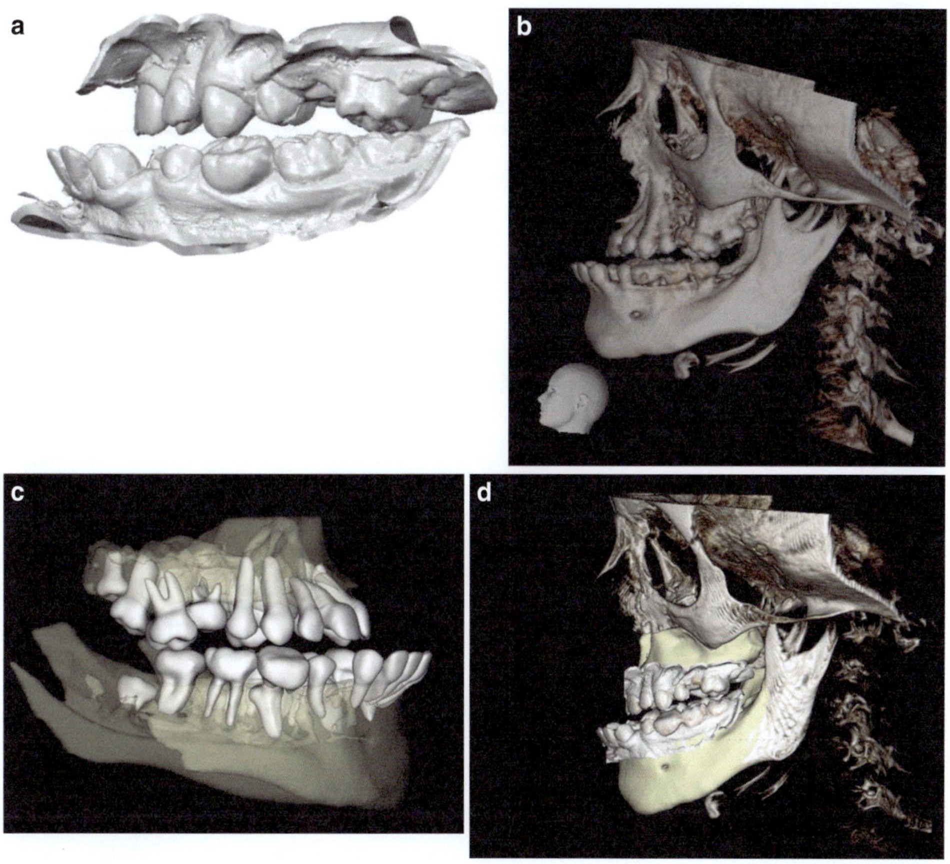

Fig. 1.24 (**a**) An STL files obtained from intraoral scan. (**b**) A CBCT of a patient. (**c**) Isolation of the dentition using the density tool in CBCT. The 3D position of the dentition is readily evident. (**d**) A fusion of STL and DICOM files

ment outcomes. These observations will enable clinicians to better recognize patterns that may have been overlooked with conventional 2D diagnostic process.

Zhao and colleagues stated "*Physicians lack systematic methods for calibrating diagnostic decisions based on feedback from their outcomes*" [86]. This statement also applies to orthodontics since most diagnostic decisions are unidirectional and based on subjective experience of treating orthodontists and treatment outcomes are not used as feedback mechanisms to improve future outcomes (Fig. 1.26).

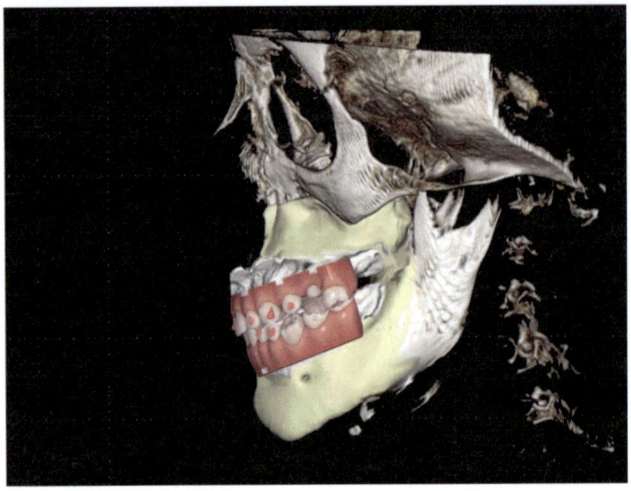

Fig. 1.25 The visualization process is initiated by manual software manipulation. Three software are superimposed but not integrated

The next frontier in digital diagnosis is to an introduction of orthodontic data mining. In the past decade, artificial intelligence (AI) and machine learning have revolutionized the use of data in medicine. "*Artificial intelligence is a branch of computer science capable of analyzing complex medical data. Their potential to exploit meaningful relationship within a data set can be used in the diagnosis, treatment and predicting outcome in many clinical scenarios*" [87]. This quote can be applied to the new 3D orthodontic diagnosis paradigm. AI uses deep learning and neural networks to predict the most probable treatment approach for a specific malocclusion. By creating layers of programming with many different and variables such as overbite, overjet, and crowding, and then assigning weight to each of these variables, AI can "learn" patterns of producing an exact diagnosis and formulating treatment options by studying very large quantity of malocclusions and their outcomes [88]. Contrary to a common misconception, machine learning needs a large amount of knowledge input and can only learn semi-repetitive and constructed patterns on its own. It lacks perception and intuition [89]. Therefore, AI requires the orthodontist's

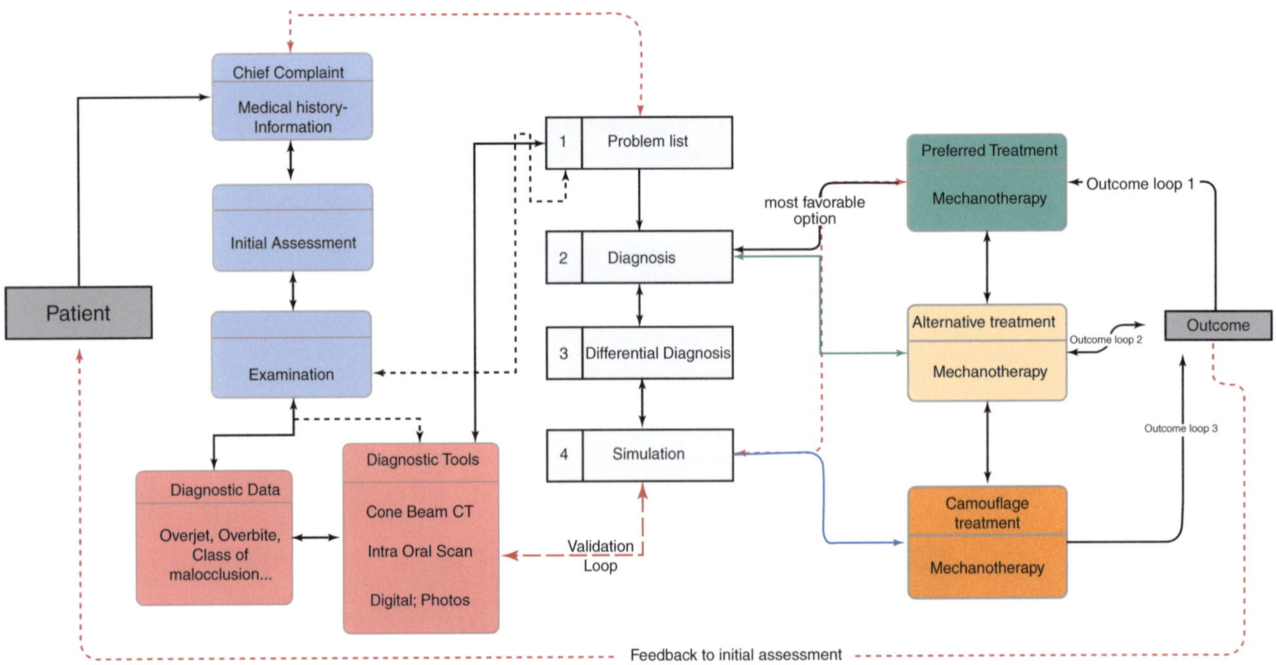

Fig. 1.26 3D diagnosis process with feedback allowing clinicians to review and assess the validity of a treatment approach

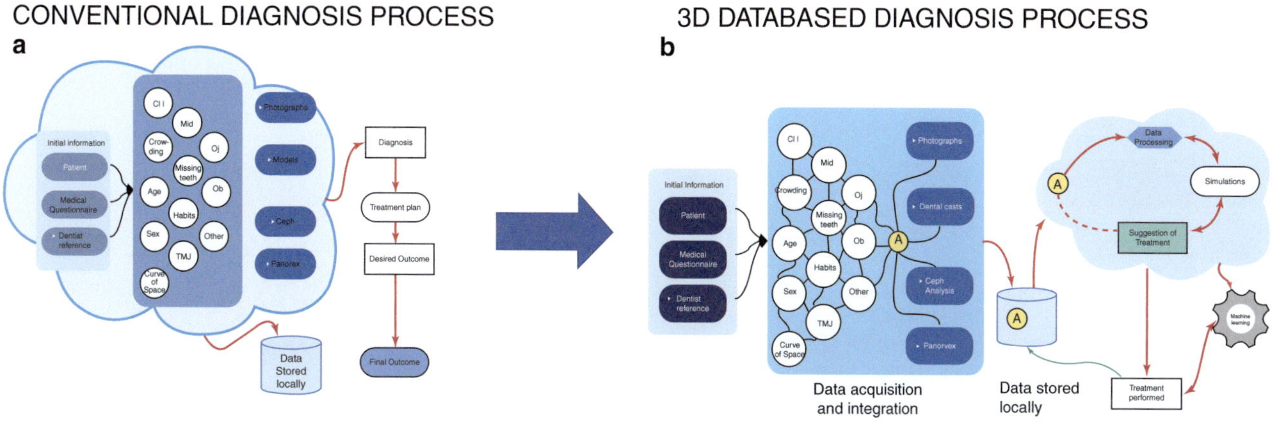

Fig. 1.27 (**a**) Conventional method to store 3D data in the cloud and design a treatment plan. (**b**) Neural network potentially used for orthodontic treatment assistance. Data is inputted into the deep learning neural network. Analyses are performed and a predicted outcome is proposed. The final outcome may be uploaded into the network to strengthen the predictions. The neural network also "learns" from the outcome of treatment and adjusts the weight of the parameters for a given malocclusion

knowledge and experience as crucial inputs into the machine learning process. AI allows orthodontists to test different probable treatment alternatives while using outcomes in a feedback mechanism to allow the construct of a deeper and more robust learning systems [90]. This new approach or back propagation which consists of constantly correcting the weights given to variables has the potential to vastly improve orthodontic treatment outcomes by allowing large amount of data to be gathered, processed, and analyzed [91]. For example, an integration of artificial intelligence (AI), and machine leaning with large amount of CBCT data may have a potential to better predict facial growth, and create a more focused treatment approach [92]. However, This process still relies on the vast knowledge and experience from orthodontists to be successful (Fig. 1.27).

1.5 Conclusions

In this chapter, a conventional diagnostic process employed in orthodontics was reviewed. The process only allows clinicians to diagnose malocclusions in a "feed forward" direction mostly driven by the operator's experience and treatment philosophy. This approach often lacks scientific basis and has mainly led to differences of opinions promoting mechanistic rather than comprehensive approaches to treatment. The introduction of the 3D diagnosis has further expanded the diagnostic capabilities of orthodontists by incorporating CBCT and intraoral scans into their armamentarium. Current technologies allow for the addition of considerable diagnostic data acquisitions. However, the orthodontic diagnosis process has by and large remained unchanged despite these technological advances. An entirely new digital diagnosis paradigm with a total integration of all 3D diagnostic data and the use of AI-machine learning is slowly emerging. Neural networks and machine learning processes already used by several aligner companies have the potential to improve diagnostic accuracy and treatment planning capabilities of orthodontists. These advances will be achieved by feeding a large amount of diagnostic data into neural networks to formulate probabilities of outcomes based on successful treatment of a large number of malocclusions. In the end, orthodontists' knowledge and experience remain very much crucial in this process. When combined with specially designed neural networks, this digitally driven statistically sound diagnostic approach will improve diagnostic and treatment planning capabilities for orthodontists (Fig. 1.28).

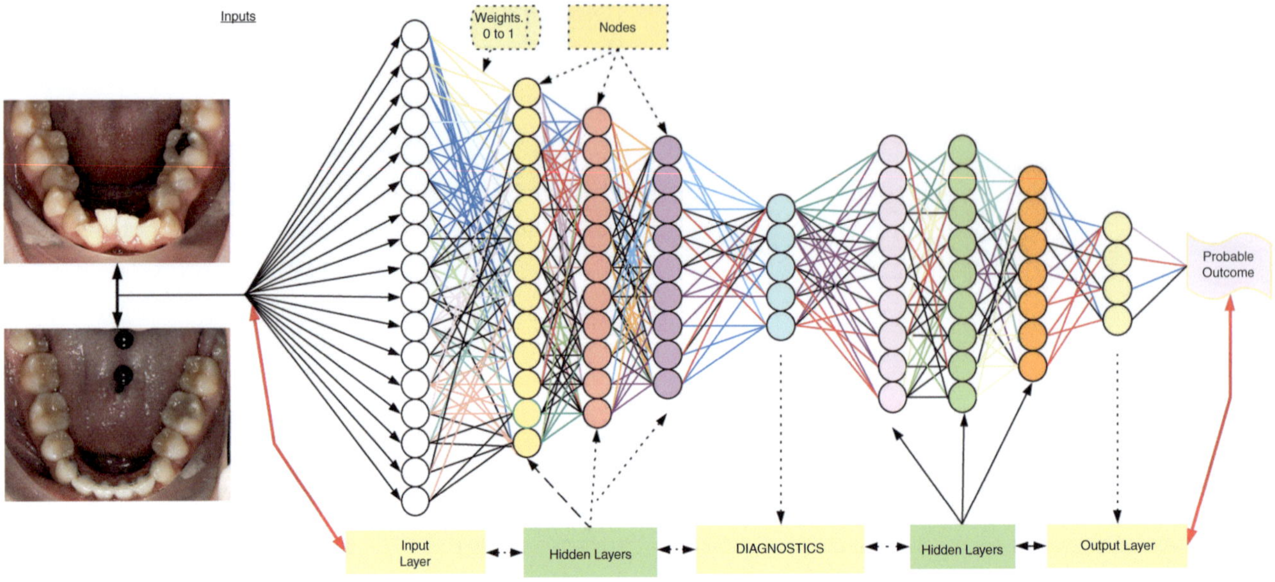

Fig. 1.28 Describes a potential neural network developed for orthodontic diagnosis using some of the most common orthodontic variables (1 to *n*) shown on the far left side of the drawing. Then connectors are used and "weighted" according to the importance of variables on the severity of malocclusion. Nodes arranged in layers are used to mimic neural activity using activation functions. Finally, back propagation happens when the neural network "learns" to recognize patterns and adjusts the "weights" accordingly. These networks can process and correlate vast amount of data that may not appear evident to orthodontists. Probable outcomes are elaborated allowing orthodontists to make the most appropriate decision

References

1. Lestrel PE. Some approaches toward the mathematical modeling of the craniofacial complex. J Craniofac Genet Dev Biol. 1989;9:77–91.
2. Harrell WE Jr, Hatcher DC, Bolt RL. In search of anatomic truth: 3-dimensional digital modeling and the future of orthodontics. Am J Orthod Dentofac Orthop. 2002;122:325–30.
3. Miller AJ, Maki K, Hatcher DC. New diagnostic tools in orthodontics. Am J Orthod Dentofac Orthop. 2004;126:395–6.
4. Nebbe B, Major PW, Prasad NGN, Hatcher D. Quantitative assessment of temporomandibular joint disk status. Oral Surg Oral Med Oral Pathol Oral Radiol Endodontol. 1998;85:598–607.
5. Lessa FCR, Enoki C, Feres MFN, Valera FCP, Lima WTA, Matsumoto MAN. Breathing mode influence in craniofacial development. Braz J Otorhinolaryngol. 2005;71:156–60.
6. Kau CH, Olim S, Nguyen JT. The future of orthodontic diagnostic records. In: Seminars in orthodontics. Elsevier; 2011. p. 39–45.
7. Sarver DM. Interactions of hard tissues, soft tissues, and growth over time,v and their impact on orthodontic diagnosis and treatment planning. Am J Orthod Dentofac Orthop. 2015;148:380–6.
8. Broadbent BH. A new X-ray technique and its application to orthodontia: the introduction of cephalometric radiography. Angle Orthod. 1981;51:93–114.
9. Mehta J. Orthodontic records: why? What? When? & how? Funct Orthod. 1993;10:44–51.
10. Abdelkarim A, Jerrold L. Orthodontic chart documentation. Am J Orthod Dentofac Orthop. 2017;152:126–30.
11. Williamson, J. Orthodontic records: more than just models and photos. Int J Orthod Milwaukee. 2003;14(1):33
12. Broadbent, B. H. The Face of the Normal Child. The Angle Orthodontist. 1937;7(4):183–208
13. Bondemark L, Jeppsson M, Lindh-Ingildsen L, Rangne K. Incidental findings of pathology and abnormality in pretreatment orthodontic panoramic radiographs. Angle Orthod. 2006;76:98–102.
14. Graber TM. Panoramic radiography in orthodontic diagnosis. Am J Orthod. 1967;53:799–821.
15. DiFranco DE, Cham T-J, Rehg JM. Reconstruction of 3D figure motion from 2D correspondences. In: Proceedings of the 2001 IEEE Computer Society conference on computer vision and pattern recognition. CVPR 2001, I-I. IEEE; 2001.
16. Han UK, Vig KWL, Weintraub JA, Vig PS, Kowalski CJ. Consistency of orthodontic treatment decisions relative to diagnostic records. Am J Orthod Dentofac Orthop. 1991;100:212–9.
17. Lee K, Torkfar G, Fraser C. An investigation into orthodontic clinical record taking. Int J Orthod Milwaukee. 2015;26:53–7.
18. McNamara JA Jr. Ordinary orthodontics: starting with the end in mind. World J Orthod. 2000;1:45–54.
19. Ejersbo LR, Leron U. Revisiting the medical diagnosis problem: reconciling intuitive and analytical thinking. In: Probabilistic thinking. Springer; 2014.
20. Harrell Jr WE. 3D diagnosis and treatment planning in orthodontics. In: Seminars in orthodontics. Elsevier; 2009. p. 35–41.
21. Hechler SL. Cone-beam CT: applications in orthodontics. Dent Clin N Am. 2008;52:809–23, vii.
22. Beuer F, Schweiger J, Edelhoff D. Digital dentistry: an overview of recent developments for CAD/CAM generated restorations. Br Dent J. 2008;204:505.
23. Hou D, Capote R, Bayirli B, Chan DCN, Huang G. The effect of digital diagnostic setups on orthodontic treatment planning. Am J Orthod Dentofac Orthop. 2020;157:542–9.
24. Palomo JM, El H, Stefanovic N, Bazina M. Diagnostic value of 3D imaging in clinical orthodontics. In: Craniofacial 3D imaging. Springer; 2019.
25. Murata S, Lee C, Tanikawa C, Date S. Towards a fully automated diagnostic system for orthodontic treatment in dentistry. In: 2017 IEEE 13th international conference on e-science (e-Science). IEEE; 2017. p. 1–8.

26. Terry DA, Snow SR, McLaren EA. CE 1-contemporary dental photography: selection and application. Compendium. 2008;29:432.
27. Claman L, Patton D, Rashid R. Standardized portrait photography for dental patients. Am J Orthod Dentofac Orthop. 1990;98:197–205.
28. Bengel W. Digital photography in the dental practice—an overview (II). Int J Comput Dent. 2000;3:121–32.
29. Pickens D. et al. Focal-plane tomography image reconstruction. IEEE Transactions on Nuclear Science. 1980;27(1):489–492
30. Maestre-Ferrín L, Carrillo-García C, Galán-Gil S, Peñarrocha-Diago M, Peñarrocha-Diago M. Prevalence, location, and size of maxillary sinus septa: panoramic radiograph versus computed tomography scan. J Oral Maxillofac Surg. 2011;69:507–11.
31. Tsolakis AI, Kalavritinos M, Bitsanis E, Sanoudos M, Benetou V, Alexiou K, Tsiklakis K. Reliability of different radiographic methods for the localization of displaced maxillary canines. Am J Orthod Dentofac Orthop. 2018;153:308–14.
32. Vandenberghe B, Jacobs R, Bosmans H. Modern dental imaging: a review of the current technology and clinical applications in dental practice. Eur Radiol. 2010;20:2637–55.
33. Steiner CC. Cephalometrics for you and me. Am J Orthod Dentofac Orthop. 1953;39:729–55.
34. Scheideman GB, Bell WH, Legan HL, Finn RA, Reisch JS. Cephalometric analysis of dentofacial normals. Am J Orthod. 1980;78:404–20.
35. Ludlow JB, Gubler M, Cevidanes L, Mol A. Precision of cephalometric landmark identification: cone-beam computed tomography vs conventional cephalometric views. Am J Orthod Dentofac Orthop. 2009;136:312.e1–12.e10.
36. Ricketts RM, Grummons D. Frontal cephalometrics: practical applications, part I. World J Orthod. 2003;4:297–316.
37. Proskauer C. The story of dentistry, from the dawn of civilization to the present, 2nd ed. In: JSTOR; 1951.
38. Yamamoto K, Hayashi S, Nishikawa H, Nakamura S, Mikami T. Measurements of dental cast profile and three-dimensional tooth movement during orthodontic treatment. IEEE Trans Biomed Eng. 1991;38:360–5.
38. Ackerman M. B. The myth of Janus: Orthodontic progress faces orthodontic history. American Journal of Orthodontics and Dentofacial Orthopedics. 2003;123(6):594–596.
39. Beglin FM, Firestone AR, Vig KWL, Beck FM, Kuthy RA, Wade D. A comparison of the reliability and validity of 3 occlusal indexes of orthodontic treatment need. Am J Orthod Dentofac Orthop. 2001;120:240–6.
40. Dolce C, Mansour DA, McGorray SP, Wheeler TT. Intrarater agreement about the etiology of Class II malocclusion and treatment approach. Am J Orthod Dentofac Orthop. 2012;141:17–23.
41. Paredes V, Gandia JL, Cibrian R. Digital diagnosis records in orthodontics. An overview. Med Oral Patol Oral Cir Bucal. 2006;11:E88–93.
42. Xiao Z, Liu Z, Gu Y. Integration of digital maxillary dental casts with 3D facial images in orthodontic patients: a three-dimensional validation study. Angle Orthod. 2020;90(3):397–404.
43. Takada K. Artificial intelligence expert systems with neural network machine learning may assist decision-making for extractions in orthodontic treatment planning. J Evid Based Dent Pract. 2016;16:190–2.
44. Yagi M, Ohno H, Takada K. Decision-making system for orthodontic treatment planning based on direct implementation of expertise knowledge. In: 2010 annual international conference of the IEEE engineering in medicine and biology, IEEE; 2010, p. 2894–97.
45. Motohashi N, Kuroda T. A 3D computer-aided design system applied to diagnosis and treatment planning in orthodontics and orthognathic surgery. Eur J Orthod. 1999;21:263–74.
46. Hennessy J, Al-Awadhi EA. Clear aligners generations and orthodontic tooth movement. J Orthod. 2016;43:68–76.
47. Eve E. Personalizing orthodontics–precision health methods in orthodontic clinical trials. UCSF; 2018.
48. Schnipper JL, Linder JA, Palchuk MB, Einbinder JS, Li Q, Postilnik A, Middleton B. "Smart forms" in an electronic medical record: documentation-based clinical decision support to improve disease management. J Am Med Inform Assoc. 2008;15:513–23.
49. Schabel BJ, Franchi L, Baccetti T, McNamara JA Jr. Subjective vs objective evaluations of smile esthetics. Am J Orthod Dentofac Orthop. 2009;135:S72–9.
50. Schaaf H, Malik CY, Howaldt H-P, Streckbein P. Evolution of photography in maxillofacial surgery: from analog to 3D photography—an overview. Clin Cosmet Investig Dent. 2009;1:39.
51. Metzger TE, Kula KS, Eckert GJ, Ghoneima AA. Orthodontic soft-tissue parameters: a comparison of cone-beam computed tomography and the 3dMD imaging system. Am J Orthod Dentofac Orthop. 2013;144:672–81.
52. Anderson PJ, Yong R, Surman TL, Rajion ZA, Ranjitkar S. Application of three-dimensional computed tomography in craniofacial clinical practice and research. Aust Dent J. 2014;59:174–85.
53. Sukovic P. Cone beam computed tomography in craniofacial imaging. Orthod Craniofac Res. 2003;6:31–6.
54. Kapila SD. Cone beam computed tomography in orthodontics: indications, insights, and innovations. Ames: Wiley; 2014.
55. Tadinada A, Schneider S, Yadav S. Role of cone beam computed tomography in contemporary orthodontics. In: Seminars in orthodontics. Elsevier; 2018. p. 407–15.
56. Van Vlijmen OJC, Maal T, Bergé SJ, Bronkhorst EM, Katsaros C, Kuijpers-Jagtman AM. A comparison between 2D and 3D cephalometry on CBCT scans of human skulls. Int J Oral Maxillofac Surg. 2010;39:156–60.
57. Bazina M, Cevidanes L, Ruellas A, Valiathan M, Quereshy F, Syed A, Wu R, Palomo JM. Precision and reliability of Dolphin 3-dimensional voxel-based superimposition. Am J Orthod Dentofac Orthop. 2018;153:599–606.
58. Lund H, Grondahl K, Grondahl HG. Accuracy and precision of linear measurements in cone beam computed tomography Accuitomo® tomograms obtained with different reconstruction techniques. Dentomaxillofac Radiol. 2009;38:379–86.
59. Cevidanes LHC, Motta A, Proffit WR, Ackerman JL, Styner M. Cranial base superimposition for 3-dimensional evaluation of soft-tissue changes. Am J Orthod Dentofac Orthop. 2010;137:S120–S29.
60. Chen M-H, Chang JZ-C, Kok S-H, Chen Y-J, Huang Y-D, Cheng K-Y, Lin C-P. Intraobserver reliability of landmark identification in cone-beam computed tomography-synthesized two-dimensional cephalograms versus conventional cephalometric radiography: a preliminary study. J Dent Sci. 2014;9:56–62.
61. Cheung LK, Chan YM, Jayaratne YSN, Lo J. Three-dimensional cephalometric norms of Chinese adults in Hong Kong with balanced facial profile. Oral Surg Oral Med Oral Pathol Oral Radiol Endodontol. 2011;112:e56–73.
62. Nada RM, Maal TJJ, Breuning KH, Berge SJ, Mostafa YA, Kuijpers-Jagtman AM. Accuracy and reproducibility of voxel based superimposition of cone beam computed tomography models on the anterior cranial base and the zygomatic arches. PLoS One. 2011;6(2):e16520.
63. Cevidanes LHS, Bailey LJ, Tucker GR Jr, Styner MA, Mol A, Phillips CL, Proffit WR, Turvey T. Superimposition of 3D cone-beam CT models of orthognathic surgery patients. Dentomaxillofac Radiol. 2014;34(6):369–75.
64. Fasbinder DJ. Computerized technology for restorative dentistry. Am J Dent. 2013;26:115–20.
65. Kassis C. CAD/CAM technology: a review. Comput Aided Des (CAD). 1980;2.

66. Luu NS, Nikolcheva LG, Retrouvey J-M, Flores-Mir C, El-Bialy T, Carey JP, Major PW. Linear measurements using virtual study models: a systematic review. Angle Orthod. 2012;82:1098–106.
67. Sinthanayothin C, Tharanont W. Orthodontics treatment simulation by teeth segmentation and setup. In: 2008 5th international conference on electrical engineering/electronics, computer, telecommunications and information technology. IEEE; 2008. p. 81–4.
68. Fleming PS, Marinho V, Johal A. Orthodontic measurements on digital study models compared with plaster models: a systematic review. Orthod Craniofac Res. 2011;14:1–16.
69. Kumar Y, Janardan R, Larson B, Moon J. Improved segmentation of teeth in dental models. Comput Aided Des Appl. 2011;8:211–24.
70. Yaqi M, Zhongke L. Computer aided orthodontics treatment by virtual segmentation and adjustment. In: 2010 international conference on image analysis and signal processing. IEEE; 2010. p. 336–9.
71. Cheng C, Cheng X, Dai N, Liu Y, Fan Q, Hou Y, Jiang X. Personalized orthodontic accurate tooth arrangement system with complete teeth model. J Med Syst. 2015;39:84.
72. Kondo T, Ong SH, Foong KW. Tooth segmentation of dental study models using range images. IEEE Trans Med Imaging. 2004;23:350–62.
73. Breuning KH, Kau CH. Digital planning and custom orthodontic treatment. Hoboken: Wiley; 2017.
74. Dickerson TE. Invisalign with photobiomodulation: optimizing tooth movement and treatment efficacy with a novel self-assessment algorithm. J Clin Orthod. 2017;51:157–65.
75. Miller RJ, Kuo E, Choi W. Validation of Align Technology's Treat IIITM digital model superimposition tool and its case application. Orthod Craniofac Res. 2003;6:143–9.
76. Robertson L, Kaur H, Fagundes NCF, Romanyk D, Major P, Mir CF. Effectiveness of clear aligner therapy for orthodontic treatment: a systematic review. Orthod Craniofac Res. 2020;23(2):133–42.
77. Jones ML, Hickman J, Middleton J, Knox J, Volp C. A validated finite element method study of orthodontic tooth movement in the human subject. J Orthod. 2001;28:29–38.
78. Tarraf NE, Ali DM. Present and the future of digital orthodontics☆. In: Seminars in orthodontics. Elsevier; 2018. p. 376–85.
79. Kwon S-Y, Kim Y, Ahn H-W, Kim K-B, Chung K-R. Computer-aided designing and manufacturing of lingual fixed orthodontic appliance using 2D/3D registration software and rapid prototyping. Int J Dent. 2014;2014(11):164164.
80. Sachdeva RCL. SureSmile technology in a patient-centered orthodontic practice. J Clin Orthod. 2001;35:245–53.
81. Widmann G, Berggren JPM, Fischer B, Pichler-Dennhardt AR, Schullian P, Bale R, Puelacher W. Accuracy of image-fusion stereolithographic guides: mapping CT data with three-dimensional optical surface scanning. Clin Implant Dent Relat Res. 2015;17:e736–e44.
82. Plooij JM, Maal TJJ, Haers P, Borstlap WA, Kuijpers-Jagtman AM, Bergé SJ. Digital three-dimensional image fusion processes for planning and evaluating orthodontics and orthognathic surgery. A systematic review. Int J Oral Maxillofac Surg. 2011;40:341–52.
83. Joda T, Wolfart S, Reich S, Zitzmann NU. Virtual dental patient: how long until it's here? Curr Oral Health Rep. 2018;5:116–20.
84. Chisari JR, McGorray SP, Nair M, Wheeler TT. Variables affecting orthodontic tooth movement with clear aligners. Am J Orthod Dentofac Orthop. 2014;145:S82–91.
85. Kunz F, Stellzig-Eisenhauer A, Zeman F, Boldt J. Artificial intelligence in orthodontics. J Orofac Orthop/Fortschritte der Kieferorthopädie. 2020;81:52–68.
86. Zhao JY, Song EAB, Schwartz D, Panesar M, Jackson GP, Elkin PL. Barriers, facilitators, and solutions to optimal patient portal and personal health record use: a systematic review of the literature. In: AMIA annual symposium proceedings, 1913. American Medical Informatics Association; 2017.
87. Ramesh AN, Kambhampati C, Monson JRT, Drew PJ. Artificial intelligence in medicine. Ann R Coll Surg Engl. 2004;86:334.
88. Kulikowski CA. Artificial intelligence methods and systems for medical consultation. IEEE Trans Pattern Anal Mach Intell. 1980;PAMI-2:464–76.
89. Ko C-C, Tanikawa C, Wu T-H, Pastewait M, Jackson CB, Kwon JJ, Lee Y-T, Lian C, Wang L, Shen D. Machine learning in orthodontics: application review. Embracing Novel Technol Dent Orthod. 2019;1001:117.
90. Martina R, Teti R, D'Addona D, Iodice G. Neural network based system for decision making support in orthodontic extractions. In: Intelligent production machines and systems. Elsevier; 2006.
91. Jung S-K, Kim T-W. New approach for the diagnosis of extractions with neural network machine learning. Am J Orthod Dentofac Orthop. 2016;149:127–33.
92. Faber J, et al. Artificial intelligence in orthodontics. APOS Trends in Orthodontics. 2019;9(4):201–205.

Use of Dental Photography in Orthodontic Diagnosis and Treatment Planning

2

Suzanne Lacombe, Marius Hack, and Shadi Samawi

2.1 Introduction

The first recorded photograph was obtained by Joseph Niepce around 1827 after an estimated 8-h exposure time [1]. In 1839, Louis Jacques Daguerre invented the light sensitive copper plates [2]. In 1888, George Eastman built the first camera to use dry films [3]. In 1974, engineers David Lewis and Steve Sasson from Kodak contributed to the creation of the first digital camera prototype and Canon commercialized the first analog electronic camera (RC-701) in 1986. Since then, photography has evolved tremendously. Since it was first used in 1850 to record "before and after" surgery photographs, photography in the dental world has gained a lot of importance (Fig. 2.1).

Photography has come to occupy a very valuable function as part of standard orthodontic record-taking [4]. It has been said that an image is worth a thousand words and in our dental photography world, Glenner and Davis (1990) said: "*Dental images transcend and supplement the written word*." What a poetic way to describe clinical dental photography! Photographs provide a faithful reproduction of soft and hard tissues and contribute significantly to the comprehensive records. They are a great help when it comes to communicate effectively with the patient or guardian. Photographs strongly support interdisciplinary treatment planning and the communication among dental professionals. They provide accurate and reliable pre-, progress and post-treatment photographic records [5]. Clinical photography is deemed effective and valuable as much by the accuracy of the information it contains as for its significance and reproducibility over time [6–8].

Clinical orthodontic photographs are invaluable because they:

- Deliver a faithful reproduction of facial soft and hard tissues.
- Allow for effective and valuable communication with the patient.
- Contribute significantly to obtaining comprehensive records.
- Support interdisciplinary planning and communication among dental professionals.
- Provide readily available, accurate and reliable pre-, progress and post-treatment photographic records.

One cannot emphasize enough the relevance of good quality clinical images. Of all the components of dental records (radiographs, study models, 3D scans), photography is the least invasive and the most visually compelling [5]. As no single tool is comprehensive in itself for establishing a valid diagnosis, photography adds to the diagnostic armamentarium of the practicing orthodontist [9] (Fig. 2.2).

2.2 Components of Digital Dental Photography Equipment

- *"A camera should be part of the standard equipment of every* ***dentist****"* [5, 7].

Digital photographs are now readily available through smartphones, tablets, "Point-and-shoot" cameras, DSLR cameras, and more recently, mirrorless camera. Clinical images are valued as diagnostic instruments, and their significant communicative power among patients and dental professionals alike is not to be underestimated. To be a useful

S. Lacombe (✉)
Department of Orthodontics, University of Missouri Kansas City, Kansas City, MO, USA
e-mail: suzanne.lacombe@umkc.edu

M. Hack
Hack Dental, Răzvad, Romania
e-mail: marius@hack.dental

S. Samawi
Samawi Dental and Orthodontic Center—SDOC, Amman, Jordan

J.-M. Retrouvey, M.-N. Abdallah (eds.), *3D Diagnosis and Treatment Planning in Orthodontics*,
https://doi.org/10.1007/978-3-030-57223-5_2

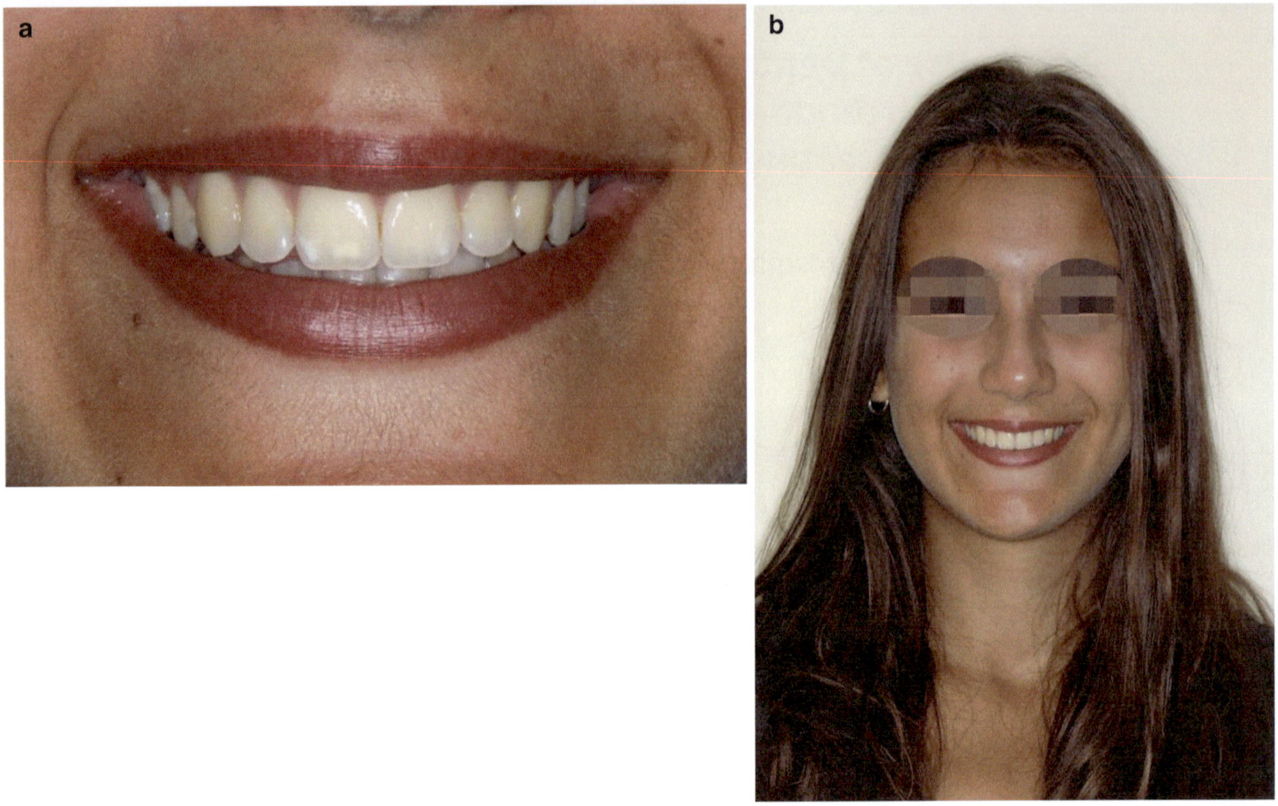

Fig. 2.1 (**a**) Close up smile; (**b**) Smiling face

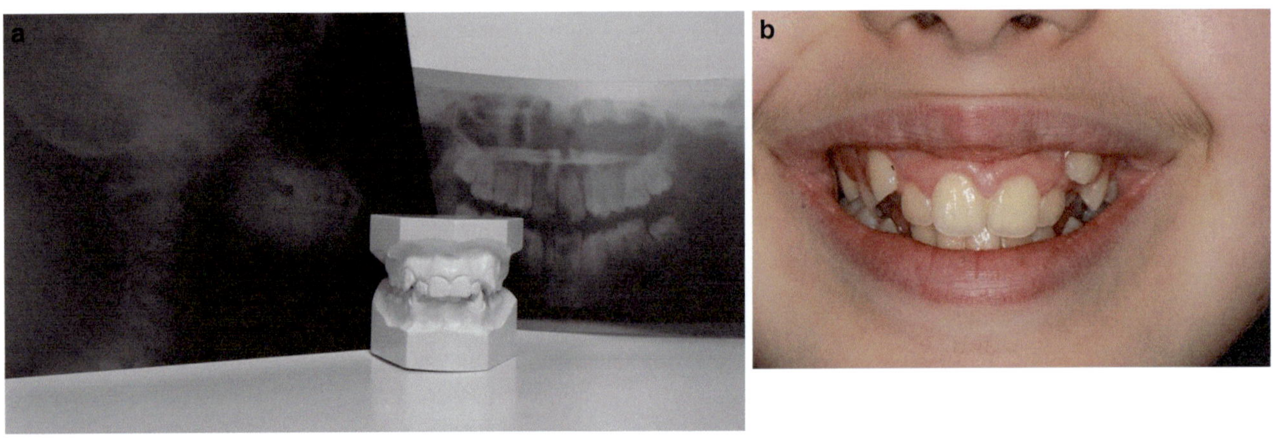

Fig. 2.2 (**a**) Dental records: panoramic film, cephalometric film, plaster models; (**b**) Photographic records

part of comprehensive orthodontic records, these photographs must be of high quality, standardized, carefully analyzed, methodically saved and stored with the confidentiality required for medical data [10].

A high-quality dental image must be sharp, bear no distortion [11] and present correct exposure of the intraoral cavity as well as facial features. It also must render the true shades and color of the dentition and the surrounding tissues, be exempt of unwanted artifacts, be calibrated, accessible and reproducible. At present, these stringent requirements can only be met through the use of Digital Single Lens Reflex (DSLR) cameras [12, 13] as well as the latest mirrorless cameras.

One must keep in mind that, in a busy orthodontic office, photographic equipment must be kept simple in its technical settings and easy to handle by the staff. The results must nonetheless be consistent, predictable, and reproducible according to pre-set rigorous protocols.

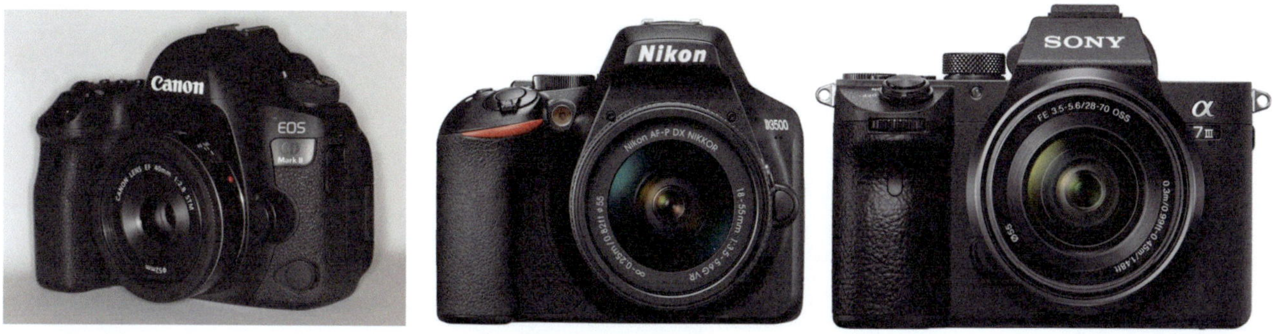

Fig. 2.3 DSLR and mirrorless cameras. From left to right: Canon, Nikon, Sony

2.2.1 Camera Body

Compact cameras became popular partly because of their simplified and automated settings and lower cost. They bear the advantage of their small size, lightweight, and ease of use among inexperienced operators. Unfortunately, compact cameras have limited macro capabilities, moderate image quality especially in low light situations and the integrated flash is inadequate for close up photography [14, 15].

Table 2.1 Advantages and disadvantages of DSLR camera in an orthodontic setup

Advantages of DSLR camera	Disadvantages of DSLR camera
Larger sensors produce better quality images	More expensive
Fine control over settings	Needs more expertise from the operator
LCD monitor screen for immediate review	Heavy
Histogram	Higher learning curve
Consistency and reproducibility of images	Somewhat intimidating for the novice user

Throughout the past decade, smartphones have become the camera everybody uses [16]. Though easy to take and to share through various applications and Wi-Fi, the photographs taken by smartphones unfortunately do not yet meet the standards needed to be considered good clinical data [17].

It is well accepted in the literature that the single lens reflex (DSLR) system and more recently the mirrorless camera (Fig. 2.3) are most suited for medical photography [7, 18]. DSLR and mirrorless cameras are strongly recommended when complete control of the photographic procedure is needed as in clinical dental photography. Yet it is not necessary to choose the most expensive equipment to achieve excellent results (Table 2.1).

2.2.2 Lens

Dental photography consists of taking photos of the dentition at close range and faces at relatively close range (1.2–1.5 m). Choosing the proper lens is of outmost importance in obtaining accurate and reproducible photographs with minimal distortion [19]. Prime macro lenses ranging from 85 to 105 mm allow for excellent intraoral photography as well as extraoral photography with the most faithful proportions and the least amount of distortion to the subject being photographed (Fig. 2.4). These lenses are short and light enough to be used without a tripod. Zoom lenses are not recommended as they offer little constancy in the magnification, provide limited macro-focusing capabilities and are less luminous with the images being somewhat less sharp than that of their prime lens counterpart (Table 2.2).

2.2.3 Flash Unit

Light is the most important factor in photography [20]. A very high focal ratio (f-stop) (very small aperture: *f* / 22 and smaller) is needed to get an adequate depth of field and achieve sharpness of the entire dentition. This requirement commands the use of accessory light units to consistently deliver the most adequate amount of light into the oral cavity.

2.2.3.1 Built-In and Pop-Up Camera Flash

The flash unit incorporated into the camera (above the lens) is a single-point flash that is not ideal in dental photography because of the large shadows created by its unfavorable position right above the lens, resulting in non-uniform light distribution over the subject. Unlike the flash integrated to the camera body, external flashes are mounted in a manner

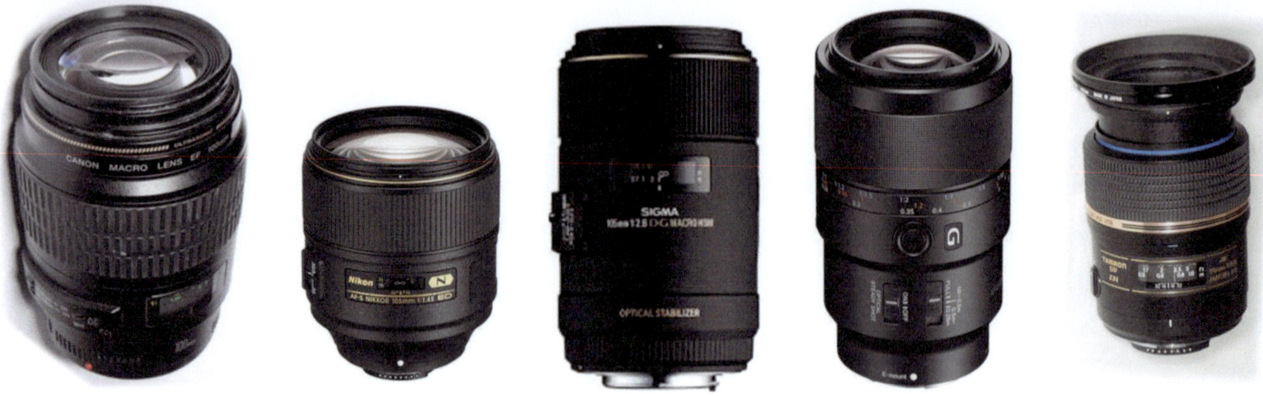

Fig. 2.4 Different macro lenses used for dental photography. From left to right: Canon™ 100 mm, Nikkor 105 mm™, Sigma 105 mm™, Sony MacroG90 mm™, Tamron 90 mm™

Table 2.2 Advantages of a macro lens in dental photography

Advantages of macro lens	Advantages of zoom lens
Best image quality	Acceptable image quality
Adjustable and improved magnification	Versatility and convenience
Good luminosity	Less equipment to carry
Good distance from subject for intraoral and extraoral photography	Variable distance
Reproducible picture	Variability in reproducing picture
Improved sharpness when compared to zoom lenses	Not as sharp as prime macro lenses

to deliver the best possible uniform and shadowless lighting of the oral cavity.

2.2.3.2 Ring Flash

The ring flash is a circular flash positioned around the lens. This flash system provides an evenly lit subject that removes any shadows thus creating a flat image, without depth. Easy to use, the ring flash is ideal for surgical, restorative, prosthetic photography and orthodontic photography that involves the posterior segment areas when shadows are not welcome. However, the overjet is poorly registered due to the very lack of shadow [8] (Fig. 2.5).

2.2.3.3 Dual Point Flash Bracket (With or Without Bouncers)

To avoid the loss of image depth caused by the lack of shadows created by the ring flash, twin flash units may be mounted and attached to the lens in the same manner as the ring flash (Fig. 2.6). The R1 system™ has two or more flash units (Fig. 2.6a). The R2 system comes with extendable arms for more lateral positioning and direction of the flash units in regard to the subject (Fig. 2.6b). Twin flashes help create softer shadows that enhance the quality of the portraiture. Bouncers, also called flash diffusers, are simple light modifiers that are usually made of white, semi-transparent plastic or reflective material and mounted onto the flash to diffuse the light of the flash unit. They soften the shadows and decrease the reflection from the flash onto the surface of the dentition. The R2 system with its extendable arms may cause shadows in the posterior segments of the oral cavity if the flash units are not positioned correctly. Dual point flashes require more manipulation and the outcome varies depending on the expertise of the operator [8].They are more geared towards the professional photographer and may be less suitable for the busy orthodontic office (Tables 2.3 and 2.4).

2.2.4 Conclusions of the Rationale to Use DSLR Cameras, Macro Lenses, and External Flashes

To achieve quality clinical dental photography in the dental office, a high-quality camera body, a macro lens, and specialized flash units suitable for macrophotography must be used [20]. The ability and knowledge to set up the camera properly is also of outmost importance. Once past the initial expense, such camera systems will last for many years without the need for upgrading and the initial investment will yield consistent results.

Clinical photographs should be downloaded and stored ideally into the same software that is used for digital radiographs as part of the comprehensive records (Table 2.5).

2.3 Dental Photography Techniques

2.3.1 Extraoral Photography

Orthodontic treatments include important esthetic components and should incorporate facial photographic

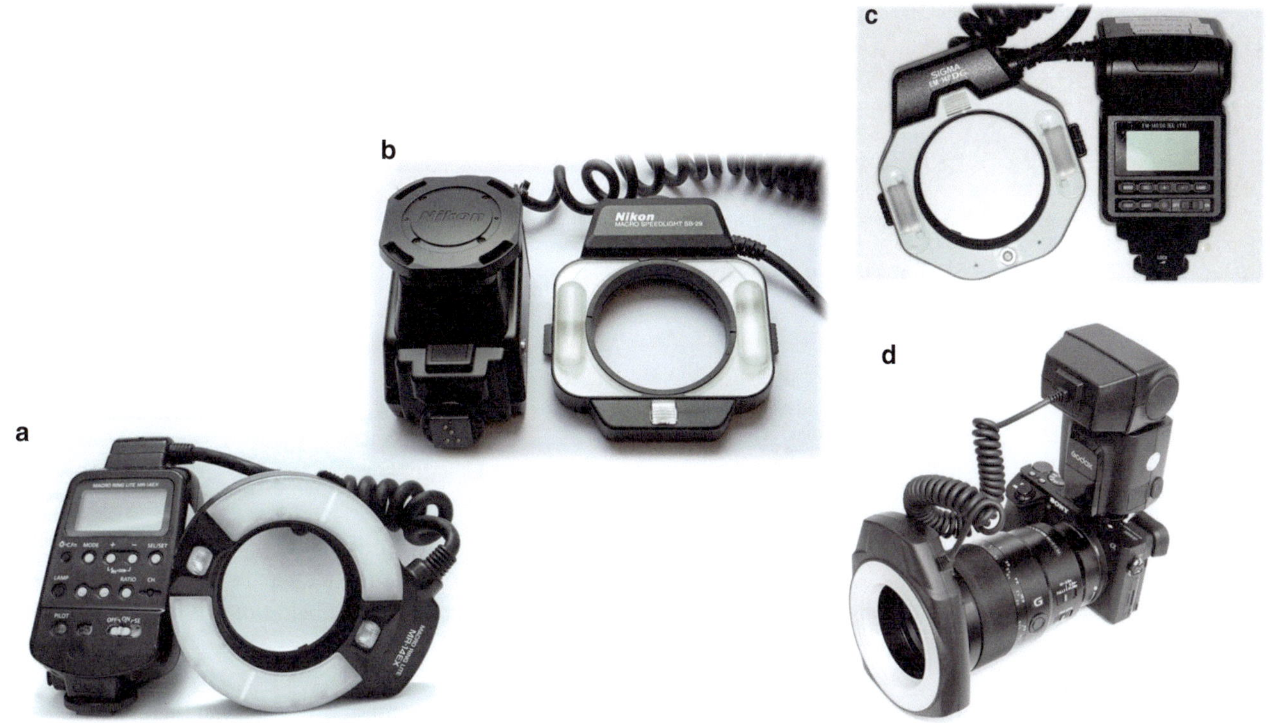

Fig. 2.5 Different ring flash used for digital dental photography. (**a**) CanonMR14EX; (**b**) Nikon SB29; (**c**) Sigma EM140; (**d**) GodoxML150

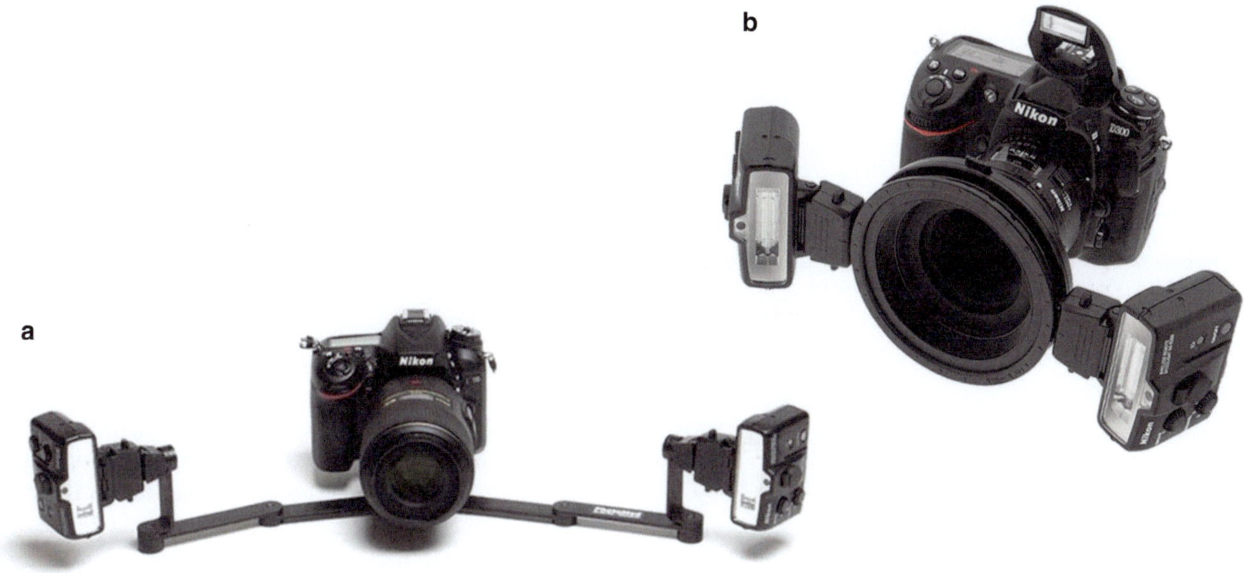

Fig. 2.6 Twin flash units. (**a**) *Nikon with R2* Dual Point Flash Bracket; (**b**) *Nikon4804 R1* wireless twin flash system

documentation as well as intraoral photographs. Portraiture photography is used in orthodontics for its clinical value. Hence, strict protocols must be applied in order to maintain quality and reproducibility. To take extraoral portraits of the patient, the same camera, lens, and flash units should be used as for the intraoral photographs [7]. The camera will be positioned vertically in portrait mode. No assistant nor special accessories are necessary. When taking extraoral photographs, the patient is standing up or sitting straight against a plain, nonreflective background and the patient/operator distance must remain constant to ensure consistency and reproducibility in the photos over time [21] (Fig. 2.7).

Table 2.3 Advantages and disadvantages of digital flash photography

The advantages of flash photography	The disadvantages of flash photography
• The flash eliminates the camera shake (no blurry pictures)	• The cost of an additional piece of equipment plus the batteries
• The great intensity of light allows for the use of small apertures needed for sharp images of entire dentition	• Proper setup is necessary to avoid blinding the subject with overpowered flash light
• The color balance of the flash is that of daylight (white balance set to "flash" results in realistic color)	• The added weight of the equipment
• The external flash is compact enough and light enough to allow for hand-held photography	• The bulkiness of the flash system specially the R1 and R2 systems may be intimidating to the patient
• It generates compelling pictures	• Operator needs additional training

Table 2.4 Flashes used for dental photography

Pop-up flash	Ring flash	Speed light flash with and/or without extensible arms
Inadequate intensity and direction of light	Uniform light	Directional light
Harsh and large shadows	Shadows are eliminated: Flatten images—Decreased 3D perception in portraiture. Eliminate overjet	Bouncers soften light and deliver softer shadows: Ideal for portraiture and creative photography; Reduce flash reflection on dentition Better overjet rendering
No control of luminosity or direction of light	Ideal for surgery and intraoral cavity	Difficult to avoid shadows when used to photograph posterior areas of the oral cavity
No adjustments possible	No adjustments needed	Adjustment of arms needed according to the subject and direction of light
Negative space (buccal corridors)	Eliminates lateral negative space	Arm adjustments needed to avoid shadows in posterior segments of the oral cavity

When a patient presents for orthodontic treatment, a series of extraoral photographs are mandated. They include but are not limited to a frontal view (repose and smiling), a right side oblique (repose and smiling), and right side full profile (repose and smiling) (Fig. 2.8). In case of asymmetry, in preparation for orthognathic surgery or when the clinical situation requires it, additional views may be indicated (Fig. 2.9).

Table 2.5 Pros and cons to using DSLR camera setup for dental photography

Advantages of the DSLR equipment	Disadvantages of DSLR camera
Excellent image quality	
Complete control over light, aperture, magnification, color	Needs more expertise from the operator
Minimal image distortion with the proper lens	
May be used for intra- and extraoral dental photography	May require assistant's help
LCD monitor screen for immediate review	Heavy and bulky
Histogram	Higher learning curve
Consistency and reproducibility of images	Somewhat intimidating for the novice user
Long-term cost-effectiveness	High initial expense

When preparing for facial photography, attention must be paid to the background and the surrounding lighting. It is important to keep the same background over time and maintain the same distance between the patient and the operator in order to ensure reproducibility and consistency so important in clinical photography [22] (Fig. 2.10).

2.3.1.1 Most Common Camera Settings for Portraiture Photography Used in Orthodontics

When the portraits are used for esthetics or marketing purposes, the rules are less stringent and artistic interests may prevail as the photographs are taken for a different purpose (Table 2.6).

2.3.2 Intraoral Photography

In orthodontics, frontal view of the dentition, teeth in occlusion, left- and right-side views with teeth in occlusion, upper and lower occlusal views are part of the standard intraoral photographic protocol [23]. The patient should be seated in the dental chair for comfort and a better control of the patient's positioning (Fig. 2.11). The camera is now positioned in landscape mode. The position of the lens of the camera should be maintained at 90° from the surface of the dentition to be photographed.

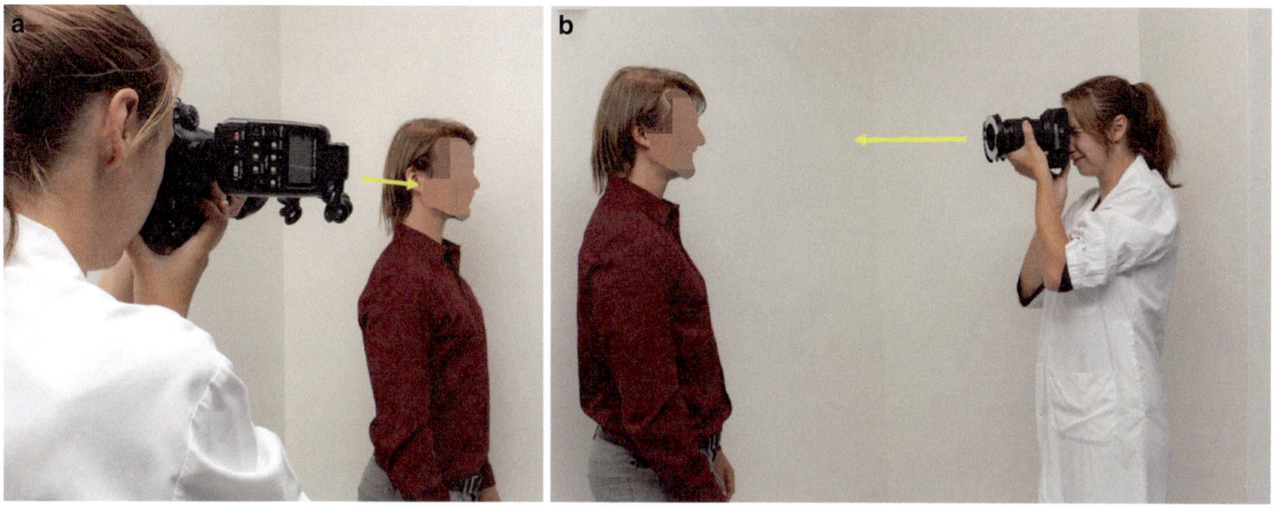

Fig. 2.7 Position of the operator while obtaining the extraoral photographs. (**a**) position of operator and camera holding; (**b**) position of lens to subject

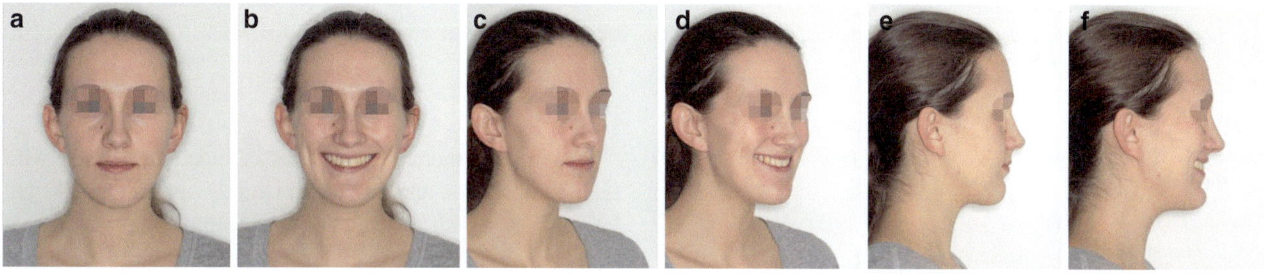

Fig. 2.8 Common poses for extraoral photographs within the content of photographic orthodontic records. (**a**) front repose; (**b**) frontal smile; (**c**) oblique repose; (**d**) repose oblique smile; (**e**) full profile repose; (**f**) full profile smile

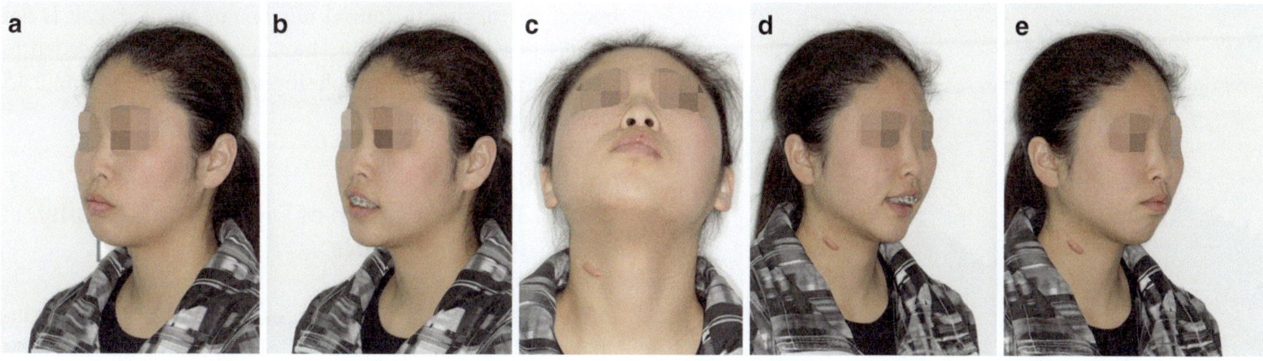

Fig. 2.9 (**a**) left side oblique; (**b**) left side smiling; (**c**) submental vertical view; (**d**) right side smiling oblique; (**e**) right side oblique

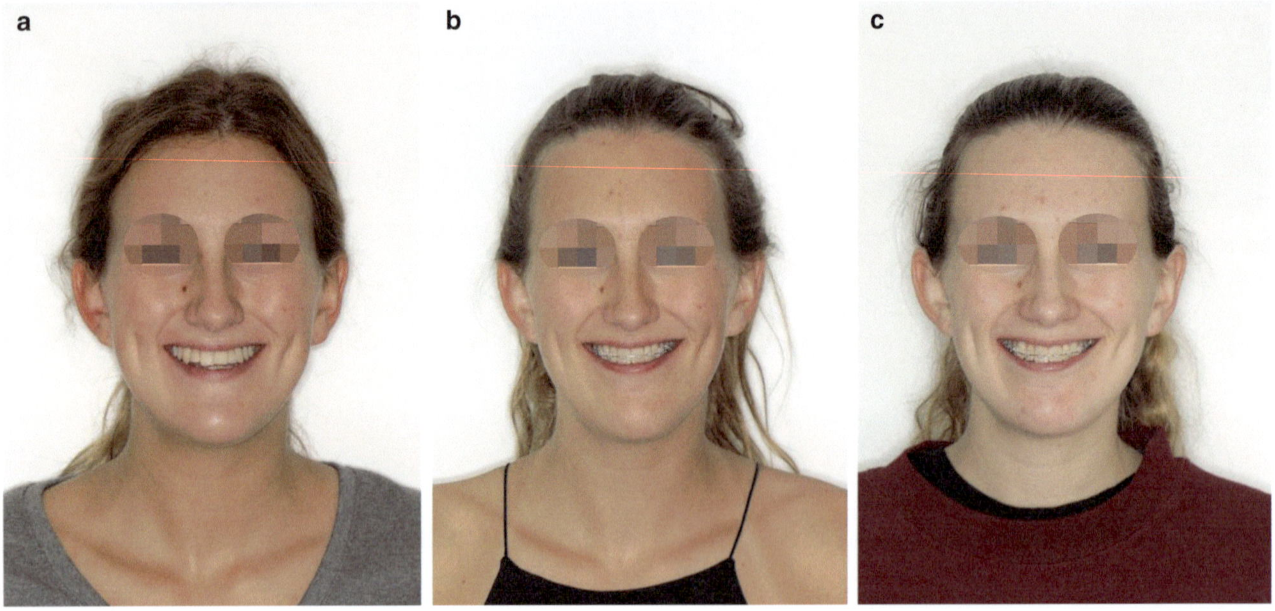

Fig. 2.10 (**a–c**) Example illustrating the importance of constant distance between operator and subject for consistent results. (**a**) Initial record, (**b**) after 12 months, (**c**) after 30 months

Table 2.6 Required camera settings for good portraiture photography in orthodontic records

Camera mode: M (manual) or Av (aperture priority) mode
F values: between f/5.6 and f/11
Shutter speed: 1/125 s (avoid camera shake)
Iso 100–400 (the lowest possible)
White balance: flash (5000–6000 K)
Flash power M: 1/1 or ETTL with flash synchronized speed in Av mode
Focus mode: manual with magnification ratio 1:10 or automatic focus with pre-set distance between patient and operator

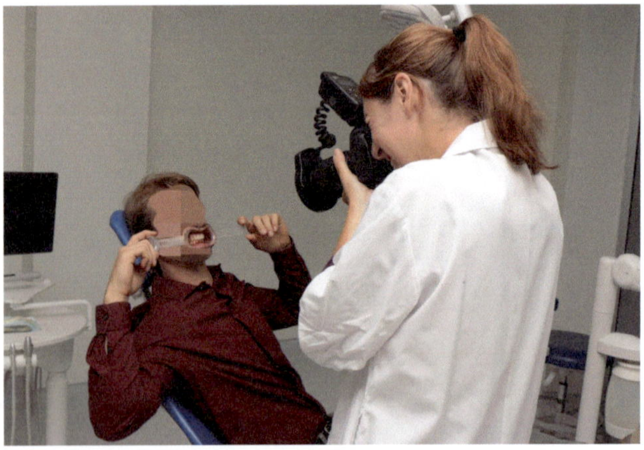

Fig. 2.11 Example of a good patient/operator positioning for intraoral photography

Standard intraoral photographs include frontal view with teeth in occlusion and with teeth slightly apart, left and right lateral views with teeth in occlusion, and lower and upper occlusal views. Additional views may be added according to the patient's clinical condition and orthodontist's preferences (Figs. 2.12 and 2.13).

Intraoral photography requires accessories to retract the soft tissues for a clear view of the dentition. Cheek retractors, buccal mirrors, and occlusal mirrors are needed as it is not always possible to open the mouth to the extent needed to obtain the desired clinical photographs (Figs. 2.14 and 2.15 and Tables 2.7 and 2.8) [7].

2.3.3 The Application of Digital Photography in Orthodontics

Photography in dentistry provides unique and highly valuable diagnostic information. A photograph that illustrates and validates the orthodontist's statement tends to increase the trust of the patient towards the dental professional. As the value and power of 2D clinical photography rest on the consistency of the views and the reproducibility of the photos, easy, simple and efficient protocols are the key to successfully implement the best photographic imaging system in the dental office. High-quality 2D intraoral and facial digital

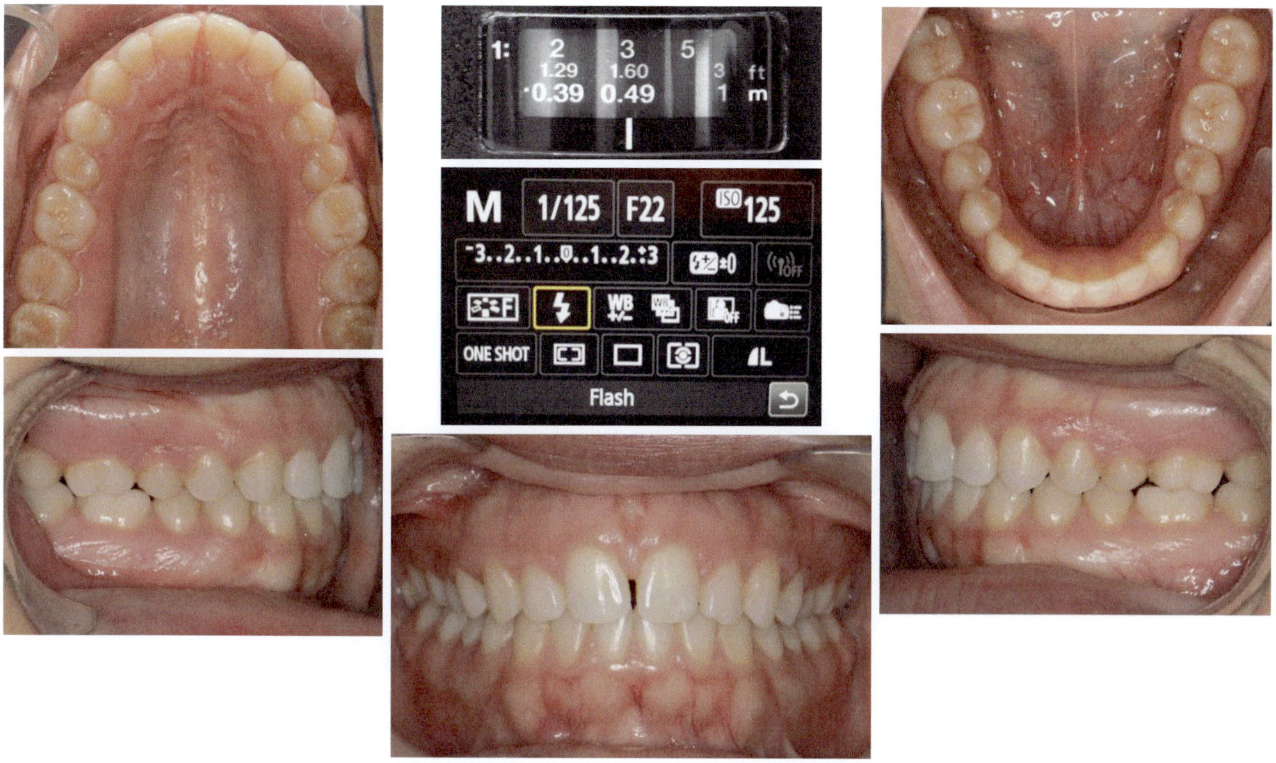

Fig. 2.12 Camera setup and most common intraoral views

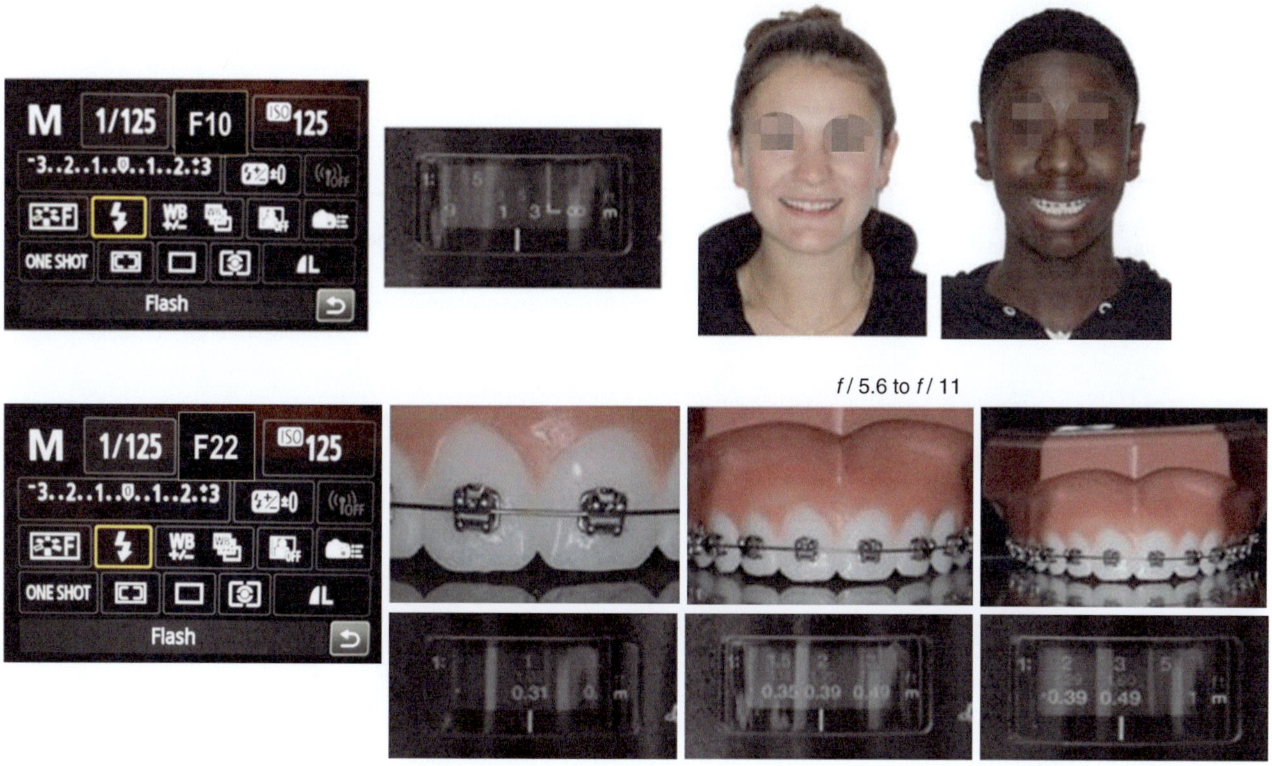

Fig. 2.13 Camera settings and magnification ratio for consistency of the views. These views may be taken either in manual (M) or aperture priority (Av) mode

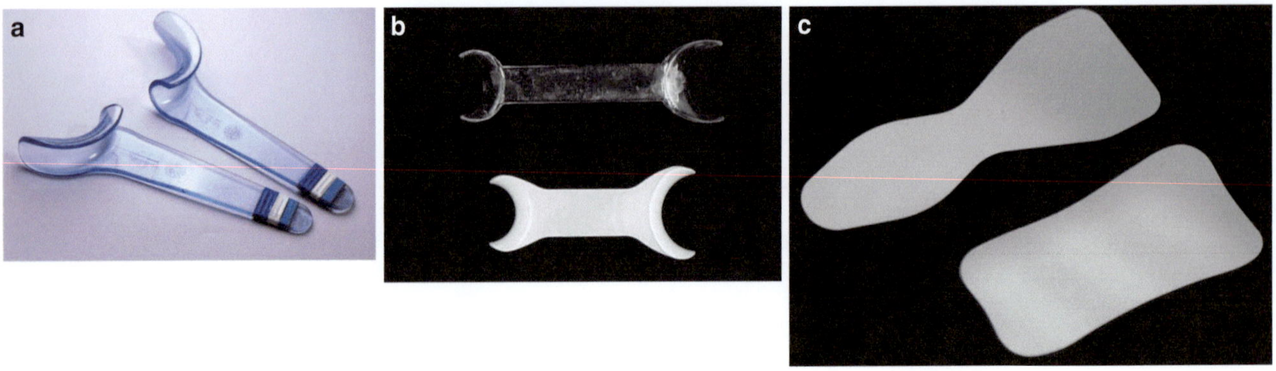

Fig. 2.14 (**a**) Lip retractor; (**b**) cheek retractors; (**c**) occlusal and buccal mirrors

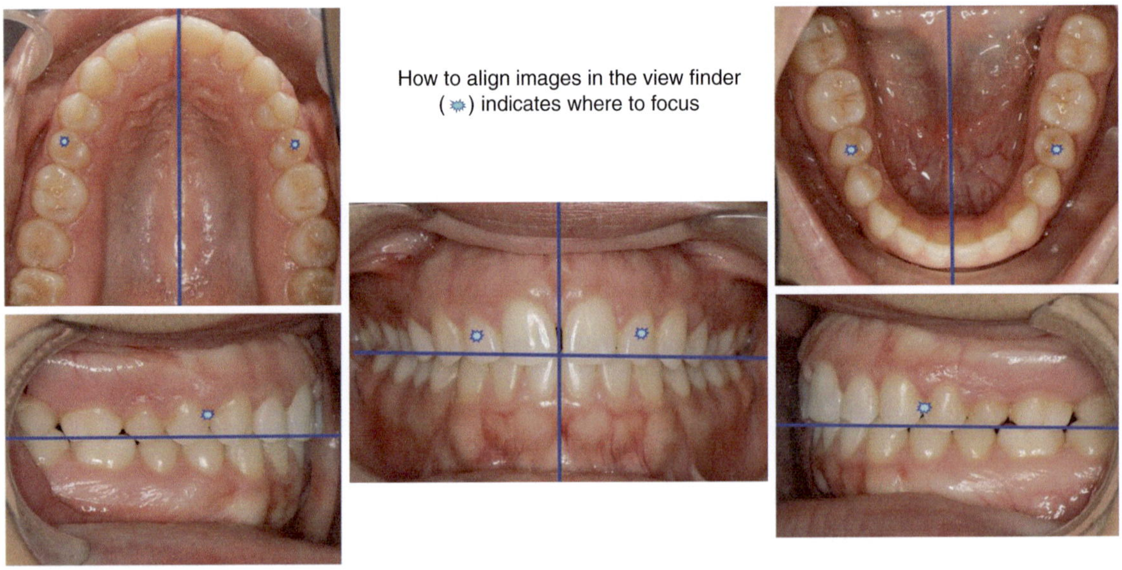

Fig. 2.15 Proper image framing and focusing points

Table 2.7 Intraoral camera and flash settings

Camera setup for intraoral dental photography
Camera mode: manual (M) or aperture priority (Av) mode with flash-sync speed in Av mode
Aperture: *f*/22 to *f*/32
Shutter speed 1/125 s or according to flash-sync speed of a given camera body in Av mode
Iso 100–400 (the lowest possible)
White balance: flash 5000–6000 K
Focus mode: manual magnification ratio 1:3. Automatic focus is not recommended as it does not allow to pre-set distance between patient and operator for adequate standardization
Flash power: M ¼ or ETTL
Camera positioned in landscape position

photographs—when associated to virtual 3D models—are also very helpful in assisting the orthodontist with the future 3D positioning of the teeth and gingival tissue contours in relation to the surrounding soft tissues, lips, and face.

Table 2.8 Protocol for patient's preparation and position for intraoral photography

Patient's and operator preparation and positioning
Patient comfortably seated (ideally in dental chair) for stability and ease of operation
Operator standing at the 9 o'clock position from seated patient
Auxiliaries necessary to obtain adequate images of the dentition and oral cavity: Retractors, occlusal mirrors, buccal mirrors if using indirect view of the buccal left and right lateral sides
The lens should be directed 90° to the surface of the teeth to be photographed to avoid any distortion
Saliva ejectors and air syringe will help control the amount of saliva on the hard and soft tissues

Patients are increasingly turning to orthodontic treatment for its esthetic value and the orthodontic discipline has moved from simply aligning the dentition and optimizing the skeletal components of the craniofacial aspects to addressing the soft tissues balance and overall facial esthetics [24]. Today, well-occluding casts and accurate cephalometric measurements are no longer considered to be the only treatment goals for the orthodontist [25].

Dr. Andre Wilson Machado has described the ten commandments of the smile esthetics [26]:

1. The smile arc
2. The ratio and symmetry of the upper central incisors
3. The proportion between the upper anterior teeth
4. No spacing between the upper anterior teeth
5. The gingival aspect and exposure
6. The buccal corridor
7. The midline
8. Tooth angulation
9. Tooth color and shape
10. Lip volume and shape

All ten aspects can readily be assessed with good quality clinical photographs and the data utilized to help create a treatment plan for obtaining the best esthetic smile for the patient.

Since visual impression plays an important role in our social environment, the smile enhancement of the patient should be given great importance in orthodontic treatment planning. Comprehensive clinical observations and record-taking in the form of clinical photographs and videos are recommended [27].

2.3.3.1 Smile Arc Analysis

The smile arc may be described as the relationship between the curve created by the edge of the upper front and side teeth to that of the lower lip at smile (Fig. 2.16). It plays an important role in determining the esthetic of the smile [27] as described by Ackerman [28].The smile arc can be readily assessed with 2D photographs and the observations collected have a considerable influence on the treatment plan, the esthetic outcome of the orthodontic treatment and ultimately, the patient's satisfaction to the treatment performed [29].

The evaluation of the smile is made through the analysis of the midlines, the smile width, the amount of gingiva showing, the position of the dentition in regard to the lips, the size of the teeth, and the amount of teeth showing at rest and when smiling (Fig. 2.17). The assessment of the changes during the orthodontic treatment is easily documented by the use of good 2D clinical photographs taken throughout the treatment.

Since we live in a highly visual world and the image that we project plays an important role in how we are perceived, the smile enhancement aspect of the treatment should be given great importance in the treatment planning and achieving a "balanced" smile is most desirable if the patient is to be satisfied [30].

2.3.3.2 Digital Smile Design

Digital Smile Design (DSD) is a treatment planning tool that uses those 2D photographs, dynamic images from short videos and software analysis to help visualize the ideal 3D positioning of the dentition in regard to the lips and face of the patient. It provides a virtual simulation of the outcome and improves communication and understanding for the patient [31].

The digital smile design tool uses eight steps to determine the optimal smile arc for a given patient [19].

- Assess the facial midline and the horizontal interpupillary line
- Analyze the shape and position of the smile curve

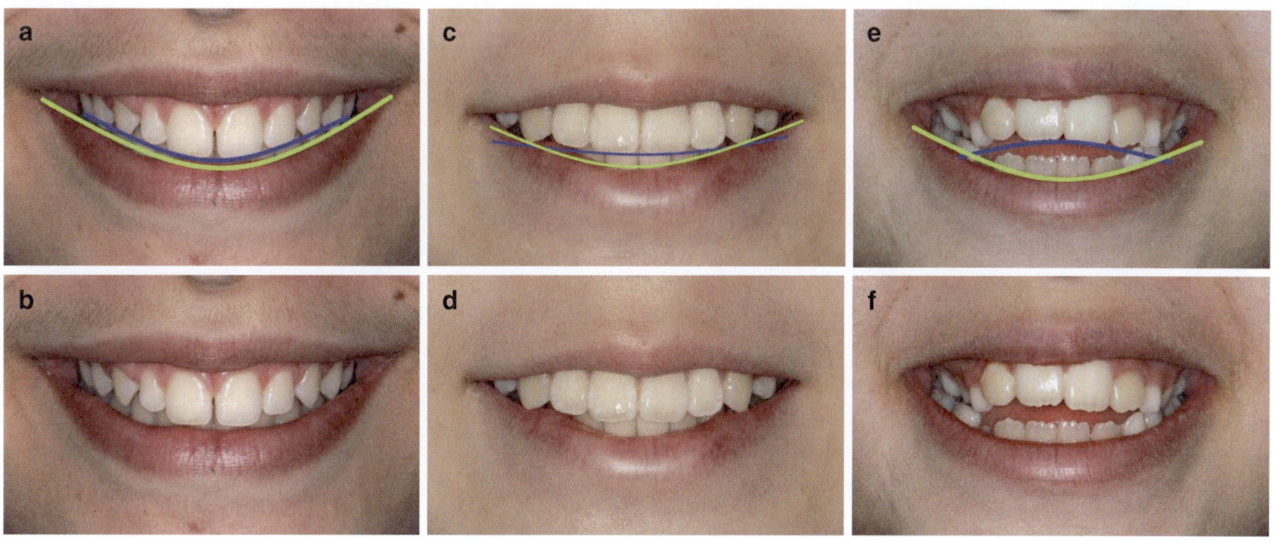

Fig. 2.16 Description of the smile arch. (**a**, **b**) Consonant smile; (**c**, **d**) flat smile; (**e**, **f**) reversed smile

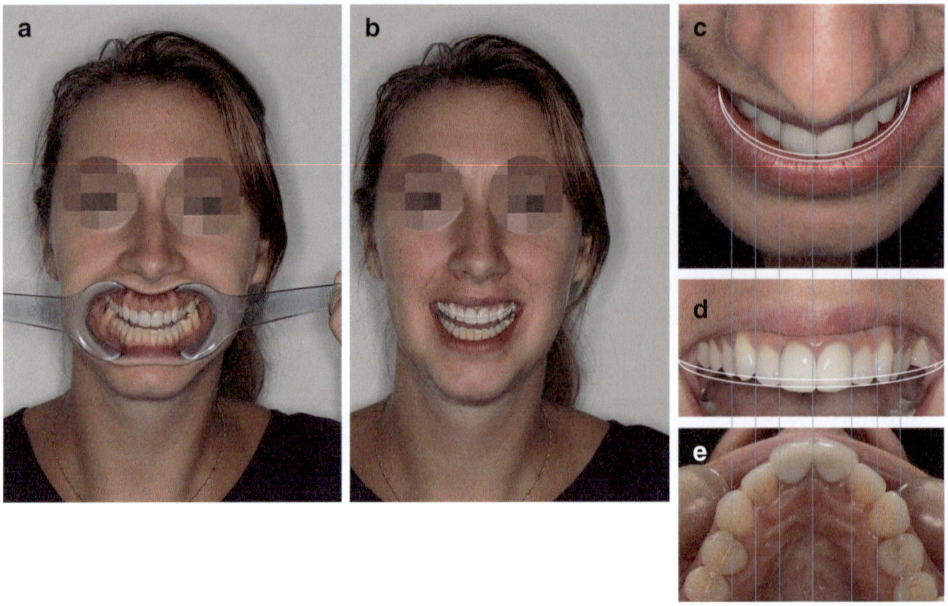

Fig. 2.17 Frontal extraoral view of the patient's smile with retracted lips (**a**) and without retracted lips (**b**); 12:00 o'clock view showing the midlines (**c**), smile curve (**d**), interdental width (**e**)

- Determine the interdental width proportion of the upper anterior teeth
- Note the central incisor width and length proportions
- Verify the gingival curve
- Evaluate the papillae curve
- Trace the vermillion curve
- Draw the arch curve

Comprehensive clinical observations combined with record-taking in the form of good clinical photographs and their analysis are of outmost importance [32].

2.3.3.3 Enhancing the Smile with Photographic Analysis and 3D Simulations

Digital Smile Design (DSD™) software allows dentists to use the latest advancements in technology to achieve excellence, improve accuracy, and increase communication. Patients are encouraged to become active participants in their own dental treatment plans, becoming co-designers of their future smiles while being able to communicate their needs and wants more effectively with their orthodontist [33].

The Digital Smile Design (DSD™) platform relies on the latest digital technologies. Some of the software used for dental improvements include but are not limited to iTero™, 3Shape™, Maestro™, SureSmile™, Onyxceph™, and OrthoClear™. Comparing the different technologies and providers will help doctors determine which option will help them achieve the best results during the course of a given treatment.

Digital smile design is much more than just a concept to improve the appearance of a smile. With this protocol, orthodontists can achieve more predictable outcomes and provide their patients with an unparalleled experience. DSD optimizes precision and efficiency for modern dental practices, ensuring more patient satisfaction towards their new and improved smiles.

Cone Beam CT

Three-dimensional Cone Beam Computer Tomography (CBCT) is making strides in the orthodontic world to improve diagnostic and treatment planning capabilities [34]. This type of tomography eliminates superimposition of structures and adds a third dimension to the views taken of a patient, which provides for more accurate diagnosis of dental problems and enables providers to come up with enhanced diagnostics and improved treatment strategies guided by the scan images [35].

With CBCT, it is easier to evaluate the direction and amplitude of tooth movement. From a single scan and depending on the size of the field of view and resolution selected, a coronal, axial, sagittal, panoramic, cephalometric, cross-sections as well as qualitative soft tissue imaging of the patients may be obtained [36]. The radiation dose delivered is much lower than that issued with a traditional CT scan and can be adjusted in function of the needs of a particular patient [34].

Intraoral Scanners

The use of the intraoral scanners has grown rapidly in the last few years and is fast becoming standard of care in orthodontics [37]. The process of using an intraoral scanner is simple and relatively comfortable for patients. Modern scanning machines are more accurate than conventional impressions and are more easily manipulated in a CAD software [38]. Options in digital scanning include Straumann™, 3Shape™, iTero™, Carestream™, Medit™, and many others. The goal of these scanners is to create an STL file that will be uploaded to a software for "cleaning" and removal of artifacts [39].

From the scans, orthodontists can produce virtual models for patients in need of comprehensive treatment such as aligner therapy, custom-made appliances or just to simulate different treatment modalities.

Many orthodontic practices now use reformatted files from intraoral digital scanners to create a more personalized treatment plan to address a given malocclusion. The iTero and 3Shape scanning systems also provide an outcome simulator that allows the patient to visualize the possible end results (Fig. 2.18).

These simulations are software driven and may be altered and improved by the orthodontist if needed. They illustrate the potential capabilities of intelligent software to use machine learning to achieve realistic simulations.

Improved Patient Outcomes

The technological advancements in the orthodontic industry have improved outcomes for millions of patients affected by malocclusions [40]. With the increase in visualization and imagery that more effectively expose the layout, dimensions, and dental movements within the oral cavity, orthodontists can design and execute more effective and realistic treatment plans and assist patients in visualizing the potential results and thus participate actively in the choices to be made in line with the proposed treatment.

Quality 2D digital photographs combined to 3D simulations allow orthodontists to use the latest advancements in technology to achieve excellence, improve accuracy, increase communication, and obtain results that will fully satisfy the patients [41]. This has allowed patients to become actively involved in their own esthetic treatment plans and the elaboration of their future smiles. These new visual tools have helped improve patients' understanding of their dental condition and enhance the communication with their orthodontic team.

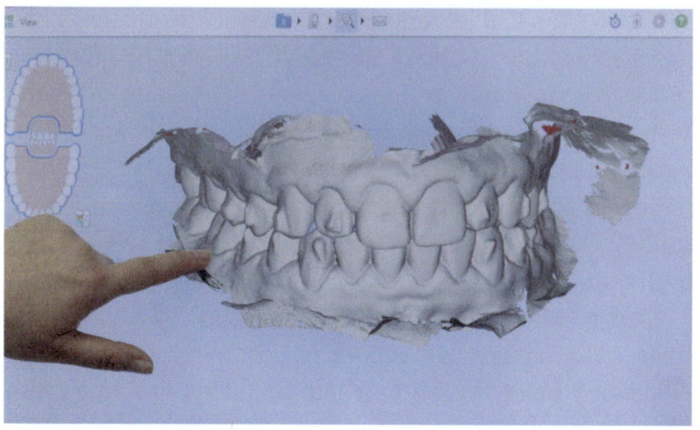

Fig. 2.18 Digital simulation of an intraoral scan using the iTero system

Computer design software combined to adequate 2D diagnostic photographs, CBCT, and intraoral scans now provide new tools to improve patients' understanding of their orthodontic condition, inform them of the possible treatment options and enable the visualization of the predicted changes in their smile.

Photos of retracted smile can be analyzed, teeth can be repositioned and/or reshaped with the use of these smile design software, and the final resulting dentition may be superimposed over the photo of the social smile to present to the patient a realistic simulation of the final results ultimately resulting in better understanding and an increased treatment outcome predictability [42].

2.3.4 Guidelines for the Alignment of Teeth in 3D Design, Starting from 2D Design

"If the esthetic parameter is not the one that will ensure the longevity of treatment, it remains the only criterion on which our patient can judge the quality of the work performed, making it an integral part of *therapeutic success*" [43].

Optimal facial esthetics is the result of the sum of all the esthetic components of the facial segments and their adjacent structures. Dental esthetics is only one aspect of the more inclusive facial esthetics [44].

Smile esthetics is an integral part of facial esthetics and is considered the most significant one when it comes to the establishment of optimum facial esthetics [45]. Basically, in designing smiles, one must consider the intimate components close to the teeth, the gums, the interdental papilla, the texture of the teeth, as well as the comprehensive components of the whole facial features, the position, dimensions, proportions, and the shape of the face and its segments [46].

The ultimate judge of the result of the orthodontic treatment is the patient. From the patient's perspective, the treatment will be assessed from a facial point of view with a forced smile representing the macroesthetics aspect of the treatment. The patient will then analyze the details of the dental arrangement in relation to the facial features (miniesthetics) and will complete his evaluation with the examination on the minute details of the dental arrangement (microesthetics) [47, 48].

All this information may be obtained and analyzed with the help of high-resolution portrait pictures of the patient either smiling or at rest. When taken separately, similarly to a puzzle, the different orthodontic elements that consist of the dental shape, color, and positioning, transmit nothing esthetically. Put together, they provide a complete picture (Figs. 2.19 and 2.20). It is quite difficult for the orthodontist to get an accurate representation about the final image when the pieces are scattered, and their rearrangement is arduous without the support of reference points.

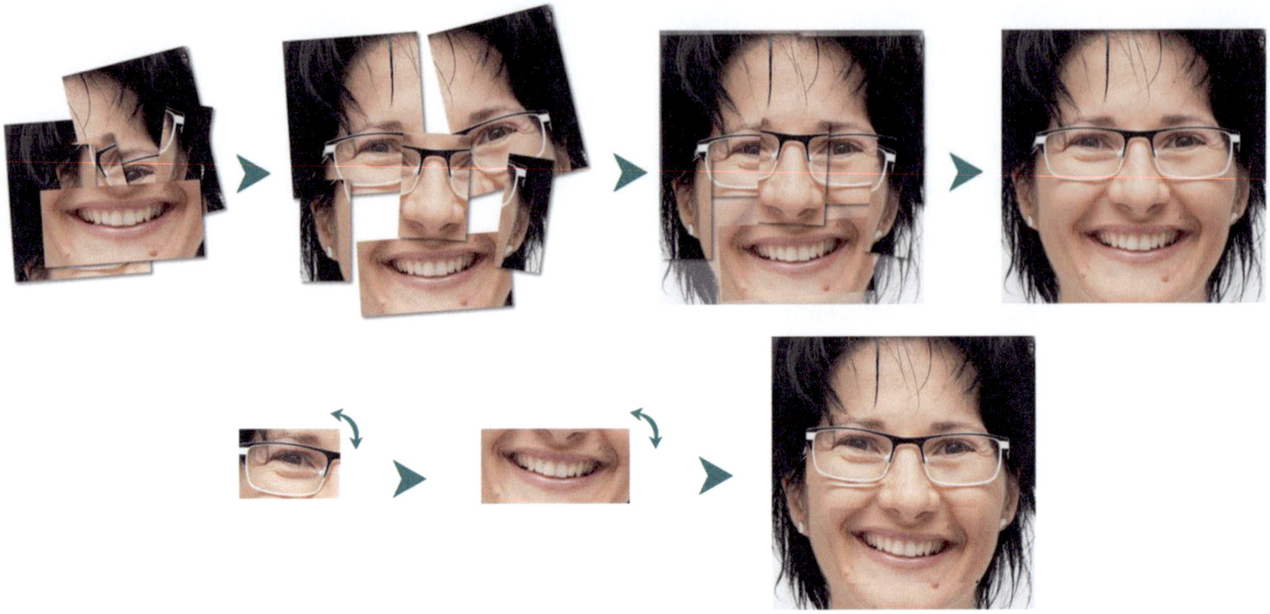

Fig. 2.19 (Upper row) Images were taken separately and each component of the facial entity provides no esthetic clue. (Lower row) Images were put together and an esthetic assessment becomes possible

Fig. 2.20 Facial components united with correction guidance

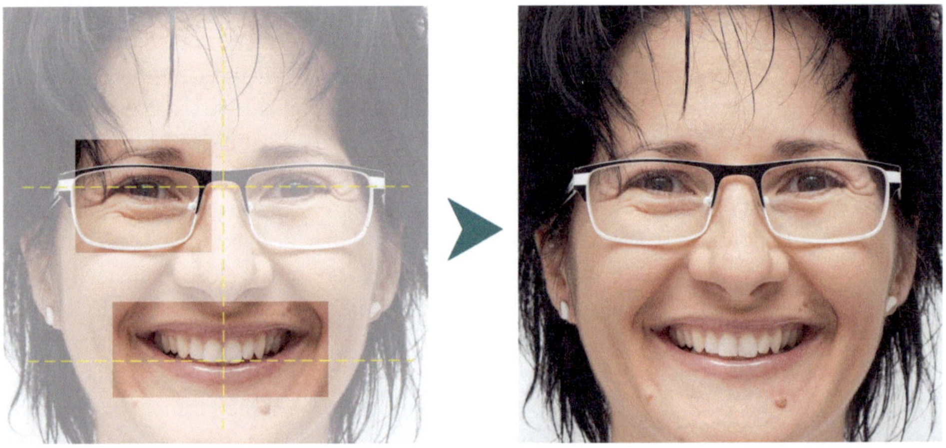

2.3.4.1 Guiding the Esthetic Plan Using Specialized Algorithms

Designing optimal dental esthetics requires a complete set of data and not just a set of models and cephalometric and panoramic radiographs.

The initial set of data studied consists of the series of portraiture photographs (rest, smiling, oblique 45°, profile) as they provide a lot of information about the positioning of the dentition in relation to the facial features. They also help establish constructive communication with the patients to better understand their expectations of the treatment.

The information present in the pictures can be immediately assessed. Once the photos are imported into specialized computer software, these images can be studied in a more systematic manner. This type of software is programmed to analyze the patient's esthetic parameters and provide a mathematical analysis such as the golden proportions [49] and several other analyses to quantify the changes needed to obtain the most esthetically appealing results (digital smile design or others). The dental software assists the orthodontist in defining esthetic goals and allows for simulations of multiple options before even initiating treatment. Several options can be tested in a controlled environment and introduced to the patient for evaluation.

Depending on the imaging software selected, the functions will either automatically or manually identify predefined points of the face and report on their interrelationship. Euclidian coordinates are used to decide on the desired amount of alteration to obtain the maximum esthetic benefits. Once accepted by the orthodontist and the patient,

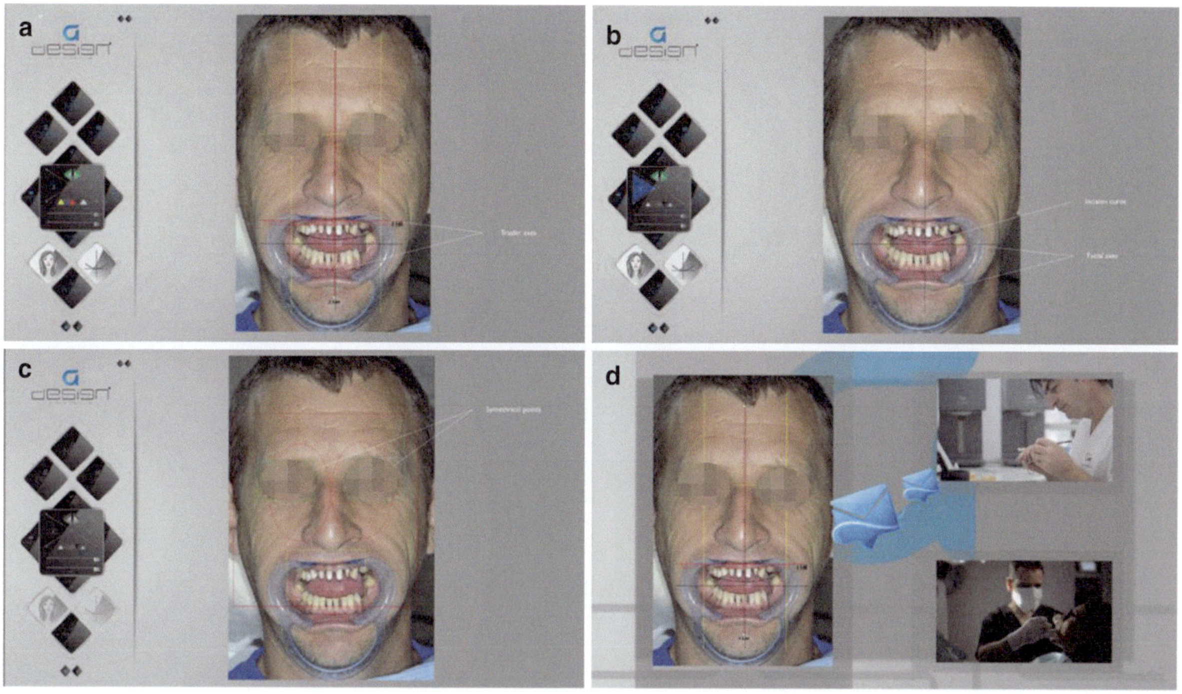

Fig. 2.21 Facial planning and alignment. (**a**) Facial axis drawn by markers; (**b**) smile arc design; (**c**) symmetrical axis of the pupils; (**d**) uprighting

the result will be incorporated into the treatment planning of the case and the modified portrait pictures of the patient uploaded into the software.

2.3.4.2 Facial Planning Through DSD Software

Specific markers are placed on the facial photograph. The first parameter to consider is establishing the facial symmetry. A first horizontal reference facial axis is drawn by linking the center of the ocular pupils. A parallel line on the lower third part of the face will determine the horizontal axis of the opening of the mouth. A perpendicular line is drawn from the middle of that horizontal line and will determine the vertical axis (Fig. 2.21).

2.3.4.3 Alignment of the Upper Anterior Teeth Without the Markers Provided by the Software

The orthodontist classically evaluates the esthetic requirements of the patient by using direct visualization of the face. The frontal positioning of the dentition is analyzed first by determining the midlines. This median line is related and compared to the philtrum and to the vertical axis of the face. Corrections are noted and this imaginary axis is now used to align the edges of the anterior teeth in relation to the imaginary horizontal axis of the face. With this method, the alignment of the dentition from a frontal perspective is determined by the facial esthetic requirements and not by dental casts or arbitrary cephalometric measurements.

The analysis of the panoramic radiograph, the lateral cephalometric radiograph, and study models can only assist marginally in the design of the smile in relation to the facial features as they are not linked to the patient's facial symmetry lines [50]. Using an antero-posterior (AP) cephalometric radiograph could also be considered to determine the facial axis by identifying left and right cranial reference points. However, this method does not take into account the soft tissues and the smile lines, which play a very important role in the making of the facial esthetics and thus, the results may not be fully predictable [51].

2.3.4.4 The Orthodontic Digital Alignment

This 3D digital design technique uses intraoral scans and imports them into a tooth-moving software such as Invisalign™, SureSmile™, Maestro™, OnyxCeph™, and others. At the moment, only the dental occlusion and the intra-arch relationship of the teeth are available to the orthodontist to design the future smile of the patient.

This type of software does not take into consideration the facial features and reference lines such as the facial axis, the lip line and curvature and the dental smile curve. Consequently, the simulation for the new alignment of the teeth is done exclusively at the level of the dental arches without any consideration for the pre and post 3D positioning of the dentition in the craniofacial structures.

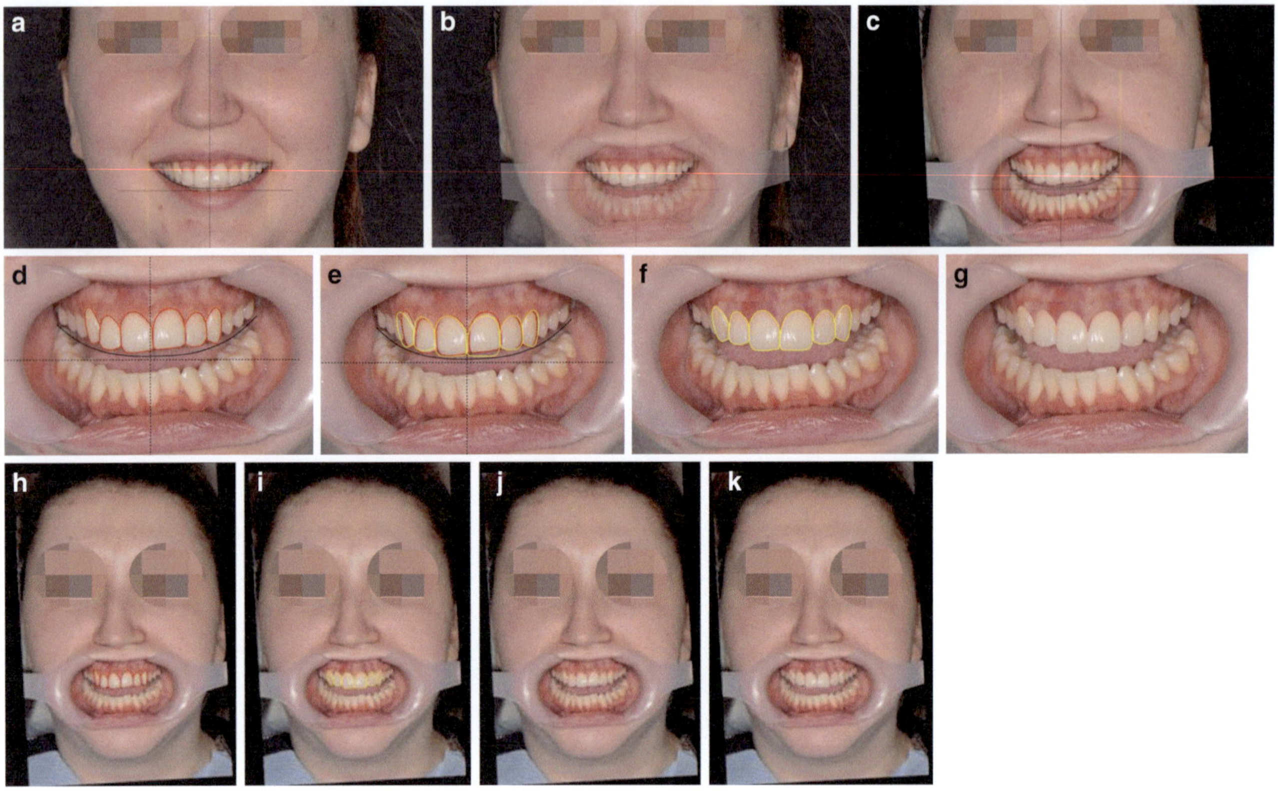

Fig. 2.22 (**a**) unretracted smile; (**b**) retracted smile arc; (**c**) retracted smile arc corrected; (**d**) initial uncorrected smile arc; (**e**) superimposition of initial and corrected smile arcs; (**f**) corrected smile arc outline; (**g**) corrected smile arc without outline; (**h**, **i**) retracted initial and corrected frontal view with outlines; (**j**, **k**) retracted initial and corrected frontal views without outlines

The referencing of the dentition is done following the instructions of the orthodontist with only minimal information on the final positioning of the dentition in the craniofacial structures. It is based on a trial and error process in a feed forward process [52] and not in the predictive manner that 3D digital planning is capable of delivering.

2.3.4.5 Planning Miniesthetics Using Digital Smile Design

Using specialized software, a digital design of the smile is elaborated by the orthodontist [33]. The input necessary for the design is extracted from 2D facial and intraoral photographs. By moving the different elements, a 2D simulation of the necessary movements is obtained which will help with the planned orthodontic treatment. This simple tool allows for a readily available simulation in the presence of the patient to visualize and better understand the course of the treatment (Fig. 2.22).

The smile design concept utilized in orthodontics uses the portrait pictures in various positions: smile, laughter, with labial retractors in place and vestibular intraoral photograph.

2.3.5 Converting 2D Images into 3D Digital Models

This digital smile design template of a 2D image is first transformed into a (pseudo) 3D design using only the frontal picture taken with the cheek retractors. Free software such as DSD CONNECT, G DESIGN, or equivalent maybe used for this procedure (Fig. 2.23).

The principle behind the transfer of information from a 2D image into a 3D digital design is based on:

- Overlapping the 2D image from the DSD design information over the 3D digital model, while the transparency is being modified.
- The superimposing and recalibrating of the 2D image within the 3D arch.
- Stitching the information obtained from the 2D design over the 3D model. The stitching will help guide the movements of the 3D design according to the 2D information provided.

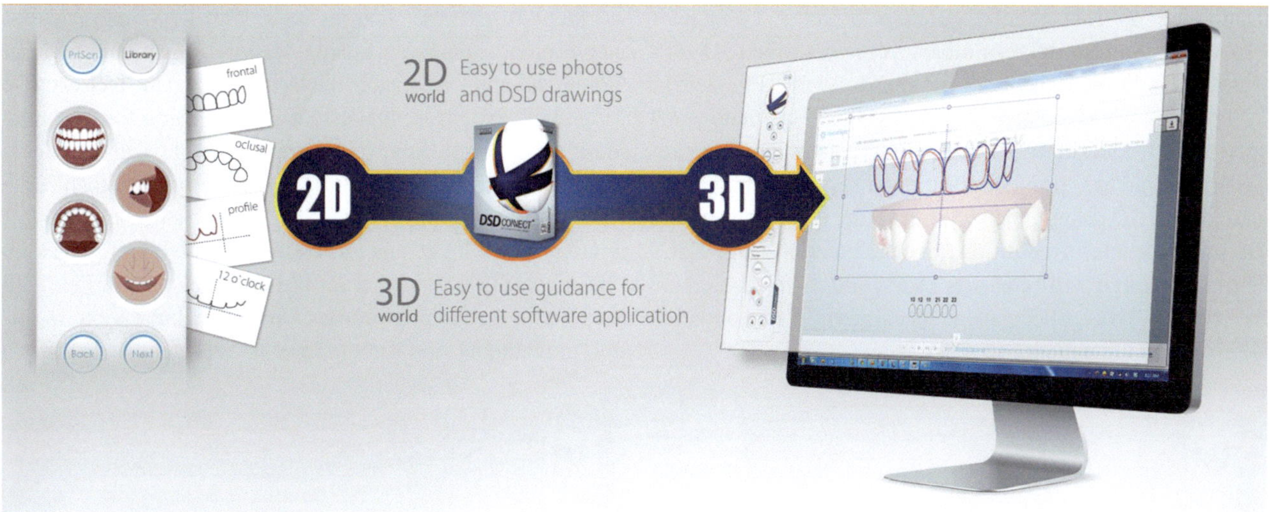

Fig. 2.23 Photographs and DSD drawings

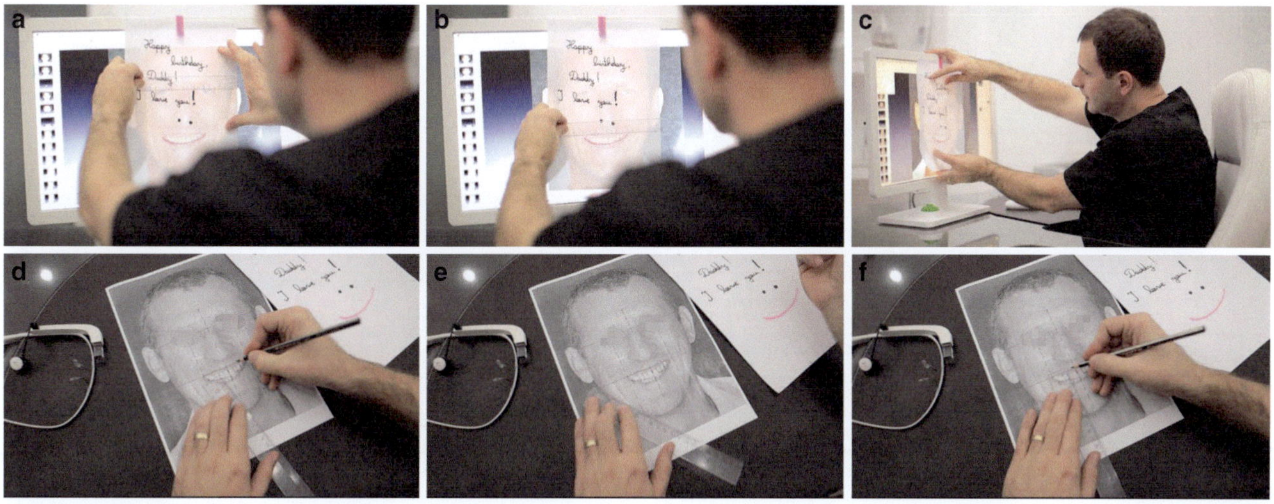

Fig. 2.24 (a-f) Example of a simple method for using the initial 2D design that was simulated and approved by the patient to calibrate and orient the 3D model

The software is designed in two parts. The first one is a summary simulation of the movements to showcase the final results for the patient and to suggest to the orthodontist some directions to treatment plan the case. The second step involves more elaborate treatment simulations and uses 3D software to refine and plan the case in a more robust and structured setting.

2.3.5.1 Digital Guidance Using Transfer Software

This software transfers all the information about the initial 2D design, simulated and approved by the patient, over the 3D model obtained either by intraoral or lab-bench scanning. The first step is to export the facial axis and teeth contours from the initial position and the approved simulation. Once the images have been imported into the software, they are calibrated over the 3D model and the repositioning is guided in the 3D orthodontic design. This information, alongside with the information obtained from the 2D design, is then imported in the 3D software which will transpose the data to 3D modeling algorithms (Fig. 2.24).

Using artificial intelligence and machine learning, the software will provide the most accurate digital orthodontic positioning of the dentition to obtain the most esthetically appropriate smile. Any tooth positioning software may be used such as Invisalign™, Clear Correct™, 3Shape™, Maestro™, SureSmile™, or others as the described 3D software is an add-on to the tooth-moving software (Fig. 2.25).

This software-assisted transfer system facilitates and speeds up the 3D design. The software automatically processes the picture, providing the necessary information for an accurate 3D design, the facial axis, the incisal curve, and the portrait picture repositioned for simulation (Fig. 2.26). Thus, 3D design will be easier, faster, and more secure, and the results will reflect more accurately the simulation approved by the patient.

Modern software such as DSD, with its simple and fast application, can automatically identify the required facial points and apply by default, the facial axis and the incisal curve (Fig. 2.27). The basic and essential information for the future design of the smile following the principles of facial esthetics is fully automated and can thus be delegated to a staff member.

The information obtained by the 2D software is automatically calibrated and transferred by overlapping over the 3D rendering obtained from the intraoral scan (Figs. 2.28 and 2.29). A stitching process allows the software to monitor movements and simulations in real time, whether in

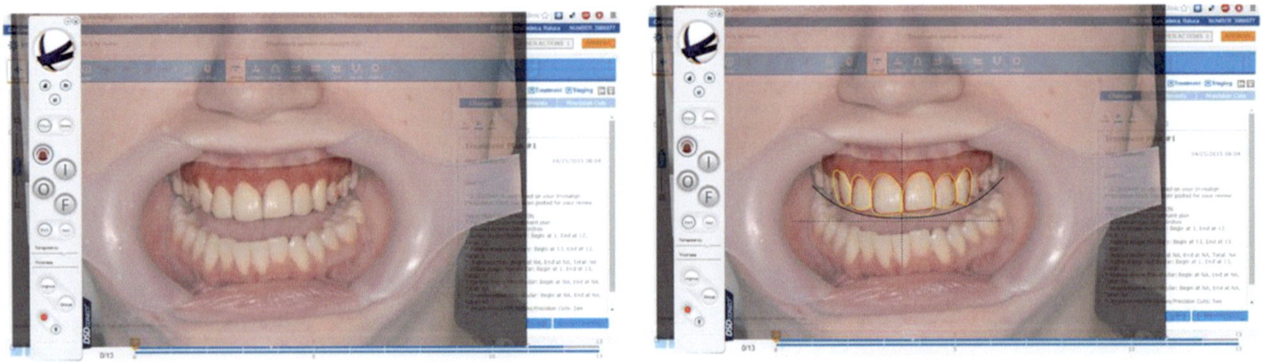

Fig. 2.25 Photo axis contour, before and after simulation

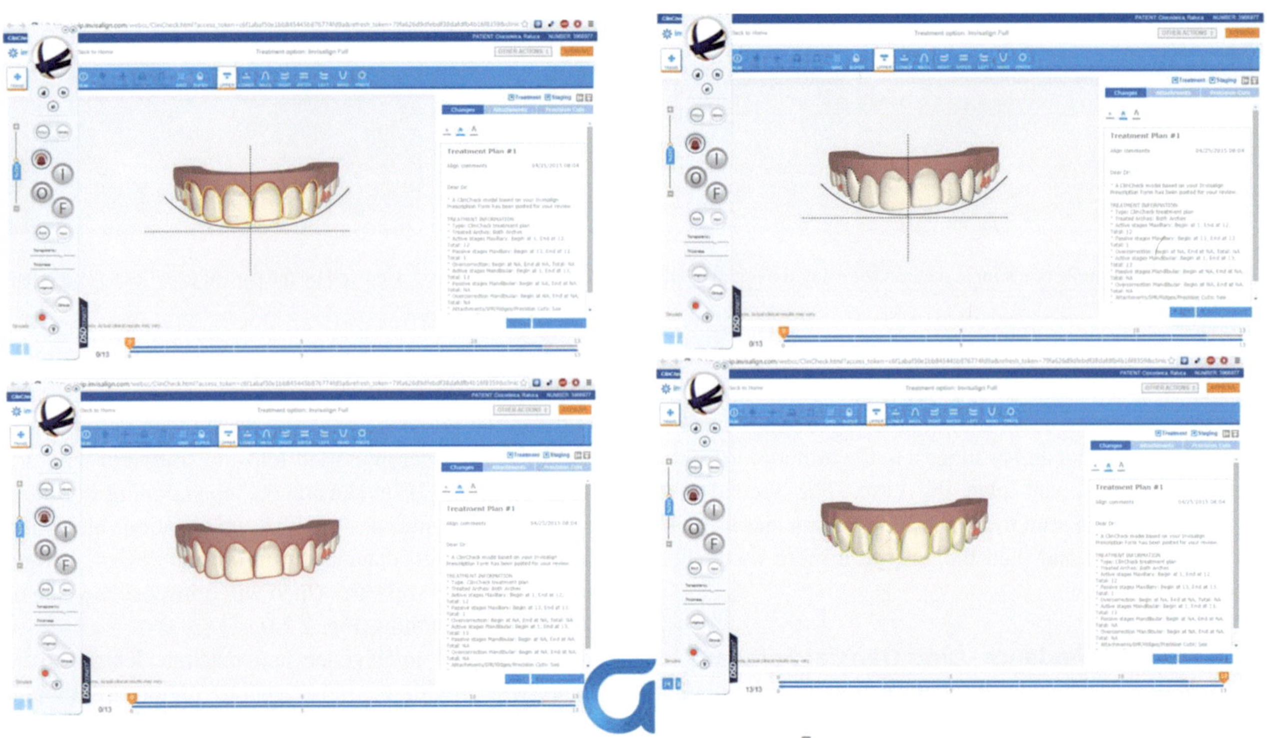

Fig. 2.26 Software repositioning of the dentition according to predetermined position obtained by 2D photographic analysis

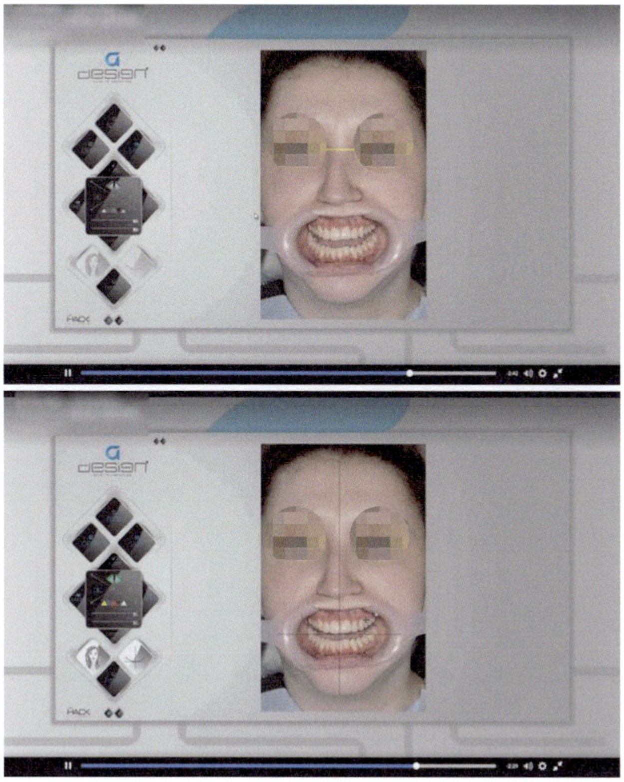

Fig. 2.27 (Upper image) line between pupils; (lower image) lower third plan and midline

Invisalign's software, or any other 3D Design software (CEREC™, Exocad™, 3Shape™, InLab™, etc.)

The 3D software (G Design) will then help verify whether the proposals for the future positioning of the teeth actually respect the parameters set by the initial smile design software. If not, then with the use of a simple "Print Screen" function, the simulation team can be instructed to review the setup in order to follow the specifications of the orthodontist.

The final position of the dentition is guided by the facial information, the expectations of the patient, in addition to the dental CAD-CAM design. The software, using the facial axis, smile line and soft tissue relationship, contributes significantly to the design of the future dental alignment and makes the results more predictable. The portrait picture on which the facial information has been processed can be captured using the print screen function of the software and forwarded to the processing team. This picture will give all the information needed for the transfer of facial axis onto the 3D model (Fig. 2.30).

2.3.6 Monitoring Treatment Results Using DSD Connect/G Design

The simulation software can also be used to monitor the intermediate stages of treatment and evaluate the final treat-

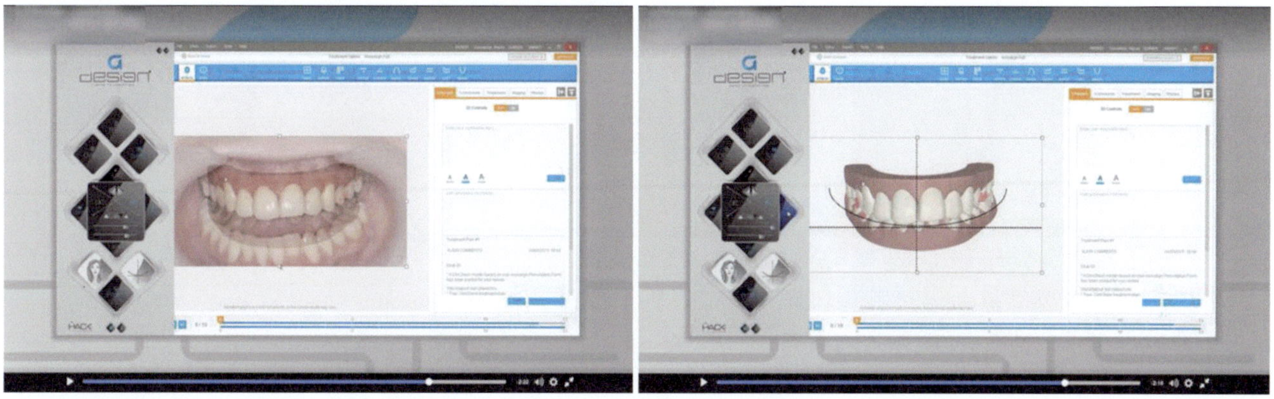

Fig. 2.28 Simulation verification

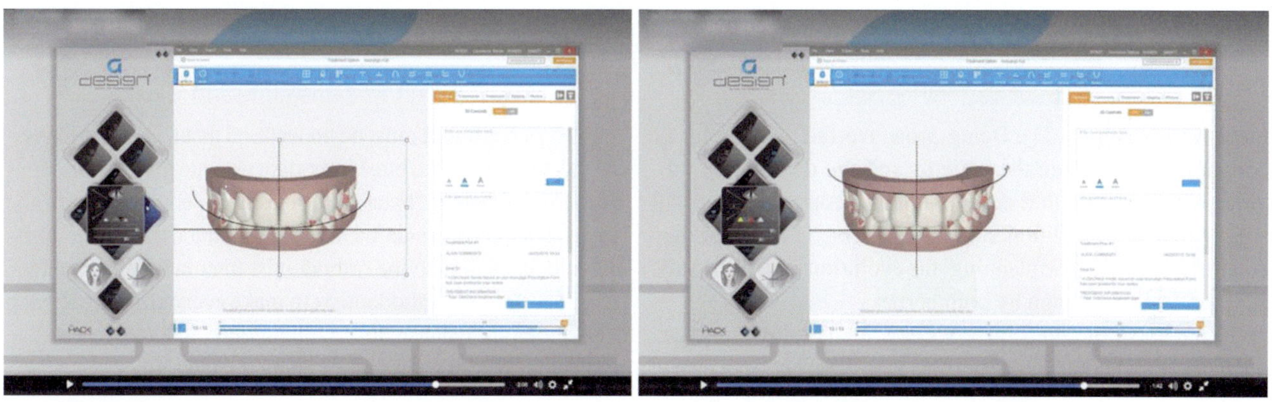

Fig. 2.29 Calibration and verification of the axis

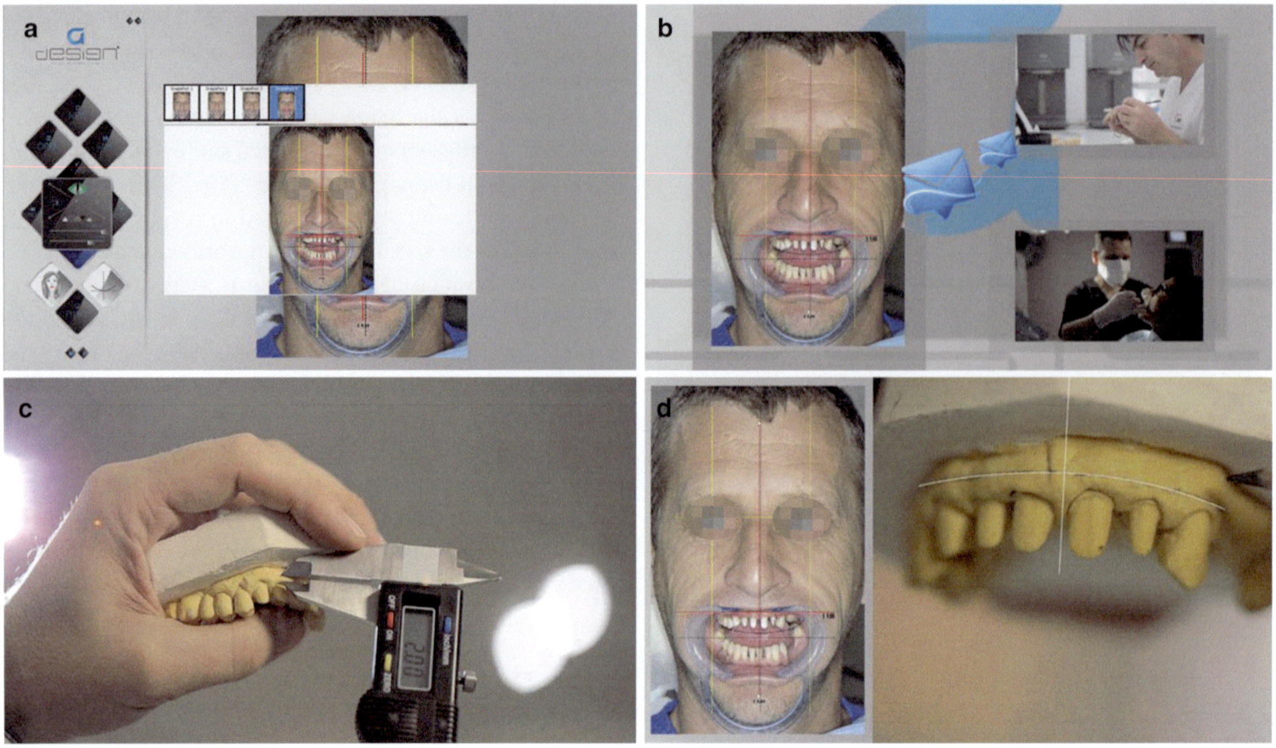

Fig. 2.30 (**a**) capture of 2D facial photograph; (**b**) transfer of information to technical team; (**c**) establishing treatment protocol; (**d**) in mouth monitoring

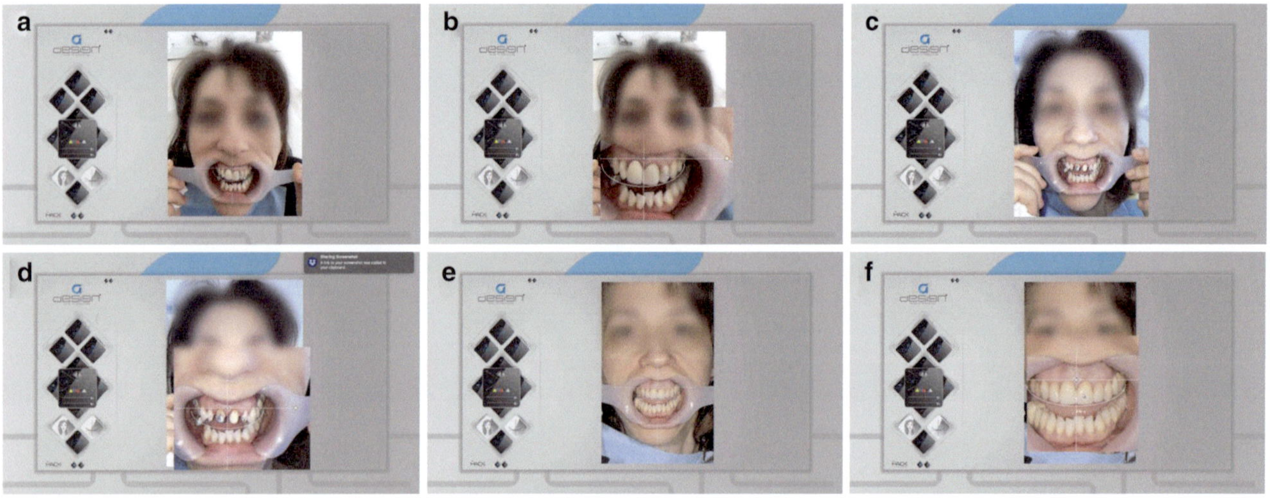

Fig. 2.31 (**a**) Portrait; (**b**) automatic application of the axis; (**c**, **d**) verification after procedure; (**e**, **f**) assessment of final results

ment results (Fig. 2.31). Being proactive facilitates a better collaboration between the patients and the dental care provider which results in a more predictable outcome that will satisfy both the practitioner and the patient. The patient may concretely witness the planning, the evolution, and the results as initially agreed upon by both parties.

In our modern competitive society, a charming smile can open doors and knock down barriers that stand between us and a fuller, richer life. It must be understood that there is no universal "ideal" smile. The most important esthetic goal in orthodontics is to achieve a "balanced" smile. The components of the smile should be considered not as rigid boundaries but as artistic guidelines to help the orthodontist treat individual patients. It is important for orthodontists to make every effort to develop a harmonious balance that will produce the most attractive smile possible for each patient being treated [30].

2.4 Conclusions

Clinical photographs are easily acquired by non-invasive methods, are readily available and relatively inexpensive to obtain and store.

A single photograph may have multiple uses as part of:

- The orthodontic examination, diagnosis, and treatment planning process
- Recording of the pre-treatment condition
- Monitoring progress records
- Communication with patient, staff and colleagues, dental technicians, academia
- Legal documentation
- Self-evaluation
- Marketing tool
- Publishing and education

Photographs allow the patient to visualize his or her orthodontic condition, treatment planning and outcome in a way that is accessible to all [53].

Good clinical photographs are very useful tools to the practitioner to assess, study, and plan the orthodontic treatment as they offer the most realistic representation of the patient's condition.

Adequate clinical images are not only informative nor are they solely used as a marketing tool. They provide the orthodontist with an ethical tool to educate their patients and lead them to a more proactive role in their decision towards their orthodontic treatment outcome. A photograph that illustrates and validates the orthodontist's statement tends to increase the trust of the patient towards him.

With photographic equipment becoming more and more efficient and less and less expensive, it is hard to imagine not incorporating clinical dental photography into everyday orthodontic practice.

References

1. Gernsheim H. A concise history of photography. North Chelmsford: Courier Corporation; 1986.
2. Barger MS. Bibliography of photographic processes in use before 1880. Their materials, processing, and conservation; 1980.
3. Jenkins RV. Technology and the market: George Eastman and the origins of mass amateur photography. Technol Cult. 1975;16(1): 1–19.
4. Neshangi S. Fundamentals of digital photography in dentistry. IJOCR. 2014;2(1):18–20.
5. Mladenović D, Mladenović L, Mladenović S. Importance of digital dental photography in the practice of dentistry. Acta Facultatis Medicae Naissensis. 2010;27(2):76.
6. Sheridan P. Practical aspects of clinical photography: part 2—data management, ethics and quality control. ANZ J Surg. 2013;83(4):293–5.
7. Bengel W. Mastering digital dental photography. New Malden: Quintessence; 2006.
8. Wander P, Ireland R. Dental photography in record keeping and litigation. Br Dent J. 2014;217(3):133–7.
9. Ahmad I. Digital dental photography. Part 1: an overview. Br Dent J. 2009;206(8):403.
10. Desai V, Bumb D. Digital dental photography: a contemporary revolution. Int J Clin Pediatr Dent. 2013;6(3):193.
11. Schoenbaum T. Digital photography enhances diagnostics, communication, and documentation. Compend Contin Educ Dent. 2011;32 Spec No 4:36–8.
12. Ahmad I. Digital dental photography. Part 4: choosing a camera. Br Dent J. 2009;206(11):575.
13. Shorey R, Moore K. Clinical digital photography: implementation of clinical photography for everyday practice. J Calif Dent Assoc. 2009;37(3):179–83.
14. Terry DA, Snow SR, McLaren EA. CE 1-contemporary dental photography: selection and application. Compendium. 2008;29(8):432.
15. Hodson NA. Clinical photography in esthetic dentistry. In: Levine JB, editor. Smile design integrating esthetics and function: essentials in esthetic dentistry, vol. 2: Elsevier; 2016. p. 89.
16. Antar F, Zebouni E. Comparative review of DSLR cameras and smartphones in dental photography: indications and limitations. Int Arab J Dent. 2018;9(3).
17. Patussi EG, Poltronieri BCG, Ottoni R, Bervian J, Lisboa C, Corazza PH. Comparisons between photographic equipment for dental use: DSLR cameras vs. smartphones. Revista da Faculdade de Odontologia-UPF. 2019;24(2):198–203.
18. Hammond BD, Romero MF, Haddock FJ. Digital dental photography, a picture is worth a thousand words, part 1. Dent Assist. 2016;85(2):6.
19. Muts E-J, Feraru M, Bichacho N. Dental visualization—a practical approach to digital photography and workflow. Tandartspraktijk. 2018;39(9):49.
20. Sheridan P. Practical aspects of clinical photography: part 1—principles, equipment and technique. ANZ J Surg. 2013;83(3):188–91.
21. Prakash A. Clinical photography in orthodontics—a diagnostic aid. Indian J Multidiscip Dent. 2012;3(1):627–32.
22. Claman L, Patton D, Rashid R. Standardized portrait photography for dental patients. Am J Orthod Dentofac Orthop. 1990;98(3):197–205.
23. Loiacono P, Pascoletti L. Photography in dentistry: theory and techniques in modern documentation. Milan: Quintessenza Edizioni; 2012.
24. Akyalcin S, Frels LK, English JD, Laman S. Analysis of smile esthetics in American Board of Orthodontic patients. Angle Orthod. 2014;84(3):486–91.
25. Passia N, Blatz M, Strub JR. Is the smile line a valid parameter for esthetic evaluation? A systematic literature review. Eur J Esthet Dent. 2011;6(3):314–27.
26. Machado AW. 10 commandments of smile esthetics. Dent Press J Orthod. 2014;19(4):136–57.
27. Sarver DM. The importance of incisor positioning in the esthetic smile: the smile arc. Am J Orthod Dentofac Orthop. 2001;120(2):98–111.
28. Ackerman MB, Ackerman JL. Smile analysis and design in the digital era. J Clin Orthod. 2002;36(4):221–36.
29. Krishnan V, Daniel ST, Lazar D, Asok A. Characterization of posed smile by using visual analog scale, smile arc, buccal corridor measures, and modified smile index. Am J Orthod Dentofac Orthop. 2008;133(4):515–23.
30. Manjula W, Sukumar M, Kishorekumar S, Gnanashanmugam K, Mahalakshmi K. Smile: a review. J Pharm Bioallied Sci. 2015;7(Suppl 1):S271.
31. Charavet C, Bernard J-C, Gaillard C, Le Gall M. Benefits of digital smile design (DSD) in the conception of a complex orthodon-

tic treatment plan: a case report-proof of concept. Int Orthod. 2019;17(3):573–9.
32. Zanardi PR, Zanardi RLR, Stegun RC, Sesma N, Costa B-N, Laganá DC. The use of the digital smile design concept as an auxiliary tool in aesthetic rehabilitation: a case report. Open Dent J. 2016;10:28.
33. Jafri Z, Ahmad N, Sawai M, Sultan N, Bhardwaj A. Digital Smile Design-An innovative tool in aesthetic dentistry. J Oral Biol Craniofac Res. 2020;10(2):194–8.
34. Kapila S, Nervina J. CBCT in orthodontics: assessment of treatment outcomes and indications for its use. Dentomaxillofac Radiol. 2015;44(1):20140282.
35. Agrawal JM, Agrawal MS, Nanjannawar LG, Parushetti AD. CBCT in orthodontics: the wave of future. J Contemp Dent Pract. 2013;14(1):153.
36. Machado GL. CBCT imaging—a boon to orthodontics. Saudi Dent J. 2015;27(1):12.
37. Kravitz ND, Groth C, Jones PE, Graham JW, Redmond WR. Intraoral digital scanners. J Clin Orthod. 2014;48(6):337–47.
38. Baheti M, Soni U, Gharat N, Mahagaonkar P, Khokhani R, Dash S. Intra-oral scanners: a new eye in dentistry. Aust J Orthop Rheumatol. 2015;2(3):1021.
39. Kravitz ND, Groth C, Shannon T. CAD/CAM software for three-dimensional printing. J Clin Orthod. 2018;52(1):22–7.
40. Larson BE, Vaubel CJ, Grünheid T. Effectiveness of computer-assisted orthodontic treatment technology to achieve predicted outcomes. Angle Orthod. 2013;83(4):557–62.
41. Coachman C, Calamita MA, Sesma N. Dynamic documentation of the smile and the 2D/3D digital smile design process. Int J Periodontics Restorative Dent. 2017;37(2):183–93.
42. Omar D, Duarte C. The application of parameters for comprehensive smile esthetics by digital smile design programs: a review of literature. Saudi Dent J. 2018;30(1):7–12.
43. Finelle G. Digital smile design in interdisciplinary and orthodontic dental treatment planning. J Dentofac Anomal Orthod. 2017;20(3):303.
44. Nold SL, Horvath S, Stampf S, Blatz M. Analysis of select facial and dental esthetic parameters. Int J Periodontics Restorative Dent. 2014;34(5):623–9.
45. Mack MR. Perspective of facial esthetics in dental treatment planning. J Prosthet Dent. 1996;75(2):169–76.
46. Sarver DM. Orthodontics & esthetic dentistry: mission possible! A broader approach to interdisciplinary esthetic treatment. J Cosmet Dent. 2016;31(4):14–26.
47. Sarver D. Facial considerations: an orthodontic perspective. In: Ronald E Goldstein's esthetics in dentistry; 2018, p. 1050–83.
48. McLaren EA, Garber DA, Figueira J. The photoshop smile design technique (part 1): digital dental photography. Compend Contin Educ Dent. 2013;34(10):772–4.
49. Levin EI. Dental esthetics and the golden proportion. J Prosthet Dent. 1978;40(3):244–52.
50. Schabel BJ, McNamara JA Jr, Baccetti T, Franchi L, Jamieson SA. The relationship between posttreatment smile esthetics and the ABO objective grading system. Angle Orthod. 2008;78(4):579–84.
51. Arnett GW, Bergman RT. Facial keys to orthodontic diagnosis and treatment planning. Part I. Am J Orthod Dentofac Orthop. 1993;103(4):299–312.
52. Lal S, Behera SK, Sethy PK, Rath AK, editors. Identification and counting of mature apple fruit based on BP feed forward neural network. In: 2017 Third International Conference on Sensing, Signal Processing and Security (ICSSS), IEEE; 2017.
53. Sandler J, Murray A. Clinical photography in an orthodontic practice environment part 1. Orthod Update. 2010;3(3):70–5.

3D Radiographic Assessment of Dental Anomalies and Management

3

Emad Eddin Alzoubi, Juliana No-Cortes,
Reinaldo Abdala-Junior,
and Arthur Rodriguez Gonzalez Cortes

3.1 Introduction

Cone beam computed tomography (CBCT) is the radiographic examination of choice when two-dimensional (2D) plain films fail to define diagnosis. CBCT has been used in several scenarios in orthodontics including diagnosis for cleft palate, impacted teeth, supernumerary tooth, resorpted roots and other pathological findings. In this context, a number of authors reported incidental findings that might require long-term follow-up; however, other situations mandate the alteration of orthodontic treatment planning.

SEDENTEX guidelines divided the CBCT view according to the field of view (FOV) size, FOV above 10 cm (craniofacial region), and small or medium FOV below 10 cm (dentoalveolar region) [1].

Although CBCT is recognized as a very powerful tool for diagnosis and treatment planning, it should be used cautiously within the radiation guidelines that facilitate the judgment of when an orthodontist should use the CBCT technology [1, 2].

E. E. Alzoubi
Department of Child Dental Health and Orthodontics, Faculty of Dental Surgery, University of Malta, Msida, Malta

Department of Restorative Dentistry, Faculty of Dental Surgery, University of Malta, Msida, Malta
e-mail: emad.alzoubi@um.edu.mt

J. No-Cortes
Department of Restorative Dentistry, Faculty of Dental Surgery, University of Malta, Msida, Malta
e-mail: jcort02@um.edu.mt

R. Abdala-Junior
Department of Radiology, UniFSP, Avaré, SP, Brazil

School of Dentistry, University of São Paulo, São Paulo, Brazil

A. R. G. Cortes (✉)
Department of Dental Surgery, Faculty of Dental Surgery, University of Malta, Msida, Malta
e-mail: arthur.nogueira@um.edu.mt

Table 3.1 Etiology of tooth impaction

Impacted tooth	
Systemic factors	Local factors
Endocrine and nutrition: • Growth disorders • Vitamin D deficiency	Trauma to deciduous teeth that displaced the permanent bud Dilacerated teeth
Syndromes: • Familial gingival fibromatosis • Cleidocranial dysostosis	Retained deciduous teeth Fibrous teeth Supernumerary teeth
Non-syndromic • Multiple supernumeraries and impacted teeth • Familial history of impaction such as canine	Thick fibrous tissue that leads to tooth impaction Premature loss of deciduous dentition Arch length deficiency

Among the most important use of CBCT in orthodontics is the impaction of a tooth, which is the retardation of the normal physiological process of eruption, keeping the tooth secured in the alveolus. Therefore, impaction was defined as the process "when the tooth is embedded in the alveolus, and eruption is impeded as it is locked in position by bone or adjacent teeth" [3]. The canine and third molars are the most common impacted teeth and can present varying challenges in their management [4]. Tooth impaction can be divided into localized and generalized etiological factors (Table 3.1).

3.2 Maxillary Impacted Canine

3.2.1 Development and Eruption Pathway of Maxillary Canine

Prior to discussing the impactions related to the maxillary canine, it is pertinent to discuss the development and eruption pathway of the maxillary canine. This is crucial to understand since the canine's path of the eruption presents differences from other teeth. The calcification of the perma-

J.-M. Retrouvey, M.-N. Abdallah (eds.), *3D Diagnosis and Treatment Planning in Orthodontics*,
https://doi.org/10.1007/978-3-030-57223-5_3

nent canine commences at 12 months of age and is initially located between the roots of the first deciduous molar. It therefore will be at the proximity of permanent first premolar roots and the first deciduous molar. Following the eruption of the first deciduous molar the permanent canine and incisor will move more anteriorly. At the age of 7 years, the crown of permanent canine is medial to the root of deciduous canine. At the age of 8 and 10 years old, the canine drift buccally and repositions distal to the lateral incisor root tip. During the so-called "ugly duckling stage" (8–12 years of age), the permanent canine crown contributes to the creation of space in the anterior teeth but as long as it begins to erupt the lateral incisors start to shift to a more upright position. It is a fact that the upper maxillary canine has a long and nonlinear path of eruption. This long and arduous path of eruption contributes directly to the maxillary canine's eruption abnormalities.

3.2.2 Etiology of Maxillary Canine Impaction

The etiology of the impacted canines is considered to be multifactorial in origin such as the presence of pathologies, which include supernumeraries, odontomas, cysts, delayed exfoliation of the deciduous canine, ankyloses, syndromes, e.g., Cleidocranial dysplasia, as well as the long path of eruption as explained previously. The two most agreed theories of canine impaction are the *Canine guidance theory* and the *Genetic theory* [5–7]. The canine guidance theory states that the canine displacement is the result of local predisposing factors such as missing lateral incisor, odontoma, supernumerary teeth, and transposition that interfere with the canine path of eruption [5]. However, Peck doubted this theory and alternatively introduced the genetic theory, which states that maxillary canine impaction often presents with other dental abnormalities such as tooth size, shape, number and structure of teeth. All of these abnormalities have genetic predisposing factors [8]. Indeed, up to 33% of maxillary impacted canine cases are reported to have 5–9 times more hypodontia than that of the general population [8]. The authors confirmed that 48% of impacted canine cases have an associated peg or diminutive lateral incisor or missing lateral incisor [9]. Patients with impacted canines tend to have hypodontia approximately 2.4 times more than the general population [7]. Evidence is unclear whether one theory is more accurate than the other; however, many authors agree that impacted canine can result from a combination of both theories.

3.2.3 Palatal Versus Labial Impaction

Impacted canines are located palataly in 85% of cases whereas the remaining 15% present labially [10]. Unilateral impaction is more common than bilateral impaction, with the latter ocurring in 8% of cases [3]. Furthermore, the incidence of palatal impaction is five times more common in Caucasians in comparison to Asians [11]. There is also gender predilection for females in comparison to males with a ratio of 2.3:1 [12].

3.2.4 Radiographic Assessment

CBCT has been used in daily practice in cases where three-dimensional (3D) imaging of oral cavity and craniofacial structures is required. CBCT is used for specific orthodontic diagnosis, as well as the evaluation of the temporomandibular joint (TMJ), which will be specifically discussed further in Chap. 7. Incidental findings might be initially discovered with conventional radiography (2D), which offers a 2D view of a 3D structure and therefore is usually not accurate enough for diagnosis and treatment planning. For this reason, the clinician might seek to visualize the structures in 3D with CBCT to perform a volumetric analysis and plan the treatment with confidence.

Although one can observe asymmetry on palpation from the age of 8 years during clinical examination, only at a later age, from 10 years and above, a lack of positive palpation will be considered abnormal [13]. It is suggested that a radiographic view assesses the status of the unerupted canine. Kurol and Ericsson suggest that the periapical view is satisfactory to visualize the canine. However, localizing the canine position using the parallax technique (Clark's) was advocated with two periapical views [13]. Parallax radiographic technique depends on a simple concept wherein if the object moves to the same direction of the x-ray cylinder, this indicates that the object is lingually positioned. However, horizontal parallax showed higher sensitivity in locating the canines (88%) in comparison to the vertical parallax (69%) [13, 14].

Due to sensitivity and accuracy issues with conventional radiography and the significant margins of error, CBCT is considered nowadays as the golden standard imaging technique. Kurol and Ericsson in 2000 reported that 2D view radiology showed moderate sensitivity in the detection of root resorption in anterior maxilla because plain radiographs cause superimposition of the incisor roots and the crown of the impacted canine. On the other hand, CBCT showed 50% more resorption [15]. Similarly, a previous study reported that Dental PantamoTomography (DPT) is a poor tool to assess the anterior teeth root forms, and six supernumeraries were missed. In addition, the DPT showed 45% sensitivity which indicates that this view presents vast limitations [16]. Ideally radiographs are required to view the impacted canines in three dimensions (vertical, mesiodistal, and buccopalatal). The impacted canines' orientation to the midline and adjacent teeth should be viewed to evaluate resorption.

Kurol and Ericson showed that in cases of impacted canines the presence of resorption of the lateral and central incisors was

38% and 9%, respectively [15]. Similarly, Walker and coworkers concluded that resorption rate was 67% and 11% for lateral incisor and central incisor, respectively [17]. The fact that the impacted canine overlap the adjacent lateral minimizes the visual sensitivity to detect resorption. This shortcoming depends on the type of imaging that was used. In 45% of the cases, the crown of the impacted canine will superimpose the lateral incisor root, which makes it very difficult to make an appropriate diagnosis [13]. Computed tomography can overcome the limitation of conventional imaging. It was reported that the resorption rate is approximately 12% when DPT was used, but this proved to be wrong when Kurol and Ericson in 2000 conducted a study using CBCT to assess the rate of resorption of lateral incisors associated with impacted canines. The percentage of resorption spiked up to 50% [15]. It is reported that the 3D imaging technique is superior over 2D, which showed a low to moderate sensitivity of 0.71% [18].

Therefore CBCT technology is a superior method to locate impacted canines accurately and minimize the invasiveness of any surgical intervention [19]. Cysts, internal resorption of the impacted tooth, external resportion of impacted adjacent teeth and migration of teeth can result as sequelae of impacted canine [7]. It was reported that females above 14 years with impacted canines more than 25° to midline have a higher risk of adjacent tooth resorption [13].

The following factors are used to assess the impacted canine prognosis [20, 21]:

1. Canine angulation to the midline (Fig. 3.1)
2. The vertical height of the canine crown
3. Anteroposterior position of the canine root apex (Fig. 3.2)
4. Canine crown overlap of the adjacent incisor
5. Root resorption of adjacent incisor
6. Labio-palatal position of the canine crown
7. Labio-palatal position of the canine apex

A canine that is angulated more toward the midline tends to show a poor prognosis of a future eruption. Angulation of 0–15° predicts a good prognosis, angulation of 16–30° an average prognosis, and angulation of 31° or more a poor prognosis (Fig. 3.1) [13, 22]. Impacted canine at the level of the cervical zone of adjacent tooth tend to show very good prognosis; however, an impacted canine positioned at the mid root level of the adjacent tooth or higher tend to show very poor prognosis [20] (Fig. 3.2). Furthermore, labiopalatal position of the crown can be a detrimental factor, for instance, if the crown is buccally positioned. In these cases, the extraction risk will be higher due to complications with keratinized mucosa [21].

Anteroposterior position of the root tip is a very important prognostic factor. If the root tip of the impacted canine is in its original place or positioned slightly distally from the first premolar, the prognostic is very good (Fig. 3.3).

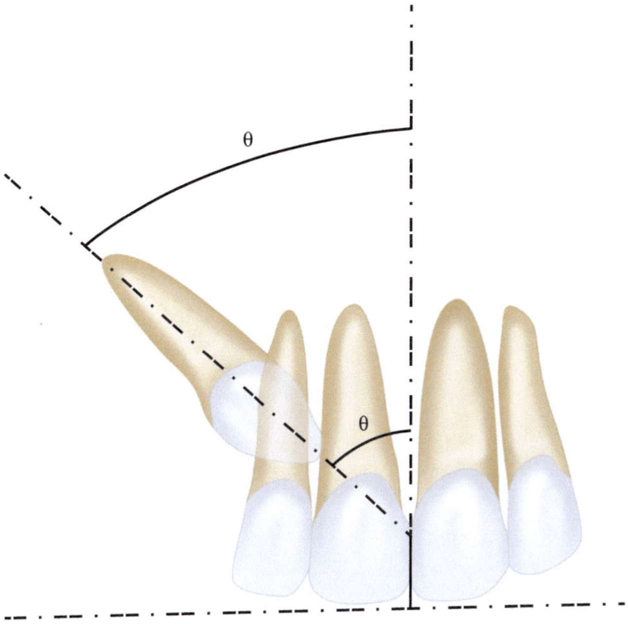

Fig. 3.1 The angulation of canine to the midline

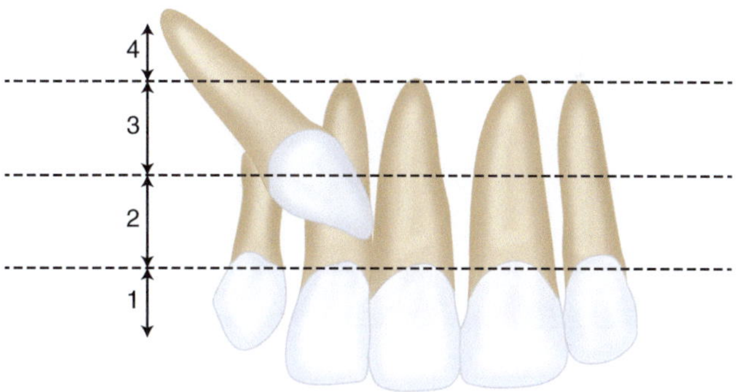

Fig. 3.2 The height of canine vertically

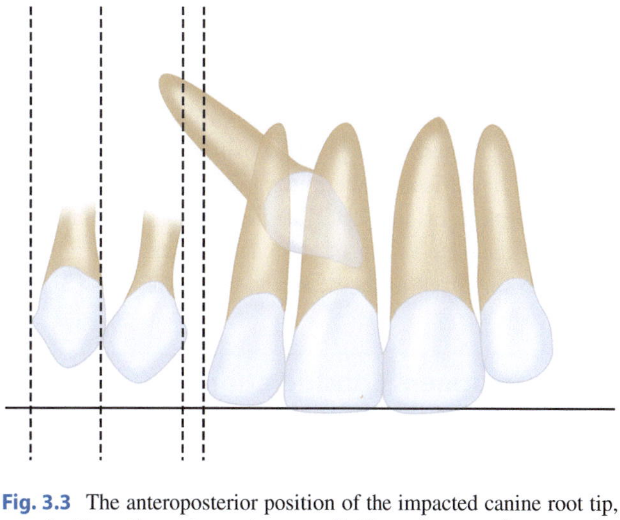

Fig. 3.3 The anteroposterior position of the impacted canine root tip, zone 1: Above the canine region; zone 2: Above the upper first premolar region; Zone 3: Above the upper second premolar regions

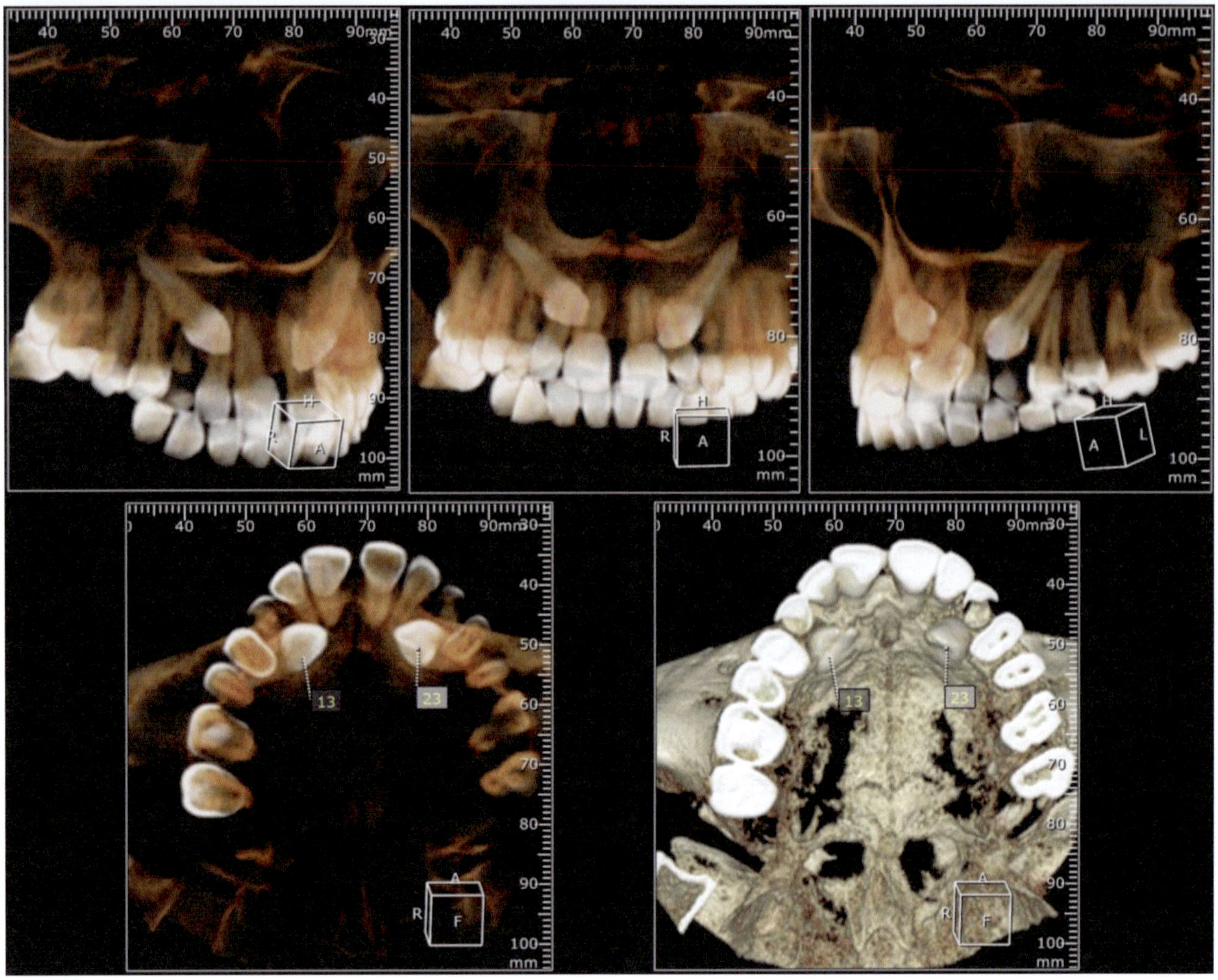

Fig. 3.4 CBCT of palatal impacted canines viewed in 3D, which facilitates the localization of their positions

DPT has proven to be unreliable to visualize the anterior maxillary teeth due to the palate superimposition with the root tips of maxillary teeth. Also, the small focal trough that prone to patients positioning error which directs the clinician toward CBCT to overcome such problems (Fig. 3.4). Clinicians can easily judge the position of the impacted canine in comparison to the midline and if there is adjacent tooth resorption or not. CBCT facilitates the assessment of the labio-palatal position of the canine apex and root tips accurately and overcomes the shortcomings of DPT [21].

3.3 Treatment Considerations for Impacted Teeth

The treatment of impacted canine can be as following:

- Monitoring
- Intervention

3.3.1 Monitoring

Observe and monitor the position of the impacted canine in relation to the space available for the eruption. Literature supports that radiographic examination should be taken place following a thorough clinical investigation. Usually radiographs are taken between 10 and 15 years of age. It has been proven that radiographic examination before the age of 10 years tends to be less reliable [13].

The guidelines state interceptive therapy must take place between 10 and 13 years of age besides the removal of any physical obstruction to allow spontaneous canine eruption [23]. Presence of any physical obstruction such as retained deciduous canine or pathology such as odontomas should be removed to allow unobstructed eruption pathway. Kurol and Ericsson concluded that 91% of the cases with spontaneous eruption happens when the deciduous canine is extracted but drops to 64% when the impacted canine lies at the level of the lateral incisor (Fig. 3.5).

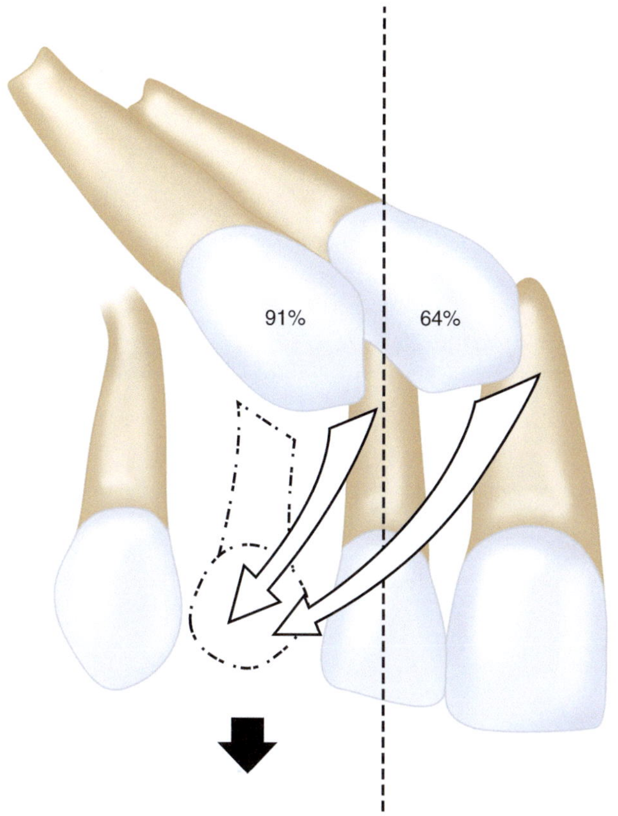

Fig. 3.5 Spontaneous eruption of permanent canine is 91% when interceptive extraction of deciduous canine is performed, versus 64% of the spontaneous eruption when the crown of the impacted canine passes the lateral incisors

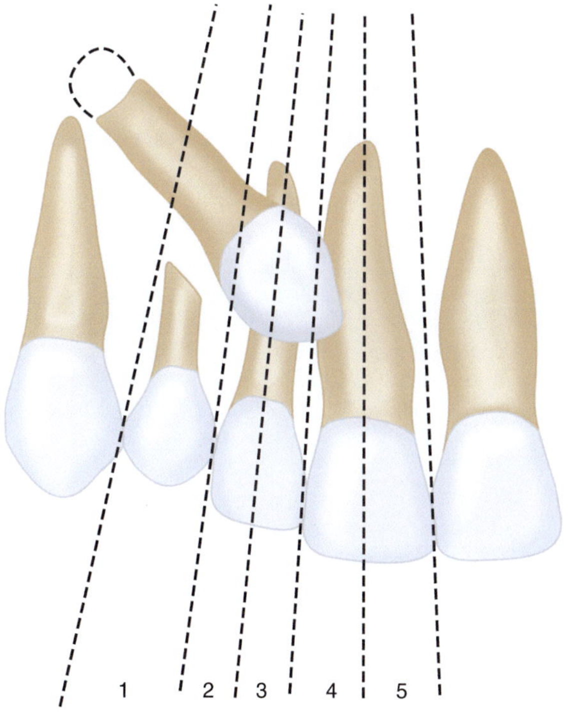

Fig. 3.6 Impacted canine sector classifications by Kurol and Ericsson

Kurol and Ericsson stated a radiological method to evaluate different degrees of impaction based on the position of canine on a method known as **sector classification** (Fig. 3.6) [13]. Basically, the more mesially oriented the canine crown is from its ideal position the less likelihood for the impacted canine to erupt by means of orthodontic treatment [13]. For instance, Figure 3.7 shows an impacted canine positioned in sector 5, which means it is very difficult to treat with orthodontic therapy only. This method can guide the orthodontist to alter the proposed treatment plan from aligning the canine, to one that incorporates an interdisciplinary approach.

3.3.2 Intervention

Intervention can be either:

1. Surgical exposure with orthodontic guidance.
2. Autotransplantation (rarely considered).

When the orthodontist interceptive approach fails, surgical exposure of the impacted canine followed by orthodontic traction is recommended. Two techniques to expose the canine can be considered. These include closed or open exposure, and both techniques are debatable among researchers. Cochrane review stated that there is no difference between closed and open exposure [24].

Autotransplantation is a less commonly used option due to complications such as resorption of the auto-transplanted tooth. In theory, the surgeon will prepare the future canine socket. For this purpose, CBCT is helpful for accurately measuring the root length, and simulating the surgery on a virtual digital model before commencing it intraorally. This approach is more complex to perform and entail more complications, thus it is rarely chosen. In difficult situations, extraction of the impacted canine might be an option and a prosthesis might be placed.

3.4 Unerupted Incisors

The eruption of upper incisors takes place approximately between 7 and 9 years of age but in some individuals, the upper incisor fails to erupt due to numerous reasons such as premature loss of deciduous incisor and consequently loss of the space, trauma, pathologies such as cysts, cleft lip, and palate and delayed exfoliation of the deciduous incisor. Unerupted central or lateral incisors can lead to a significant facial and dental aesthetic impact (Fig. 3.8). Since conventional imaging techniques have a considerable limitation in the anterior teeth region, CBCT can be useful for diagnosis and treatment planning.

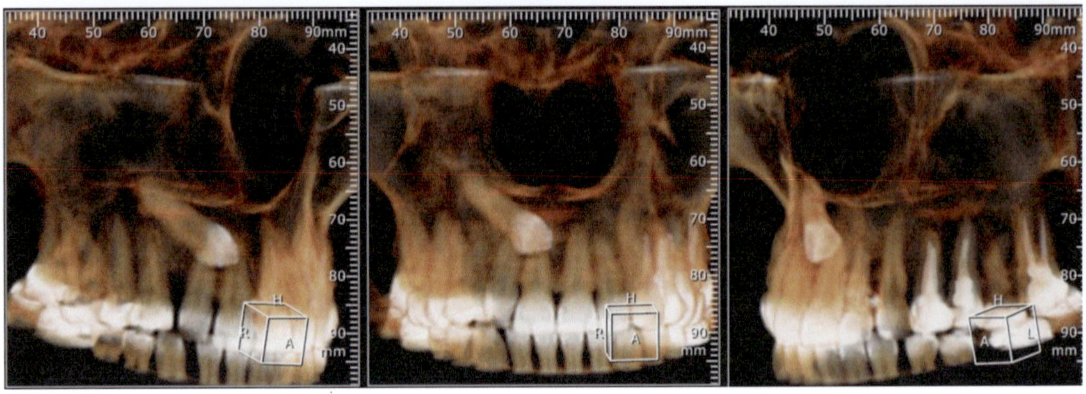

Fig. 3.7 Impacted canine positioned toward dental midline

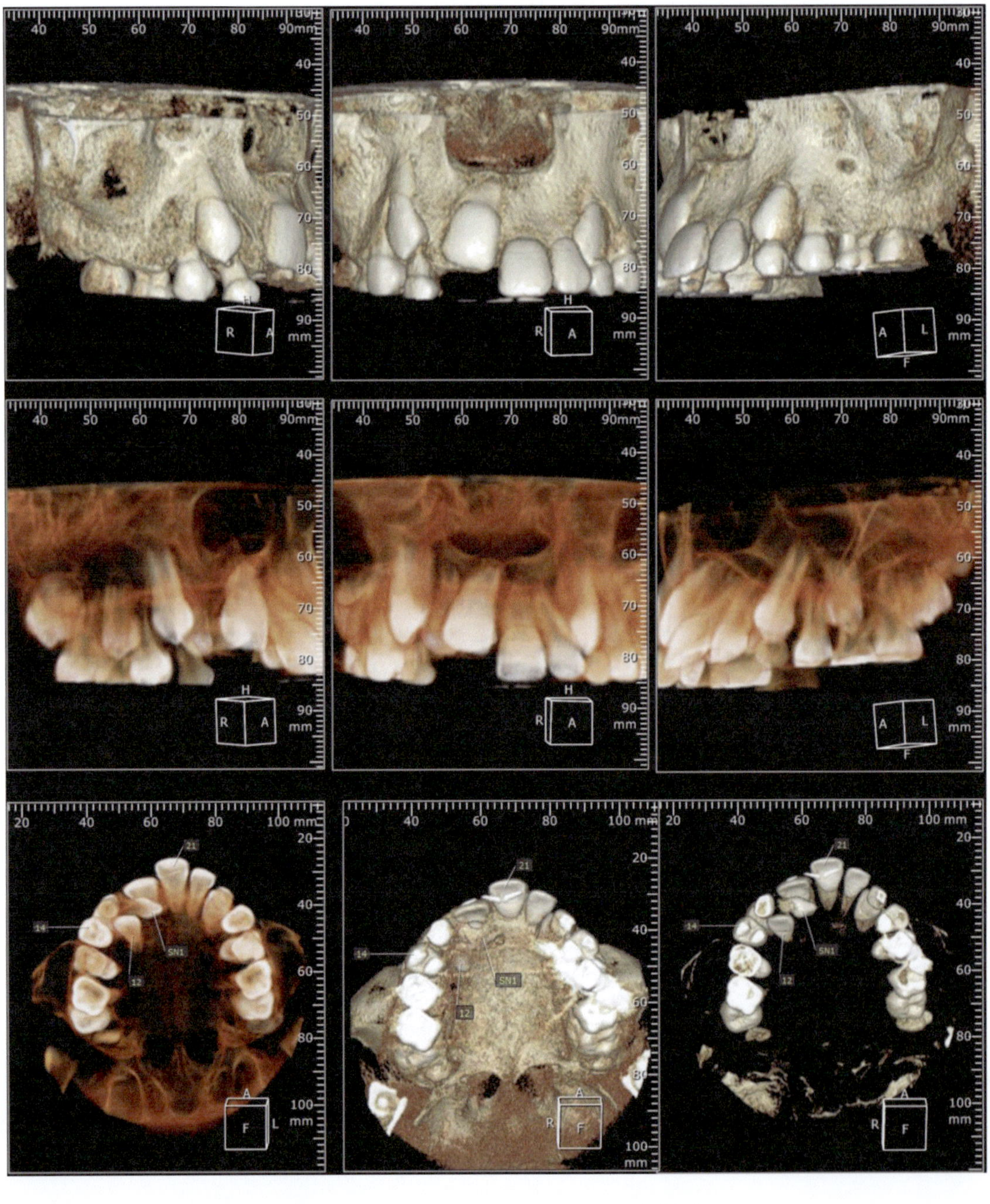

Fig. 3.8 Impacted upper central incisors [11] due to the presence of a supernumerary tooth (SN1)

3.4.1 Diagnosis and Management

Clinicians should look carefully during the examination of unerupted incisors in relation to the contralateral tooth. If there is a discrepancy of more than 6 months, this suggests that there is a problem in the eruption process. Clinicians should investigate whether the maxillary incisors remained unerupted for more than 6–12 months—following the eruption of lower permanent incisors. Examine thoroughly if there is any eruption abnormality, i.e., eruption of canine or lateral incisors before central [25].

Periapical or standard maxillary occlusal views can aid in determining the position or presence of any abnormality [25]. Furthermore, vertical and horizontal parallax techniques can be used to localize the position of an unerupted tooth or any associated pathology such as cyst, odontomas, or supernumerary teeth. The vertical parallax technique in such cases can carry a considerable margin of inaccuracy, which takes us to CBCT as a golden standard technique. European guidance and SEDENTEXCT guidelines recommend using a small field of view CBCT in case the conventional radiographic views are not helpful; in cases of dilacerations of incisors, root CBCT view is helpful. Current British Orthodontic Society (BOS) guidelines state that no rationale for routine CBCT, in situations where the clinician in a dilemma whether or not to take CBCT view opinion of oral maxillofacial radiology should be sought [2].

3.4.2 Treatment of Unerupted Central Incisor

3.4.2.1 Removal of any Physical Obstruction

The delay of eruption might be attributed to physical obstruction such as odontoma or supernumerary tooth. The presence of mesiodens tends to delay the eruption of permanent incisor unlike tuberculate, which tends to impede eruption. Impaction of the permanent central incisor is common (28–60%). The removal of supernumerary tooth tends to allow self-correction and spontaneous eruption of the impacted central incisors [26, 27]. Furthermore, creating enough space for the eruption of the incisors along with the removal of obstruction would facilitate the eruption of incisors. Authors showed that when enough space is created spontaneous eruption took place [26, 28]. Similarly Pavoni et al. stated that spontaneous eruption rate following the removal of the obstruction is 82%. Simple space creation can be achieved with removable or fixed appliances [29].

3.4.3 Surgical Intervention

In cases where the obstruction is removed with no signs of spontaneous eruption, surgical exposure of the maxillary incisor may be indicated. The surgical exposure facilitates traction and guidance of incisor to its desired position. In the case of supernumerary tooth surgical removal, there is no scientific evidence to clearly show the best approach regarding the impacted incisor, whether to bond the incisor immediately or wait for spontaneous eruption [25]. Removal the obstruction or supernumerary tooth will result in 30–50% spontaneous eruption of the impacted incisor, which gives 50:50 chance that the same patient might go under general anesthetic again thus it is wiser to start exposure of the impacted incisor on the same appointment of removal of the supernumerary tooth [26].

3.5 Dentigerous and Maxillary Sinus Cysts

Odontogenic cysts usually represent a chronic condition that might be asymptomatic or demonstrate sequels of pain and flare-ups. Many types of cysts can form in the jaws and a high percentage of them are coincidental discoveries. Dentigerous cysts are the most common odontogenic of the jaws, sometimes prevent the eruption of the tooth [30, 31]. Usually dentigerous and maxillary sinus cysts are visible on panoramic radiography (2D) when it is taken before the commencement of orthodontic treatment. The limitation of the orthopantomography (DPT) view is that cysts will be shown in two dimensions as a circle without enabling the clinician to estimate the proper extension of the lesion and the related damage. CBCT will enable the clinician to assess the cysts in-depth to determine the appropriate treatment plan. CBCT will aid in planning surgery in case the pathology is near a vital structure, for instance, if the lower third molars are displaced due to dentigerous cyst, CBCT will enable the surgeon to estimate the extension of the lesion in 3D to avoid vital structures such as inferior alveolar nerve bundle. Dentigerous cysts can be treated either surgical enucleation or marsupialization, which does not guarantee the spontaneous eruption of the tooth, which in turn leads to surgical tooth extraction [32]. When marsupialization is successful and spontaneous tooth eruption happens, this enables the orthodontist to bond the newly erupted tooth and align it in the line of the arch.

Maxillary sinus cysts incidence is reported to range from approximately 10.9% and 69.1% [33]. Maxillary sinus pathologies tend to be inflammatory in nature, they might not appear on DPT due to artifacts associated with this type of images but an indication of abnormality should be evident. CBCT facilitates the visualization of mucus retention cysts which tend to fade by themselves with no consequences on orthodontic treatment (Fig. 3.9).

Odontogenic related pathology can involve the maxillary sinus and manifest itself as a maxillary pathology. Thus, an appropriate clinical examination should be carried out to reach the appropriate diagnosis and treatment plan. CBCT enables the clinician to use multiplanar reconstructions in 3D to determine which tooth is associated with the maxillary pathology (Fig. 3.10). Sometimes tooth extraction is the only solution to treat the periapical pathology that extended to the

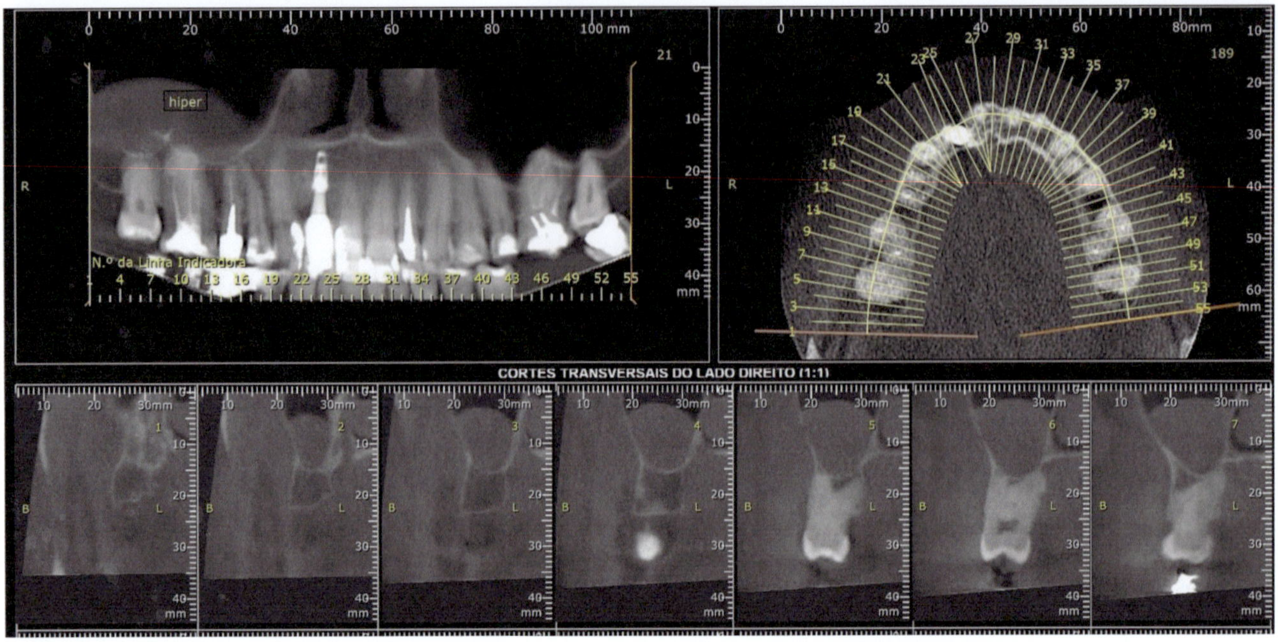

Fig. 3.9 Mucus retention cyst in the maxillary sinus, usually discovered by coincident during a routine examination

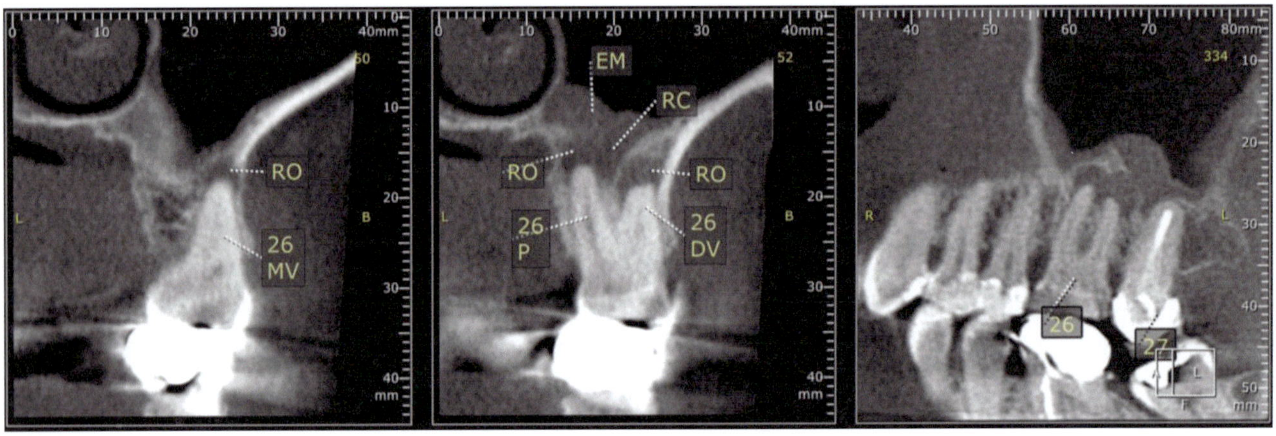

Fig. 3.10 Maxillary sinus infection with an odontogenic origin. The upper first molar has a periapical infection which penetrated the maxillary sinus floor

maxillary sinus. An interdisciplinary approach must be sought in such cases if the extraction space can be closed orthodontically or implant-supported prosthesis should be placed.

3.6 Odontomas

Odontomas are considered the most common benign odontogenic tumors of epithelial and mesenchymal origin [35]. Odontomas constitute approximately 22% of all odontogenic tumors [35].

Odontomas are two types compound and complex, the majority of compound odontomas are found in the anterior segment of the jaws (61%) while the complex odontomas are found in the posterior segment of the jaws (34%) [34, 35].

The etiology of odontomas is poorly understood; however, it has been linked to pathological conditions such as local trauma, inflammatory or infectious causes, or hereditary anomalies such as Gardner's syndrome. It was suggested that odontomas are inherited due to mutagens with genetic control of tooth development [34].

The conventional views with panoramic or occlusal maxillary radiographs (2D) aid in the diagnosis of odontomas; however, the dimension and type of the lesion are hard to determine in 2D views. On the other hand, CBCT can show the lesion in 3D which will allow the clinician to measure its extention and determine its type accurately (Fig. 3.11a, b).

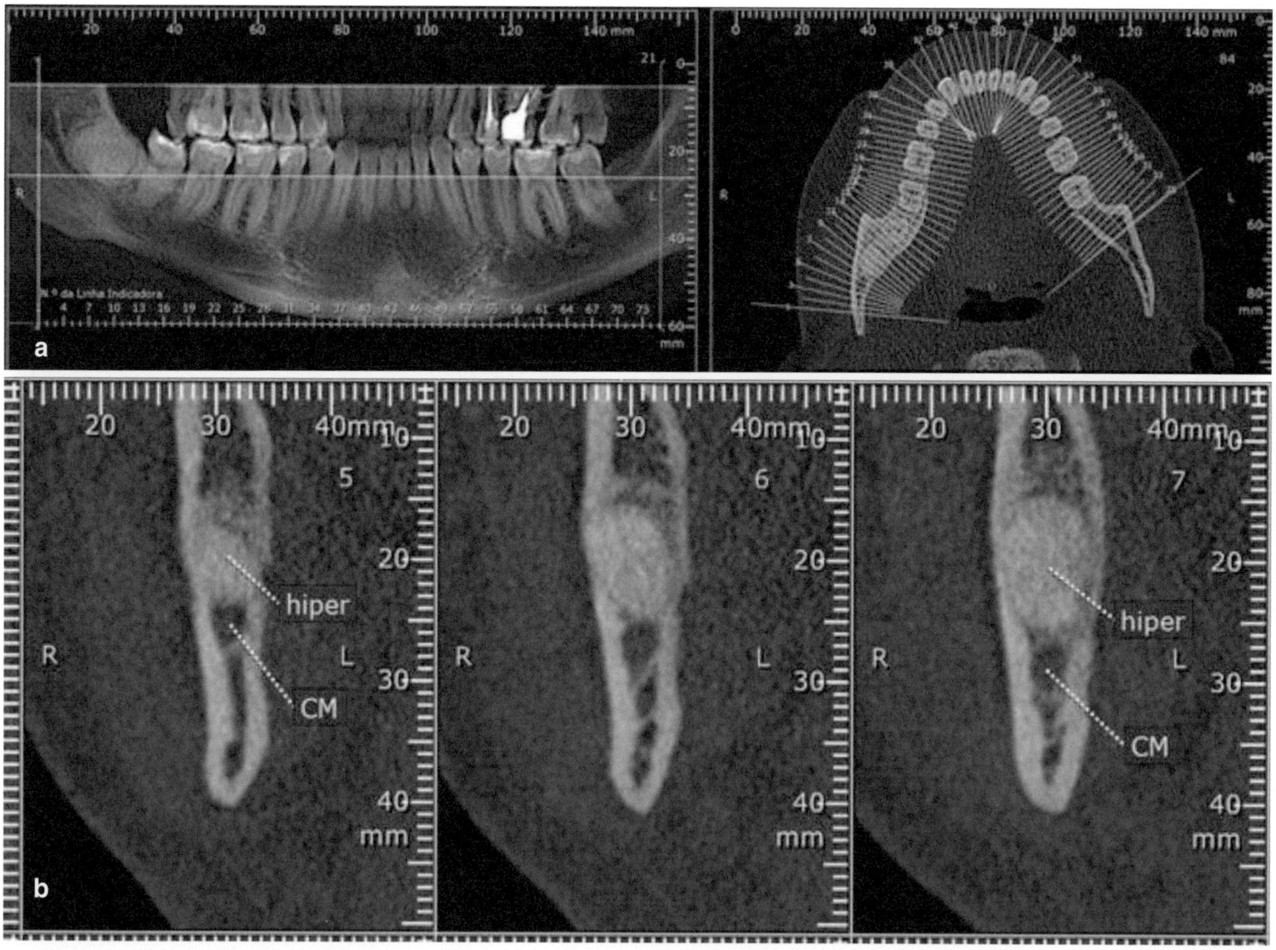

Fig. 3.11 (a) The odontoma size is evaluated along with how close to vital structures in 3D. (b) Odontoma is sliced in the transverse section and shows proximity with the inferior alveolar nerve

Histopathology examination is essential consequent to lesion removal to confirm the clinical findings.

3.7 Transposition

Tooth transposition is considered to be a form of ectopic eruption, where two adjacent teeth interchange position or development and the eruption of a tooth in a position that normally occupied by another tooth [36].

The etiology of dental transposition is still not well understood; however, there is increasing evidence suggesting a genetic basis [37]. Dental transposition is usually found in association with other congenital dental anomalies, such as hypodontia and peg lateral maxillary incisors [36]. Transposition cases show a tendency for female predilection and unilateral left-sided dominance [36].

Environmental factors can also play an important role in dental transposition such as a retained deciduous tooth.

Transposition is divided into true and pseudo-transpositions. True transposition is defined as when the whole tooth is transposed in a new position; however, the pseudo-transposition is described as when the transposed tooth root is still in the original position while the crown overlaps the adjacent tooth [38].

Conventional 2D radiographs, such as periapical and panoramic, have enough accuracy to assist dentists to diagnose the type of transposition. CBCT view offers higher quality and better visualization of the teeth to formulate a treatment plan. CBCT aids to visualize the bone overlying the roots. This is valuable if there is dehiscence or thin buccal cortical bone, which will affect the orthodontic treatment plan.

Treatment of tooth transposition can be achieved with orthodontic appliances and it depends whether it is a true transposition or pseudo-transposition. Ideally, orthodontists accept the true transposition; for example in the case of canine lateral incisor transposition, the orthodontist accepted the transposition (Fig. 3.12).

In the case of pseudo-transposition usually it is corrected by tipping back the tooth to its original position and aligning it in the line of the arch.

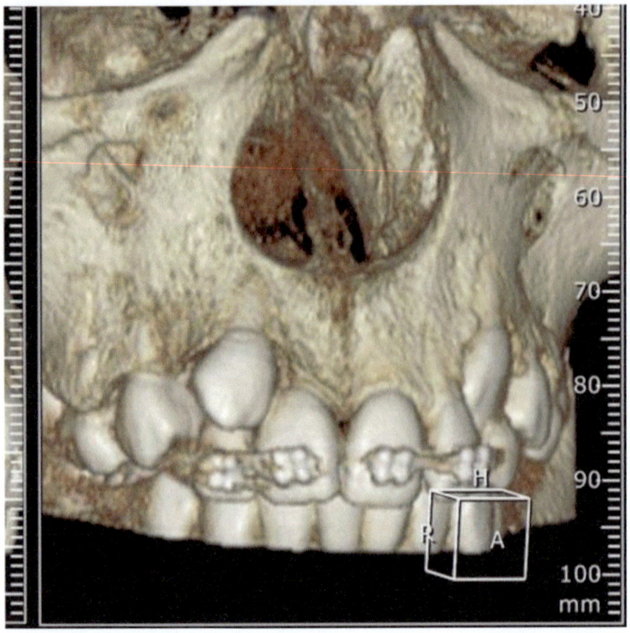

Fig. 3.12 A transposed upper right canine in the lateral incisor position, with a thin buccal bone plate

3.8 Supernumerary Teeth

A supernumerary tooth is defined as any tooth or odontogenic structure that is formed from tooth germ in excess to the usual number of teeth in that particular region [39]. The supernumerary teeth could occur at any region of the dental arch but most commonly in the premaxilla. Several hypotheses proposed explanation on their formation but the etiology remains equivocal [39]. There are environmental and genetic factors that play an important role in their formation [39, 40]. Females are twice more at risk of having a supernumerary tooth in comparison to males; however, it has also been reported that some forms of supernumerary teeth are site-specific related to gender. For instance, males are commonly affected in midline and premolar regions and incisor and canine regions have had females predilection [28].

Supernumerary teeth may occur in permanent and primary dentitions. These extra teeth may occur as a unilateral or bilateral, single tooth or two or multiple teeth, and in the maxilla, the mandible, or both the arches. The supernumerary teeth have different classification based on the morphology, orientation, position, and location (Table 3.2).

Table 3.2 Classification of supernumerary teeth

Supernumerary teeth		
	Location	Mesiodens Para-molar Para-premolar Disto-molar
	Morphology	Conical Tuberculate Supplemental Odontome
	Position	Buccal Transverse Palatal
	Orientation	Vertical or normal Inverted Horizontal

Mesiodens and tuberculate supernumeraries are found in the maxillary anterior region. Mesiodens may occur as single, multiple, unilateral or bilateral. Prevalence is estimated between 0.15 and 1.9% with a higher prevalence in males compared to females [41]. It has been reported that in 9-year-old children in Italy, the prevalence of this defect has increased from 0.64 to 1.06 in recent years [41, 42]. Mesiodens are conical or small peg-shaped tooth and it usually presents between the maxillary central incisors as a mesiodens [41, 42]. Tuberculate is larger in size than the conical, barrel-shaped with several tubercles or cusps, and may have incomplete or abnormal root formation compared to permanent incisors.

During clinical examination when there is a delay of the eruption of the centrals or laterals on one side in comparison to the contralateral side, the clinician would ask for radiographic views to assess the diagnosis. Conventional DPT view is the method used to assess the whole dentition; however, due to the small focal trough and the overlap of upper anterior root apices with the palate the anterior maxillary region will not be clear to visualize. The maxillary anterior teeth usually need a supplementary view such as maxillary occlusal to compensate for the latter disadvantage. DPT demonstrated a poor ability to detect anterior teeth root form and in many cases, the supernumerary teeth were missed when it was not supplemented with an upper standard maxillary view [16]. Thus, CBCT will fill a huge void and help the clinician to view the anterior maxilla in 3D. The dentist can choose either a small or medium field of view which allows visualization of the supernumerary and at the same time avoid unnecessary radiation for the unwanted maxilla.

In conclusion, the use of CBCT in dentistry made a very significant impact and upgraded the level of diagnosis and treatment planning. Nevertheless, CBCT should be used when 3D imaging is required, according to guidelines and protocols. Safeguarding the patient's interest should be always a priority, according to Isaacson where the conventional view is not sufficient then a small field of view for the desired region can be obtained [2].

References

1. Sedentexct. Radiation protection 172: cone beam CT for dental and maxillofacial radiology—evidence-based guidelines. Eur Communities. 2012;156.
2. Scarfe WC, Azevedo B, Toghyani S, Farman AG. Cone Beam Computed Tomographic imaging in orthodontics. Aust Dent J. 2017;62(1):33–50
3. Shapira Y, Kuftinec MM. Early diagnosis and interception of potential maxillary canine impaction. J Am Dent Assoc. 1998;129(10):1450–4.
4. Elsey MJ, Rock WP. Influence of orthodontic treatment on the development of third molars. Br J Oral Maxillofac Surg. 2000;38(4):350–3.
5. Becker A. In defense of the guidance theory of palatal canine displacement. Angle Orthod. 1995;65(2):95–8.
6. Peck S, Peck L, Kataja M. Prevalence of tooth agenesis and peg-shaped maxillary lateral incisor associated with palatally displaced canine (PDC) anomaly. Am J Orthod Dentofac Orthop. 1996;110(4):441–3.
7. Bishara SE, Ortho D. Impacted maxillary canines: a review. Am J Orthod Dentofac Orthop. 1992;101(2):159–71.
8. Peck S, Peck L, Matti K. Impacted canines pecker 1994.pdf. Angle Orthod. 1994;4(64):249–56.
9. Brin I, Becker A, Shalhav M. Position of the maxillary permanent canine in relation to anomalous or missing lateral incisors: a population study. Eur J Orthod. 1986;8:12–6.
10. Ericson S, Kurol J. Radiographic assessment of maxillary canine eruption in children with clinical signs of eruption disturbance. Eur J Orthod. 1986;8(3):133–40.
11. Abron A, Mendro RL, Kaplan S. Impacted permanent maxillary canines: diagnosis and treatment. N Y State Dent J. 2004;70(9):24–8. http://europepmc.org/abstract/MED/15683219.
12. Dachi SF, Howell FV. A survey of 3,874 routine full-mouth radiographs. I. A study of retained roots and teeth. Oral Surg Oral Med Oral Pathol. 1961;14(8):916–24.
13. Ericson S, Kurol J. Radiographic examination of ectopically erupting maxillary canines. Am J Orthod Dentofac Orthop. 1987;91(6):483–92.
14. Armstrong C, Johnston C, Burden D, Stevenson M. Localizing ectopic maxillary canines—horizontal or vertical parallax. Eur J Orthod. 2003;25(6):585–9.
15. Ericson S, Kurol J. Resorption of incisors after ectopic eruption of maxillary canines: a CT study. Angle Orthod. 2000;70(6):415–23.
16. Witcher TP, Brand S, Gwilliam JR, McDonald F. Assessment of the anterior maxilla in orthodontic patients using upper anterior occlusal radiographs and dental panoramic tomography: a comparison. Oral Surgery, Oral Med Oral Pathol Oral Radiol Endodontol. 2010;109(5):765–74.
17. Walker L, Enciso R, Mah J. Three-dimensional localization of maxillary canines with cone-beam computed tomography. Am J Orthod Dentofacial Orthop. 2005;128(4):418–23.
18. Ericson S, Kurol J, Kurol J. Longitudinal study and analysis of clinical supervision of maxillary canine eruption. Community Dent Oral Epidemiol. 1986;14(3):172–6.
19. Mah J, Enciso R, Jorgensen M. Management of impacted cuspids using 3-D volumetric imaging. J Calif Dent Assoc. 2003;31(11):835–41.
20. Pitt S, Hamdan A, Rock P. A treatment difficulty index for unerupted maxillary canines. Eur J Orthod. 2006;28(2):141–4.
21. Stivaros N, Mandall NA. Radiographic factors affecting the management of impacted upper permanent canines. J Orthod. 2000;27(2):169–73.
22. Counihan K, Al-Awadhi EA, Butler J. Guidelines for the assessment of the impacted maxillary canin. Dent Update. 2013;40:770–7.
23. Husain J, Burden D, McSherry P, Morris D, Allen M. Clinical standards committee of the faculty of dental surgery, Royal college of surgeons of England. National clinical guidelines for management of the palatally ectopic maxillary canine. Br Dent J. 2012;213(4):171–6.
24. Parkin N, Bazargani F, Benson PE, Atwal A. Interventions for promoting the eruption of palatally displaced permanent canine teeth,

without the need for surgical exposure, in children aged 9 to 14 years. Cochrane Database Syst Rev. 2017;2017(10):CD012851.
25. Abdelkarim A. Cone-Beam Computed Tomography in Orthodontics. Dent J (Basel). 2019;7(3):89. Published 2019 Sep 2. https://doi.org/10.3390/dj7030089.
26. Foley J. Surgical removal of supernumerary teeth and the fate of incisor eruption. Eur J Paediatr Dent. 2004;5(1):35–40.
27. Leyland L, Batra P, Wong F, Llewelyn R. A retrospective evaluation of the eruption of impacted permanent incisors after extraction of supernumerary teeth. J Clin Pediatr Dent. 2006;30(3):225–31.
28. Mitchell L, Bennett TG. Supernumerary teeth causing delayed eruption—a retrospective study. Br J Orthod. 1992;19(1):41–6.
29. Pavoni C, Franchi L, Laganà G, Baccetti T, Cozza P. Management of impacted incisors following surgery to remove obstacles to eruption: a prospective clinical trial. Pediatr Dent. 2013;35(4):364–8.
30. Contar CMM, Thomé CA, Pompermayer A, Sarot JR, Vinagre RO, Machado MÂN. Marsupialization of dentigerous cyst: report of a case. J Maxillofac Oral Surg. 2015;14:4–6.
31. Meningaud JP, Oprean N, Pitak-Arnnop P, Bertrand JC. Odontogenic cysts: a clinical study of 695 cases. J Oral Sci. 2006;48(2):59–62.
32. Aoki N, Ise K, Inoue A, Kosugi Y, Koyama C, Iida M, et al. Multidisciplinary approach for the treatment of a dentigerous cyst—marsupialization, orthodontic treatment, and implant placement: a case report. J Med Case Rep. 2018;12(1):1–7.
33. Raghav M, Karjodkar FR, Sontakke S, Sansare K. Prevalence of incidental maxillary sinus pathologies in dental patients on cone-beam computed tomographic images. Contemp Clin Dent. 2014;5(3):361–5.
34. Sharma R, Satish V, Prabhadevi MC. Odontome: a brief overview. Int J Clin Pediatr Dent. 2011;4(3):177–85.
35. Or S, Yücetaş Ş. Compound and complex odontomas. Int J Oral Maxillofac Surg. 1987;16(5):596–9.
36. Peck L, Peck S, Attia Y. Maxillary canine-first premolar transposition, associated dental anomalies, and genetic basis. Angle Orthod. 1993;63(2):99–109.
37. Leonardi R, Farella M, Cobourne MT. An association between sella turcica bridging and dental transposition. Eur J Orthod. 2011;33(4):461–5.
38. Chattopadhyay A, Srinivas K. Transposition of teeth and genetic etiology. Angle Orthod. 1996;66(2):147–52.
39. Omer R, Anthonappa RP, King NM. Determination of the optimum time for surgical removal of unerupted anterior supernumerary teeth. Pediatr Dent. 2010;32(1):14–20.
40. Brook AH. A unifying aetiological explanation for anomalies of human tooth number and size. Arch Oral Biol. 1984;29(5): 373–8.
41. Alberti G, Mondani PM, Parodi V. Eruption of supernumerary permanent teeth in a sample of the urban primary school population in Genoa, Italy. Eur J Paediatr Dent. 2006;7(2):89–92.
42. Van Buggenhout G, Bailleul-Forestier I. Mesiodens. Eur J Med Genet. 2008;51(2):178–81.

Cone Beam Computerized Tomography Imaging for Orthodontic Diagnosis

4

Normand Boucher, Muralidhar Mupparapu, and Kensuke Matsumoto

4.1 Introduction to a 3-Dimensional Approach for Orthodontic Diagnosis

The commercial availability of the first CBCT unit occurred approximately 21 years ago. Up to that point, orthodontic diagnosis was largely limited to sagittal and vertical dento-skeletal relationships. Efforts at rendering a meaningful transverse skeletal diagnosis with a two-dimensional posterior-anterior cephalometric radiograph has not been universally accepted due to head positioning issues and extensive overlapping of structures reducing diagnostic quality. CBCT imaging provides the orthodontist with a tool to evaluate dental-skeletal relationships in the third plane of space (Fig. 4.1).

Radiographic evaluation of the temporomandibular joints is also limited with two-dimensional orthodontic records. CBCT coronal and sagittal views of the temporomandibular joint (TMJ) spaces provide insight on internal soft tissue derangements and condylar remodeling which can impact the potential of maxillary and mandibular growth in adolescents or the stability of the occlusion in adults.

CBCT imaging of the nasal cavity, the nasopharyngeal, oropharyngeal, and the hypopharyngeal areas provides the orthodontist with a screening tool to evaluate the structures of the airway that can adversely affect the orofacial development of adolescents and the systemic health of adult patients.

N. Boucher (✉)
Department of Orthodontics, University of Pennsylvania, Philadelphia, PA, USA

M. Mupparapu
Division of Oral and Maxillofacial Radiology Department of oral Medicine, University of Pennsylvania, Philadelphia, PA, USA

N. Matsumoto
Department of Periodontics and Orthodontics, University of Pennsylvania, Philadelphia, PA, USA

4.2 CBCT Imaging Characteristics

4.2.1 Field of View (FOV)

The Field of View (FOV) in cone beam CT imaging refers to the proposed imaging field within a patient's head and neck anatomy that has been designated to give the maximum information needed for the orthodontist and at the same time exposing them to the lowest possible radiation dose [1]. Typically, this is a cylindrical shape with a height (H) and a width (W) component (Fig. 4.2).

This FOV determines the volume that will be captured during the acquisition of basis images and eventually the dose imparted to the patient. There is a range of FOVs, starting from 4 × 4 cm to as large as 20 × 20 cm, and medium FOVs within the range of 10 × 10 cm. In orthodontic practice, small and medium volumes can be used for diagnosis of the relationships of impacted teeth to the neighboring teeth and for diagnostic applications related to the maxillary expansion, positioning of temporary anchorage devices, and similar tasks that require higher resolutions. For cephalometric needs and for visualization of TMJ area, a large volume CBCT is recommended (Fig. 4.3) [2].

4.2.2 Resolution

Resolution of the CBCT image depends on several physical parameters that are used to acquire the volume. Essentially, the FOV determines the basic resolution, as most of the CBCT machines have built-in algorithms to manage the CBCT acquired volume for storage and display and hence the resolution is adjusted by the acquisition computer [3]. The resolution is the sharpness with which one can see and interpret an image. Traditional radiographs have high line pair resolution (lppm) with poor contrast resolution. CBCT and CT modalities have poor line pair resolution (anatomic) but very good contrast

J.-M. Retrouvey, M.-N. Abdallah (eds.), *3D Diagnosis and Treatment Planning in Orthodontics*,
https://doi.org/10.1007/978-3-030-57223-5_4

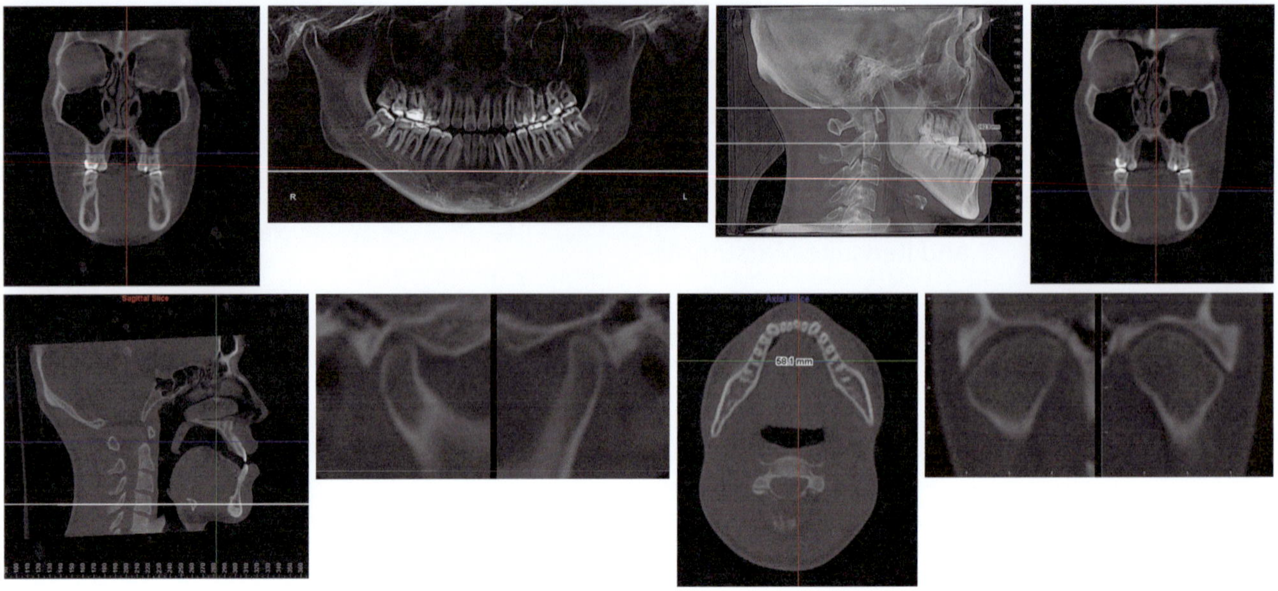

Fig. 4.1 Examples of CBCT-derived images for orthodontic diagnosis

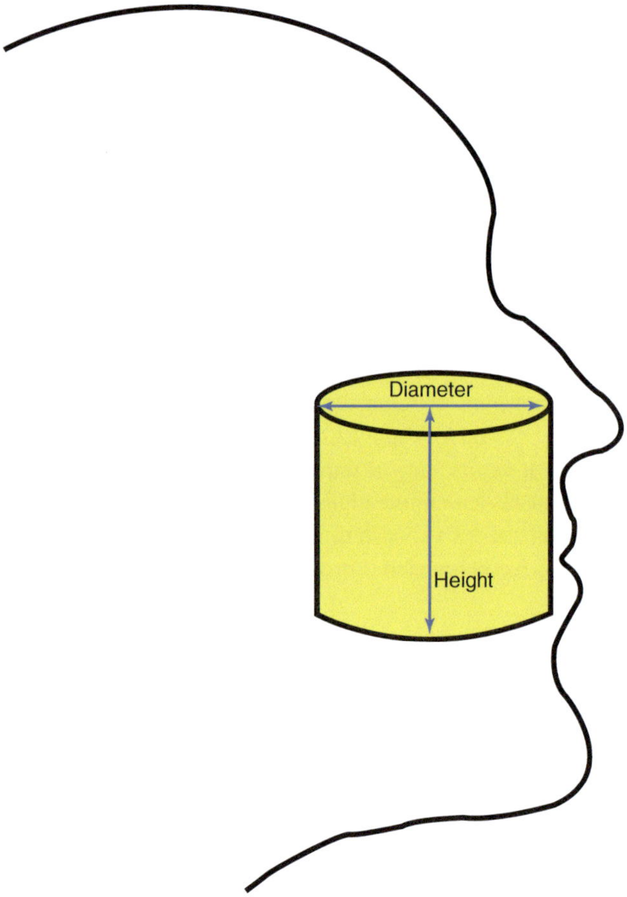

Fig. 4.2 Schematic showing the characteristics of the field of view (FOV)

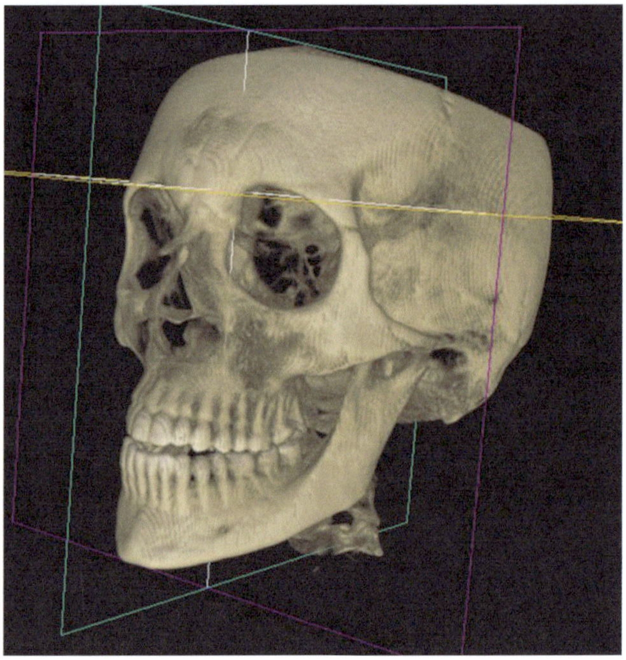

Fig. 4.3 Reconstructed full volume from the original CBCT data

resolution. The anatomic resolutions are measured in micrometers (μm) or mm. For instance, if the anatomic resolution is 200 μm, it is equivalent to 0.2 mm. This essentially becomes the native resolution. The thinnest cut can be made at the thickness of one-pixel depth. Bone morphology demands slightly thicker cuts, for example, 1- or 2-mm thickness, so that noise can be minimized by adding thickness.

4.2.3 Radiation Overview

Generally speaking, in the traditional CT scanners, the radiation dose goes up as the tube current (mA) and the associated voltage (kVp) goes down if the section thickness, voxel size, or pitch (incremental patient movement through the gantry controlled by the machine) is increased. With everything else being constant, an increased radiation dose leads to decrease in the noise, creating a better contrast [4].

Although by convention, the CT dose index (CTDI) and dose length product (DLP) are measured in grays (Gy), and the effective doses are measured in sieverts (Sv), these methods are not adapted for CBCT dose measurement purposes, as the beam geometry and the scattered radiation profile are much different. Commercial CBCT scanners are designed and manufactured with individual proprietary variations in their equipment and operators can alter patient doses by adjusting beam collimation (FOV), image quality (number of basis images, resolution, and arc of trajectory), and exposure parameters (milli amperage and kilovoltage); hence, there will be significant dose variation among various machines for the similar FOVs. For instance, a 15 × 15 cm large FOV CBCT might impart a dose of 52 μSv [5] to 680 μSv when another machine was used [6]. Similarly, with a small volume CBCT (4 × 4 cm), patients can receive as low as 31 μSv [7] or as high as 166 μSv [8]. Although the internal variation in doses within CBCT seems quite high, when compared with MSCT doses in the ranges of 430–1410 μSv [9], the doses are much lower.

4.2.4 Perspective Vs. Orthogonal Review

4.2.4.1 Perspective

Perspective views are essentially CBCT volumes that are made to look like planar (plain) x-ray images. Examples are lateral and posterior/anterior cephalograms. Although these perspective views are extracted from CBCT volumes, they essentially mimic the plain two-dimensional cephalometric views. There is no added advantage to using these, other than the fact that they are digitally available and easily imported to cephalometric software for cephalometric analysis (Fig. 4.4). The perspective views attempt to replicate the magnification of traditional cephalometric radiographs with the accompanying undesirable distortions due to the divergence of the beam as it traverses the left side of the skull to the right side of the skull. The availability of this feature allows the clinician to compare images generated from CBCT machines to that of traditional two-dimensional radiographic machines.

4.2.4.2 Orthogonal

Orthogonal images have no magnification or distortion and project "anatomic truth." Orthogonal views are created at a right angle to the original anatomy. They are frequently referred to as cross-sectional views. Orthogonal views are frequently used to assess the bucco-lingual dimension of maxillary and mandibular alveolar processes. This advantage over 2D planar images has begun to redefine the Ackerman–Proffit envelope

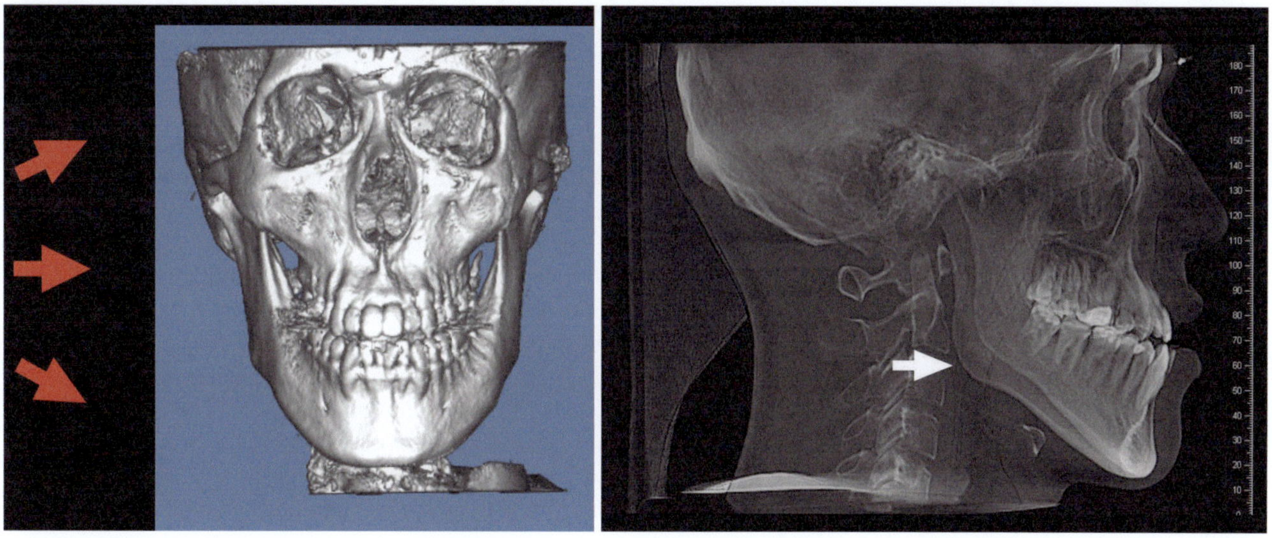

Fig. 4.4 Perspective view from Dolphin Imaging—note the exaggerated appearance of mandibular asymmetry at the base of the body of the mandible as well as along the posterior border of the ramus. The radiation emanates from the center of emitter. There is magnification and distortion (above and below the center beam of radiation)

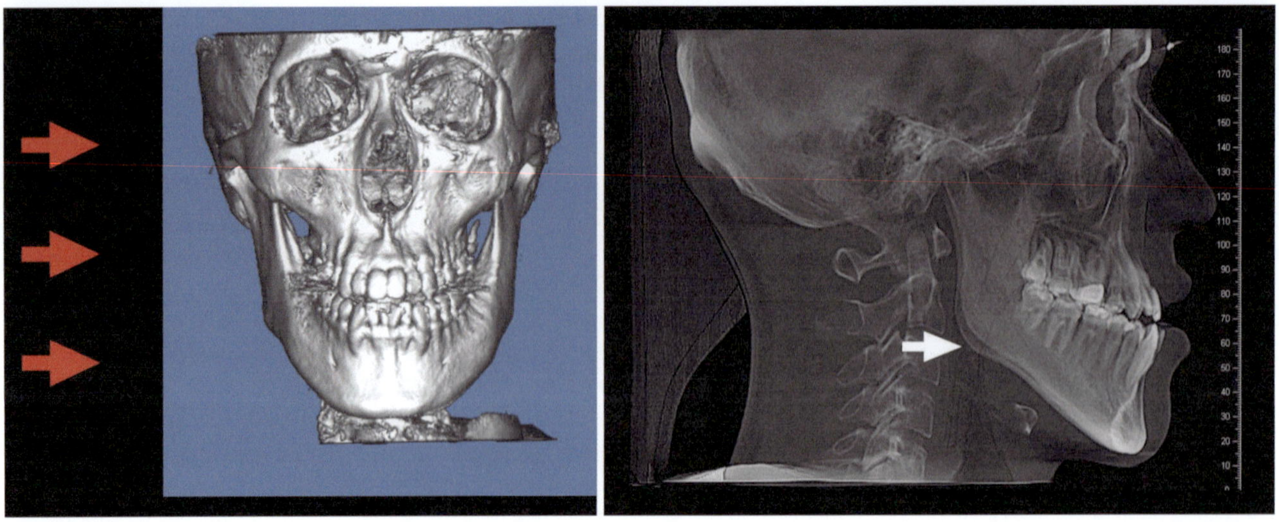

Fig. 4.5 Orthogonal view from Dolphin imaging with true anatomy and 0% distortion. There is no magnification nor distortion and the beams of radiation are parallel

of treatment to avoid adverse periodontal outcomes as a result of orthodontic treatment [10]. Sagittal, coronal, and axial orthogonal views are used for diagnostic purposes (Fig. 4.5).

4.3 Image Reconstruction from CBCT Data

4.3.1 Head Orientation

Two-dimensional planar images only allow orientation of the sagittal view. For enhanced visualization and perspective, CBCT images are oriented in three planes of space. A step by step approach begins with the "tipping orientation," where the most inferior point of the right and left orbits of the eye are parallel to a horizontal reference point. The "yaw" orientation is achieved by orienting the sagittal view so that the most posterior point of the right and left orbits of the eye overlap perfectly. The "pitch" of the sagittal is oriented to a vertical plane tangent to glabella, so that the horizontal distance of the center of the most prominent clinical crown is the distance estimated clinically when visualizing the head in adjusted natural head position [11].

The outcome of orientation provides the orthodontist with views that reduce distorted visual perception. Proper orientation enhances the ability to identify areas of asymmetry (Fig. 4.6).

4.3.2 Segmentation

CBCT software can provide soft tissue, hard tissue, and translucent renderings to enhance anatomic landmark identification (Figs. 4.7 and 4.8).

4.3.3 Stepwise Building of Orthodontic Diagnostic Images

The stepwise instructions on building diagnostic images with Dolphin Imaging 11.95 Premium 3D software are detailed in Appendices 1–5:

1. Building a lateral cephalometric radiograph
2. Building panoramic radiograph
3. Building transverse radiograph
4. Building TMJ radiograph
5. Building airway studies

4.4 Integration of Digital Models with CBCT Images

Digital models from intraoral scans can be merged with CBCT. Visualizing the roots allows the orthodontist to treatment plan occlusal changes with well-positioned roots within the alveolar process.

The orthodontist can treatment plan to a periodontally driven envelope of treatment to potentially reduce iatrogenic complications, such as gingival recession and root sensitivity.

Merging the crowns of digital models with the crowns of a CBCT image allows the orthodontist to relate the morphology and position of the crowns of teeth to the shape and position of the roots. Posterior root inclinations and anterior root angulations can be evaluated from a frontal perspective. Anterior root inclinations and posterior root angulations can be assessed from a buccal perspective (Fig. 4.9).

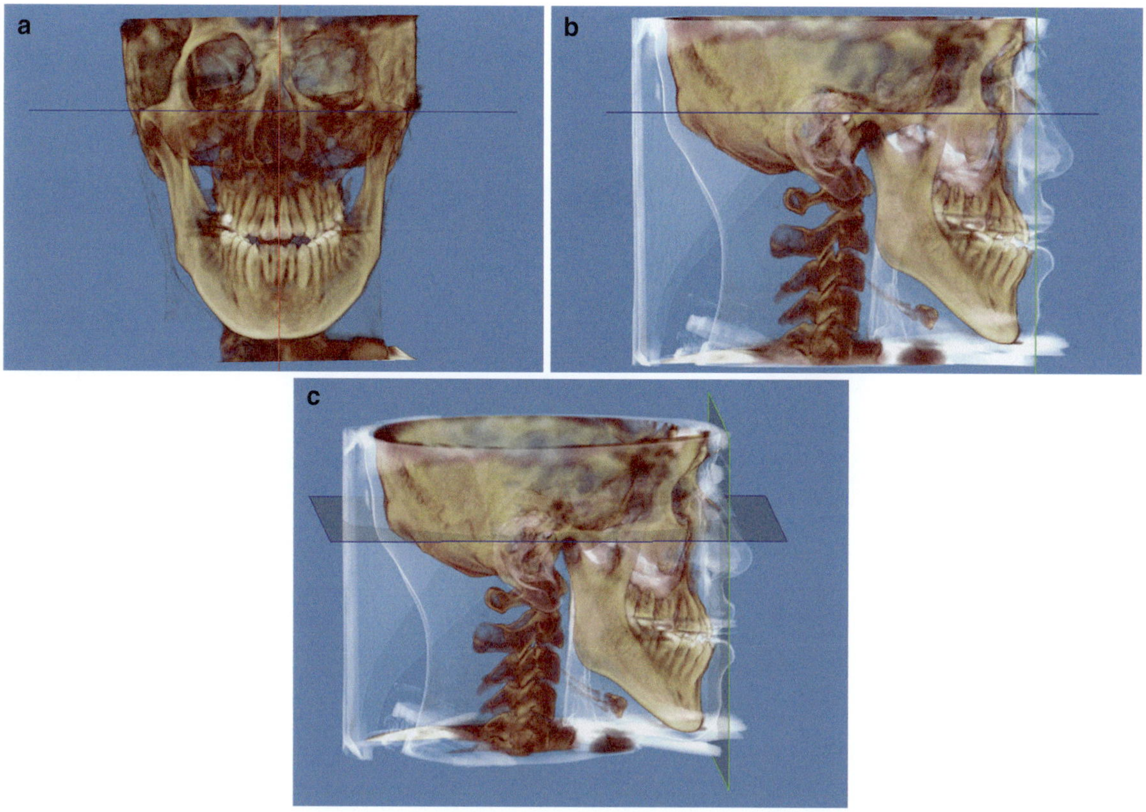

Fig. 4.6 (**a**) Coronal-horizontal view: the most inferior points of the orbits of the eyes are in contact with the horizontal plane; (**b**) Sagittal view: the vertical plane is tangent to the inner aspect of glabella and the head is rotated to replicate adjusted natural head position; (**c**) Combined planes

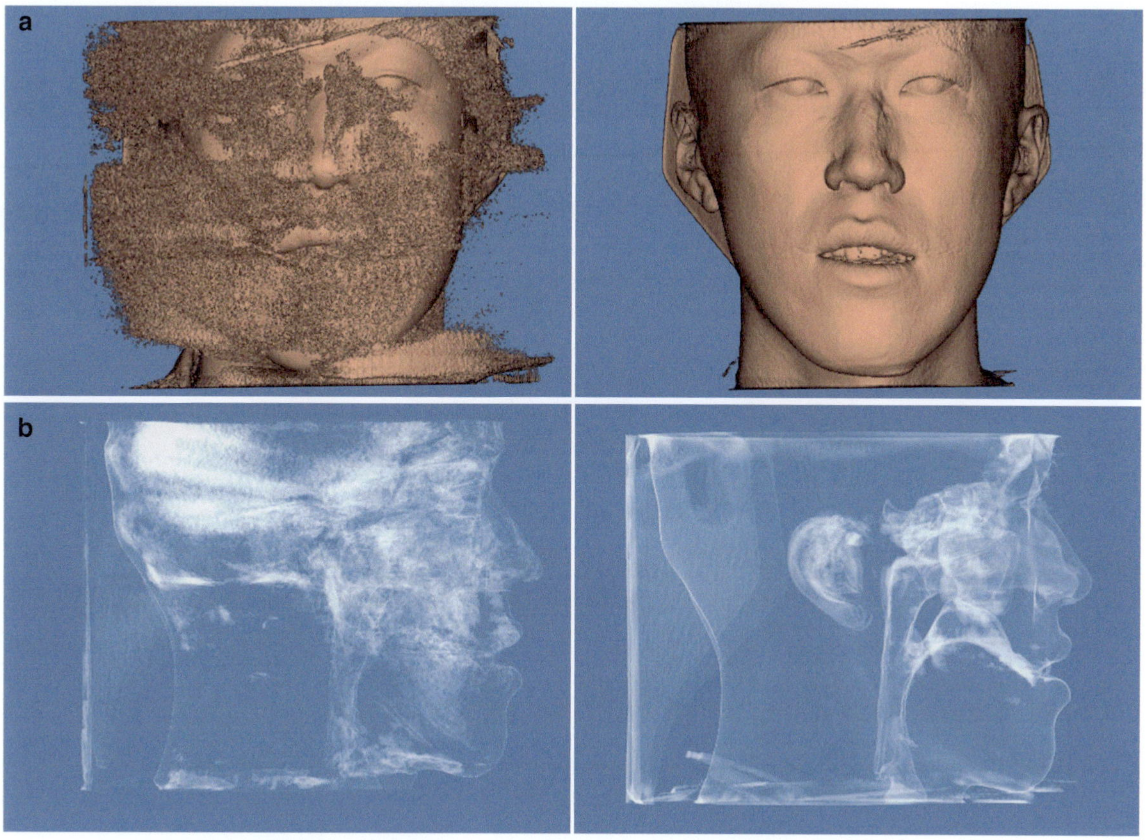

Fig. 4.7 (**a**) An example of soft tissue rendering; (**b**) An example of translucent rendering

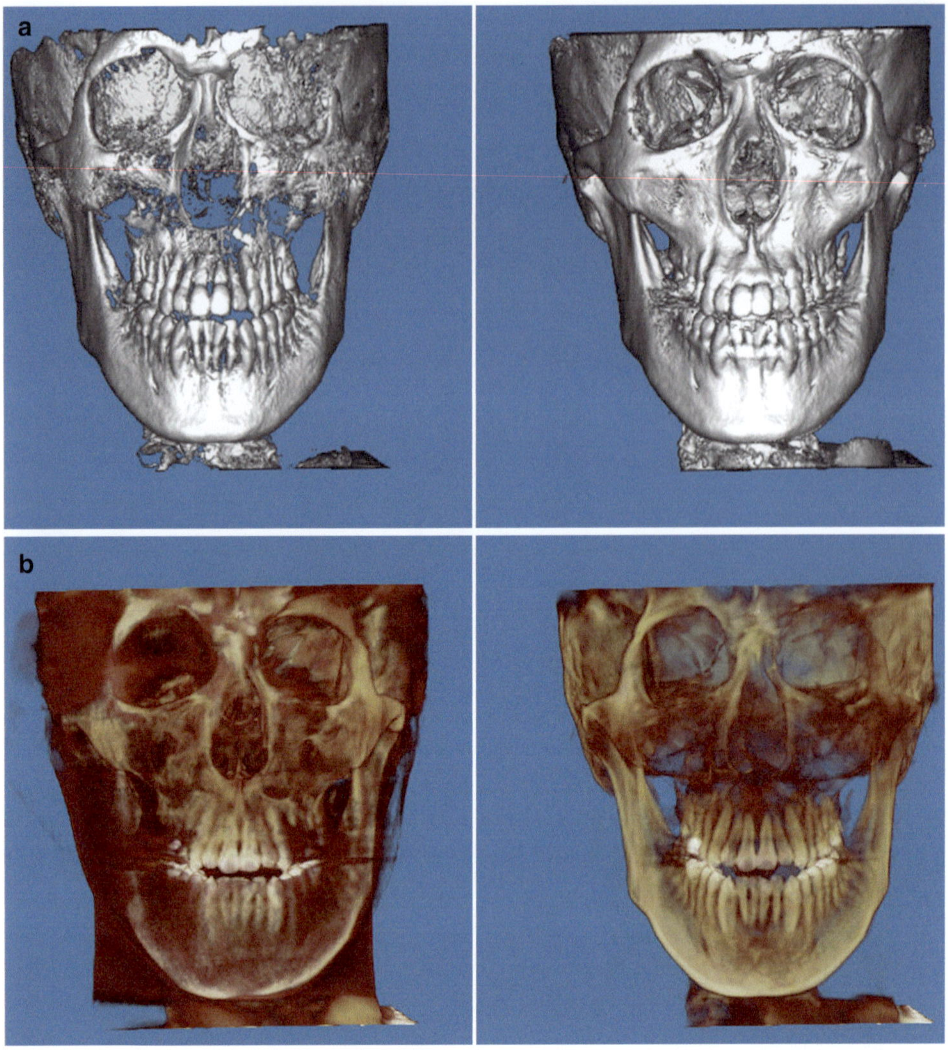

Fig. 4.8 (**a**, **b**) Examples of hard tissue rendering

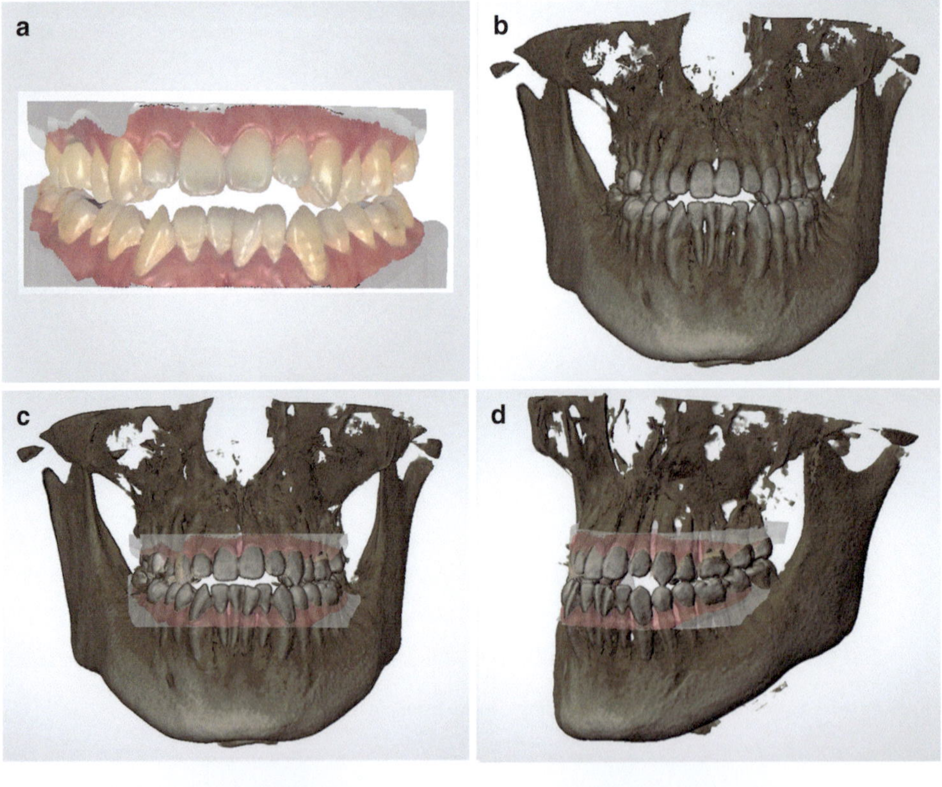

Fig. 4.9 Integration of digital models with CBCT images. (**a**) Digital simulations of an intraoral scan; (**b**) CBCT 3D model; (**c**, **d**) integrated dental digital model with the CBCT 3D model

4.5 Orofacial Orthodontic Diagnosis

4.5.1 Sagittal-Vertical

With a CBCT volume, the sagittal perspective can include the entire skull, a right and left half skull with the Dolphin clipping feature to identify asymmetry, and a 2 mm median slice to evaluate the quality of the upper and lower anterior alveolar processes (Fig. 4.10).

4.5.1.1 Mandibular Symphysis

Excessive maxillary and mandibular vertical development of the lower third of the face results in elongation and narrowing of the alveolar processes supporting the roots of the upper and lower anterior teeth [12]. This can be particularly significant for the mandibular symphysis. Two-dimensional planar images project the entire chin, which exaggerates the volume of the symphysis. A 2-mm sagittal CBCT image provides a cross-sectional view to accurately assess the bucco-lingual volume of bone (Fig. 4.11). The volume of the symphysis is a consideration when targeting the anteroposterior position of the anterior teeth.

4.5.2 Transverse Dimension

Many cephalometric analyses of the sagittal and vertical dento-skeletal dimensions have been anecdotally created, championed by orthodontic opinion leaders, and over time, accepted as orthodontic diagnostic dogma. Analyses of the transverse dimension with CBCT coronal and axial views are undergoing gradual acceptance. The most credible, yet unvalidated, approach is an adaptation of the Andrews Element III analysis adapted for CBCT [11, 13]. The step by step approach is as follows (Fig. 4.12):

1. Coronal slice at the sagittal depth of the mesio-buccal cusp of the upper first molars
2. Axial slice at the vertical level of the furcation of the upper first molars
3. Measure the linear distance of the buccal bone over the mesio-buccal cusp of the upper first molars (*X* mm)
4. Coronal slice at the sagittal depth of the midpoint between the mesial and distal roots of the lower first molars
5. Axial slice at the vertical level of the furcation of the lower first molars

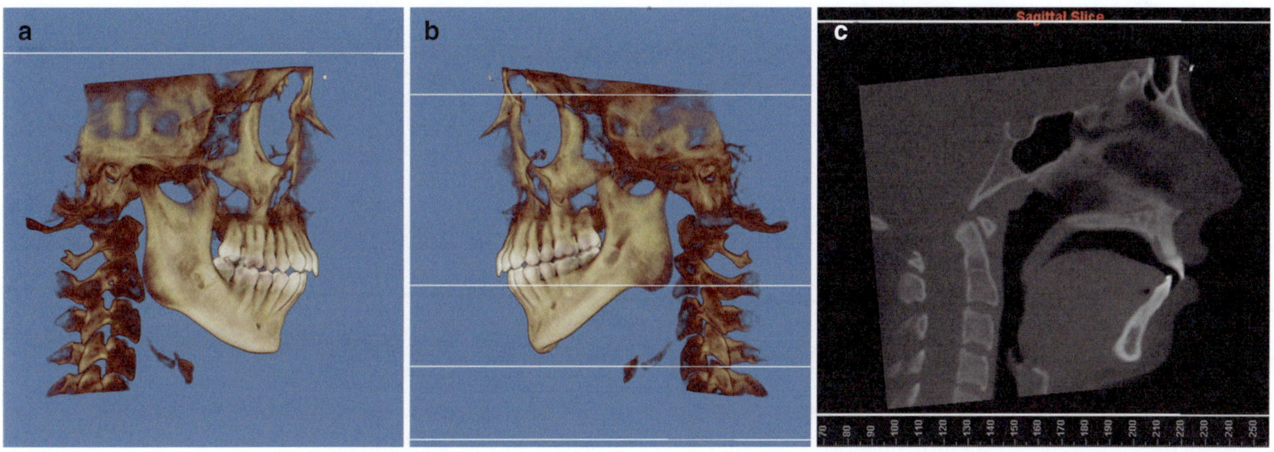

Fig. 4.10 (**a**) Sagittal view of the right side; (**b**) Sagittal view of the left side; (**c**) Sagittal view showing the upper and lower anterior alveolar processes

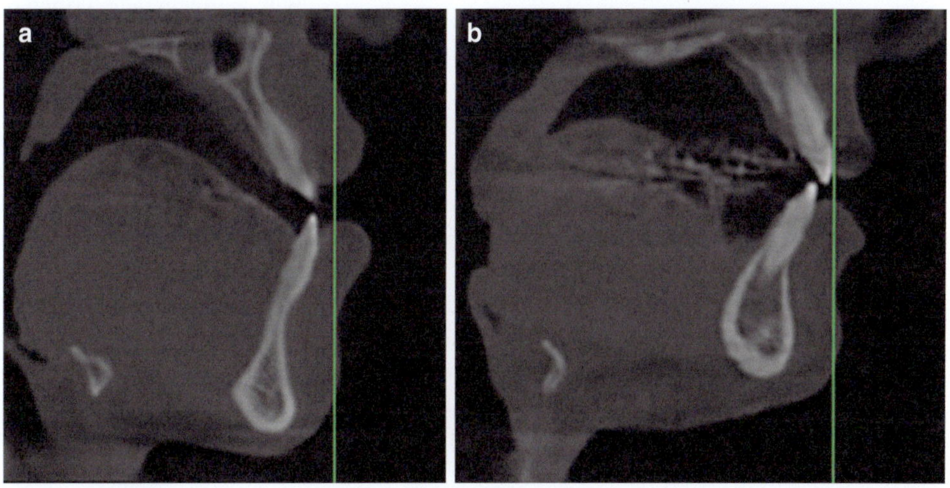

Fig. 4.11 (**a**) Dolichocephalic facial pattern resulting in elongated and narrow symphysis; (**b**) Brachycephalic facial pattern with short, wide symphysis

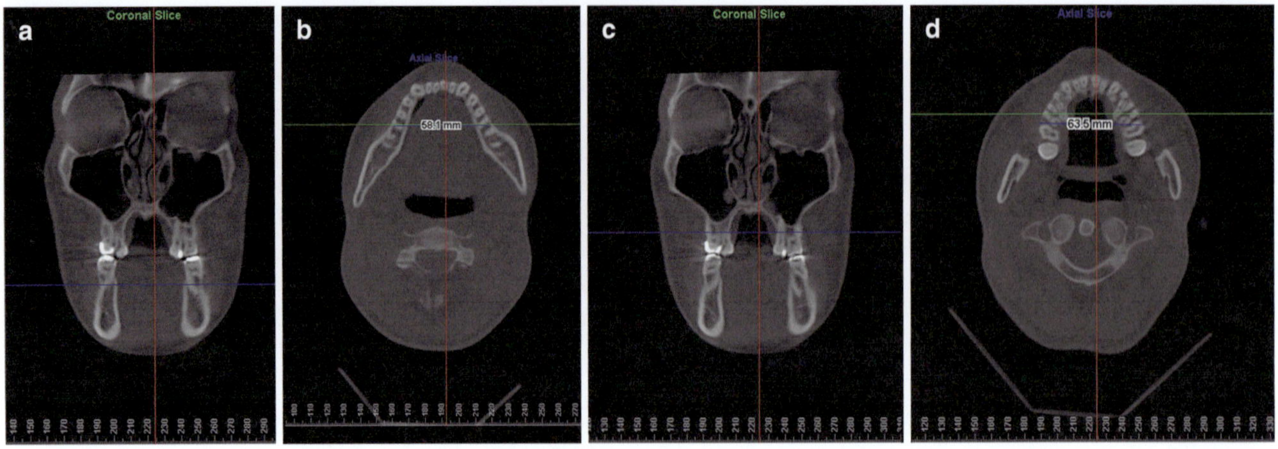

Fig. 4.12 (**a**) Coronal slice at the sagittal depth of the midpoint between the mesial and distal roots of the first molar. (**b**) Axial cut at the vertical level of the furcation of the lower first molars. (**c**) Coronal slice at the sagittal depth of the mesio-buccal cusp of the upper first molar. (**d**) Axial slice at the vertical level of the furcation of the upper molars

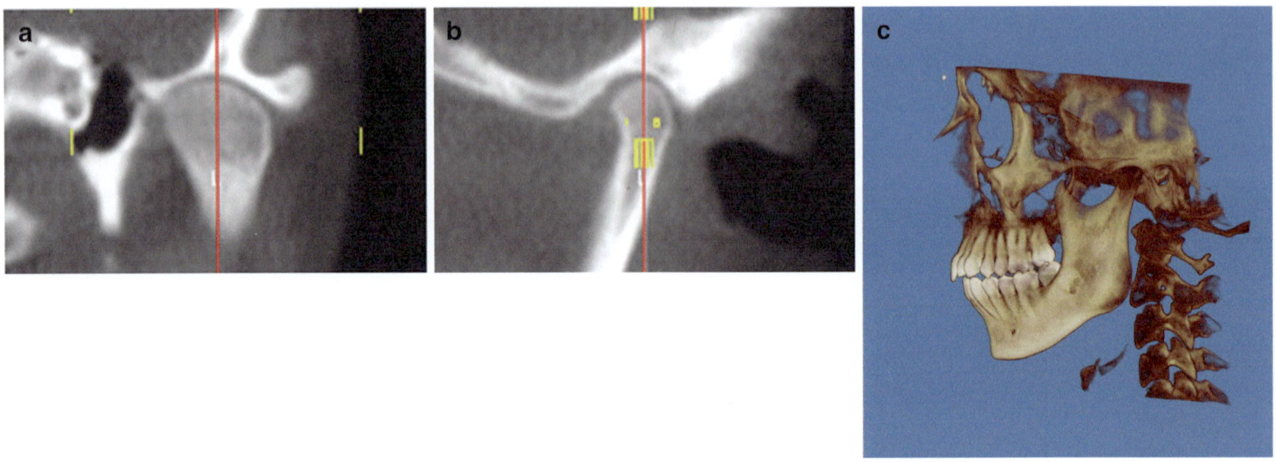

Fig. 4.13 (**a–c**) Altered joint spaces indicative of discal displacement resulting in reduced sagittal growth of the maxilla and mandible

6. Measure the linear distance between the mesial and distal roots from the inner aspect of the buccal bone (*Y*)
7. Ideal width of the maxilla relative to the width of the mandible is calculated as follows: *X* mm + 5 mm = *Y*

4.5.3 TMJ Diagnosis

There are risk markers associated with temporomandibular joint disorders (TMD) that can be identified on CBCT. Studies identifying good growers (counterclockwise) versus bad growers (clockwise) recognize that a normal versus compromised temporomandibular joint (TMJ) is an important etiologic factor associated with bad growth (Figs. 4.13 and 4.14) [14]. With adults, the traditional perspective that the end of growth results in stable skeletal morphology has been challenged when consideration has been given to the status of the temporomandibular joints (Fig. 4.15). The loss of condylar vertical dimension results in regional adaption and altered spacial relationships of the structure of the head and neck [15, 16].

Several studies have reported a high prevalence of temporomandibular joint disc displacement in pre-orthodontic adolescents [17, 18]. Disc displacement has been associated with a growth deficit often referred to as a “growth penalty” [18]. The severity of the growth deficit is directly proportional to the severity of the joint insult and indirectly proportional to the age of the onset [19]. Joint insults damage the condylar growth site, limiting endochondral bone formation and growth of the affected ipsilateral half of the mandible. Unilateral joint insults can lead to a mandibular asymmetry while regional adaptions resulting from bilateral joint insults can be associated with a dolicofacial growth pattern and possibly an anterior open bite [20–22].

4.5.3.1 Joint Spaces

CBCT assessment of temporomandibular joint spaces is important for every orthodontic patient.

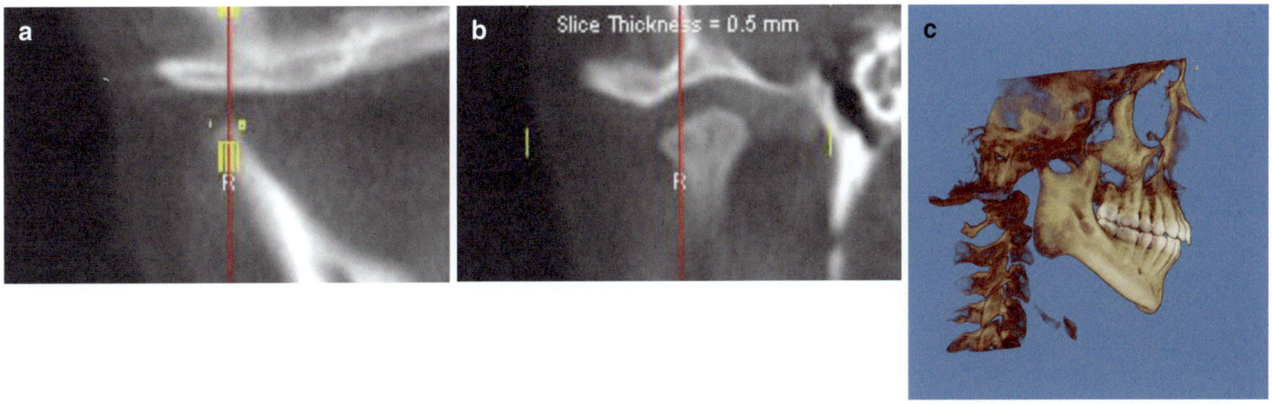

Fig. 4.14 (**a–c**) Severe condylar degenerative resorbtion resulting indownward and backward displacement of the mandible

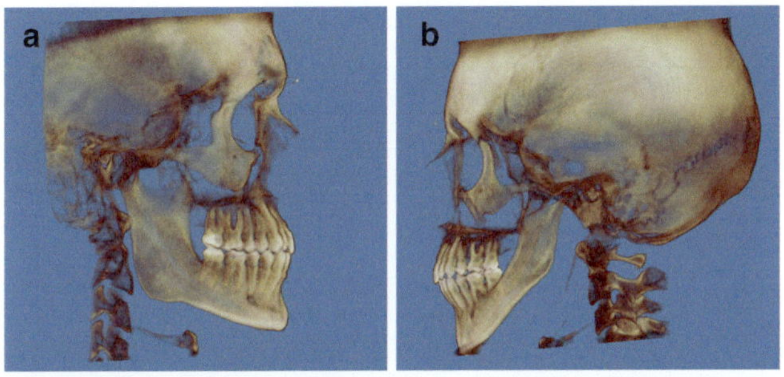

Fig. 4.15 (**a**) Normal TMJ and counterclockwise growth and development of the maxilla and mandible. (**b**) Degenerative joint disease of the TMJ resulting in clockwise downward and backward displacement of the maxilla and mandible

Optimal TMJ Spaces

An orthodontic dento-skeletal sagittal diagnosis begins with the condyle in centric relation (CR) with anterior, superior, and posterior joint spaces meeting the criteria established by Ikeda on sagittal TMJ CBCT images [23] (Figs. 4.16 and 4.17). According to Okesson, the centric relation (CR) position is a necessary factor in establishing an orthopedically stable occlusion [24]. It can be defined as seating the condyle in the antero-superior regions of the fossa with the disc interposed and at the same time the teeth are in maximum intercuspation.

When the morphology and/or spacial relationships of TMJ structures is less than optimal, the concept of CR is replaced with a clinical entity established by Dawson and referred to as Adaptive Centric Posture (ACP). Dawson has taken the anecdotal position that ACP can also meet the criteria of an orthopedically stable occlusion. He states that this position is clinically acceptable but may not be as stable [25].

4.5.3.2 Joint Space Alteration: Large Anterior Joint Space on Sagittal CBCT

The most common joint space alteration from the Ikeda normal is a larger anterior joint space, larger superior joint space, and a smaller posterior joint space (Fig. 4.18). There are three prevailing, although anecdotal, explanations for this condyle to fossa altered relationship that are significant for the orthodontist. The first, adopted by most clinicians, is the presence of a premature posterior contact resulting in an anterior open bite that fulcrums to a maximum intercuspal position when the anterior teeth are coupled at the expense of the posterior/inferior displacement of the condyles. The result is a larger anterior joint space and a diminished posterior joint space. Resolving the fulcrum with occlusal appliances results in a reduced posterior face height and increased anterior face height. A second explanation for a large anterior joint space is based on anterior displacement of the disc resulting in the thick posterior band of the disc being situated downward and forward on the eminence, causing a posterior displacement of the condyle. Dr. Mariano Rocabado provides the third explanation for a large anterior joint space. He contends that cranio-cervical abnormalities can alter the position of the condyle in the fossa [26–30]. Kyphosis of the cervical spine with forward head posture and backward rotation of the head results in retraction of the mandible and distal movement of the condyle in the glenoid fossa [26].

The large anterior and reduced posterior joint space can press the condyle to the posterior wall of the fossa and may be associated with "regressive remodeling" characterized by a loss of condylar volume along its posterior surface without a corresponding loss of vertical dimension. Regressive remodeling can be the result of therapy that posteriorly displaces the proximal segment of the mandible, such as inter-arch elastics, and BSSO orthognathic surgery.

4.5.3.3 Joint Space Alterations: Superior Joint Space Narrowing on Sagittal CBCT

Superior joint space narrowing can occur following disc displacement and subsequent thinning or perforation of the articular tissues interposed between the condyle and the opposing temporal bone. Perforations can occur in the disc when it is optimally positioned. Perforations of retrodiscal tissues can occur when the disc is displaced. Perforation of the soft tissues frequently results in bone erosions which

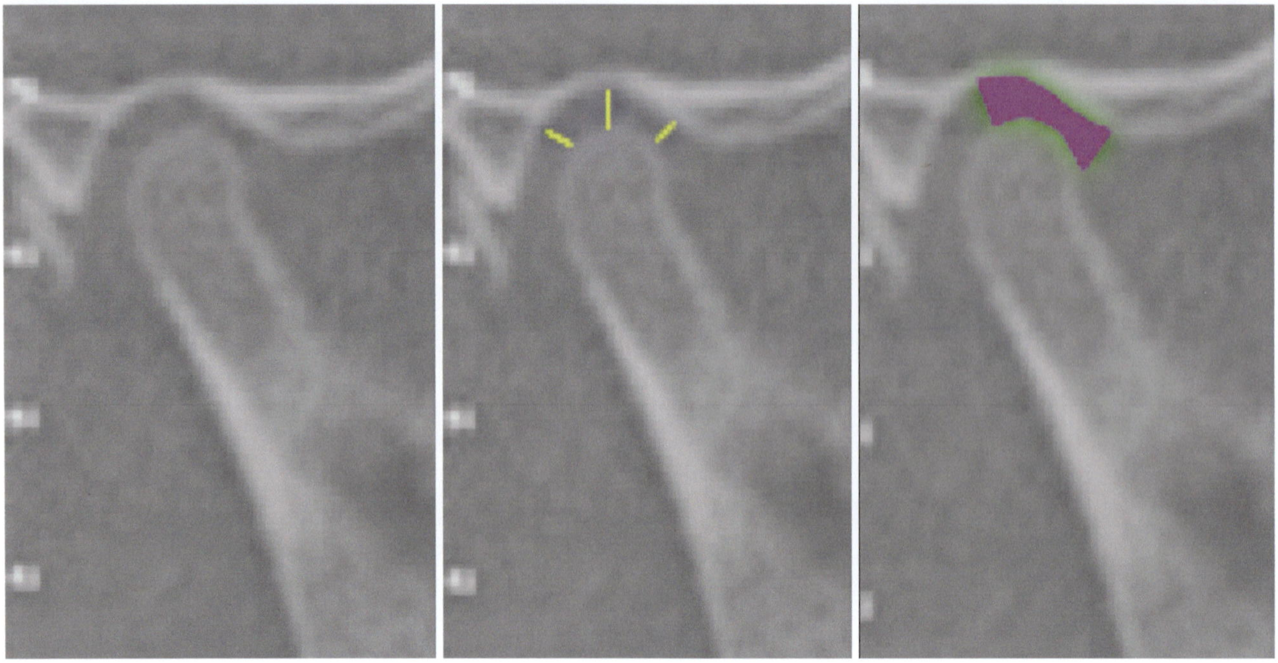

Fig. 4.16 An ideal TMJ space

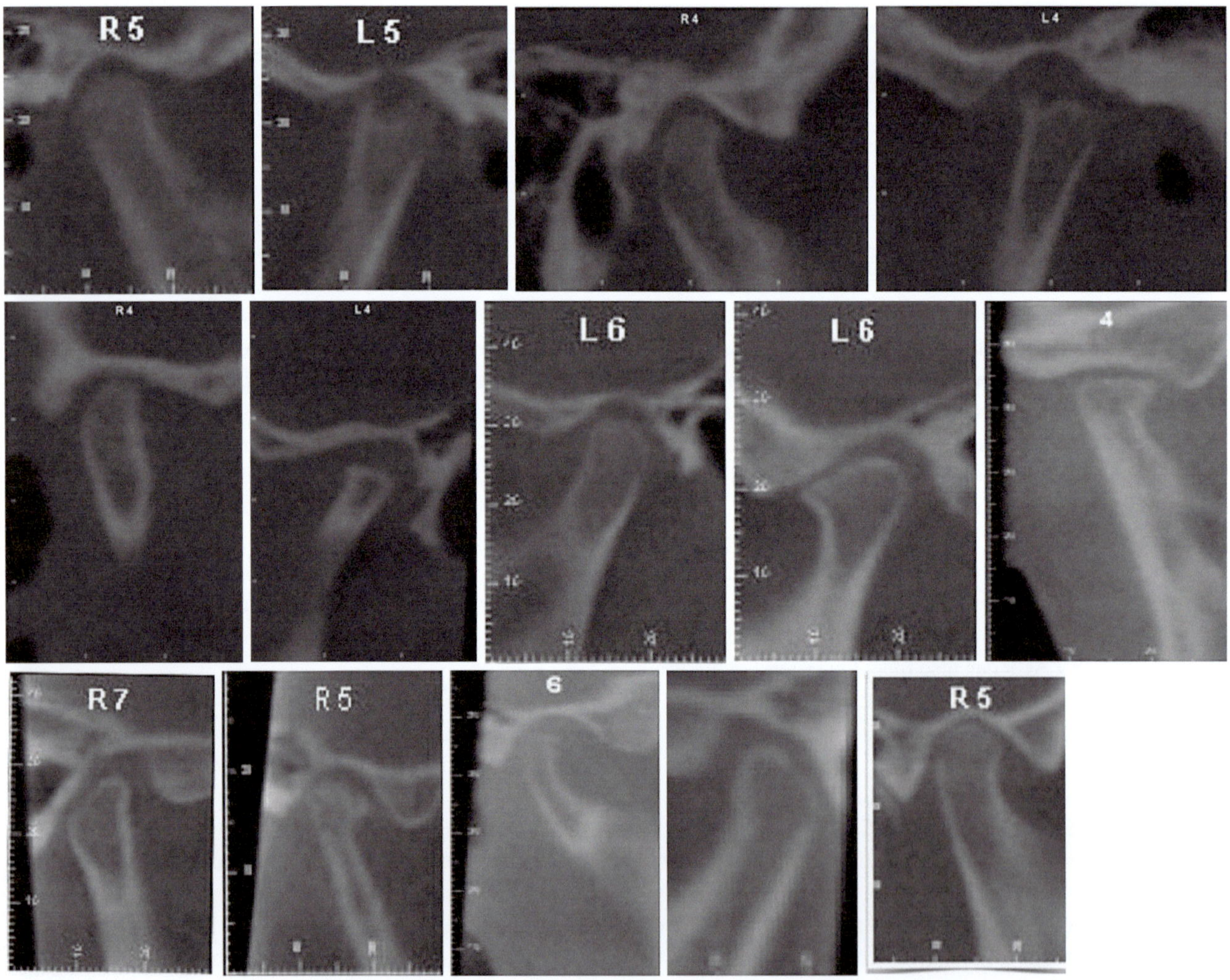

Fig. 4.17 Examples of an altered TMJ space

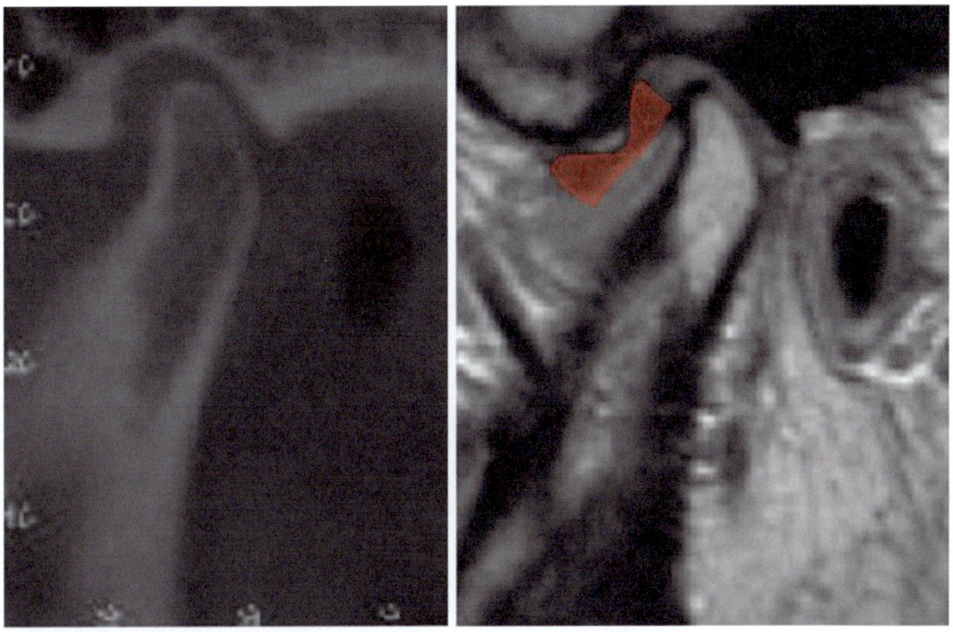

Fig. 4.18 Large anterior joint space and diminished posterior joint space. The mandible is driven to the back of the fossa resulting in a class two malocclusion. Note: Regressive remodeling of the posterior border of the head of the condyle due pressure against the posterior wall of the fossa

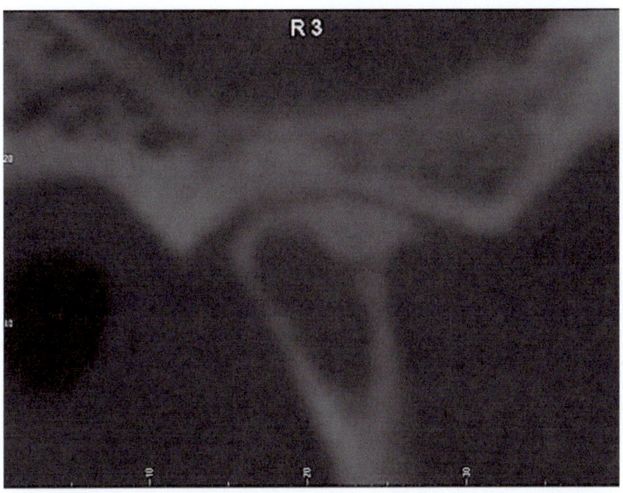

Fig. 4.19 Decreased superior joint space as a result of discal displacement followed by perforation of retrodiscal tissues

eventually undergo sclerotic repair and develop congruent surfaces with diminished joint spaces (Fig. 4.19). Loss of vertical condylar dimension is referred to as "degenerative" remodeling of the condyle and can result in "distal drift" of the mandible with increased anterior face height, decreased posterior face height, a steeper mandibular plane, and a class two molar/canine relationship (Fig. 5.31, left). The presence of active degenerative remodeling during orthodontic treatment can result in a less predictable outcome.

4.5.3.4 CBCT Diagnosis of Skeletal Asymmetry

The diagnosis of skeletal asymmetry is complex and is summarized in the Hatcher diagnostic tree where the most common etiologic condition listed is a unilateral insult to the TMJ with subsequent arthritides resulting in "regional adaptation" of the mandible and maxilla [15, 16, 31]. A unilateral insult can result in the following characteristics on the affected side (Figs. 4.20, 4.21, 4.22, and 4.23):

- there is a short ramus.
- short condyle.
- increased mandibular plane angle.
- the occlusal plane is elevated.
- the mandible is inset.
- the skeletal buccal corridor is reduced.
- the distance between the ramus and maxilla in the frontal view is reduced.
- Menton deviates to the affected side.
- the fossa is down on the affected side.
- the body of the mandible is more lingually inclined on the affected side.
- the roots of the lower posterior teeth begin to deflect to the affected side.
- there is a posterior bend of the condylar process on the affected side.
- there is a steeper concavity on the distal surface of the ramus on the affected side.
- the distance of the sigmoid notch to the dental arch is reduced on the affected side.
- the coronoid process is relatively large on the affected side.
- in the body of the mandible, the amount of bone under the roots of the molar teeth is less on the affected side.
- there is a more prominent antigonial notch on the affected side.

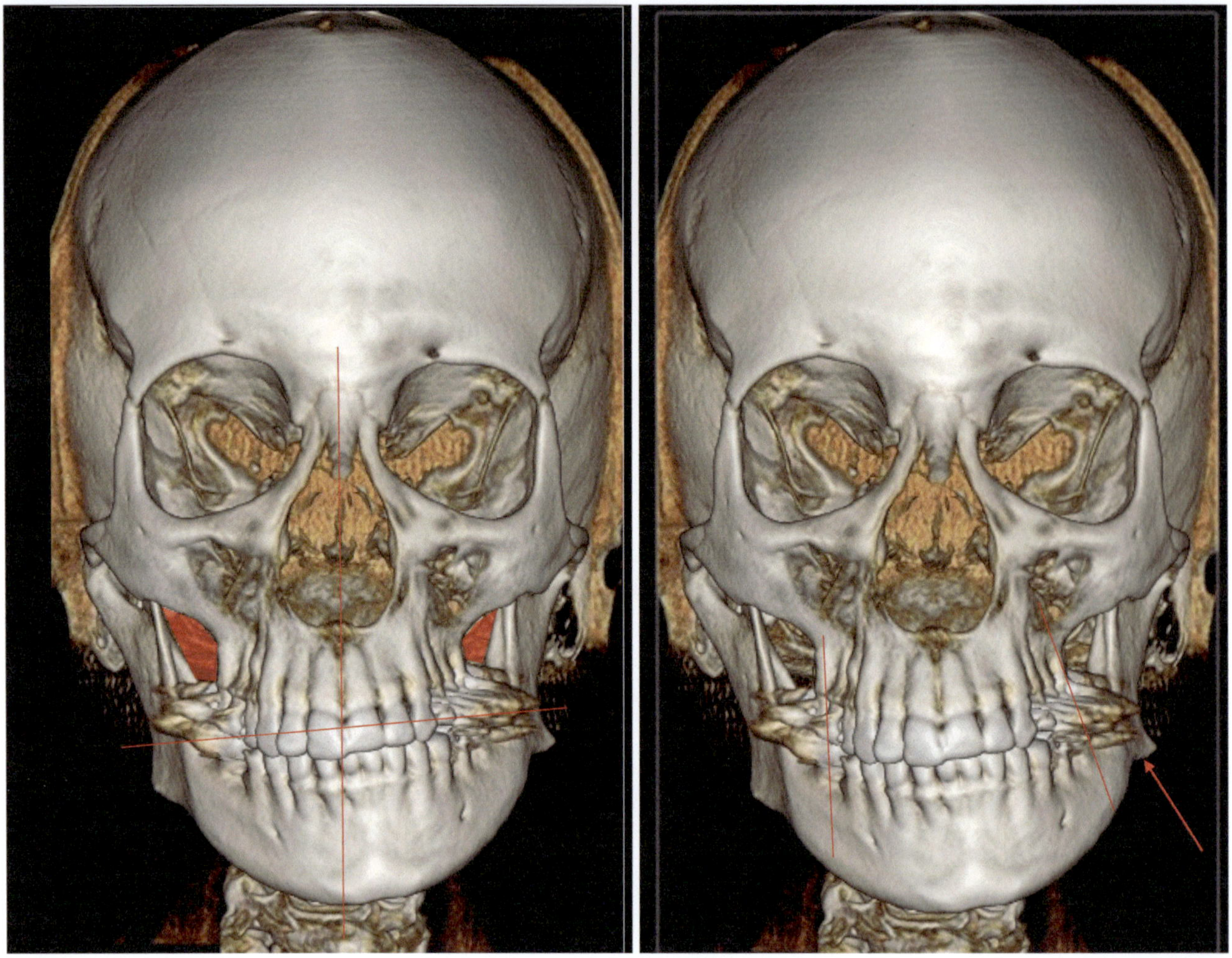

Fig. 4.20 Occlusal plane elevated; skeletal buccal corridor is reduced; deviated menton; narrow maxilla and mandible; body of the mandible is more lingually inclined; and more prominent antegonial notch

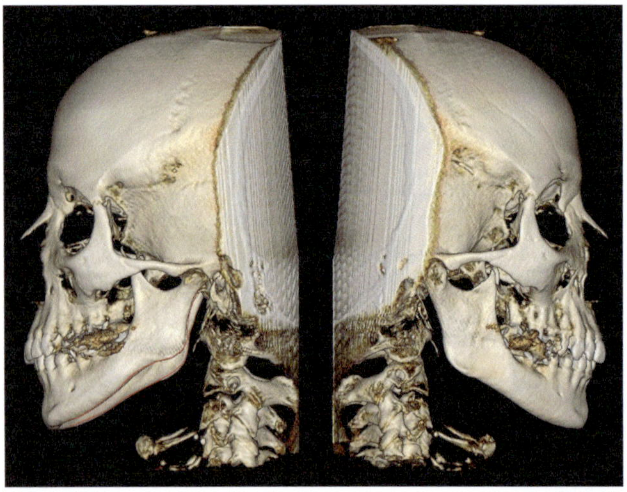

Fig. 4.21 Short ramus; short condyle; and increased mandibular plane angle

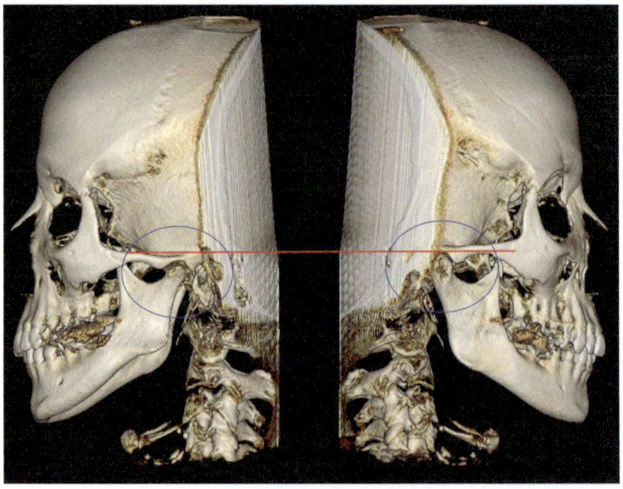

Fig. 4.22 Remodeling of fossa at lower position

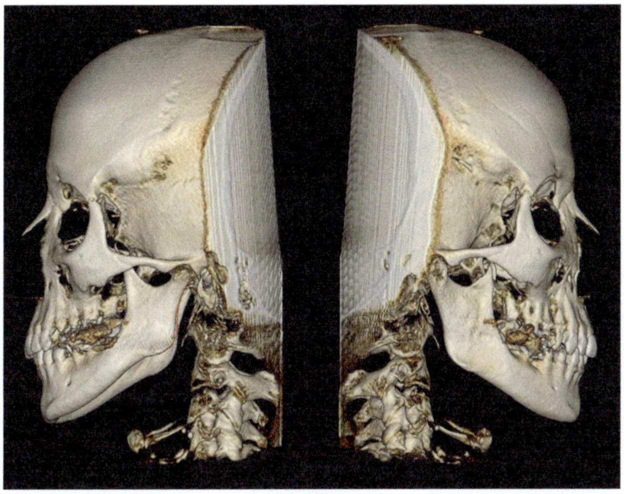

Fig. 4.23 Posterior bend of the neck of the condyle; deeper concavity on the distal surface of the ramus

In summary, asymmetry of the maxilla and mandible provides insight into the significant impact that a failing temporomandibular joint can have on the stomatologic system and the importance of rendering a diagnosis on the status of each temporomandibular joint.

4.5.4 CBCT Airway Diagnosis

The increased awareness of obstructive sleep apnea in children and adults has driven the assessment of the airway to the forefront of orthodontic diagnostic importance [31]. The upper airway is defined by the anatomy of the skeleton and soft tissues. It begins with the opening of the nares and extends to the pharyngeal bifurcation of the trachea and esophagus. Areas of constriction lead to increased airway resistance and are referred to as "airway valves." The nasal valve is at the junction of the anterior and middle thirds of the nasal passageway and is frequently associated with a deviated septum. The soft palate, tongue, and epiglottis are soft tissues that can also create areas of constriction resulting in an airway valve. Anatomic anomalies of these tissues such as enlarged turbinates, hypertrophied adenoids and tonsils, a large tongue, and deviated septum can lead to increased airway resistance and can contribute to obstructive sleep disturbed breathing (OSDB).

CBCT volumetric, area, and linear measurements are not adequate to render a definitive diagnosis of OSDB. Nevertheless, CBCT imaging can identify phenotypes that are at risk of obstruction due to anatomic characteristics associated with OSDB [32–39].

4.5.4.1 Limitations of CBCT Imaging of the Airway

The most significant limitation of CBCT studies assessing the airway is body, head, jaw, and tongue position at the time of the scan acquisition [40, 41]. The stage of inhalation and exhalation also has a significant influence on upper airway dimension. To mitigate inaccuracies the following protocol has been proposed: The patient must be still; must avoid swallowing; hold their breath; be seated in an upright position with Frankfurt plane parallel to the ground; guided to centric relation; and the lips relaxed [42–44].

The "sensitivity" of CBCT imaging of empty space is also a limitation. CBCT scans do not provide absolute Hounsfield Unit (HU) value like that obtained with a medical CT scan. A CBCT machine is not calibrated to actual HU numbers. The CBCT HU numbers vary from manufacturer to manufacturer, from machine to machine, and even from scan region to scan region [45, 46]. Denser tissue will have higher numbers, but they are not correctly calibrated to the actual HU scale.

With Dolphin imaging software, the adjustment of image sensitivity determines how the seed point in the airway responds to the HU reading of the airway. Increased sensitivity requires a wider range of the HU scale. Sensitivity should be the same for the scans of the same exposure protocol on the same patient. As a rule, the sensitivity is adjusted until the airway is meeting the nasal airway and pharyngeal walls, but not seeping into the wall tissues. Although selection of threshold sensitivity value has poor intra-examiner and inter-examiner reliability, it has been reported to improve with examiner experience and is excellent for the oropharynx, which is most often the area of greatest constriction [47].

4.5.4.2 CBCT Airway Segmentation

(a) **Nasal boundaries**
(b) **Pharyngeal boundaries**

Nasal Boundaries

Nasal airway obstruction (NAO) affects up to one-third of Americans and is one of the most common complaints by patients to otolaryngologists, head and neck surgeons, and primary physicians [48]. In a healthy patient, adequate nasal airway size offers a normal nasal breathing pattern. However, when obstructed, nasal breathing becomes difficult and patients may divert to predominantly mouth breathing. Studies have shown that NAO not only significantly impairs one's quality of life, but is linked to negative consequences such as obstructive sleep apnea (OSA) and altered craniofa-

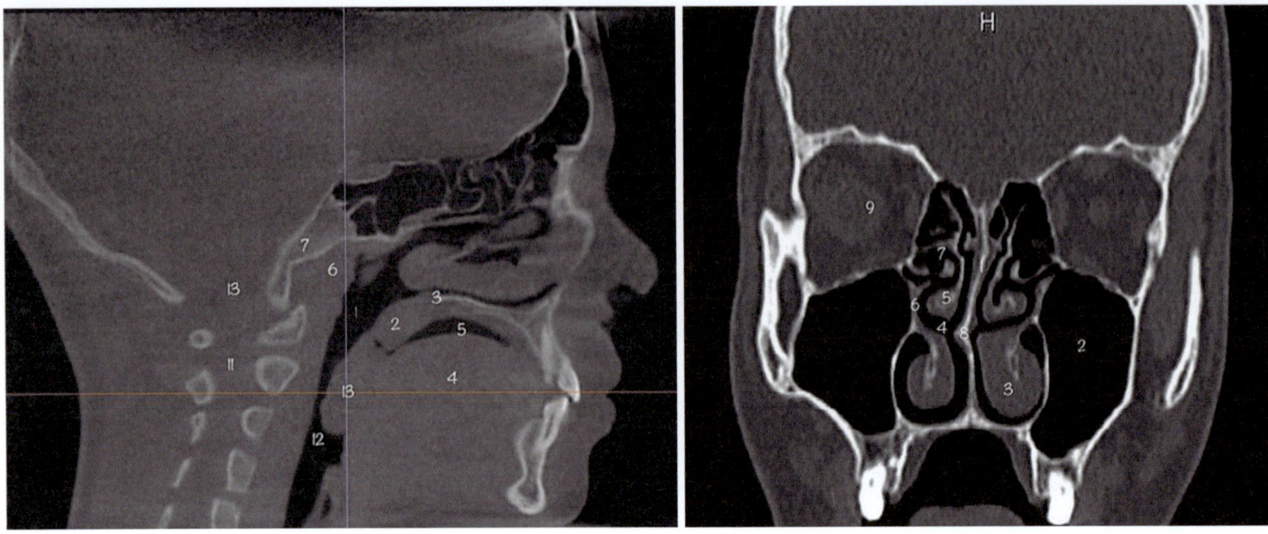

Fig. 4.24 (Left) sagittal CBCT image (bone windows) showing no significant pathology in this section; (Right) coronal CT (bone windows) showing hypertrophic left inferior concha (3), deviated nasal septum (8)

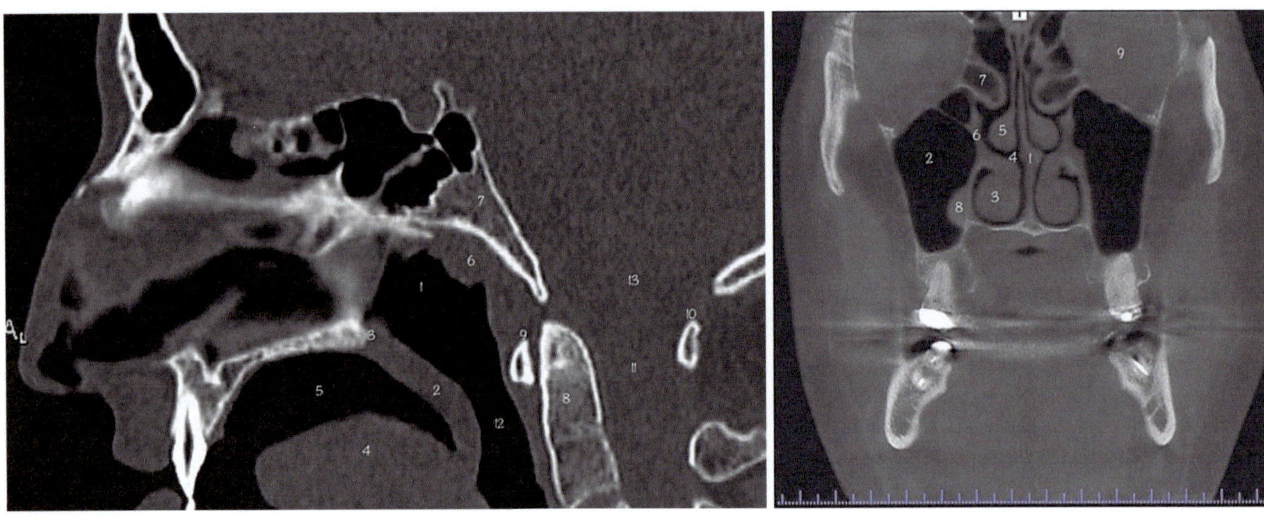

Fig. 4.25 (Left) Sagittal CT (bone windows) showing ethmoid air cell mucositis, mildly enlarged pharyngeal tonsils (6); (Right) coronal CBCT (bone windows) showing a mucous polyp along the medial wall of the right maxillary sinus (8) with everything else being normal

cial development [49, 50]. For the nasal airway specifically, CBCT has become a useful modality to diagnose nasal polyps, masses, turbinate hypertrophy, concha bullosa, septal deviation, and other anatomical variations (Figs. 4.24, 4.25, and 4.26) [51].

Coronal Images

1. Nasal septum is deviated impairing breathing on one side of the nasal cavaity
2. Maxillary sinus—normal, disease (ostium patent and not)—comment saying the need to scroll through
3. Inferior nasal concha (comment on the differences between concha and turbinates)
4. Middle meatus
5. Middle nasal concha (normal and abnormal)
6. Uncinate process
7. Ethmoid sinus
8. Nasal spine (in DNS 2, it is a mucous polyp)—comment that with this specific issue, obstruction becomes more complicated
9. Orbit

Sagittal Images

1. Nasopharynx
2. Uvula
3. Posterior nasal spine
4. Tongue
5. Oral cavity

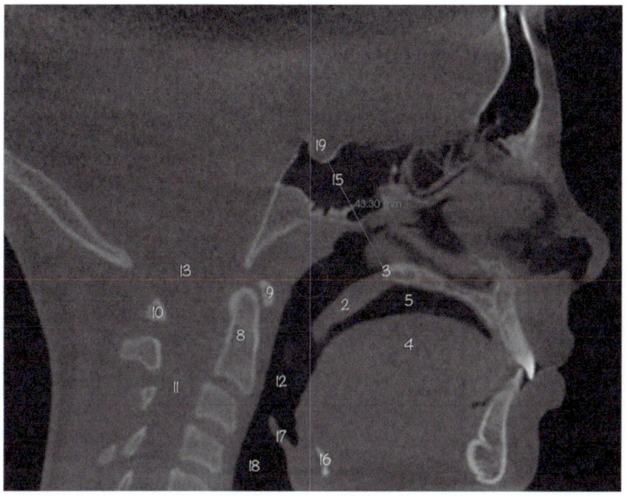

Fig. 4.26 Sagittal view numerically identifying airway anatomy and boundaries

6. Pharyngeal tonsil (Adenoids)
7. Clivus
8. Odontoid process
9. Anterior arch of Atlas
10. Posterior arch of Atlas
11. Spinal canal
12. Oropharynx
13. Foramen magnum (in one image, it is palatine tonsil)
14. Right palatine tonsil
15. Line connecting the center of sella to the posterior nasal spine
16. Hyoid bone
17. Epiglottis
18. Hypopharynx
19. Sella

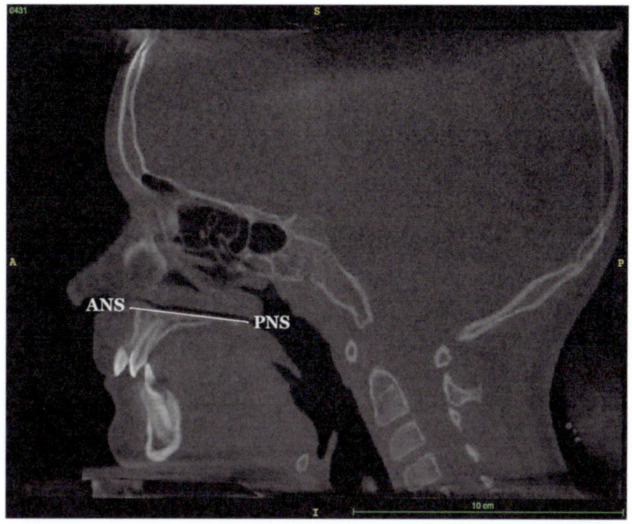

Fig. 4.27 The inferior border is defined by the ANS-PNS line

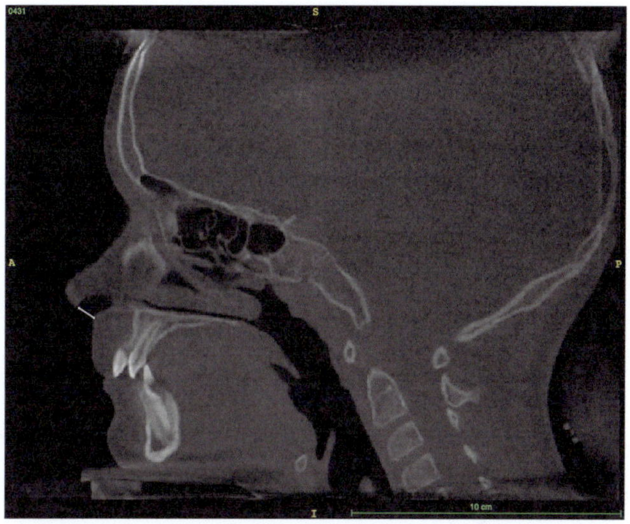

Fig. 4.28 The anterior border is defined by the anterior nares

4.5.4.3 Anatomical Boundaries for the Segmentation of Nasal Airway Using Three-Dimensional CBCT

The nasal cavity and nasopharynx are distinct anatomical areas. The pharyngeal airway, different from the nasal airway, is made up of the nasopharyngeal, oropharyngeal, and laryngopharyngeal (common pharynx) airway spaces. The upper airway is defined as the combination of the nasal airway and the pharyngeal airway above the axial plane of the base of the epiglottis. If sinuses and nasal airway are both considered, then the term "sinonasal" airway is most appropriate.

The following proposal focuses towards a gold standard on the anatomical boundaries of the nasal airway for the consistent segmentation and quantification using three-dimensional CBCT. The boundaries are organized as follows: (1) the inferior ANS-PNS border (Fig. 4.27), (2) anterior nares border (Fig. 4.28), (3) posterior S-PNS border (Fig. 4.29), and (4) superior border in alignment with the base of the skull excluding the ostia and the paranasal air sinuses including frontal, ethmoidal, sphenoidal and occipital air cells (Fig. 4.30).

Inferior ANS-PNS border

Consistent with most previous studies, the inferior border for nasal airway segmentation is defined by the axial plane that includes the line formed by the anterior nasal spine (ANS) and posterior nasal spine (PNS) [52, 53].

Anterior Nares Border

Air enters the nose starting at the openings, or anterior nares; thus, the definition of the anterior border is right to the open-

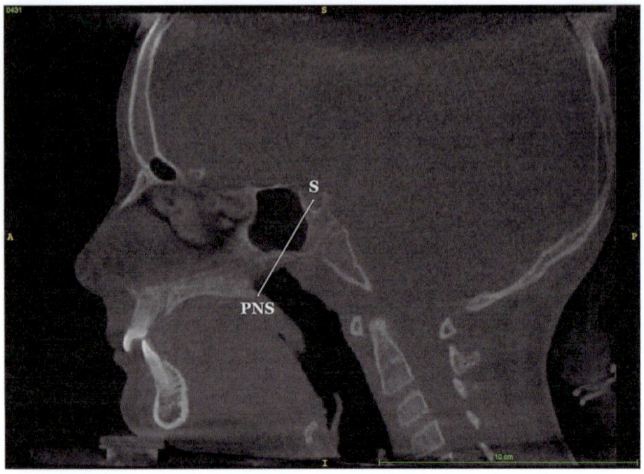

Fig. 4.29 The posterior border is defined on the mid-sagittal plane with the line extending from center of sella (S) to posterior nasal spine (PNS) as hard tissue landmarks for the location of the posterior choanae

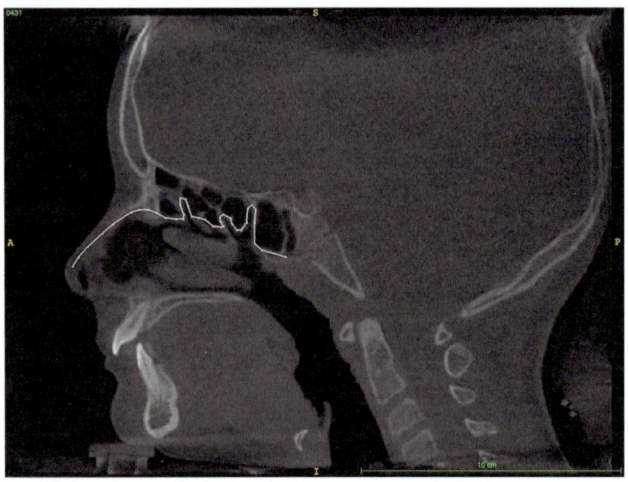

Fig. 4.30 The superior border is defined as in alignment with the base of the skull excluding the ostia and the paranasal air sinuses including frontal, ethmoidal, sphenoidal, and occipital air cells

ings anteriorly and any air within the boundaries of the soft tissue anteriorly. Including this portion of air in the anterior is significant, as lateral wall collapse contributes to NAO, and although a factor that can be easily detected without the use of CBCT, it should still be considered.

Posterior Center of S-PNS Border

The true anatomical delineation between the nasal airway and the nasopharyngeal airway is with the posterior nares, also known as the posterior choanae. However, there is a great complexity of structures and defining the choanae can be challenging, especially in cases of choanal atresia and stenosis that may contribute to NAO. The great variation in relation to the posterior anatomy can be exemplified by the assorted posterior boundaries defined by previous studies from using structures like the anterior arch of the atlas [54], dens of axis tip [55], posterior nasal plane [56], and even including the nasopharynx itself [57]. Thus, with the complexity of the posterior nasal anatomy, there is a need for hard tissue landmarks that will provide for more reproducible results for quantitative analysis. The center of sella turcica (S) and posterior nasal spine (PNS) are a reliable and easily obtained metric for identifying the region of the posterior choanae.

Superior Base of Skull Excluding Ostia and Paranasal Sinuses Border

In order to ensure accurate anatomical inclusion of the nasal airway for segmentation, the superior border is defined as in alignment with the base of the skull, excluding the ostia and the paranasal air sinuses including frontal, ethmoidal, sphenoidal, and occipital air cells.

4.5.4.4 Using ITK-SNAP® to Demonstrate and Assess the Proposed Standardized Segmentation [58]

There is currently a lack of a gold standard using CBCT technology for the segmentation of the nasal airway. The ITK-SNAP®, a DICOM imaging software [59], was developed at the University of Pennsylvania and the University of Utah to address this need and offer recommendations towards:

1. Improving anatomical boundaries for the nasal airway in three-dimensional CBCT.
2. Creating a more reliable and precise three-dimensional CBCT segmentation of the nasal airway for assisting diagnosis, treatment, and monitoring of NAO and identification of abnormalities.

ITK-SNAP® provides reliable results in volume segmentation of the upper airway, though omitting the nasal airway, with less than 2% error in volumes compared to gold standard [42]. After importing CBCT DICOM slices (.dcm) into the software, the process of labelling the nasal airway by the operator is completed with semi-automatic segmentation algorithms and manual segmentation (Fig. 4.31). The careful process starts with semi-automatic segmentation, also known as "Active Contour Segmentation Mode" on ITK-SNAP®, in which there are three stages: (1) Pre-segmentation, (2) Initialization, and (3) Evolution. Pre-segmentation first requires the determination of the region of interest. In this step, the goal is to differentiate and only label the one type of structure at hand from the rest of the image. This is achieved using the thresholding function that allows for selecting the range of intensities of the voxels that belong to the desired structure; in this case, air. The result is a speed image that

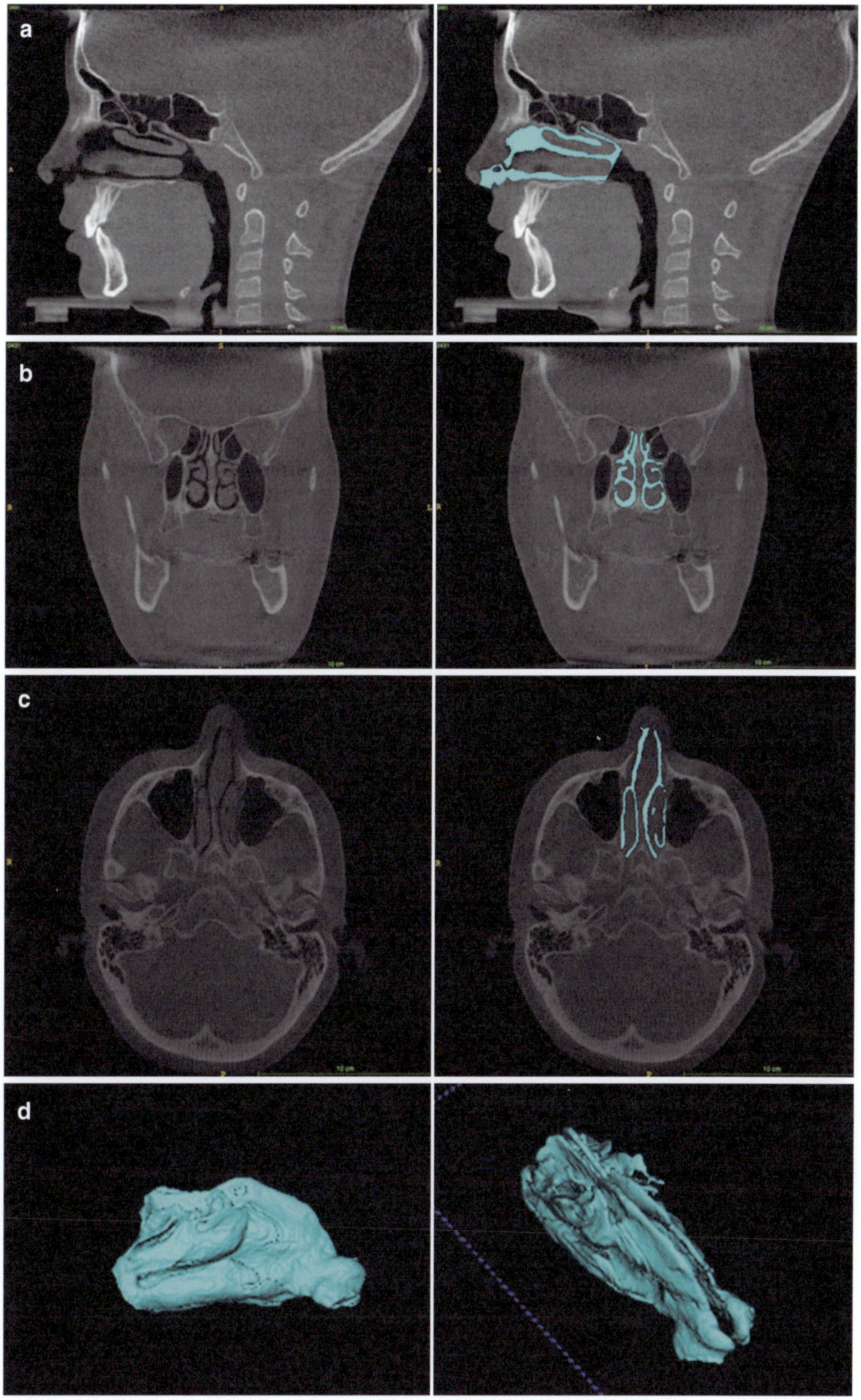

Fig. 4.31 Using ITK-SNAP®, example CBCT segmentations of the nasal airway are displayed with light blue in the (**a**) sagittal plane, (**b**) coronal plane, (**c**) axial plane, and (**d**) 3D reconstruction

displays the selected airway as white, and all unselected structures as blue. Once the desired structure is adequately selected, initialization is manually completed by adding seeding points to the desired structure. These seeds are three-dimensional in nature and ultimately expand into the final segmentation. This expansion is termed evolution. During this final stage, the seeds expand uniformly to fill the white selected structures and recede from blue unselected structures. After labels are completed in this fashion, each slice (sagittally, coronally, and axially) is reviewed and manually revised. Volumetric and intensity data is available using ITK-SNAP to determine the volume of the nasal airway and mean and standard deviation of the Hounsfield unit intensity.

The borders of the airway are standardized between patients with the following parameters in sagittal view: (1) anteriorly by the opening of the nares, (2) posteriorly center of S-PNS line, (3) inferiorly by the ANS-PNS line, and (4) superiorly in alignment with the base of the skull, excluding the ostia and the paranasal air sinuses including frontal, ethmoidal, sphenoidal, and occipital air cells.

4.5.4.5 Pharyngeal Airway

Relevance of Airway Volume to Orthodontic Diagnosis

The volume of the airway has been shown to be proportionally related to dento-facial growth. The total upper airway volume in class three patients is larger than class one or two patients [60]. Counterclockwise growth of the maxilla and mandible results in a larger airway than clockwise growth. Predominant mouth breathing, as opposed to nasal breathing, can be detrimental to the growth and development of the stomatological system [61–64]. Impaired nasal airflow can induce a clockwise growth pattern characterized by a long lower face height, steep mandibular and occlusal planes, a high and narrow palatal vault [65, 66]. The volume of the airway continues to grow from 7 to 18 years of age, but more so in males than females. Male patients have larger airways than female patients [67].

Relevance of Airway Cross Section Area and Radius to Orthodontic Diagnosis

A reduction in airway radius increases airflow resistance according to Poiseuille's Law. Airflow maintenance requires increased inhalation effort resulting in a greater differential pressure between the nasopharyngeal area and the lungs. The generation of a large pressure gradient can lead to collapse of the nasal and/or pharyngeal air passageway. The following relationship between cross-sectional airway area and a higher risk for OA has been established: high probability—minimal axial area between <52 mm^2; intermediate probability—minimal axial area between 52 and 110 mm^2; low probability—minimal axial area >110 mm^2. It is noteworthy that the pharyngeal valve (minimal axial area) is most often located in the oropharynx [65]. The oropharynx has excellent intra-examiner and inter-examiner reliability of airway assessment [47]. The smallest cross-sectional area increases in size with aging but at a faster rate in males after 12 years of age. The following anatomic abnormalities can result in upper airway cross-sectional area reductions resulting in airway obstruction: hypertrophy of adenoids and tonsils; allergic and chronic rhinitis; congenital nasal deformities; trauma to the nose; nasal septum deviation; polyps and tumors in the nasal cavity; sinus disease altering the flow in and out of the sinuses with a detrimental impact on air quality reaching the upper airway. These anatomic aberrations can lead to functional changes resulting in mouth breathing, which, in turn, can result in adverse facial growth patterns, altered dental arch forms, and malocclusion [32, 61–64].

Although polysomnography remains the gold standard for diagnosis of SDB and OSA, the phenotypical dento-skeletal information derived from CBCT by an orthodontist, coupled with validated adolescent and adult sleep questionnaires, is a potential screening strategy to identify individuals at risk for OSA. Nevertheless, it behooves the orthodontist to be aware that quantitative airway measurements from CBCT images do not necessarily play a significant diagnostic role in the development of OSA. It is possible that physiologic compensation by dilation of the airway during inspiration reduces the significance of anatomic risk factors [68, 69].

4.6 Summary

There are findings in the literature suggesting CBCT could be the standard of care for specific clinical conditions. It is our opinion that the clinical examination and health history are important in deciding between standard two-dimensional versus CBCT orthodontic imaging. Consider a patient who presents with a minor malocclusion with a favorable skeletal pattern; no sign or symptoms of TMD; a normal periodontal attachment apparatus; a normal sleep index based on a validated sleep questionnaire. This patient could be diagnosed and treatment planned from two-dimensional images. Alternatively, consider a patient with a severe dento-skeletal malocclusion possibly benefitting from orthognathic surgery; with advanced periodontal disease; with signs and symptoms of TMD; with a validated sleep index suggesting a high risk of sleep disturbed breathing. Any of these clinical findings suggest the patient might benefit from CBCT imaging for diagnosis since it might alter the treatment plan.

Going forward the orthodontic community will be challenged to establish guidelines where three-dimensional imaging is indicated versus two-dimensional imaging.

Appendix 1: Building Radiographs (X-rays) in Dolphin 3D

Lateral Cephalogram

- Confirm the desired orientation of the volume
- Confirm which type of lateral cephalogram will be created through "Options"
  - Orthogonal
    NO magnification
    NO distortion
    Parallel beams of radiation
  - Perspective
    Magnification
    Distortion (above and below the center beam of radiation)
    Radiation emanates from the center of emitter

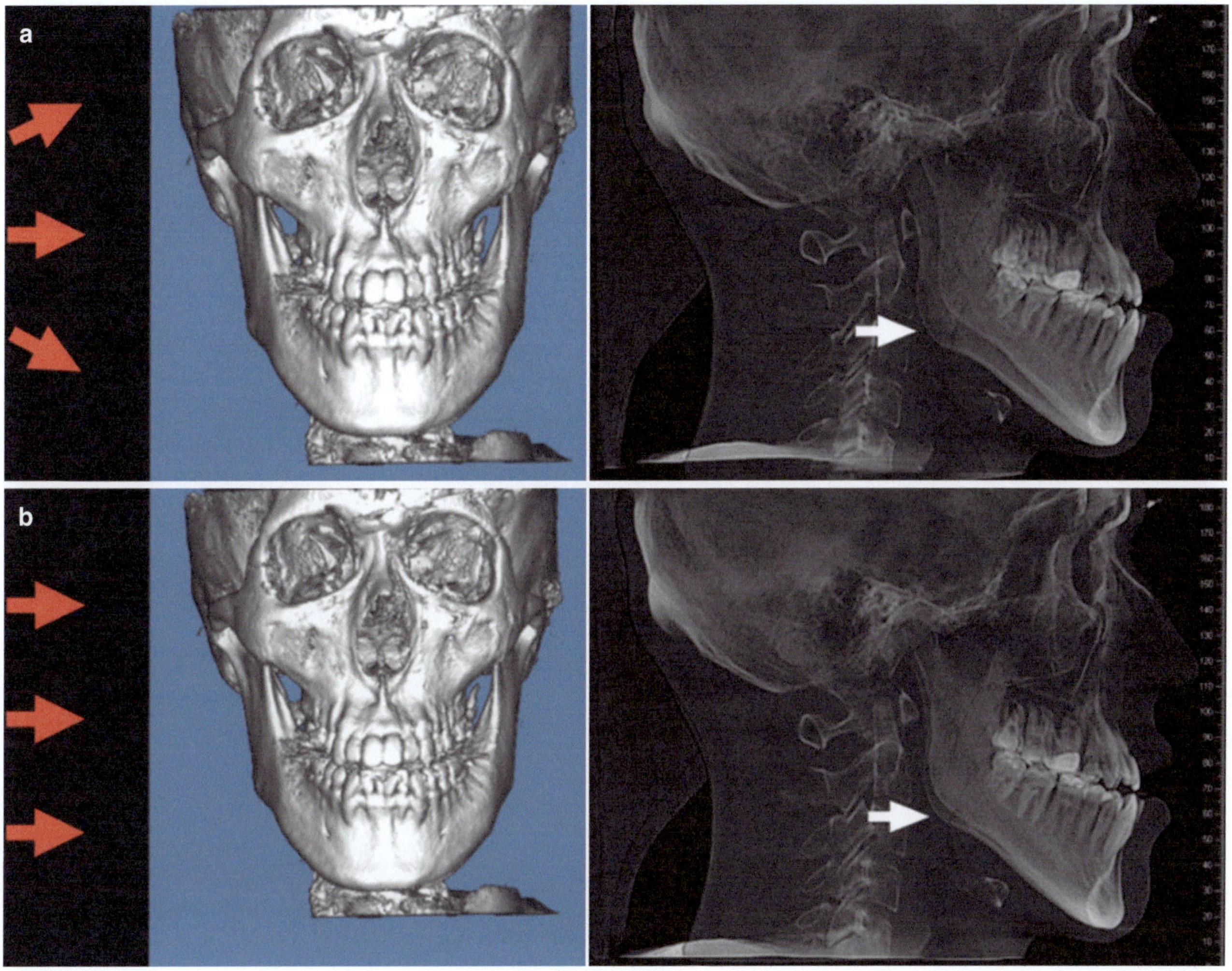

*For perspective view, select the center of the projection, typically through porion

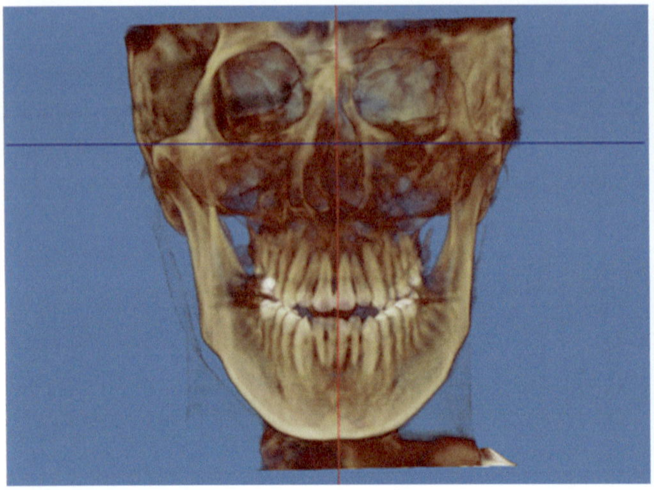

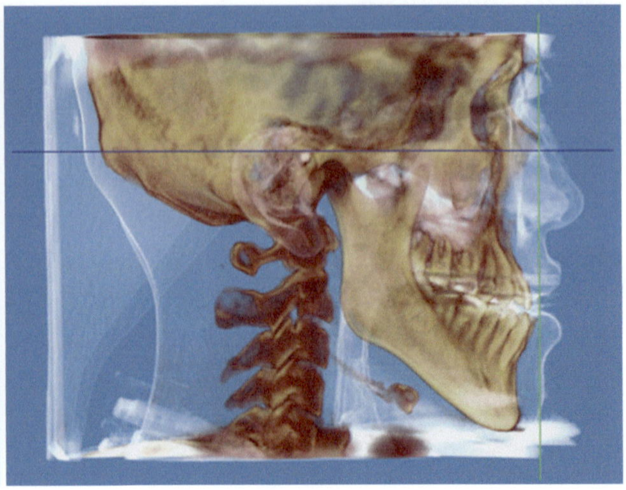

- Select a ruler option
  - Tickmarks or 100 mm bar
    - Tickmarks are preferred
  - Location
    - Left is preferred in this case
  - If the volume is very large, select to add a margin to the x-ray image, and select the size of the border
  - The selection of a ruler will also allow for labelling of the image as to Perspective or Orthogonal as well as the magnification included in the image.
- Through Preferences, the magnification of the orthogonal image can be set, and also the distances from emitter to mid-plane and mid-plane to film for perspective images

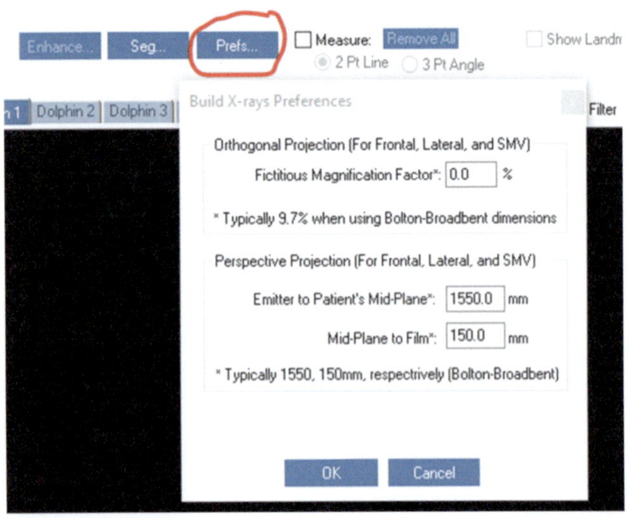

- Click APPLY to create the image. Once the image is generated, each level of the projection should be idealized BEFORE saving the image to the Dolphin Layout.
  - Dolphin 1—Dolphin default level
    - Set the Dolphin 1 level (most lateral projections are best at +2)
    - Adjust the sharpen slider for the best image

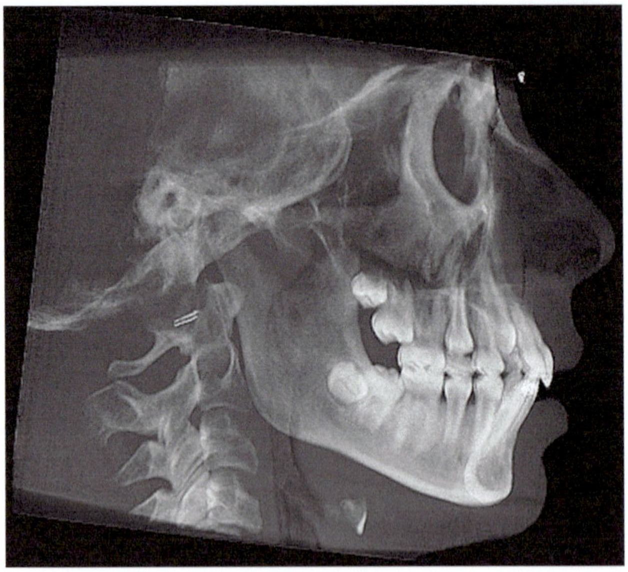

  - Dolphin 2—Soft tissue emphasis
    - Adjust the sharpen slider for the best image

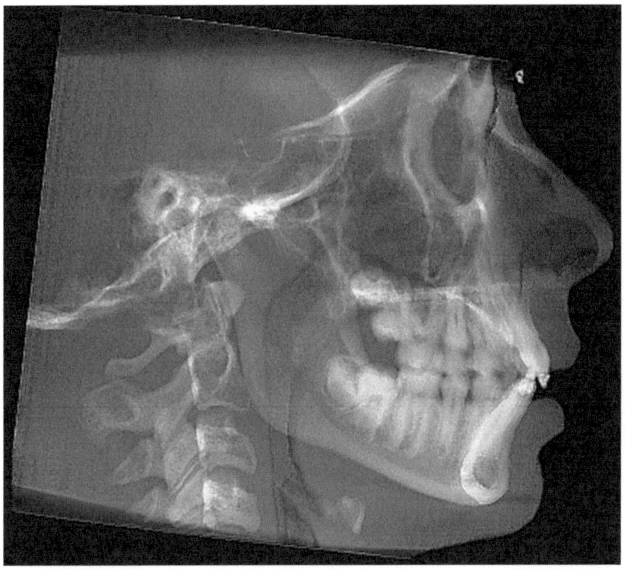

- Dolphin 3—Hard tissue emphasis
  Adjust the sharpen slider for the best image

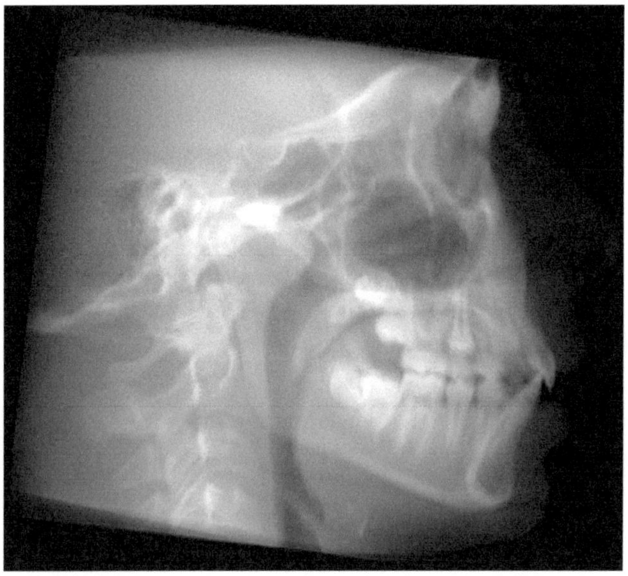

- Emboss—emboss-style image.
  Adjust the sharpen slider for the best image

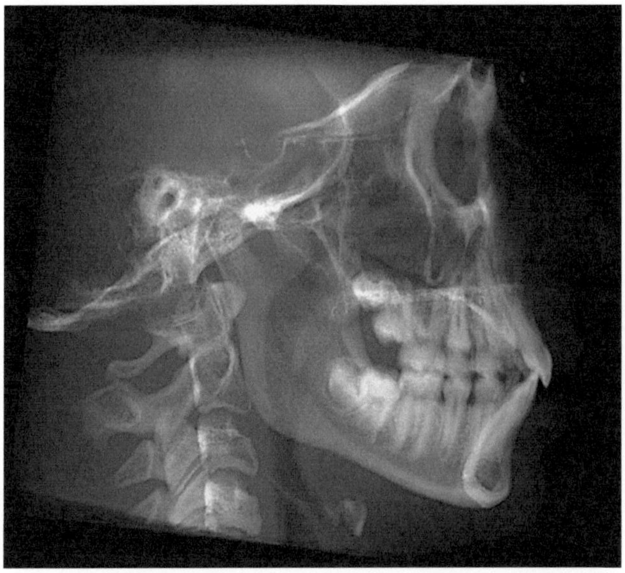

- Ray Sum—Film-based image emulation
  Adjust the sharpen slider for the best image

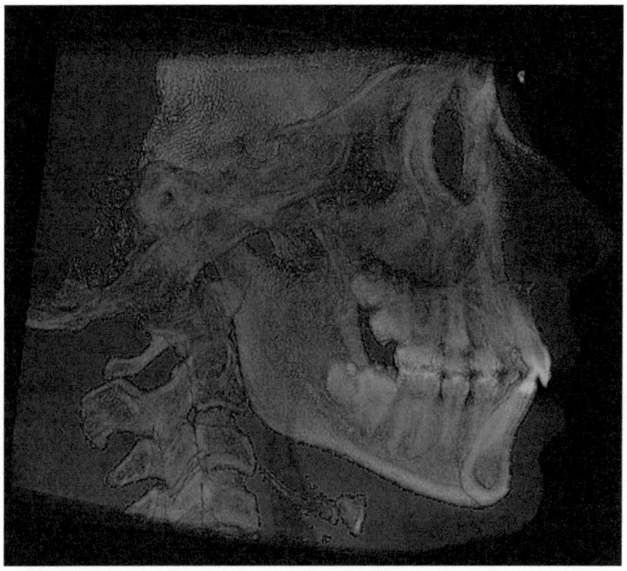

- MIP—Maximum Intensity Projection, surface-focused
  Adjust the sharpen slider for the best image

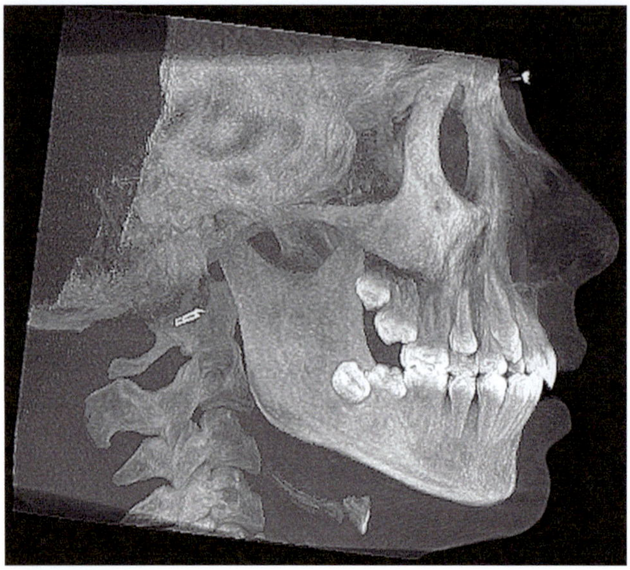

– Traced—Optional tracing-based image
Adjust the sharpen slider for the best image

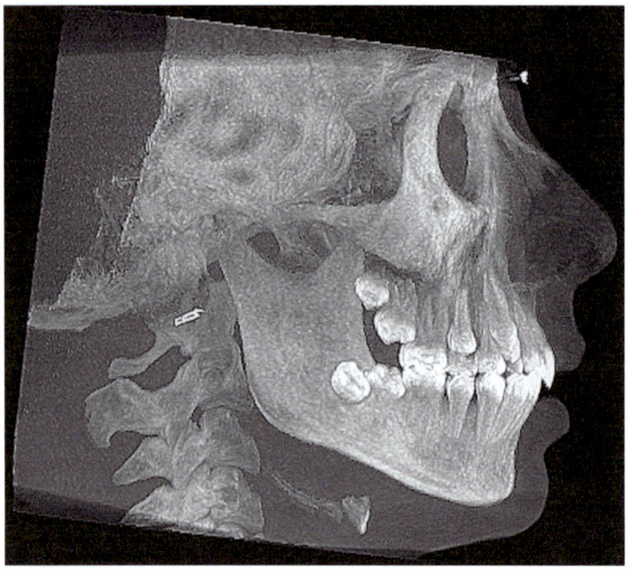

- Brightness and contrast can be adjusted by clicking and dragging vertically or horizontally on any image. When all levels are adjusted, save the image to the Dolphin Layout/Database via the "Send Snapshot" button
- All filters will be available for viewing in Dolphin 2D by clicking the icon in the upper-right corner of each image, to cycle through the various filters.

Appendix 2: Building Radiographs (X-rays) in Dolphin 3D

Panoramic

- Confirm the desired orientation of the volume
- Adjust the field of view for the radiograph

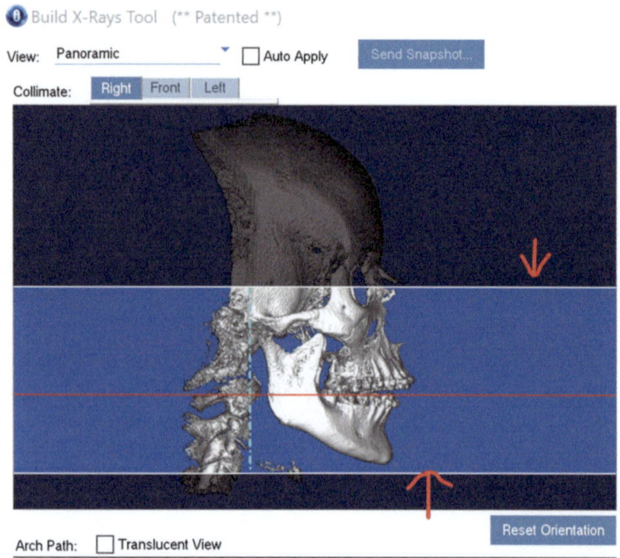

- Place the dotted blue line at the distal aspect of the condyle
- Select the slice location (red line)
  – Typically through the lower anterior incisal tips

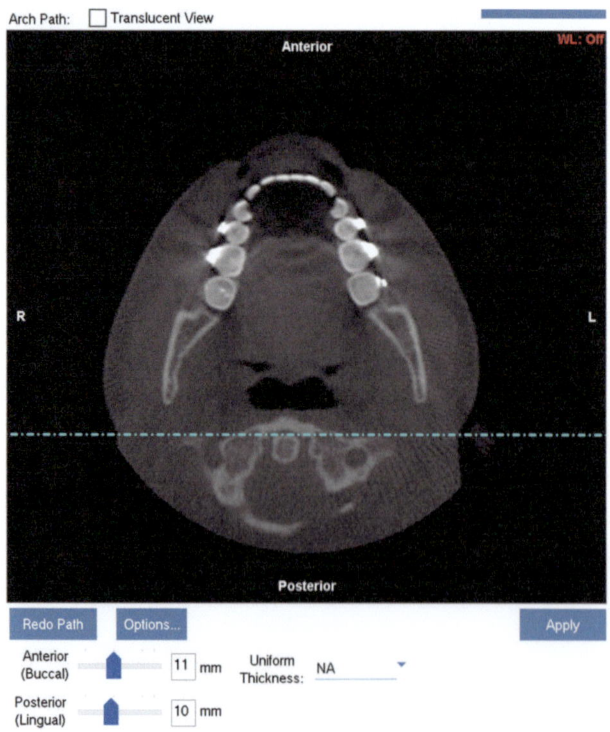

- Define the path for the panoramic radiograph in the slice view
  - Start at the right condyle (near the blue line) and select the next point on the lower first molar, then the canine, several points through the incisors (average the curvature of the teeth if there is crowding), followed by the left canine, left molar, and out to the condyle
  - Double-click to end the path
  - The trough will appear once the path is completed

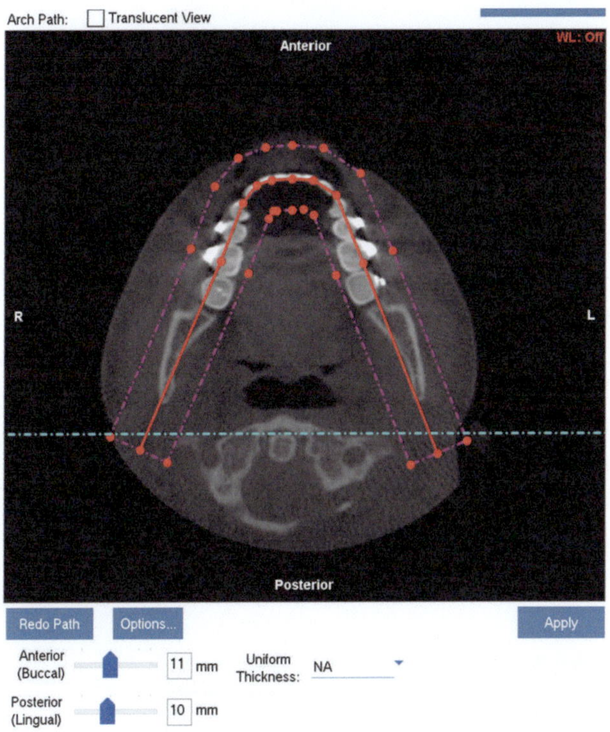

- Confirm that all of the required anatomy is included in the trough
  - If the trough is excluding any anatomy, the resultant panoramic image will have a void

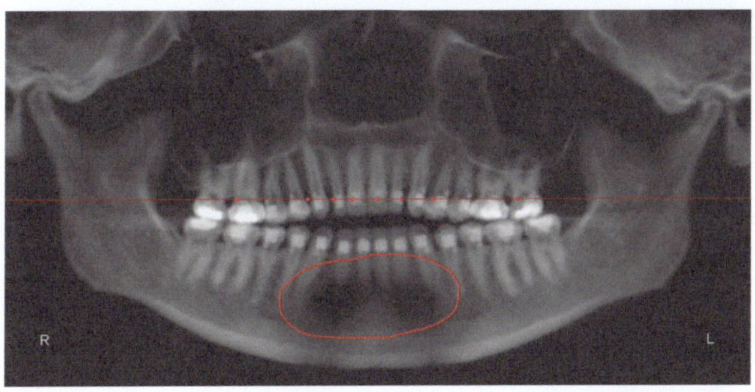

  - Use the "Translucent View" to validate the tough width and anatomy inclusion

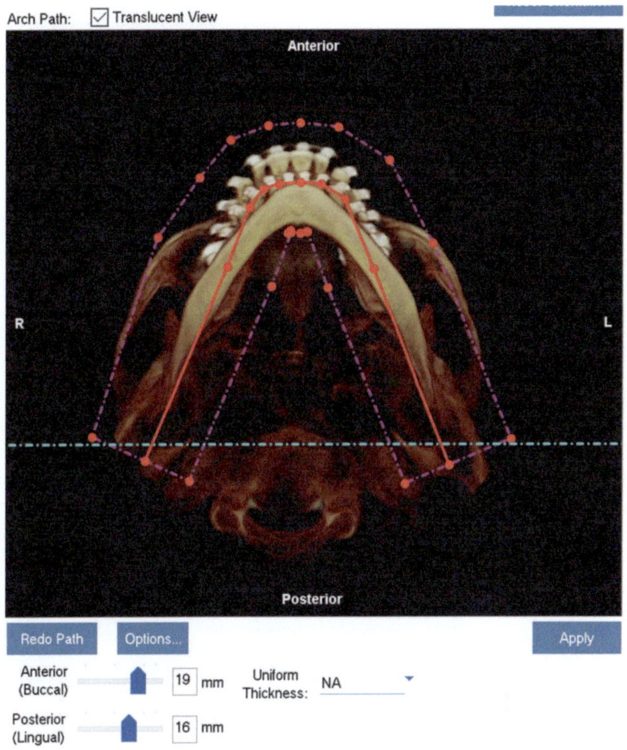

  - Widen the overall trough using the Anterior (Buccal) and Posterior (Lingual) sliders
  - Individual points can be clicked and dragged to adjust a specific area
- Click APPLY to create the image. Once the image is generated, each level of the projection should be idealized BEFORE saving the image to the Dolphin Layout.
  - Dolphin 1—Dolphin default level

    Set the Dolphin 1 level (most panoramic projections are best at +1)

    Adjust the sharpen slider for the best image

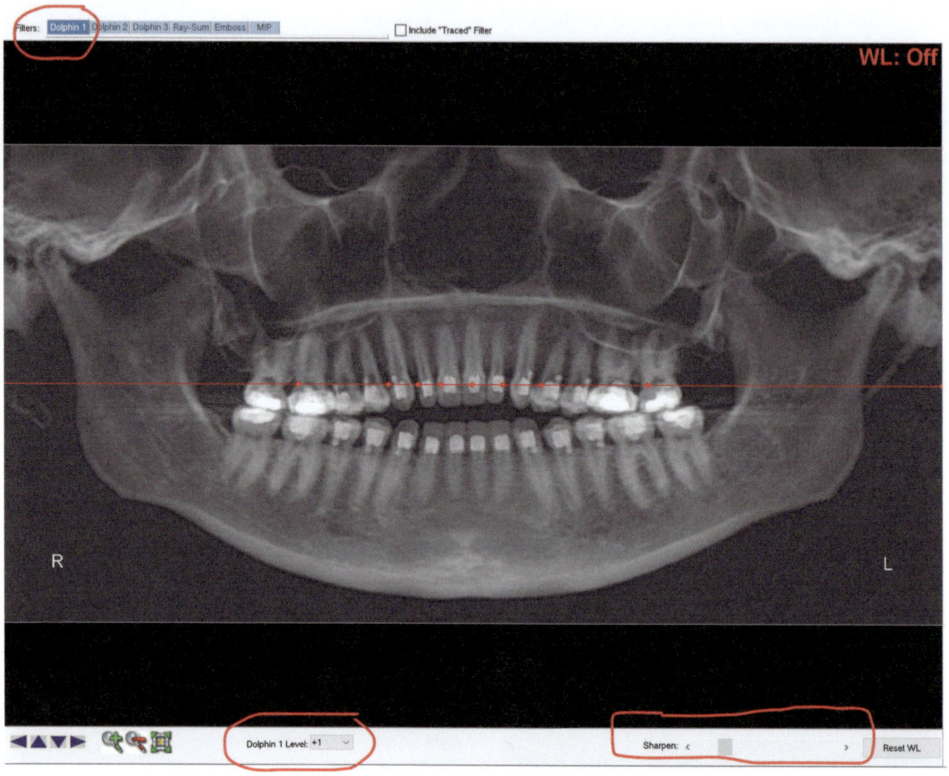

– Dolphin 2—Soft tissue emphasis
  Adjust the sharpen slider for the best image

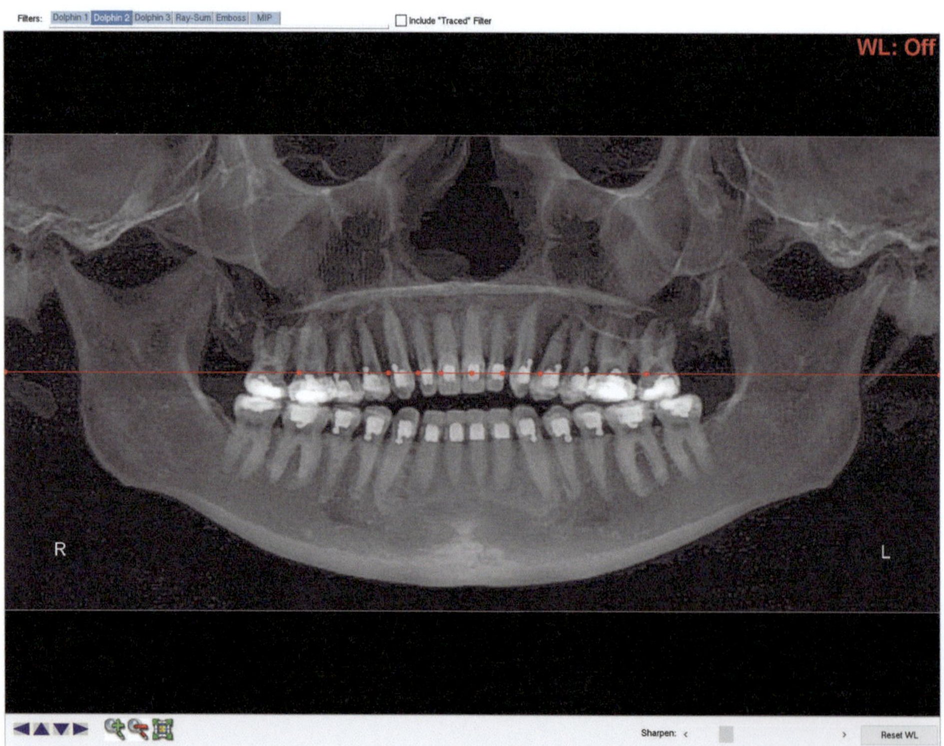

- Dolphin 3—Hard tissue emphasis
  Adjust the sharpen slider for the best image

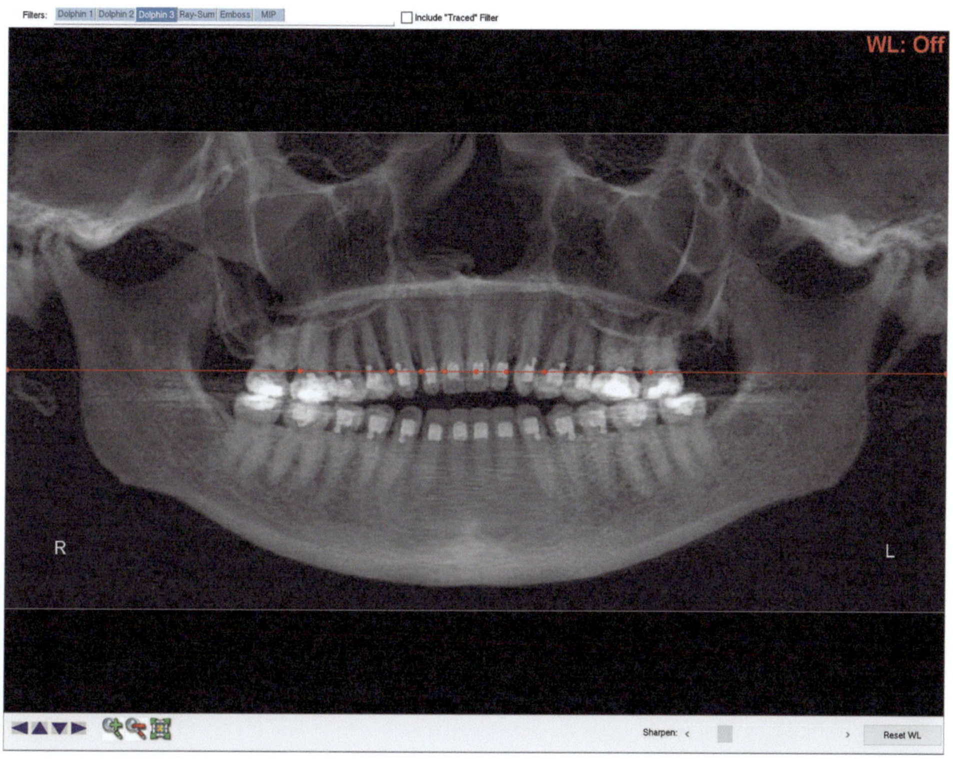

- Ray Sum—Film-based image emulation
  Adjust the sharpen slider for the best image

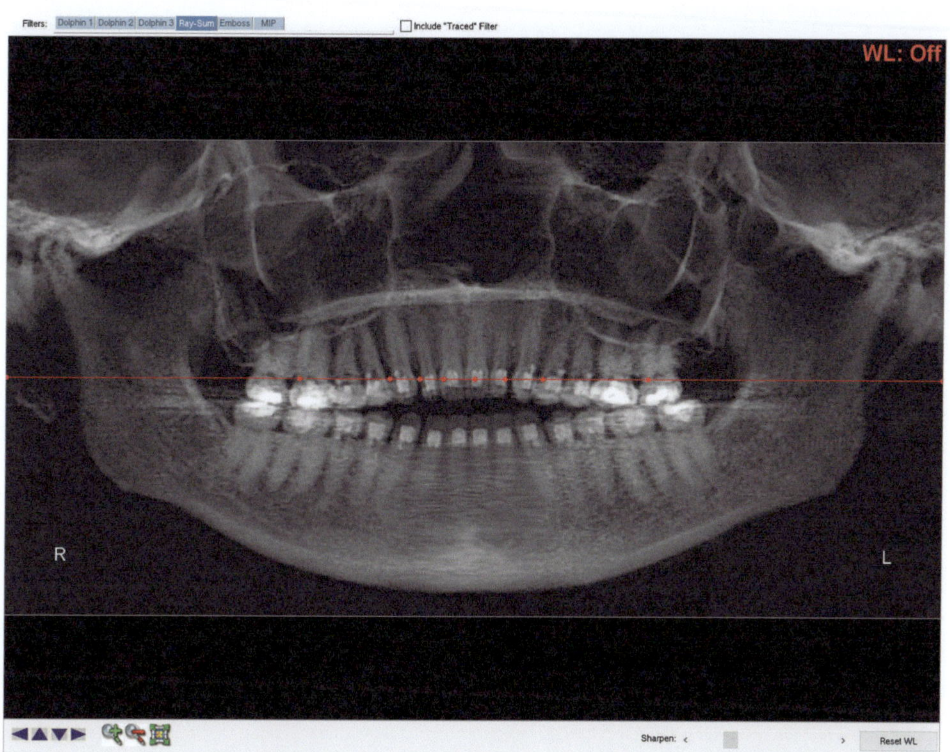

– Emboss—emboss-style image
  Adjust the sharpen slider for the best image

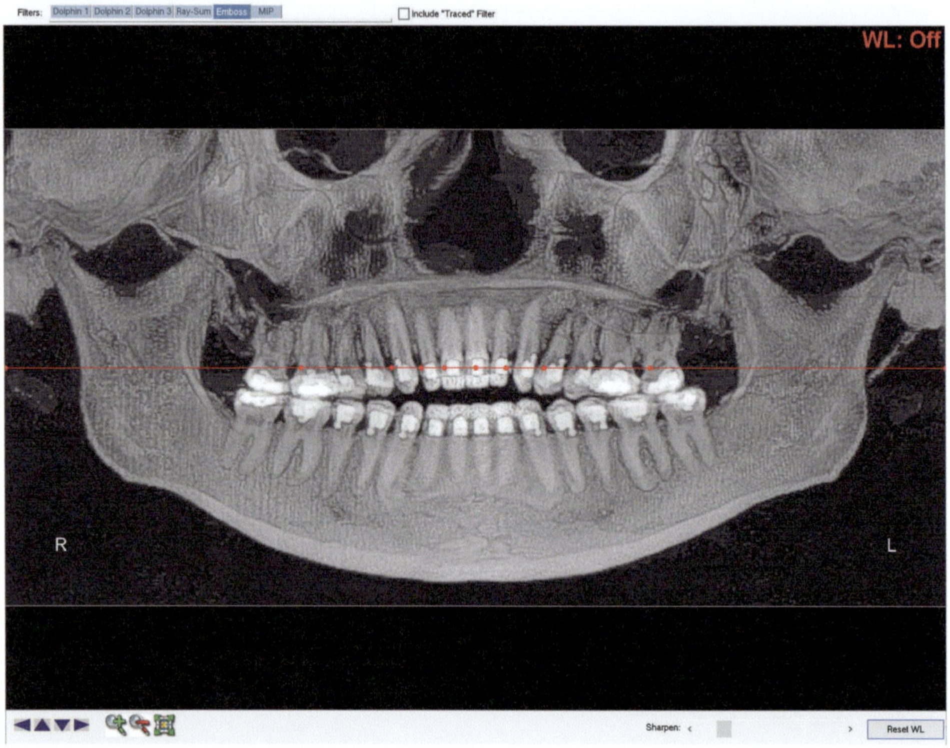

– MIP—Maximum Intensity Projection, surface-focused
  Adjust the sharpen slider for the best image

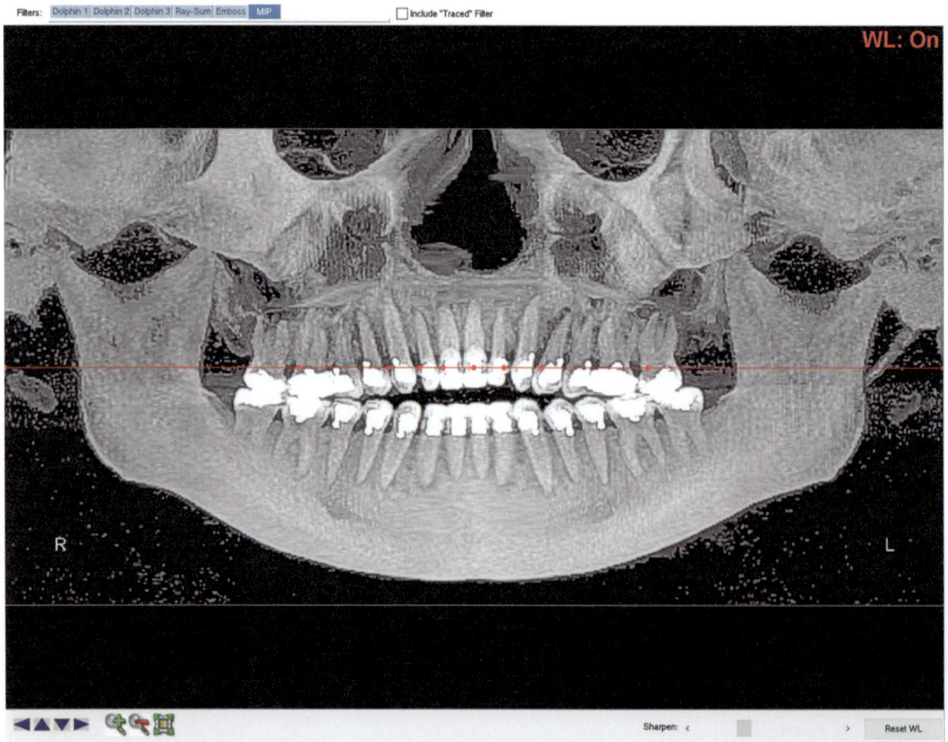

- Traced—Optional tracing-based image
  Adjust the sharpen slider for the best image

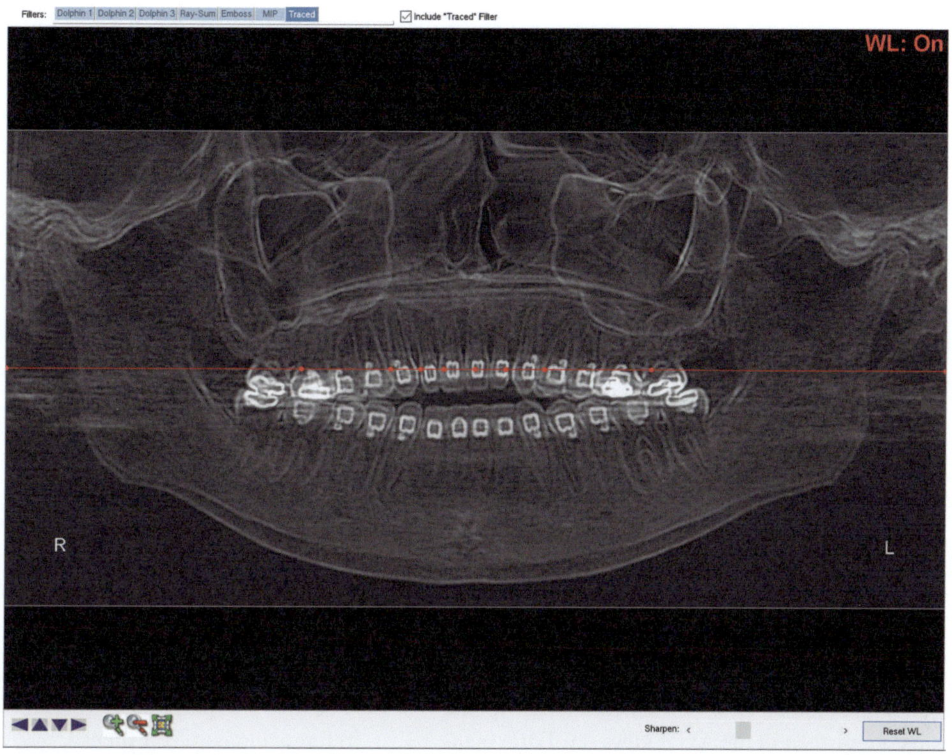

- Brightness and Contrast can be adjusted by clicking and dragging vertically or horizontally on any image. When all levels are adjusted, save the image to the Dolphin Layout/Database via the "Send Snapshot" button
- All filters will be available for viewing in Dolphin 2D by clicking the icon in the upper-right corner of each image, to cycle through the various filters.

Appendix 3: Building Transverse Studies in Dolphin 3D

- Select the "Coronal Slice" view
- Scroll through to the maxillary first permanent molars, and send snapshot to Dolphin 2D

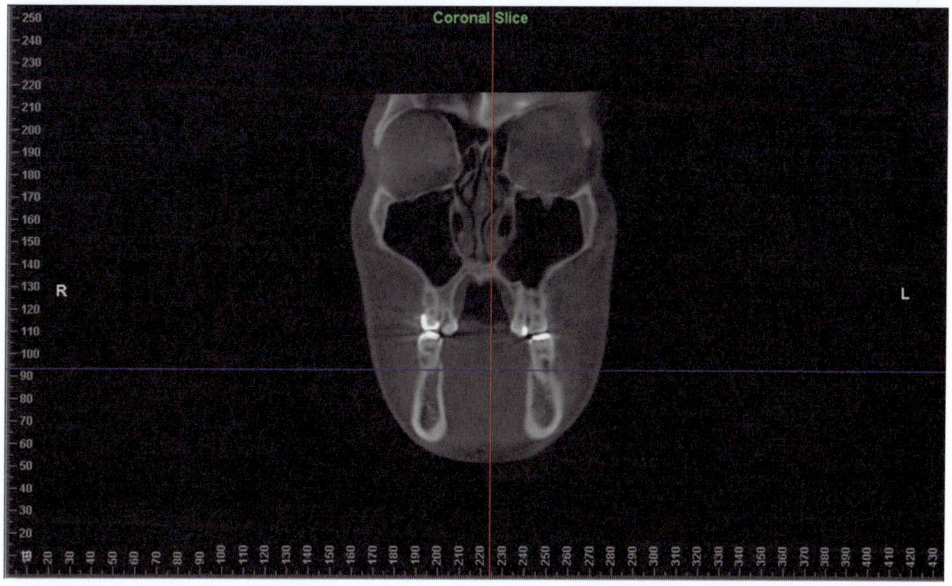

- Select the "Axial Slice" view
- Scroll to the maxillary first permanent molar furca, and send snapshot to Dolphin 2D
  – Use the "4-Equal Slices-Volume View" to allow cross-referencing between slices

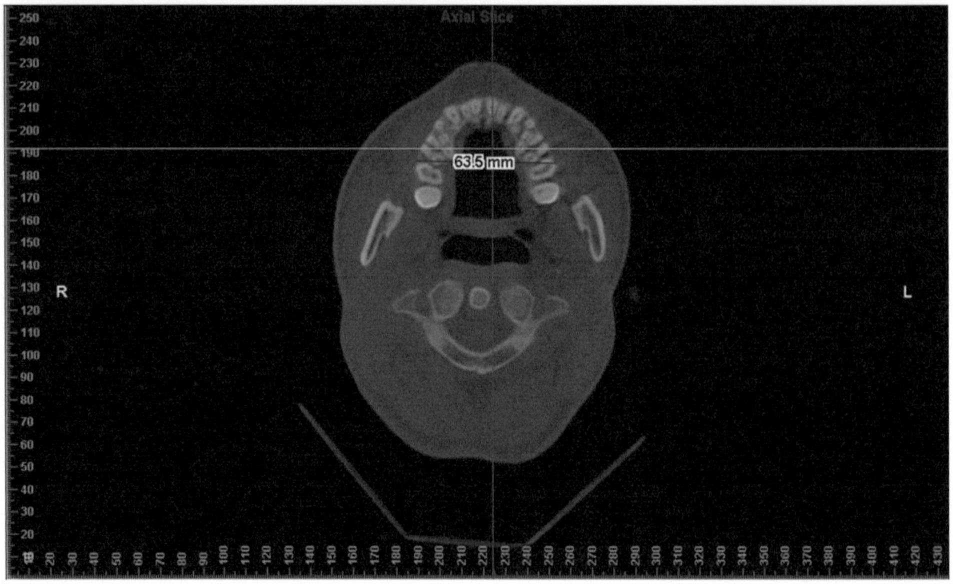

- Scroll to the mandibular first permanent molar in the Coronal slice view, then in the Axial view scroll the mandibular furca, and send snapshot to Dolphin 2D
  – Use the "4-Equal Slices-Volume View" to allow cross-referencing between slices

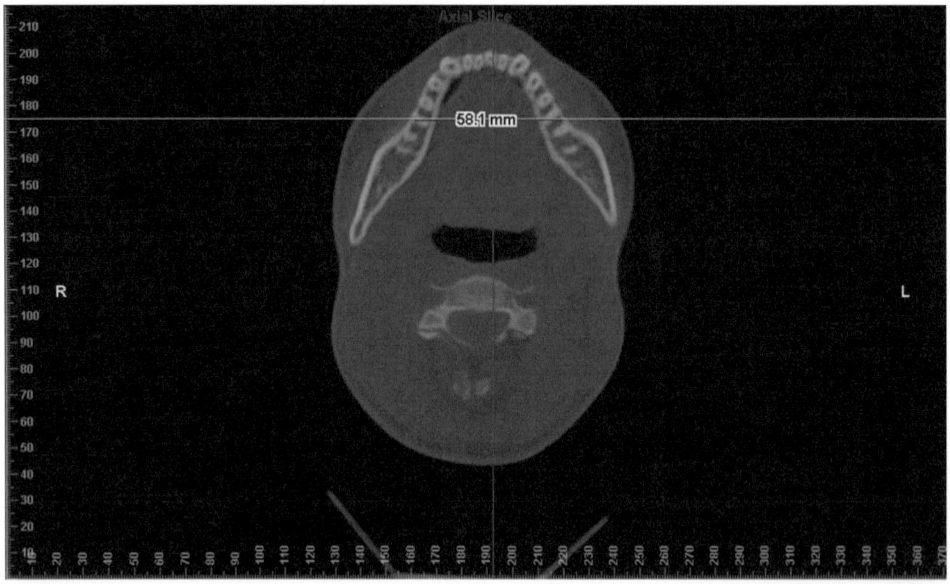

- Close out from Dolphin 3D, and return to the 2D patient screen
- Click on the Mandibular Axial Slice image
- Right click on the image, and select "Annotations and Measurements"
- Calibrate to "DPI" as this image will be accurately calibrated to the CBCT resolution

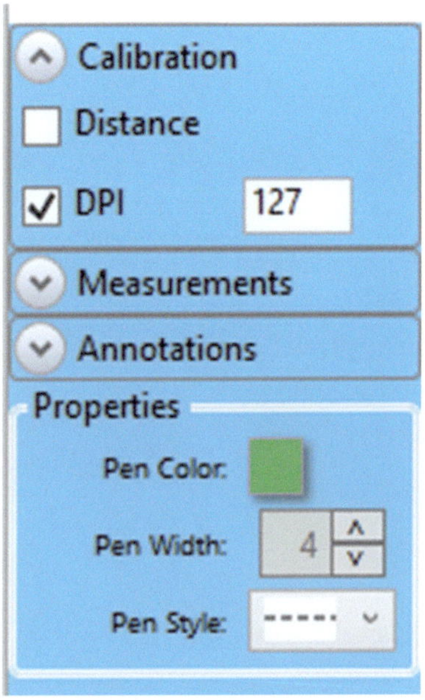

- Click on "Measurements" and select "Distance"
- Measure the mandibular width from the internal ridge on each side, at the furca
- Click on the Maxillary Axial Slice image
- Right click on the image, and select "Annotations and Measurements"
- Calibrate to "DPI" as this image will be accurately calibrated to the CBCT resolution
- Click on "Measurements" and select "Distance"
- Measure the mandibular width from the internal ridge on each side, at the furca
- NOTE: Proper placement of the plane lines will ensure accurate and repeatable measurements

Appendix 4: Building Radiographs (X-rays) in Dolphin 3D

TMJ

- Confirm the desired orientation of the volume
- Adjust the field of view for the radiograph

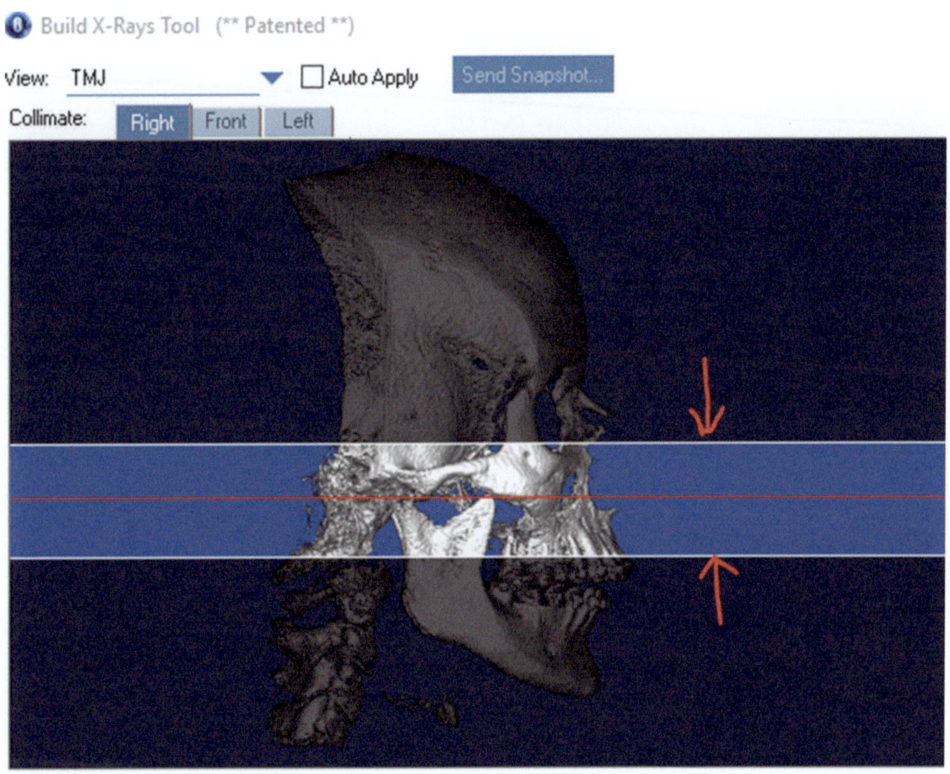

- Set the slice location (red line)
  - Typically through the lateral poles of the condyle
  - Head position may need to be adjusted so that both condyles sit equally on the horizontal plane of the slice line
    - Confirm by view from the right and also the left view
- Using the Coronal direction, set the box over each condyle, centering the condyle within the cut box
- Rotate the box using the upper red dot (toggle) to approximate the long axis of the condyle through the length of the cut box

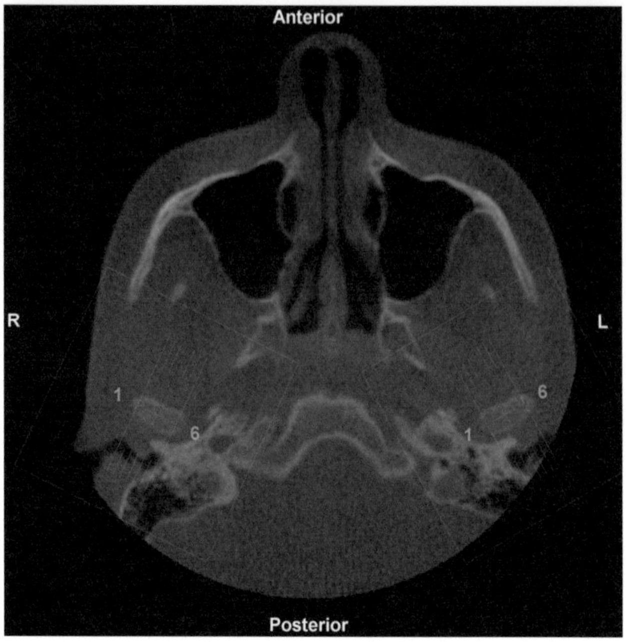

- Click APPLY to create the image. Once the image is generated, each level of the projection should be idealized BEFORE saving the image to the Dolphin Layout. NOTE that the Dolphin levels apply only to the upper orientation image, and not to the slice view. The slice view has a dedicated Sharpen slider to clarify the images

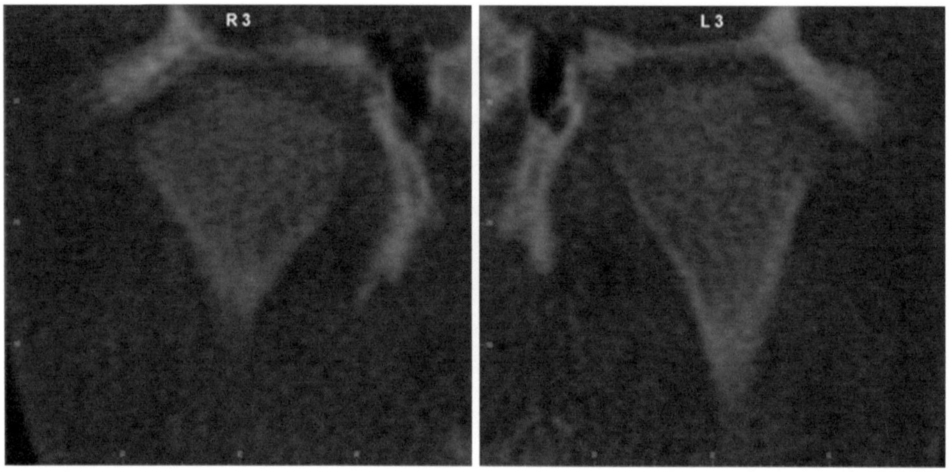

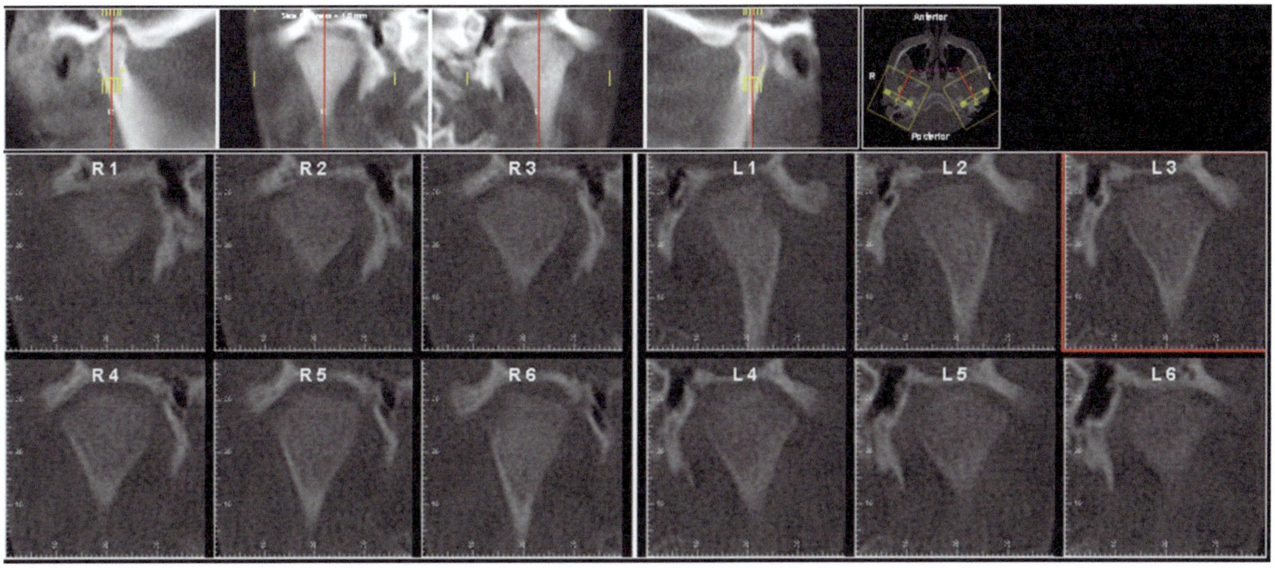

- Select the number of cuts, the thickness, and width of the cuts

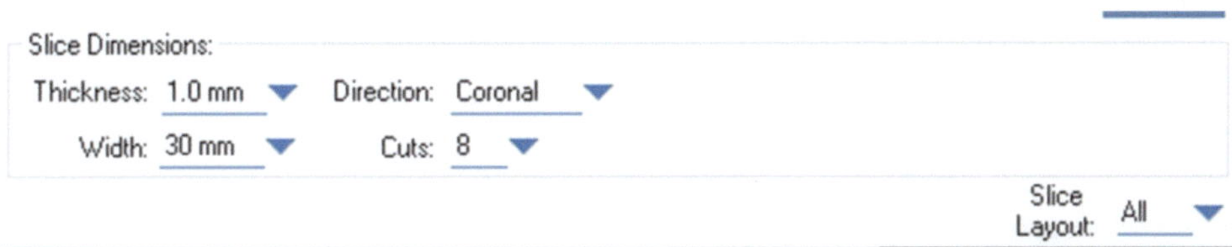

- Brightness and Contrast can be adjusted by clicking and dragging vertically or horizontally on any image. When all levels are adjusted, save the image to the Dolphin Layout/Database via the "Send Snapshot" button.
- To create the sagittal view, change the direction to "Sagittal" and click APPLY to create the image. Once the image is generated, each level of the projection should be idealized BEFORE saving the image to the Dolphin Layout. NOTE that the Dolphin levels apply only to the upper orientation image, and not to the slice view. The slice view has a dedicated Sharpen slider to clarify the images.
  - Adjust the number of cuts, the thickness, and the width of the cuts.
  - Center the cuts to create the desired images.

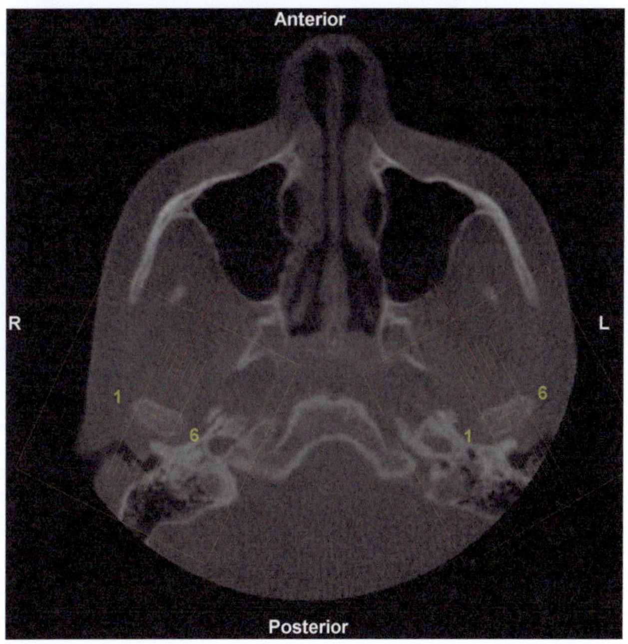

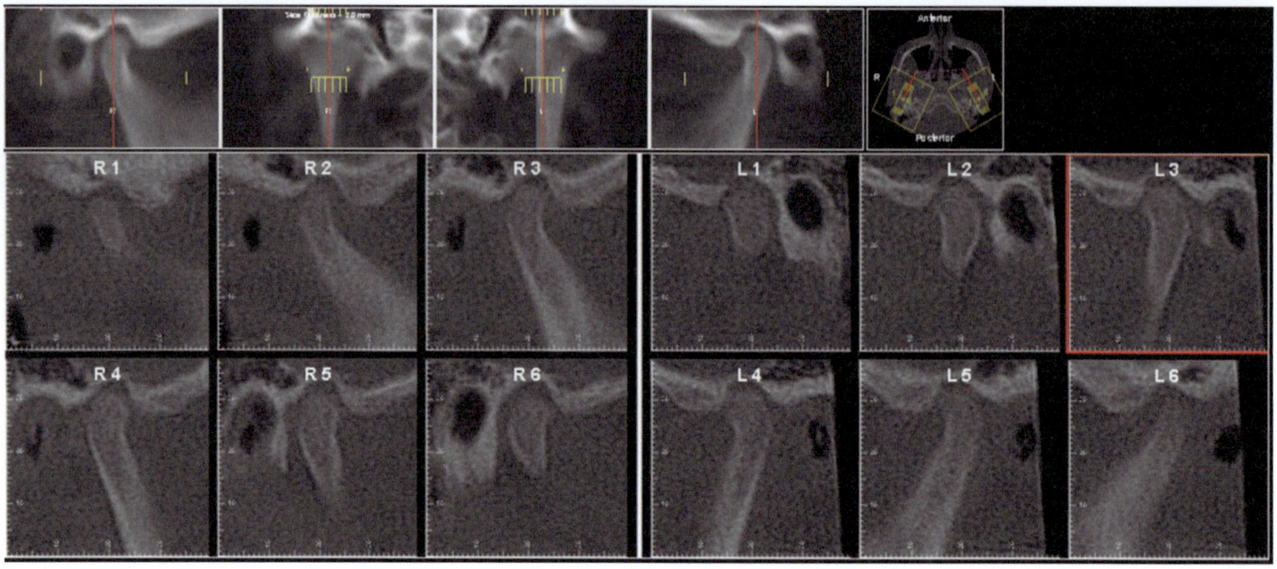

- Brightness and Contrast can be adjusted by clicking and dragging vertically or horizontally on any image. When all levels are adjusted, save the image to the Dolphin Layout/Database via the "Send Snapshot" button.
- To view slices in a side-by-side comparison, double click on any of the slice views to bring up the side-by-side view.
- Use the mouse wheel to scroll through the slices.
  - NOTE: make sure to note the slice number at the top of the image.
  - Refer to the upper guide image to reference the slices that are in view.

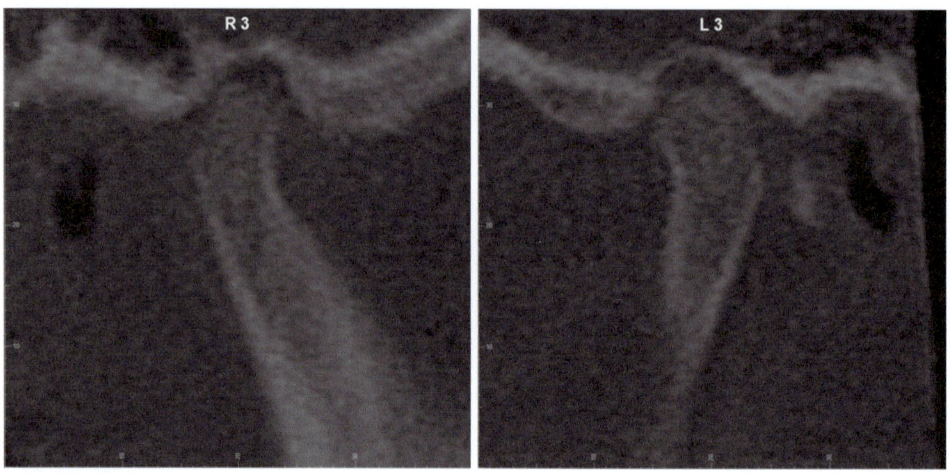

Appendix 5: Building Airway Studies in Dolphin 3D

Sinus/Airway

Pharyngeal Boundaries According to Zimmerman [47]

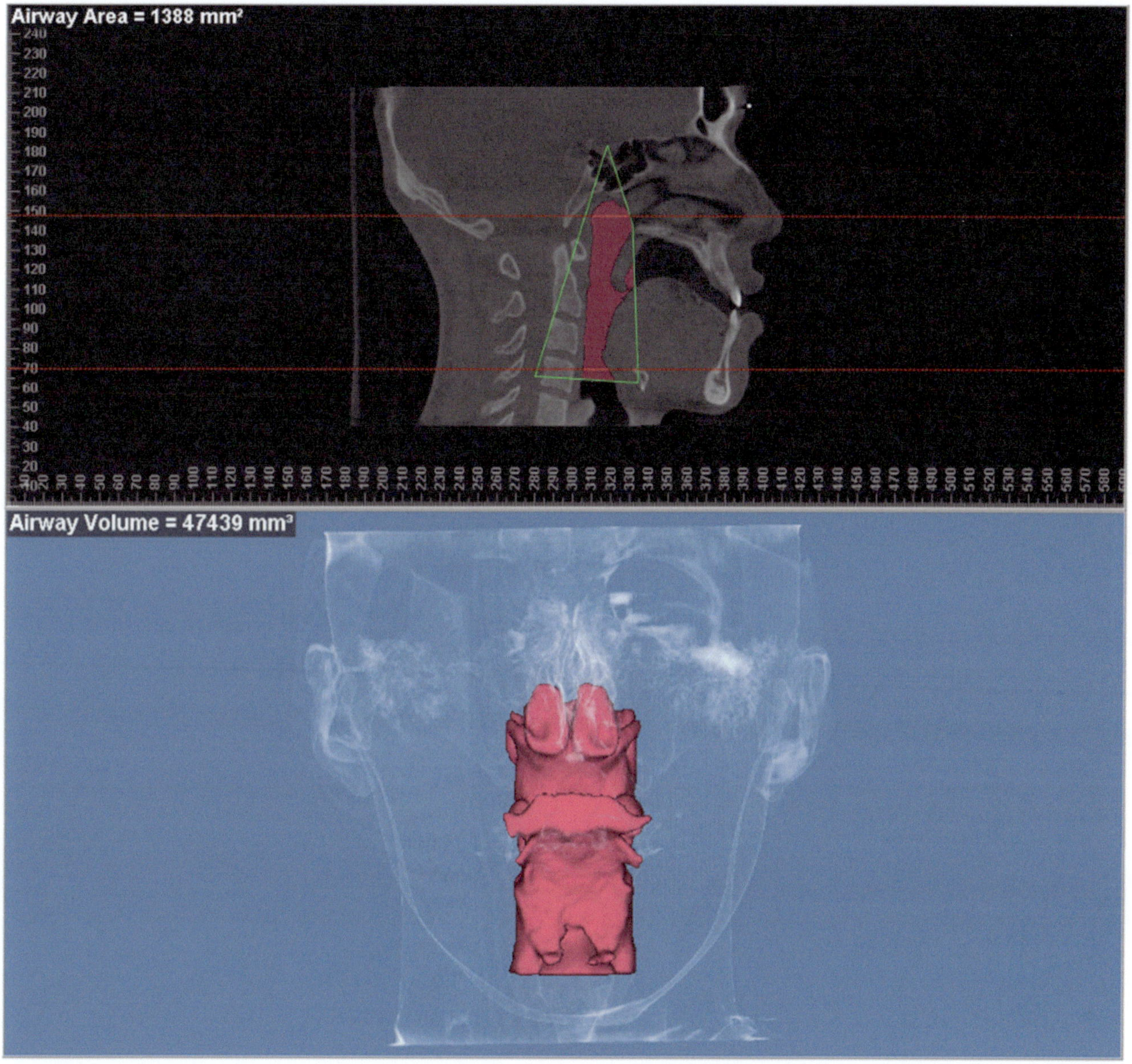

- Select the boundaries of the area to be measured on the Draft side
  - If studying upper airway or sinus, boundaries may need to be set in each of the slice views (Sagittal, Coronal, and Axial)
- Place a Seed Point in the airway area
  - Depending on the study being completed, more than 1 airway Seed Point may be required
  - Adjust the airway sensitivity, using the Quick or HU method

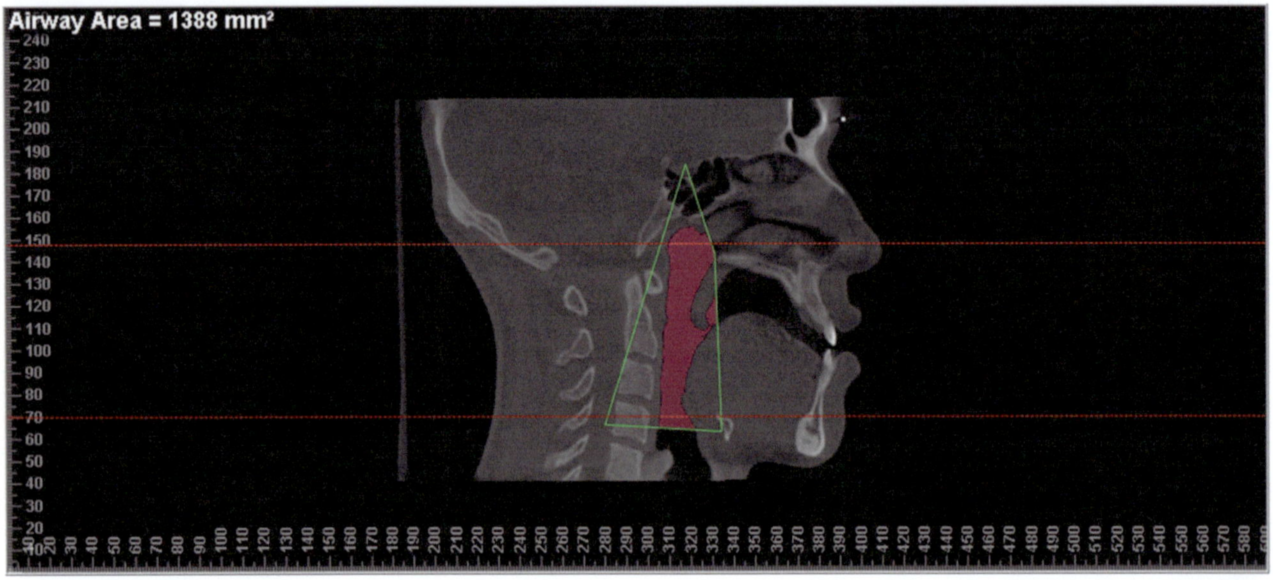

- Click Update Airway to create the airway image
  - Slice view
    - All three slices can be displayed individually
  - Volume view
    - View the airway as a Surface or a Solid
    - Select the desired color for the airway
    - Soft Tissue and Hard Tissue can be added to the volume view

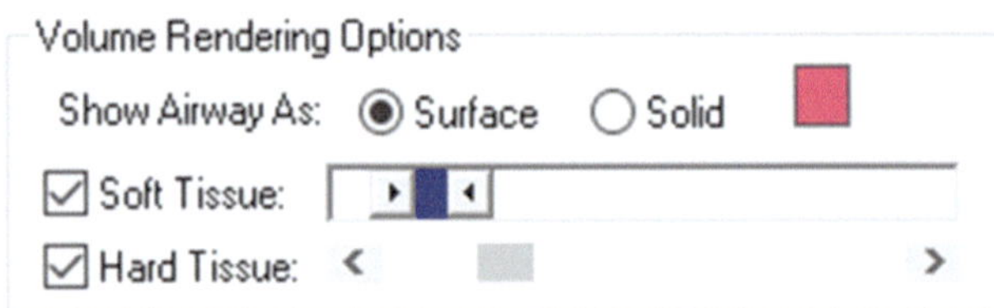

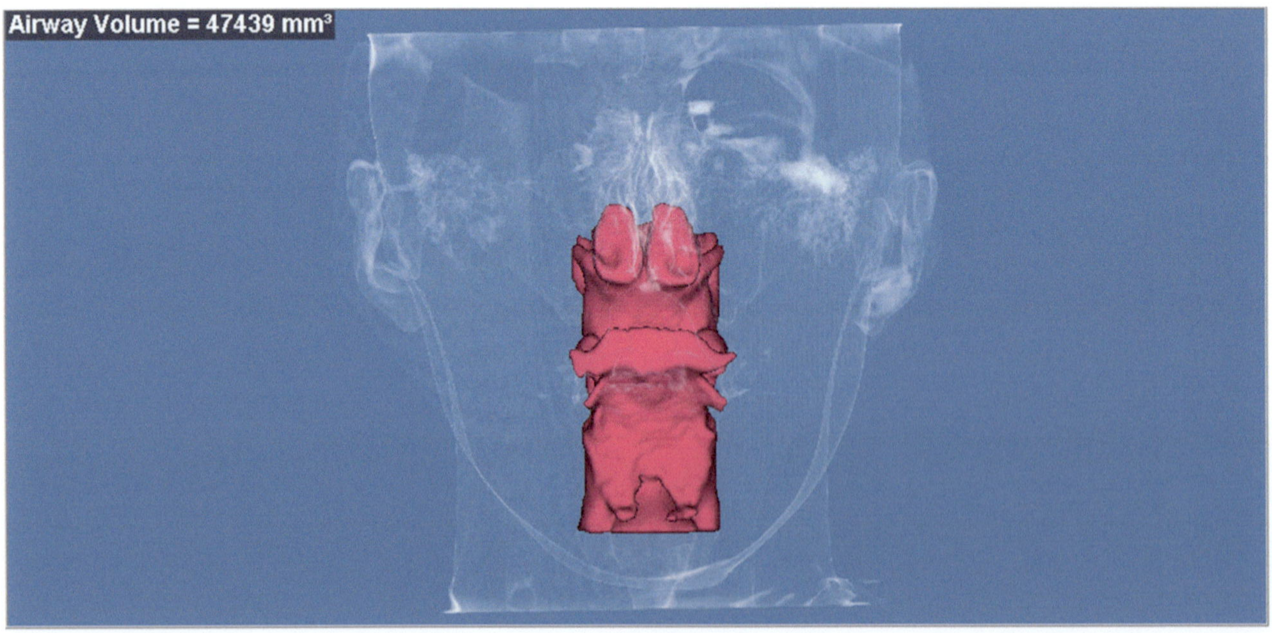

- Select the tick box to determine the "Minimum Axial Area"
- Click and drag the red lines to the upper and lower limit of the area that will be used to determine the minimum axial area
- Click FIND to calculate the minimum axial area in both the slice and volume view

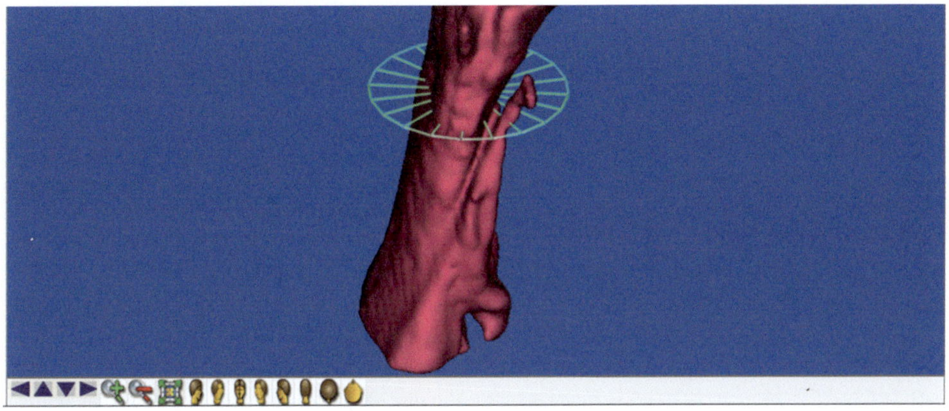

- Click SAVE to save the workup in an available slot

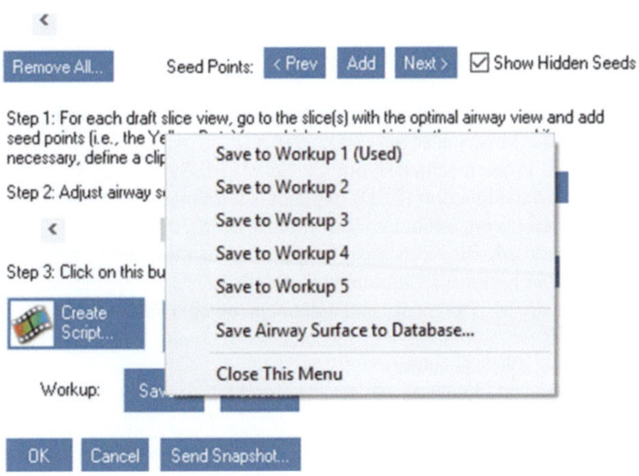

- Workups can be saved and restored as needed

Upper Constricted Airway (with Colormap)

- Define the airway to be studied with a series of clicks
  - Click twice to end the airway
  - Adjust the airway sensitivity, using the Quick or HU method
- Click Update Airway to create the airway image, and determine the minimum axial area
  - Slice view

    All three slices can be displayed individually
  - Volume view

    Airway is displayed as a colormap as per the volume of the airway at any particular point
- Soft Tissue and Hard Tissue can be added to the volume view
- NOTE: The Sinus/Airway method samples the airway constriction horizontally across the screen while the Upper Constricted Airway method samples the airway constriction perpendicular to the airway path as defined by the user.
- Click SAVE to save the workup in an available slot

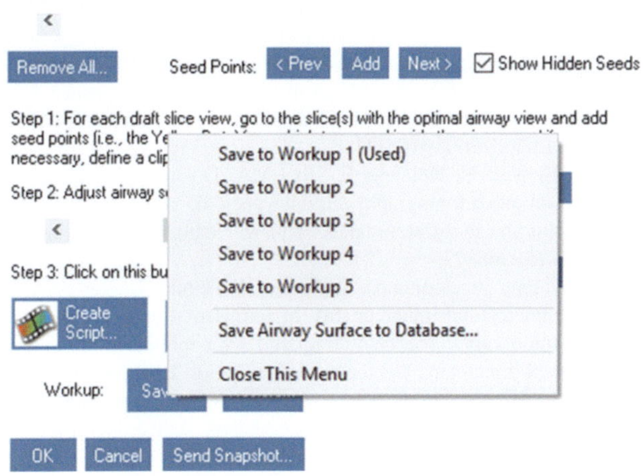

- Workups can be saved and restored as needed
- Airway volume is indicated at the top of the "Result Half" screen
- Left and right side of the airway can be studied individually (as separate studies) for comparison
- Click SAVE to save the workup in an available slot

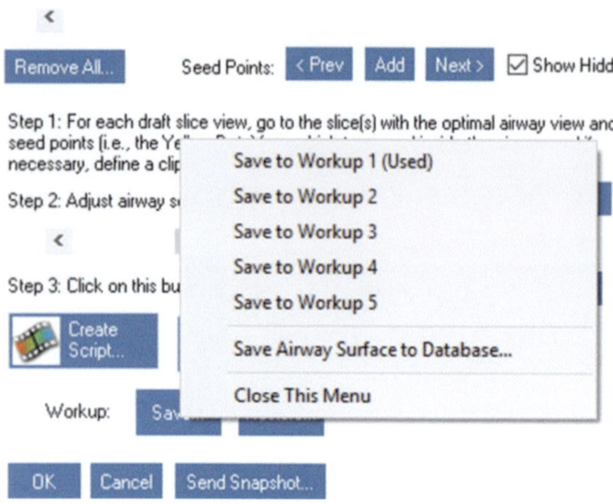

- Workups can be saved and restored as needed

References

1. The American Academy of Oral and Maxillofacial Radiology. Clinical recommendations regarding use of cone beam computed tomography in orthodontics. Position statement by the American Academy of Oral and Maxillofacial Radiology. Oral Surg Oral Med Oral Pathol Oral Radiol. 2013;116(2):238–57.
2. Mupparapdu M, Creanga AG, Singer SR. Interpretation of cone beam computed tomography volumetric data: how to report findings? Quintessence Int. 2017;48(9):733–41.
3. Abramovitch K, Rice DD. Basic principles of cone beam computed tomography. Dent Clin N Am. 2014;58(3):463–84.
4. Miracle AC, Mukherji SK. Conebeam CT of the head and neck, part 1: physical principles. AJNR Am J Neuroradiol. 2009;30(6):1088–95.
5. Ludlow JB, Ivanavic M. Comparative dosimetry of dental CBCT devices and 64-slice CT for oral and maxillofacial radiology. Oral Surg Oral Med Oral Pathol Oral Radiol Endod. 2008;106(1):106–14.
6. Palomo JM, Rao PS, Hans MG. Influence of CBCT exposure conditions on radiation dose. Oral Surg Oral Med Oral Pathol Oral Radiol Endod. 2008;105:773–82.
7. Hirsh E, Wolf U, Heinicke F, Silva MA. Dosimetry of the cone beam computed tomography veraviewpocs 3D compared with the 3D accuitomo in different fields of view. Dentomaxillofac Radiol. 2008;37(5):268–73.
8. Suomalainen A, Kiljuinen T, Käser Y, Peltola J, Kortesniemi M. Dosimetry and image quality of four dental cone beam computed tomography scanners compared with multislice computed tomography scanners. Dentomaxillofac Radiol. 2009;38:367–78.
9. Miracle AC, Mukherji SK. Conebeam CT of the head and neck, part 2: clinical applications. AJNR Am J Neuroradiol. 2009;30(7):1285–92.
10. Matsumoto K, Sherrill-Mix S, Boucher N, Tanna N. A cone-beam computed tomographic evaluation of alveolar bone dimensional changes and the periodontal limits of mandibular incisor advancement in skeletal Class II patients. (Accepted for publication in the Angle Orthodontist in Dec 2019).
11. Andrews LF. The six elements of orofacial harmony. Andrews J. 2000;1:13–22.
12. Hoang N, Nelson G, Hatcher D, Oberoi S. Evaluation of mandibular anterior alveolus in different skeletal patterns. Prog Orthod. 2016;17:22.
13. Tamburrino RK, Boucher NS, Vanarsdall RL, Secchi A. The transverse dimension: diagnosis and relevance to functional occlusion. RWISO J. 2010:13–21.
14. Bjork A. Prediction of mandibular growth rotation. Am J Orthod. 1969;55(6):585–99.
15. Hatcher DC, Faulkner MG, Hay A. Development of mechanical and mathematic models to study temporomandibular joint loading. J Prosthet Dent. 1986;55(3):377–84.
16. McEvoy SP. Effects of facial morphology or TMJ loading (thesis). Edmonton: Univ. of Alberta; 1989.
17. Nebbe B, Major PW. Prevalence of TMJ disc displacement in a pre-orthodontic adolescent sample. Angle Orthod. 2000;70(6): 454–63.
18. Flores-Mir C, Nebbe B, Heo G, Major PW. Longitudinal study of temporomandibular joint disc status and craniofacial growth. Am J Orthod Dentofac Orthop. 2006;130(3):324–30.
19. Hatcher DC. Progressive condylar resorption: pathologic processes and imaging considerations. Semin Orthod. 2013;19(2):97–105.
20. Legrell PE, Isberg A. Mandibular length and midline asymmetry after experimentally induced temporomandibular joint disc displacement in rabbits. Am J Orthod Dentofac Orthop. 1999;115(3):247–53.
21. Bryndahl F, Eriksson L, Legrell PE, Isberg A. Bilateral TMJ disc displacement induces mandibular retrognathia. J Dent Res. 2006;85(12):1118–23.
22. Bryndahl F, Warfvinge G, Eriksson L, Isberg A. Cartilage changes link retrognathic mandibular growth to TMJ disc displacement in a rabbit model. Oral Maxillofac Surg. 2011;40(6):621–7.
23. Ikeda K, Kawamura A. Assessment of optimal condylar position with limited cone-beam computed tomography. Am J Orthod Dentofac Orthop. 2009;135(4):495–501.
24. Okeson JP. Management of temporomandibular disorders and occlusion. 8th ed. St. Louis: Elsevier; 2020. 512 p.
25. Dawson P. Functional occlusion, 1st ed. From TMJ to smile design. St. Louis: Mosby Elsevier; 2006. 648 p.
26. Fink M, Tschernitschek H, Stiesch-Scholz M. Asymptomatic cervical spine dysfunction (CSD) in patients with internal derangement of the temporomandibular joint. Cranio. 2002;20(3):192–7.
27. Rocabado M. Biomechanical relationship of the cranial, cervical, and hyoid regions. J Craniomandibular Pract. 1983;1(3):61–6.
28. Rocabado M. Diagnosis and treatment of abnormal craniocervical and craniomandibular mechanics. Tacoma, WA: Rocabado Institute; 1981. (Lecture).
29. Rocabado M, Johnston BE Jr, Blakney MG. Physical therapy and dentistry: an overview. J Craniomandibular Pract. 1982;1(1):46–9.
30. Wright EF, Domenech MA, Fischer JR Jr. Usefulness of posture training for patients with temporomandibular disorders. J Am Dent Assoc. 2000;131(2):202–10.
31. Behrents RG, Shelgikar AV, Conley RS, Flores-Mir C, Hans M, Levine M, et al. Obstructive sleep apnea and orthodontics: an American Association of Orthodontists white paper (Amended 3-15-19). Am J Ortho Dentofac Orthop. 2019;156(1):13–28.e1.
32. de Berry-Borowiecki B, Kukwa A, Blanks RH. Cephalometric analysis for diagnosis and treatment of obstructive sleep apnea. Laryngoscope. 1988;98(2):226–34.
33. Enciso R, Nguyen M, Shigeta Y, Ogawa T, Clark GT. Comparison of cone-beam CT parameters and sleep questionnaires in sleep apnea patients and control subjects. Oral Surg Oral Med Oral Pathol Oral Radiol Endod. 2010;109(2):285–93.
34. Finkelstein Y, Wexler D, Horowitz E, Berger G, Nachmani A, Shapiro-Feinberg M, et al. Frontal and lateral cephalometry in patients with sleep disturbed breathing. Laryngoscope. 2001;11(4 Part 1):634–41.
35. Jamieson A, Guilleminault C, Partinen M, Quera-Salva MA. Obstructive sleep apneic patients have craniomandibular abnormalities. Sleep. 1986;9(4):469–77.

36. Partinen M, Guilleminault C, Quera-Salva MA, Jamieson A. Obstructive sleep apnea and cephalometric roentgenograms. The role of anatomic upper airway abnormalities in the definition of abnormal breathing during sleep. Chest. 1988;93(6):1199–205.
37. Pittayapat P, Bornstein MM, Nozu Imada TS, Coucke W, Lambrichts I, et al. Accuracy of linear measurements using three imaging modalities: two lateral cephalograms and one 3D model from CBCT data. Eur J Orthod. 2015;37(2):202–8.
38. Poirier AL, Pire S, Raskin S, Limme M, Poirrier R. Contributions of posterior-anterior cephalometry in obstructive sleep apnea. Laryngoscope. 2012;122(10):2350–4.
39. Riley R, Guilleminault C, Herran J, Powell N. Cephalometric analysis and flow volume loops in obstructive sleep apnea patients. Sleep. 1983;6(4):303–11.
40. Ono T, Otsuka R, Kuroda T, Honda E, Sasaki T. Effects of head and body position on two- and three-dimensional configurations of the upper airway. J Dent R. 2000;79(11):1978–84.
41. Gurani SF, Di Carlo G, Cattaneo PM, Thorn JJ, Pinholt EM. Effect of head and tongue posture on the pharyngeal airway dimensions and morphology in three-dimensional imaging: a systematic review. J Oral Maxillofac Res. 2016;7(1):e1.
42. Weissheimer A, Menezes LM, Sameshima GT, Enciso R, Pham J, Grauer D. Imaging software accuracy for 3-dimensional analysis of the upper airway. Am J Orthod Dentofac Orthop. 2012;142(6):801–13.
43. Alvis M, Baratieri C, Mattos CT, Brunetto D, Fontes Rda C, Santos JR, et al. Is the airway volume being correctly analysed? Am J Orthod Dentofac Orthop. 2012;141(5):657–61.
44. Brunetto DP. Prediction of 3-dimensional airway changes after orthognathic surgery: a preliminary study. Am J Orthod Dentofac Orthop. 2014;146(3):299–309.
45. Pauwels R, Jacobs R, Singer SR, Mupparapu M. CBCT-based bone quality assessment: are Hounsfield units applicable? Dentomaxillofac Radiol. 2015;44:20140238.
46. Pauwels RL, Araki K, Siewerdsen JH, Thongvigitmanee SS. Technical aspects of dental CBCT: state of the art. Dentomaxillofac Radiol. 2015;44(1):20140224.
47. Zimmerman JN, Vora SR, Pliska BT. Reliability of upper airway measurement using CBCT. Eur J Orthod. 2019;41(1):101–8.
48. Schuman TA, Senior BA. Treatment paradigm for nasal airway obstruction. Otolaryngol Clin N Am. 2018;51(5):873–82.
49. Chambi-Rocha A, Cabrera-Dominguez ME, Dominguez-Reyes A. Breathing mode influence on craniofacial development and head posture. J Pediatr. 2018;94(2):123–30.
50. Awad MI, Kacker A. Nasal obstruction considerations in sleep apnea. Otolaryngol Clin N Am. 2018;51(5):1003–9.
51. Parks ET. Cone beam computed tomography for the nasal cavity and paranasal sinuses. Dent Clin N Am. 2014;58:627–51.
52. El H, Palomo JM. Measuring the airway in 3 dimensions: a reliability and accuracy study. Am J Orthod Dentofac Orthop. 2010;137(4 Suppl):S50.e1–9.
53. Cui DM, Han DM, Nicolas B, Hu CL, Wu J, Su MM. Three-dimensional evaluation of nasal surgery in patients with obstructive sleep apnea. Chin Med J. 2016;129(6):651–6.
54. Gupta JV, Makhija PG, Gupta KC. Does a correlation exist between nasal airway volume and craniofacial morphology: a cone beam computed tomography study. Indian J Dent Res. 2016;27(4):359–63.
55. Zaoui K, Kuehle R, Baumann I, Scheussler DL, Ristow O, Plath M, Freudlsperger C. Impact of Le-Fort I osteotomy on anatomical and functional aspects of the nasal airway and on quality of life. Eur Arch Otorhinolaryngol. 2019;276(4):1065–73.
56. Kim YJ, Hong JS, Hwang Y, Park YH. Three-dimensional analysis of pharyngeal airway in preadolescent children with different anteroposterior skeletal patterns. Am J Orthod Dentofac Orthop. 2010;137(3):306.e1–11.
57. De Water VR, Saridin JK, Bouw F, Murawska MM, Koudstaal MJ. Measuring upper airway volume: accuracy and reliability of dolphin 3D software compared to manual segmentation in craniosynostosis patients. J Oral Maxillofac Surg. 2014;72(1): 139–44.
58. Shi K, Mupparapu M. Three-dimentional standardization for segmentation and quantification of nasal airway: ITK-SNAP-CBCT study. Presented at International Congress of IADMFR/70th annual session of AAOMR. Philadelphia, Pennsylvania. 2019;22–5. https://iadmfr2019.org.
59. Zhang C, Bruggink R, Baan F, Bronkhorst E, Maal T, He H, Ongkosuwito EM. A new segmentation algorithm for measuring CBCT images of nasal airway: a pilot study. PeerJ. 2019;7: e6246.
60. Shokri A, Miresmaeili A, Ahmadi A, Amini P, Falah-kooshki S. Comparison of pharyngeal airway volume in different skeletal facial patterns using cone beam computed tomography. J Clin Exp Dent. 2018;10(10):e1017–28.
61. Woodside D, Linder-Aronson S, Lundstrom A, McWilliam J. Mandibular and maxillary growth after changed mode of breathing. Am J Orthod Dentofac Orthop. 1991;100(1):1–18.
62. Yamada T, Tanne K, Miyamoto K, Yamauchi K. Influences of nasal respiratory obstruction on craniofacial growth in young Machaca fuscata monkeys. Am J Orthod Dentofac Orthop. 1997;111(1):38–43.
63. Solow B, Siersbaek-Nielsen S, Greve E. Airway adequacy, head posture, and craniofacial morphology. Am J Orthod. 1984;86(3):214–23.
64. Vargervik K, Miller AJ, Chierici G, Harvold E, Tomer BS. Morphiologic response to changes in neuromuscular patterns experimentally induced by altered modes of respiration. Am J Orthod. 1984;85(2):115–24.
65. Schendel SA, Jacobson R, Khalessi S. Airway growth and development: a computerized 3-dimensional analysis. J Oral Maxillofac Surg. 2012;70(9):2174–83.
66. Stutzmann JJ, Petrovic AG. Role of the lateral pterygoid muscle and menisco temporomandibular frenum in spontaneous growth of the mandible and in growth stimulated by the postural hyperpropylsor. Am J Orthod Dentofac Orthop. 1990;97(5):381–92.
67. Chiang CC, Jefferies MN, Miller A, Hatcher DC. Three-dimensional airway evaluation in 387 subjects from one university orthodontic clinic using cone beam computed tomography. Angle Orthod. 2012;82(6):985–92.
68. Barrera JE. Sleep magnetic resonance imaging: dynamic characteristics of the airway during sleep in obstructive sleep apnea syndrome. Laryngoscope. 2011;121(6):1327–35.
69. Cheng S, Brown EC, Hatt A, Butler JE, Gandevia SC, Bilston LE. Healthy humans with a narrow upper airway maintain patency during quiet breathing by dilating the airway during inspiration. J Physiol. 2014;592(21):4763–74.

3D Cephalometry

5

Juan Martin Palomo, Hakan El, Neda Stefanovic, Manhal Eliliwi, Tarek Elshebiny, and Fernando Pugliese

5.1 Introduction

The Western Reserve University roentgenographic craniostat was developed by Broadbent and T. Wingate Todd in Cleveland, which allowed for acquisition of standardized lateral and anteroposterior planar radiographs of the human skull and mandible (Fig. 5.1) [1–6]. Refinements to this device would result in the Broadbent-Bolton cephalometer in 1931 (Fig. 5.2). This imaging approach also became a standard part of orthodontic records for confirming diagnosis and evaluating treatment outcomes. A main drawback of cephalometry is that it relies on a 2-dimensional (2D) projection of a 3-dimensional (3D) object, leading to projection and magnification errors [7, 8]. The advent of Cone Beam Computed Tomography (CBCT) completely revolutionized orthodontic imaging allowing the clinician to see the patient as what they really are, 3D structures. The purpose of this chapter is to illustrate techniques that go beyond the regular diagnosis, and provide further information for the treatment planning and outcome assessment of the orthodontic patient.

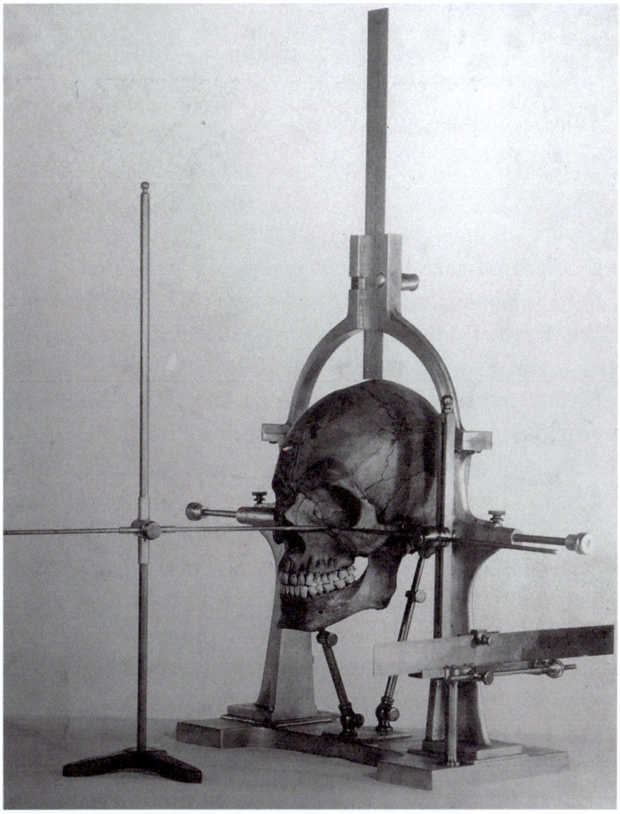

Fig. 5.1 Craniostat developed by Broadbent and Todd as a precursor to the first cephalometric head holder

J. M. Palomo (✉) · M. Eliliwi · T. Elshebiny · F. Pugliese
School of Dental Medicine—Department of Orthodontics, Case Western Reserve University, Cleveland, OH, USA
e-mail: jmp5@case.edu; mxe181@case.edu; tme18@case.edu; fdp10@case.edu

H. El
School of Dental Medicine—Department of Orthodontics, Hacettepe University, Ankara, Turkey
e-mail: hakanel@hacettepe.edu.tr

N. Stefanovic
Faculty of Dental Medicine—Department of Orthodontics, University of Belgrade, Belgrade, Serbia

5.2 Accuracy and Reliability of 3D Cephalometric Landmarks

With a single acquisition that can be taken in few seconds CBCT can generate panoramic, cross-sectional and reconstructed images of the labial and lingual bone plates, which are not apparent in conventional two-dimensional x-rays due to image superimposition. In addition, views not previously available can be created—axial, coronal, sagittal, and sepa-

J.-M. Retrouvey, M.-N. Abdallah (eds.), *3D Diagnosis and Treatment Planning in Orthodontics*,
https://doi.org/10.1007/978-3-030-57223-5_5

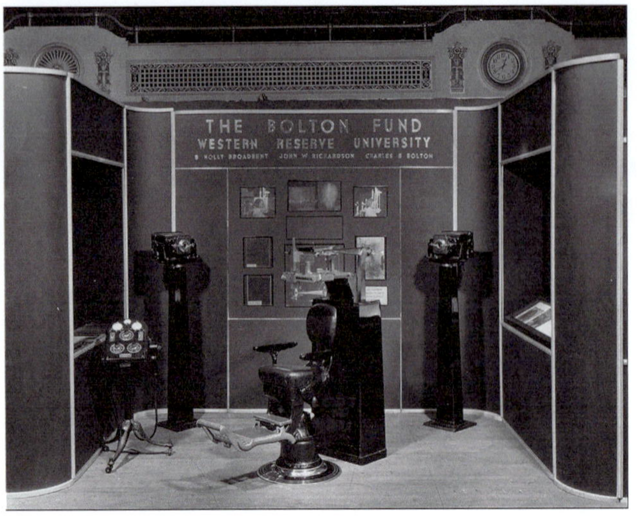

Fig. 5.2 The first cephalometer on display on the third floor of the School of Dental Medicine in the Bolton Brush Growth Study Center, Cleveland, Ohio, ca 1970

rate views of the right and left sides of the head. Several studies compared measurements derived directly from a 3D CBCT cephalogram with traditional 2D cephalograms. Zamora et al. [9] found no statistical differences between the measurements of one versus the other. Lagravere et al. [10] evaluated the reliability and accuracy in locating several different foramina in the cranial base by CBCT images for establishing reference coordinate systems to show that all landmarks provided high intra-examiner reliability and accuracy, and can be considered acceptable landmarks to use in establishing reference coordinate systems for future 3D superimposition. De Oliveria et al. [11] evaluated reliability in 3D landmark identification using CBCT to conclude that intra- and inter-observer reliability was excellent. 3D landmark identification using CBCT can offer consistent and reproducible data if a protocol for operator training and calibration is followed.

3D landmarks can be identified in the actual 3D image, each landmark must be identified in three dimensions: anteroposteriorly, vertically, and transversely

5.3 3D Assessment of Facial Asymmetry

Appropriate symmetry is an essential factor in facial esthetics. It is generally accepted today that a small degree of bilateral asymmetry exists in essentially all normal individuals and that perfect bilateral symmetry is largely a theoretical concept. As the human face is not always symmetric over the facial midline, asymmetries and deviations within limits are recognized as normal [12]. However, moderate, severe, or pathologic asymmetry of the craniofacial complex is not acceptable and needs orthodontic treatment alone or combined with surgical treatment. Facial appearance is basically composed of both the hard and soft tissues. Consequently, not only the skeletal structure but also the soft tissues of the craniofacial region must be evaluated for adequate diagnosis of asymmetry [12].

Traditionally, facial asymmetry has been diagnosed primarily with posteroanterior cephalometric radiograph and clinical pictures. The reliability of posteroanterior cephalometric measurement for the evaluation of facial asymmetry, however, is limited because some landmarks are difficult to identify due to the overlapping of the complex anatomical structures in the skull [13]. The incomplete assessment of soft tissues is another limitation of the posteroanterior cephalometric. Therefore, it may be difficult to determine whether hidden asymmetries in the posterior regions are caused by dental factors, skeletal factors, or both. Also, head positioning, which is usually determined by the position of the external auditory meatus, may modify the symmetric features of some landmarks and natural head position cannot be always ensured, especially in these asymmetric patients [13].

The development of CBCT has greatly reduced errors of posteroanterior cephalometric radiograph and improved our ability to diagnose asymmetry and other craniofacial deformities. 3D CBTC CBCT images are uniquely suited to assess asymmetry. These images use a built-in reconstruction algorithm to correct known distortions due to projection geometry, and allow clinicians to assess skull anatomy either through 1 to 1 ratio 3D surface renderings or through accurate 2D slices through the skull [14].

For more accurate evaluation of asymmetry, 3D digital image diagnosis data go through a process called reorientation [15], which involves the adjustment of the head position on software images (Fig. 5.3). After reorientation, asymmetry can be assessed by different quantitative methods. Comparisons with bilateral linear measurements or using mirror images have been reported recently [13].Both methods are critically based on which planes are to be used in the assessment. An appropriate midsagittal reference plane based on the anatomy of the cranial base is needed to evaluate facial asymmetry [16]. In order to determine this reference plane, landmark positioning is necessary, which is an accurate and reproducible method when using 3D images.

There are some studies showing a relationship between malocclusion and skeletal asymmetry. One relationship frequently cited is the Class II subdivision patient, with both skeletal and dental asymmetries described. The Class III malocclusion is also sometimes related to a mandibular deviation [14]. It is also known that facial asymmetry is more frequently identified in the lower third of the face [12]. The fact

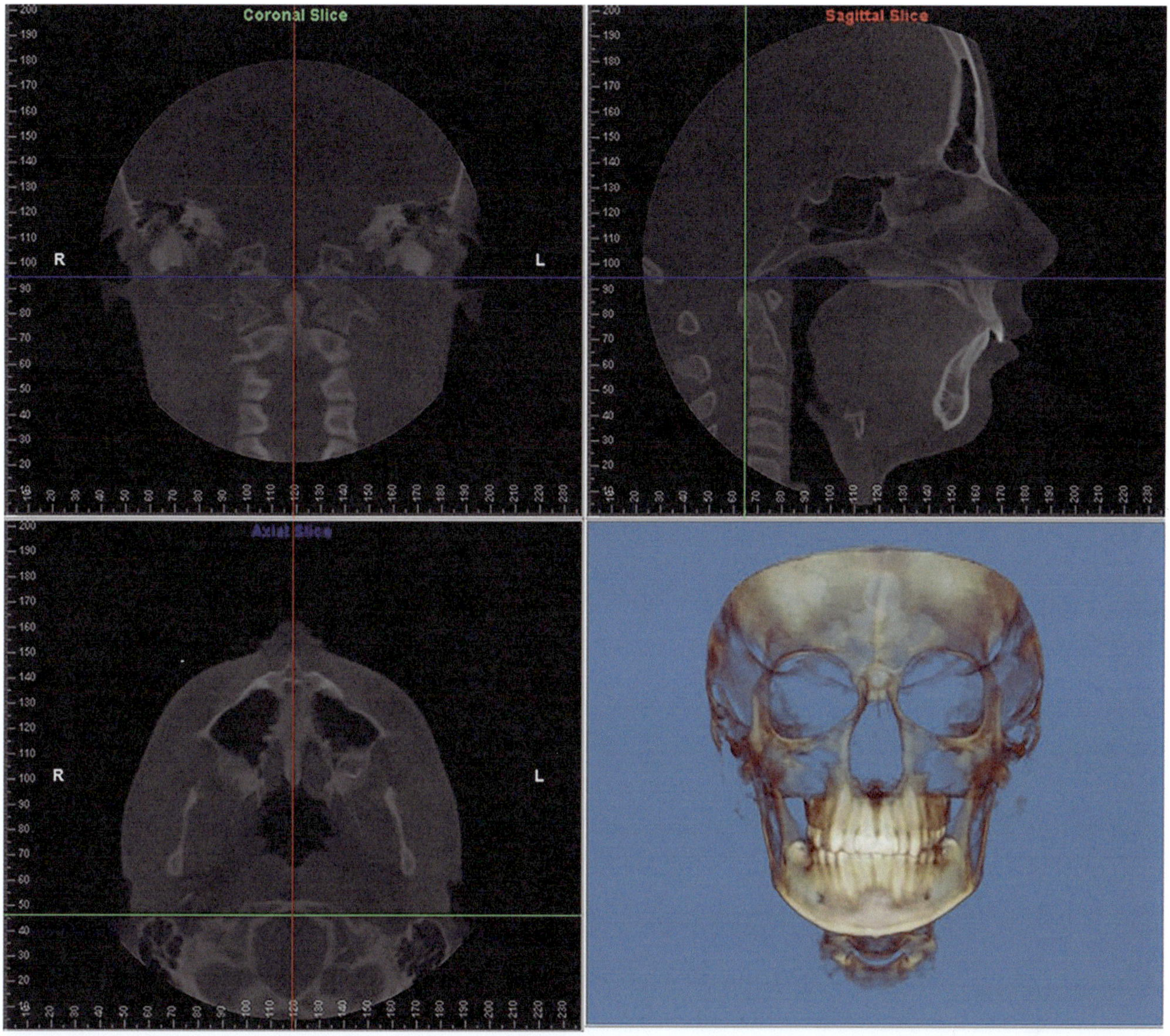

Fig. 5.3 Reorientation method using Dolphin 3D Imaging Software

that the mandible is a mobile bone that grows over a longer period than the maxilla has been reported as the reason for the increased frequency of lower facial asymmetry. Although asymmetry is more significant in the mandible, there can also be different levels of asymmetry in the maxilla [17].

Imaging software can be a helpful tool for asymmetry assessment. With mirroring or superimposition methods, it is possible to easily visualize the differences between right and left sides of the skull (Fig. 5.4). Another method to visualize and quantify hard and soft tissue asymmetry is using mirrored images and color map quantification [17].This is a very useful method not just to plan the orthodontic treatment but also to simplify the communication with patient, since it is a very clear way to visualize the differences between facial sides. After reorientation, the right side of the 3D skull is mirrored using a midsagittal plane as a reference (Fig. 5.5). The original 3D skull is superimposed on the new 3D mirrored skull by best-fit methodology using the right side as a reference. The asymmetry quantification can be assessed by color map (Fig. 5.6).

Regardless of the assessment method, the correct diagnosis of the tissues and regions with craniofacial asymmetry leads to better treatment plans [12]. 3D evaluation is very important to understand the complex nature of craniofacial asymmetry and CBCT analysis allows evaluation of asymmetry via linear and colormap measurements, which can demonstrate morphological differences between sides more realistically.

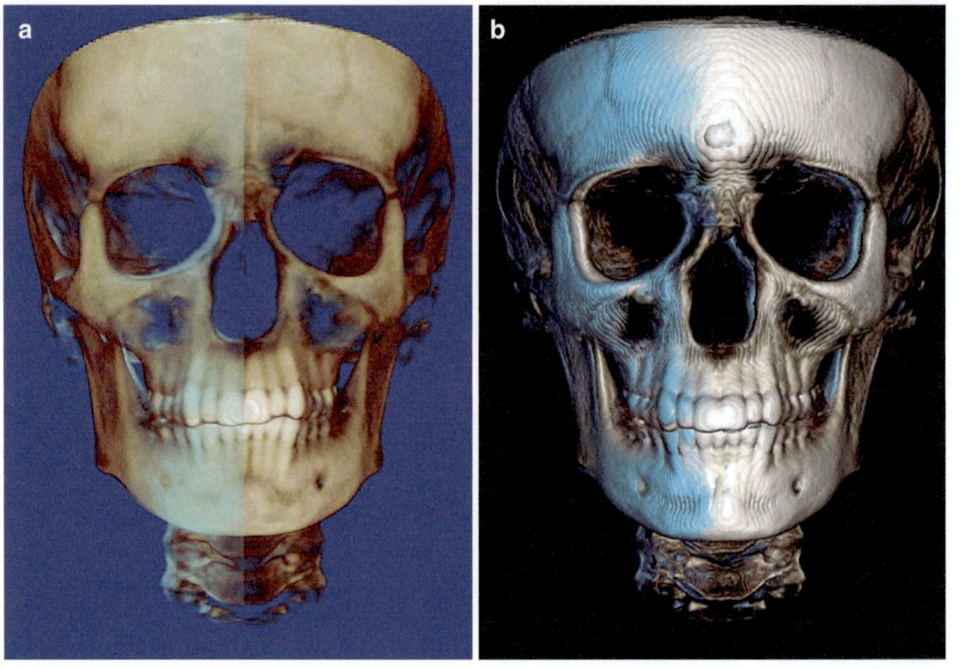

Fig. 5.4 Asymmetry assessment using mirroring and superimposition methods. (**a**) Dolphin 3D Imaging Software. (**b**) InVivo 3D Imaging Software

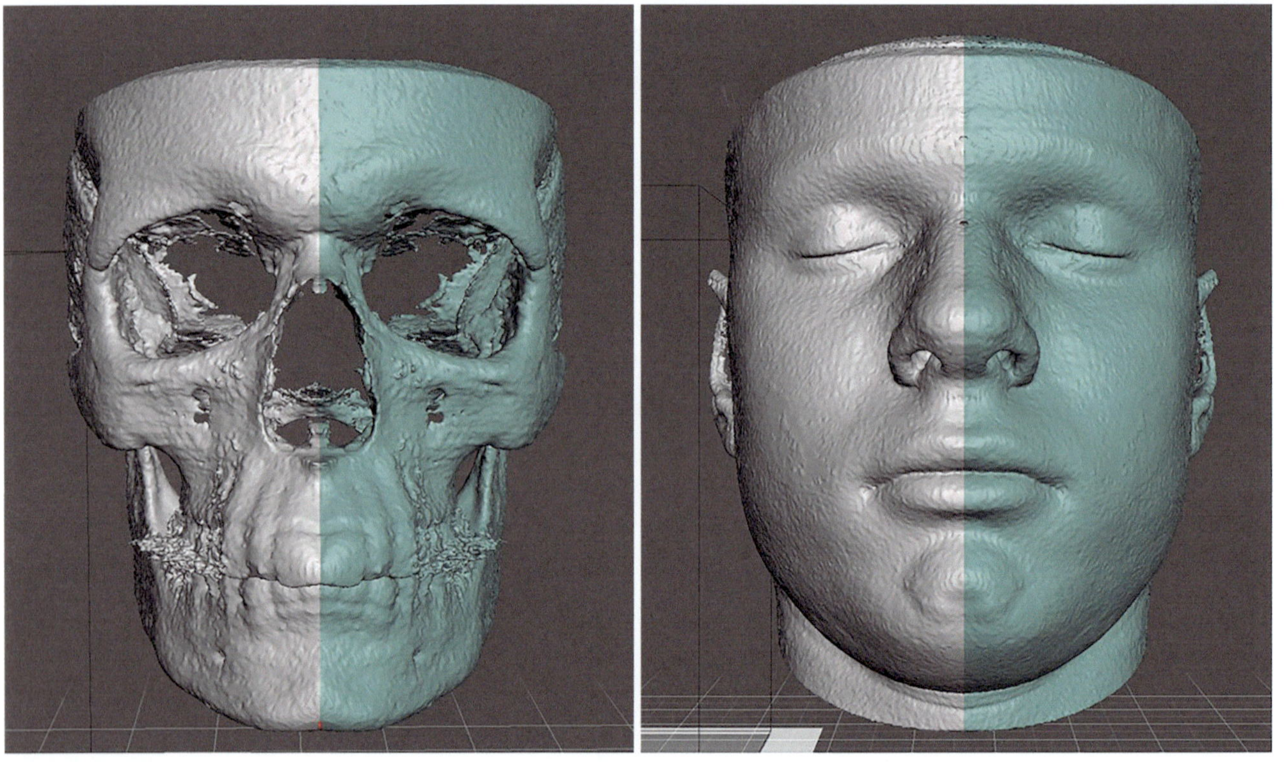

Fig. 5.5 Hard and soft tissue right side mirroring

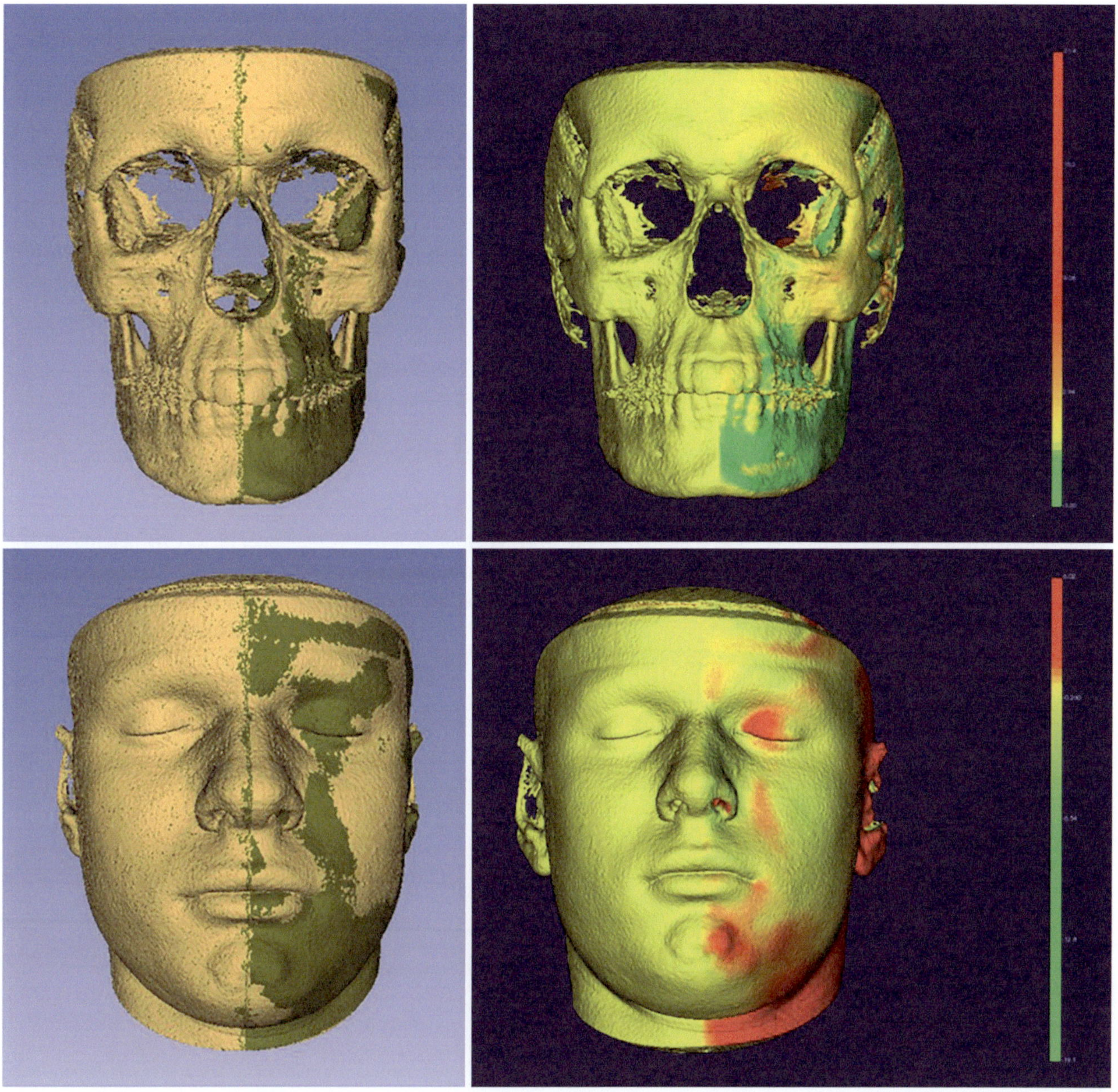

Fig. 5.6 Superimposition and colormap quantification for asymmetry assessment

5.4 3D Assessment of the Upper Airway

Human airways can be divided into the upper and lower airway. The upper airway consists of the oral and nasal cavities, pharynx, and larynx. Pharyngeal airway obstruction and breathing disorders during the most intensive growth period may result in significant long-term negative effects on the dentition and dentofacial development. Narrow upper jaw with increased palatal depth, increased overjet, anterior open bite, posterior cross-bite, and steep mandibular plane angle are some of the most important dentofacial changes associated with airway obstruction and disordered breathing [18–21]. Dentofacial structures are the main focus of the specialty of orthodontics and dentofacial orthopedics. Various orthodontic and orthopedic treatment procedures, like maxillary expansion [22, 23], functional treatment [24, 25], and orthognathic surgery [26, 27] have a direct effect on the size and shape of the upper airway. Therefore, it is easy to understand why airway analysis has become a part of the standard orthodontic diagnostic protocol.

The airway is a movable 3D structure that can only be properly represented with 3D imaging. Even though lateral cephalograms have been used for many years to measure the airway, the lack of medio-lateral information render 2D information useless and at times misleading. No study of the upper airway can be performed using a lateral cephalogram, unless it is used for adenoid assessment [28–31]. It has to be taken under consideration that a CBCT of the airway only provides a static image, and the airway is not static. For this reason, CBCT is not an appropriate diagnostic imaging method at this time, since it cannot assess the function or collapsibility of the airway, which are the essential when performing risk assessment for sleep apnea. CBCT may be used for outcome assessment and monitoring treatment approaches, but does not replace, or is as complete as a sleep study.

5.4.1 Software Programs and Methods for Measuring the Upper Airway

There is a wide range of software programs currently available in the market that can be used for airway analysis. The most commonly used are the proprietary Dolphin 3D (Dolphin Imaging & Management Solutions, Chatsworth, CA) and InVivo 6 (Anatomage Inc., San Jose, CA), as well as the open-source alternatives like ITK-SNAP (http://www.itksnap.org) for segmenting the airway. These software programs are intuitive, easy to use, and do not require extensive training.

5.4.1.1 Dolphin 3D

Following image orientation, the automatic airway segmentation is done in the Sinus/Airway section. Two methods are available for obtaining upper airway measurements.

Method #1 (Fig. 5.7)

(a) The operator marks the upper airway by placing several points down the airway path, from the upper border (most commonly the posterior nasal spine) through to the lower border (most commonly the most anteroinferior part of the third cervical vertebra—CV3).

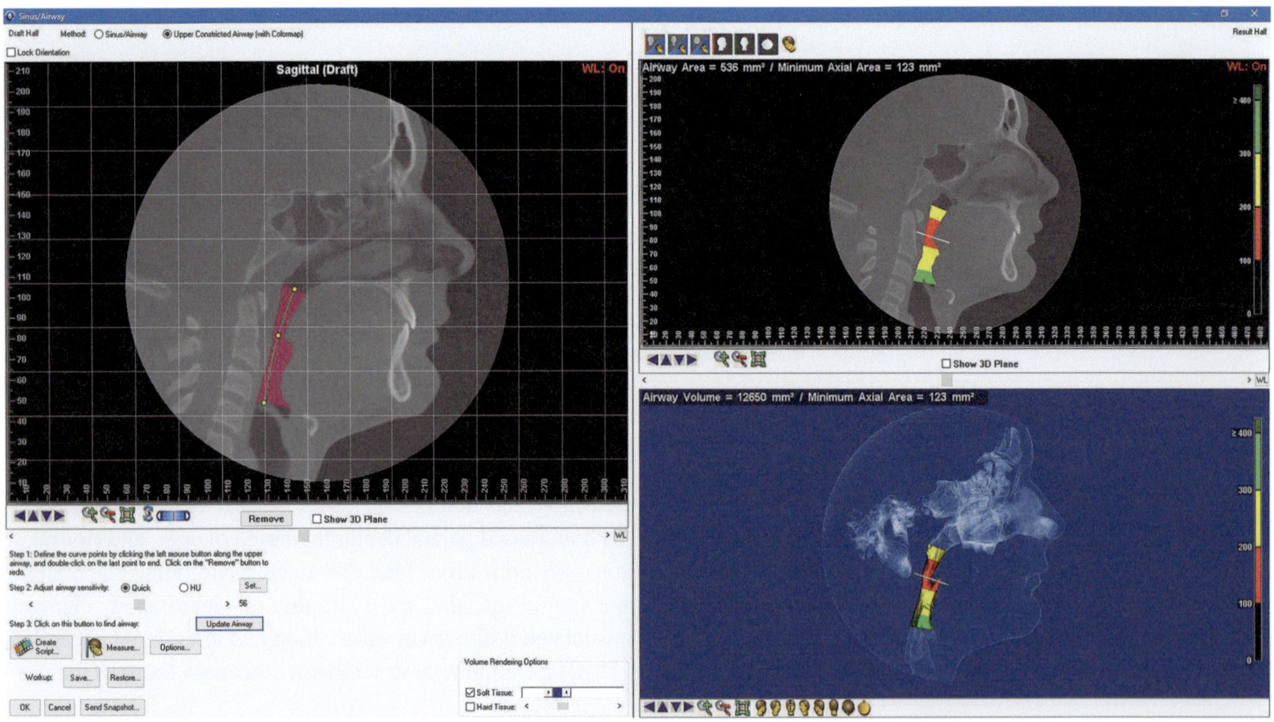

Fig. 5.7 The operator marks the upper airway by placing several points down the airway path, from the upper border (most commonly the posterior nasal spine) through to the lower border (most commonly the most anteroinferior part of the third cervical vertebra—CV3). Once the airway is segmented, the airway volume and area measurements are presented at the top of the screen. This method also provides a color-coded presentation with an explanatory scale on the right side. 3D reconstruction of the airway can be moved in all three planes of space

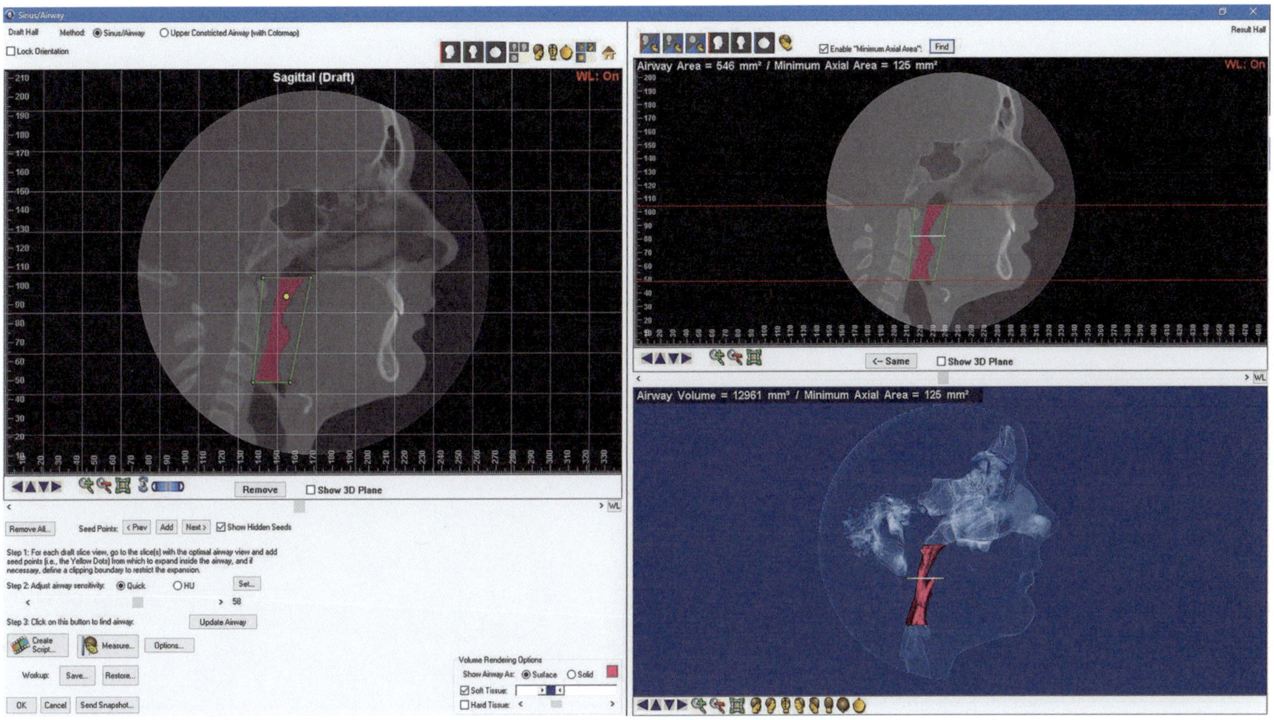

Fig. 5.8 Sagittal (anterior and posterior to the airway) and vertical (upper and lower) borders of the upper airway are marked, after which threshold seed points are places inside the airway. Upon airway segmentation, the airway volume and area measurements are presented at the top of the screen. No color-coded presentation is available when using this method

(b) Once the airway is segmented, the airway volume and area measurements are presented at the top of the screen. This method also provides a color-coded presentation with an explanatory scale on the right side.
(c) 3D reconstruction of the airway can be moved in all three planes of space.

Method #2 (Fig. 5.8)
(a) Sagittal (anterior and posterior to the airway) and vertical (upper and lower) borders of the upper airway are marked, after which threshold seed points are places inside the airway.
(b) Upon airway segmentation, the airway volume and area measurements are presented at the top of the screen. No color-coded presentation is available when using this method.
(c) Three-dimensional reconstruction of the airway can be moved in all three planes of space.

5.4.1.2 InVivo 6

Following image orientation, the automatic airway segmentation is done in the Airway section.

(a) The upper airway border is marked at the level of the posterior nasal spine and the lower border at the level of the most anteroinferior part of the CV3 (Fig. 5.9a).
(b) Once the airway is segmented, the airway volume and area measurements are presented next to the color-mapped image. The explanatory scale for the color map is located at the bottom of the screen. A diagram of the AP and RL distances and the cross-section area are available on the right side. Three-dimensional reconstruction of the airway can be moved in all three planes of space (Fig. 5.9b).
(c) Minimum cross-sectional area and diagrams (Fig. 5.10).

5.4.1.3 ITK-SNAP

ITK-SNAP open-source software is used to segment the airway.

(a) Following image orientation, the region of interest (ROI) is determined on the axial, sagittal, and coronal slices (Fig. 5.11).
(b) The picture is reversed by setting the threshold. The lower threshold is reduced to zero, and the upper threshold is adjusted until for best airway presentation. After the adjustments, the airway is presented in white, and the surrounding structures in blue (Fig. 5.12).
(c) Threshold bubbles are added to fill the airway space (it does not need to be filled completely) (Fig. 5.13).
(d) Once the bubbles have been placed, the "play" button is pressed, segmentation updated, and the airway is segmented (Fig. 5.14).

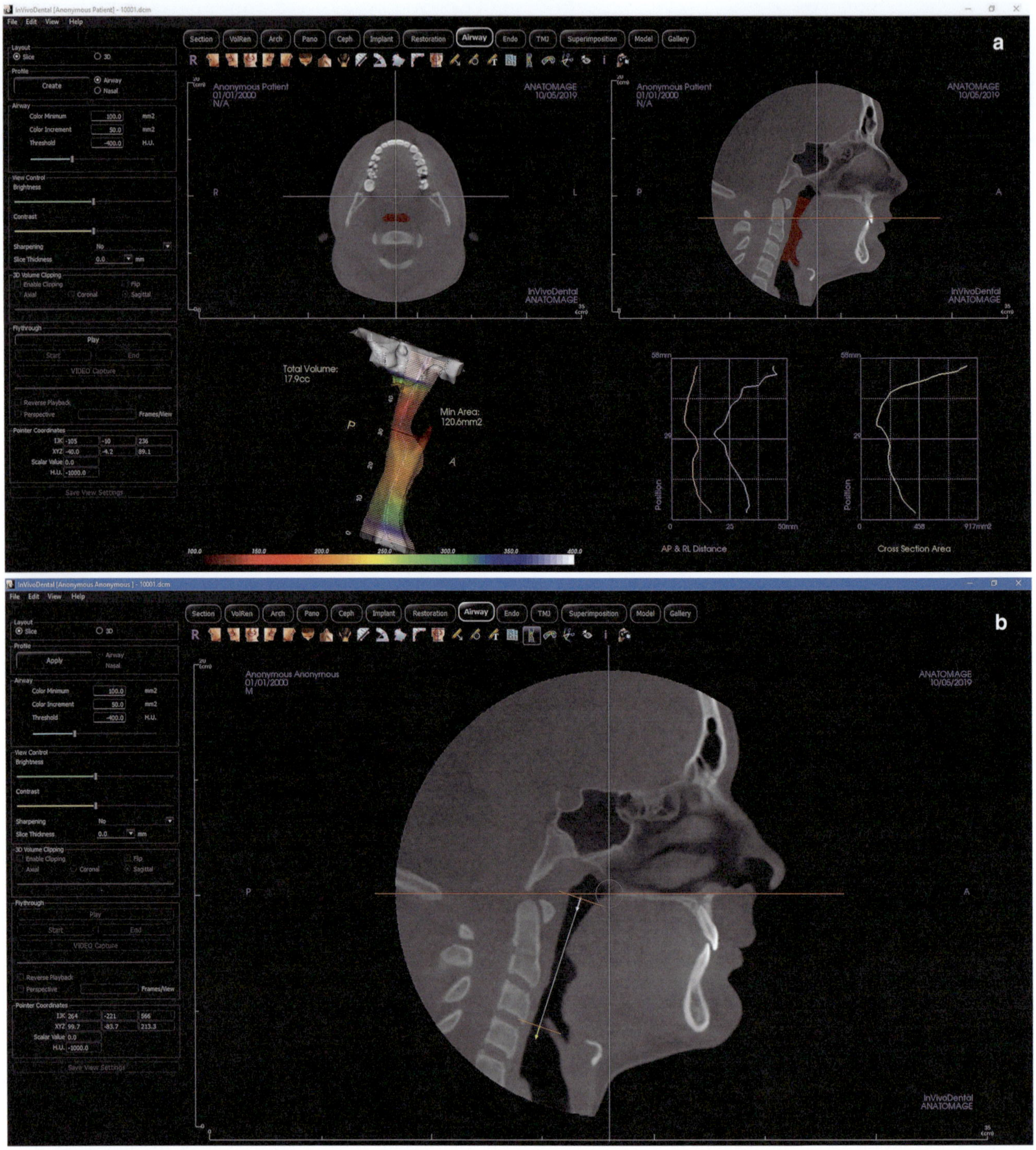

Fig. 5.9 (**a**) The upper airway border is marked at the level of the posterior nasal spine and the lower border at the level of the most anteroinferior part of the CV3. (**b**) A diagram of the AP and RL distances and the cross-sectional area are available on the right side. Three-dimensional reconstruction of the airway can be moved in all three planes of space

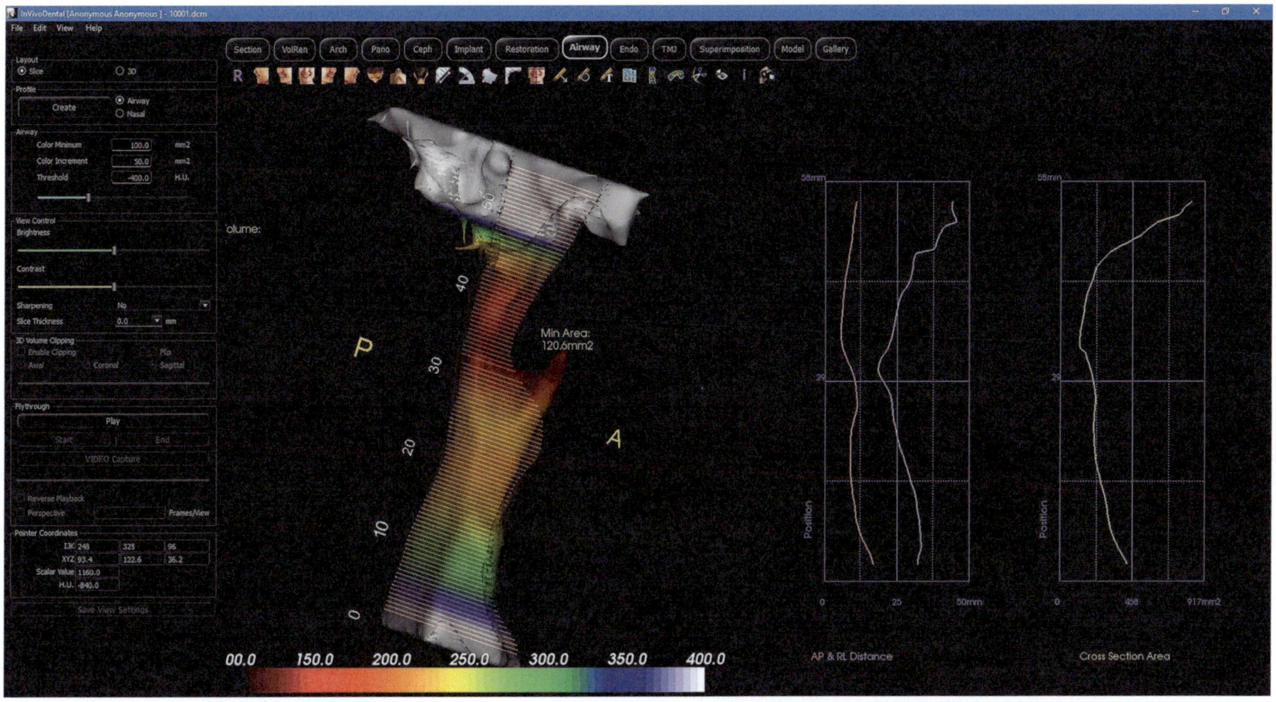

Fig. 5.10 Minimum cross-sectional area and diagrams

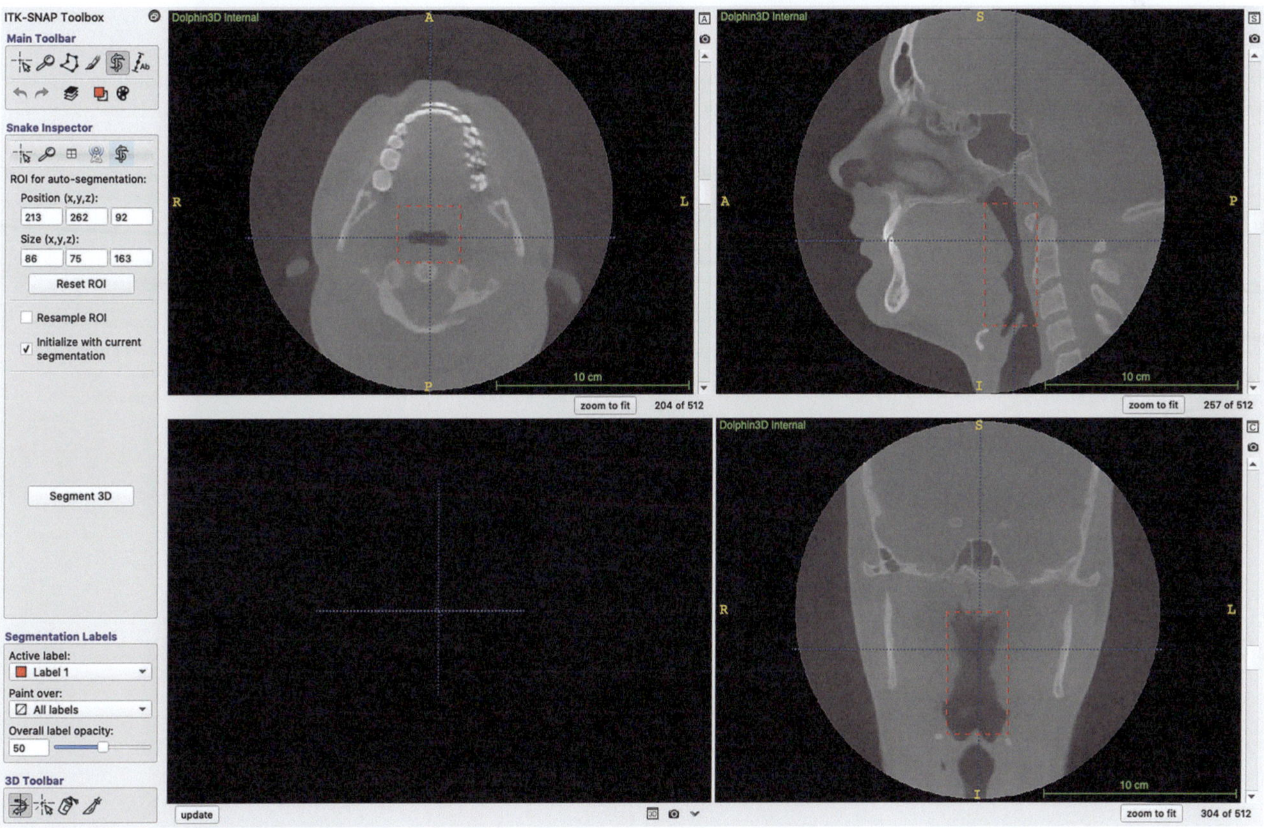

Fig. 5.11 The region of interest (ROI) is determined on the axial, sagittal, and coronal slices

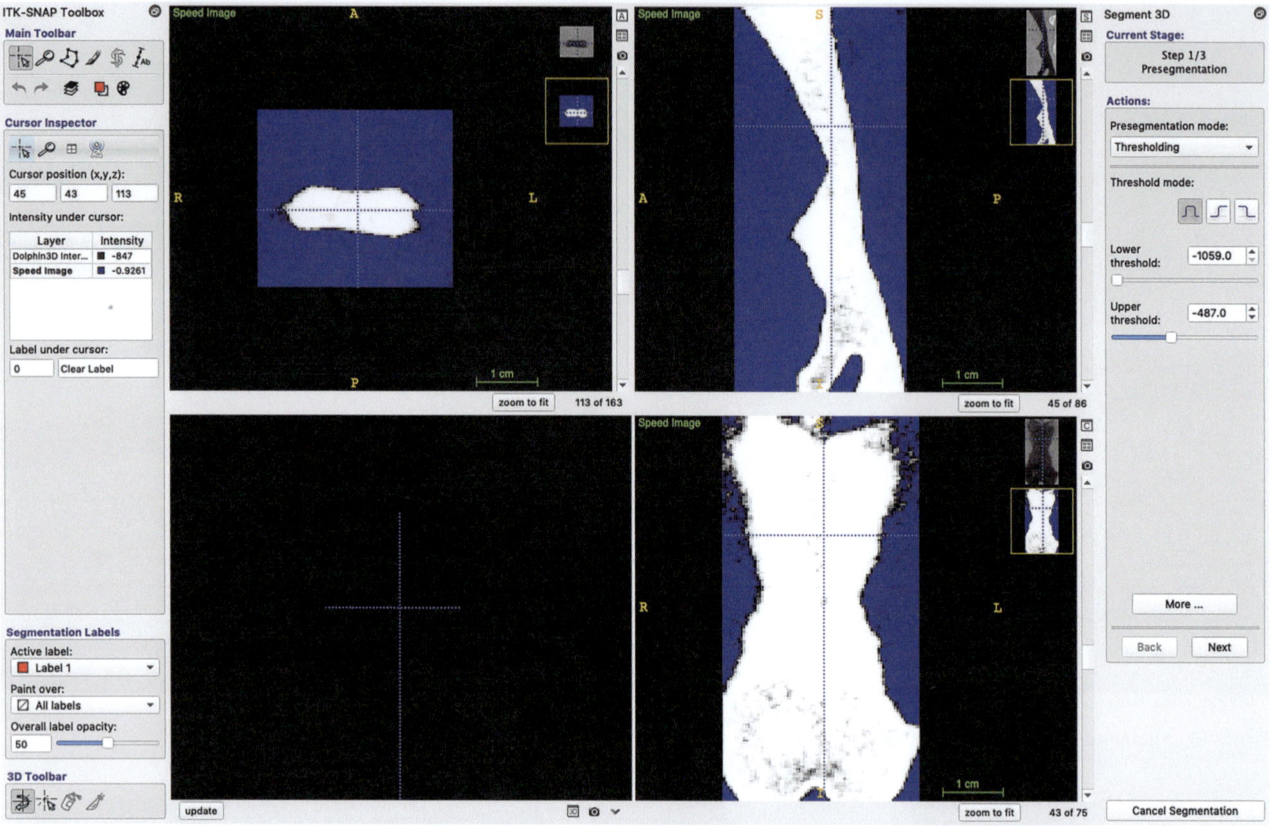

Fig. 5.12 The picture is reversed by setting the threshold. The lower threshold is reduced to zero, and the upper threshold is adjusted until for best airway presentation. After the adjustments, the airway is presented in white, and the surrounding structures in blue

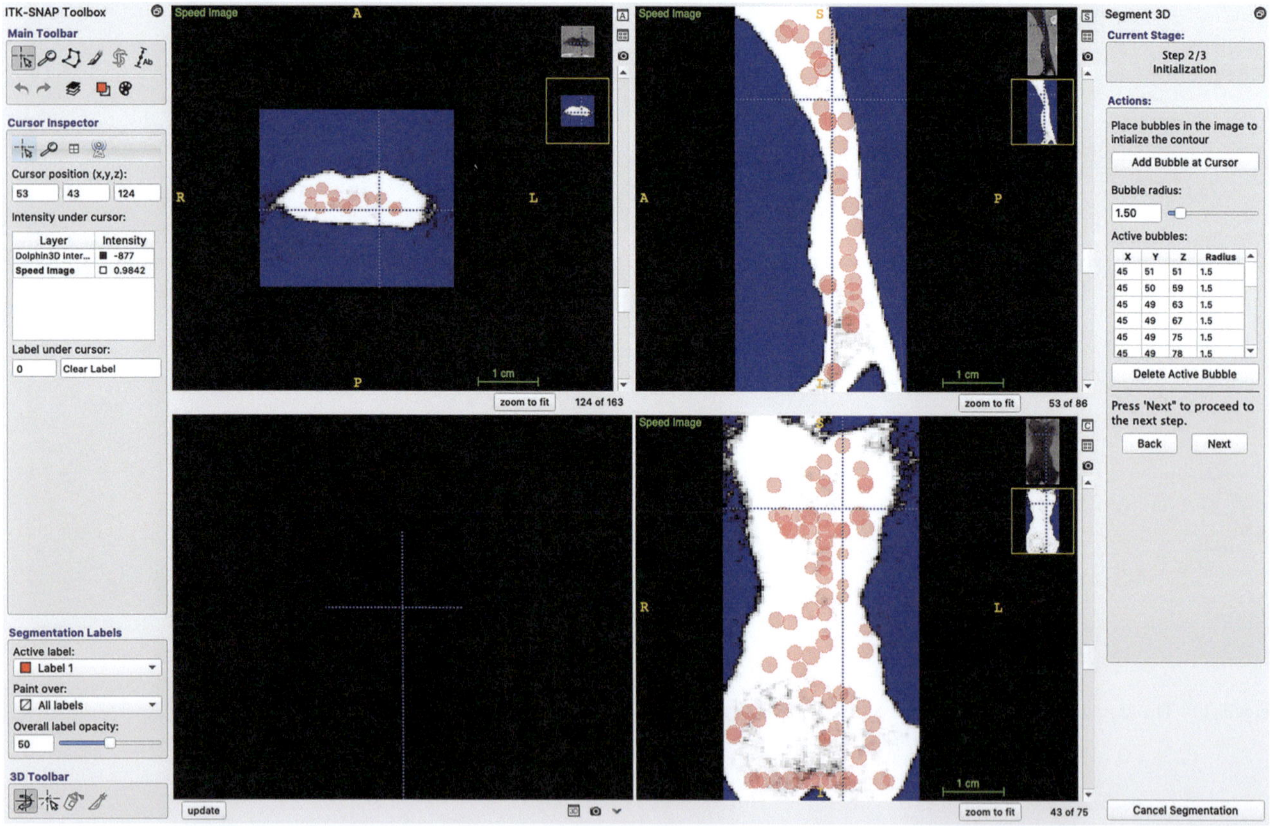

Fig. 5.13 Threshold bubbles are added to fill the airway space (it does not need to be filled completely)

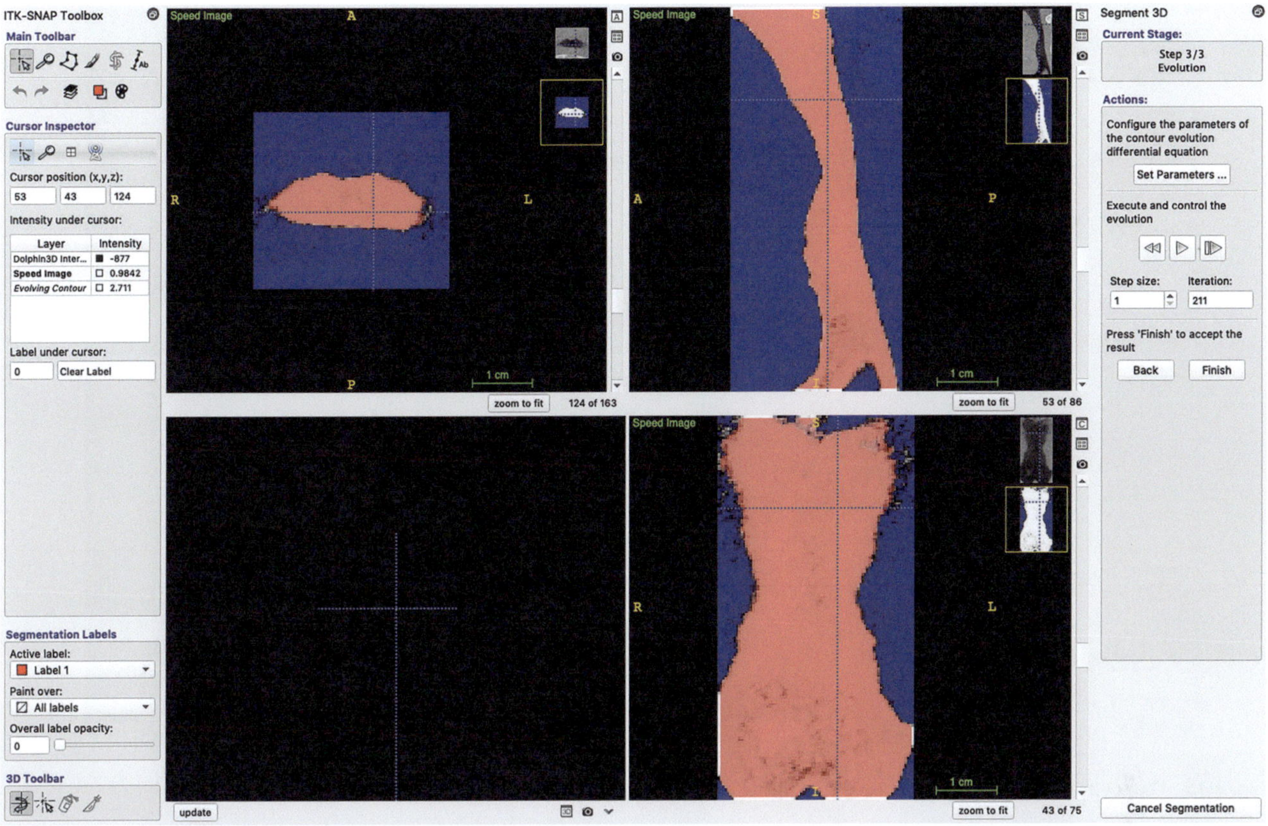

Fig. 5.14 Once the bubbles have been placed, the "play" button is pressed, segmentation updated, and the airway is segmented

(e) The segmented airway can be observed on the axial, sagittal, and coronal slices, in addition to the 3D reconstruction (Fig. 5.15).

5.4.2 Accuracy and Reliability of Airway Imaging

The accuracy and reliability of upper airway measurements obtained from CBCT scans using different software programs were frequently investigated over the past decade. Most studies have concluded that CBCT measurements were accurate and reliable [29, 32]; however, significant differences were found between values obtained using different software programs [33, 34]. El and Palomo [33] looked at 30 CBCT scans to test the reliability and accuracy of 3 commercially available software programs (Dolphin 3D, InVivo, and OnDemand). They found that all three software programs were highly reliable in airway calculations and showed high correlation of results, but poor accuracy, suggesting systematic errors. Weissheimer et al. [34] assessed the accuracy of six imaging software programs for measuring upper airway volumes in 33 growing patients. Semi-automatic and segmentations with interactive and fixed threshold protocols were performed by using Mimics, ITK-SNAP, OsiriX, Dolphin3D, InVivo, and OnDemand3D software programs. They concluded that all software programs were reliable but had errors in the volume segmentations of the oropharynx. However, it has been shown that under current scanning protocols volumetric measurements show significant variability [35], which makes the minimum cross-sectional area a more useful measurement in upper airway assessment.

Even though there are currently no standard or minimal values for airway volumes and minimum cross-sectional areas, the difference in airway size before and after treatment can easily be appreciated by looking at the pre- and post-treatment segmentation (Figs. 5.16 and 5.17).

5.5 CBCT and Obstructive Sleep Apnea (OSA)

OSA is a common disorder characterized by collapse of the upper airway during sleep resulting in hypoxemia and arousal [36]. CBCT can be employed to assess the location of obstruction in OSA patients. One study compared the upper airway structure in OSA patients and control subjects using CBCT images [37]. It was shown that OSA subjects presented lower total airway volume, smaller anterior-posterior dimension of the minimum cross-sectional seg-

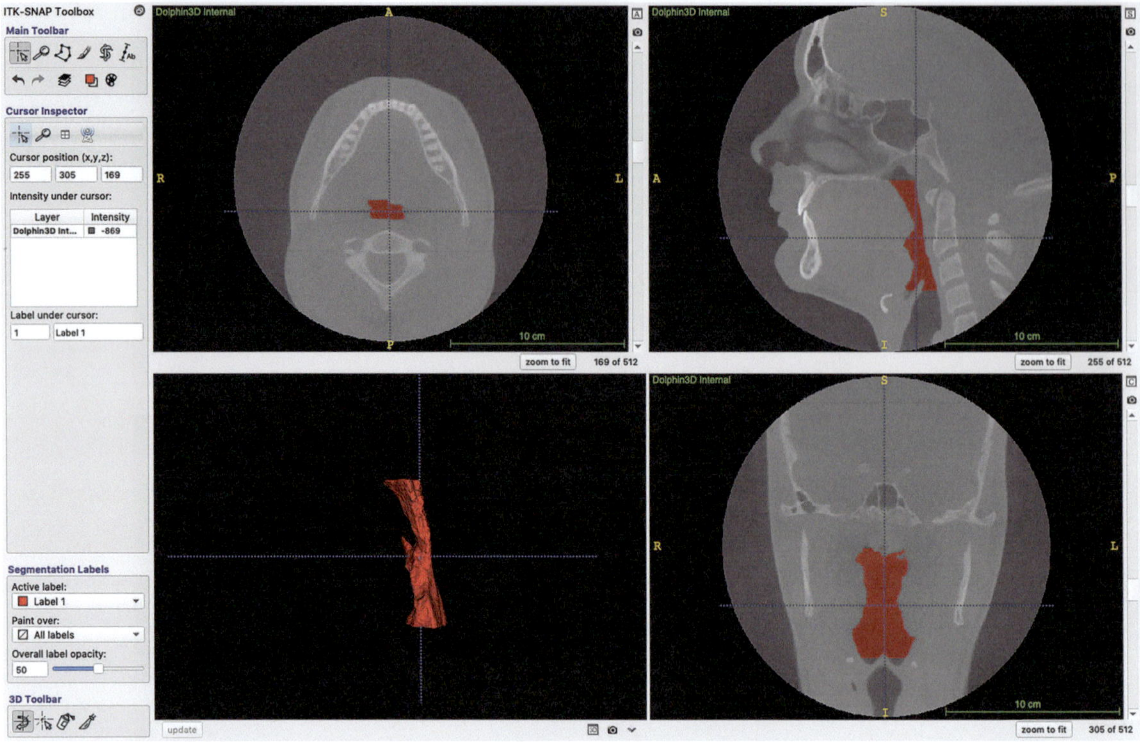

Fig. 5.15 The segmented airway can be observed on the axial, sagittal, and coronal slices, in addition to the 3D reconstruction

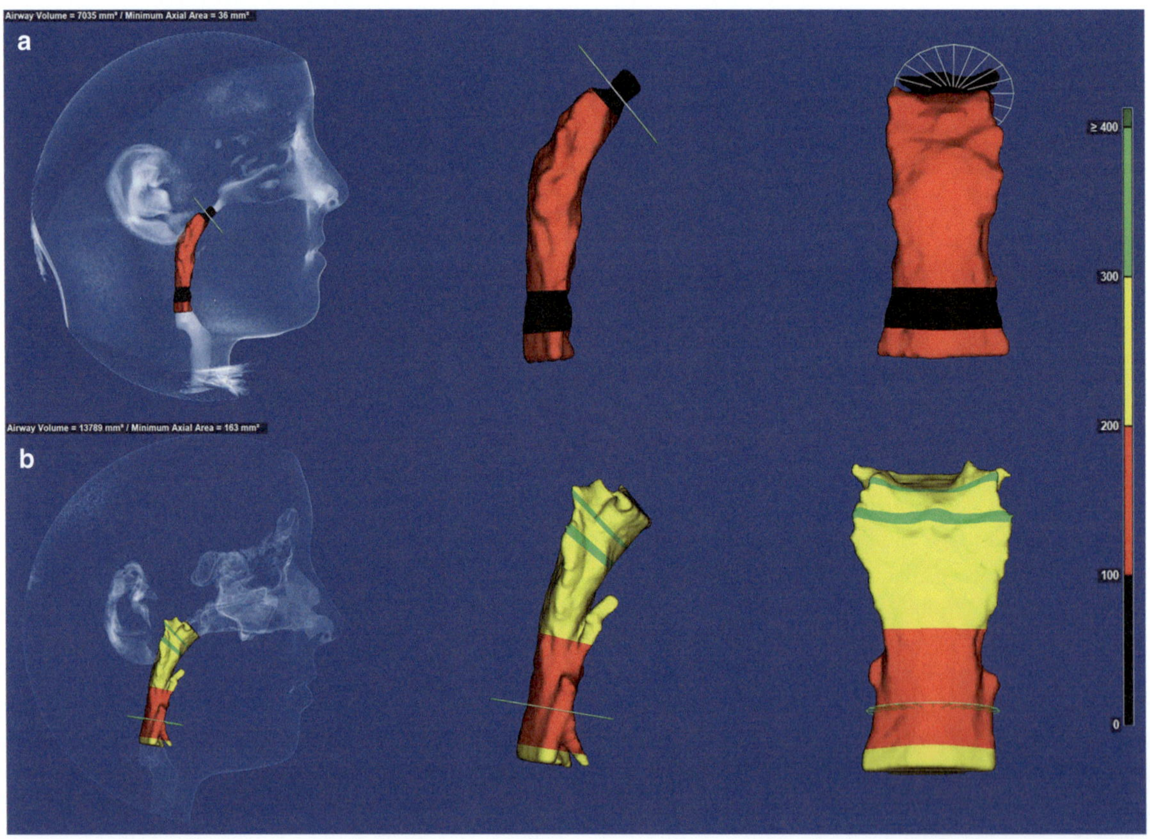

Fig. 5.16 Herbst patient description. (**a**) The pre-treatment color-coded airway segmentation indicates reduced airway size (red and black) and the location of the minimum cross-sectional area at the level of the CV2 lower border. (**b**) The post-treatment segmentation shows an increase in the airway size (green), especially of the minimum cross-sectional area (yellow)

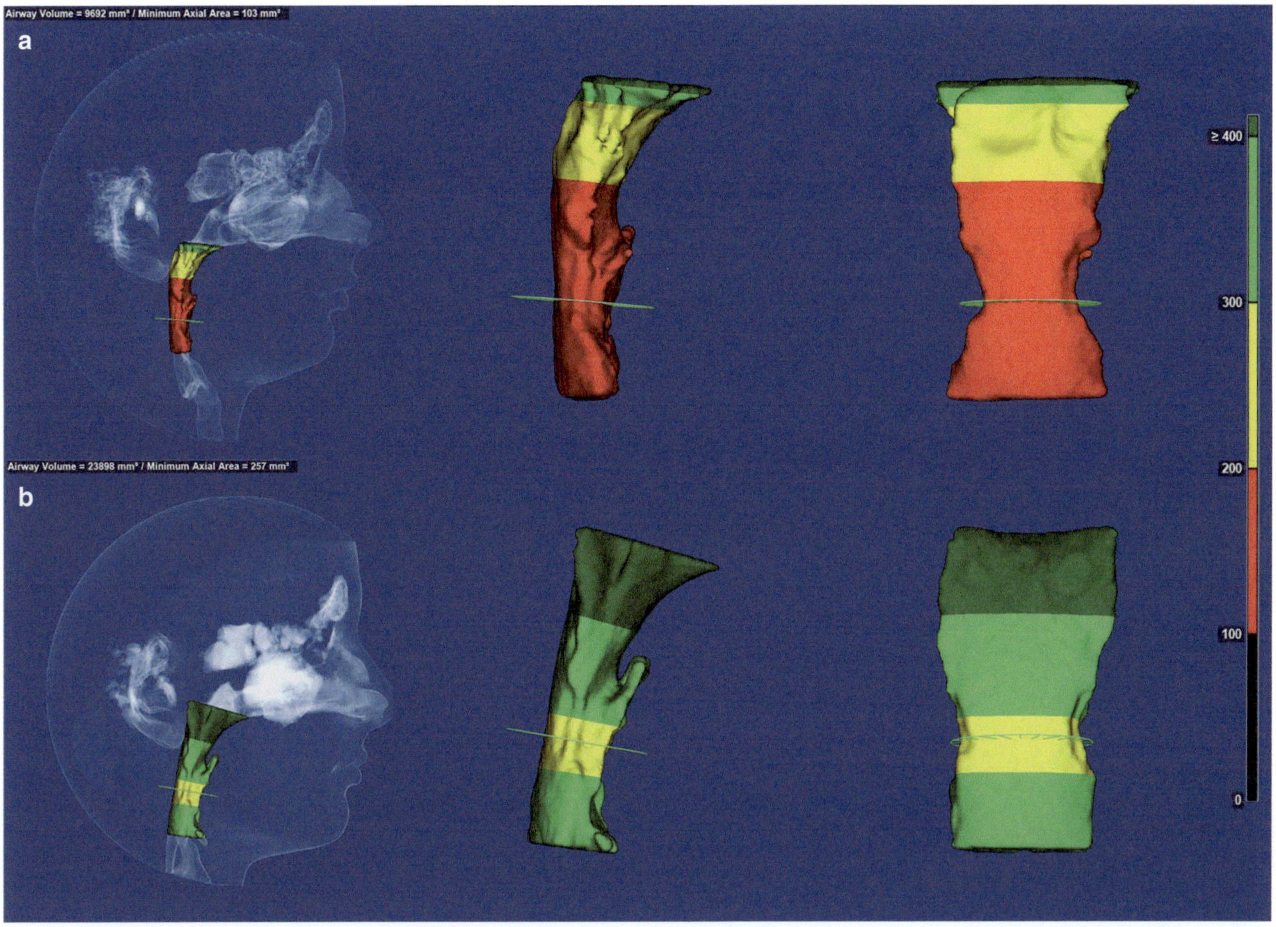

Fig. 5.17 FaceMask patient description. (**a**) The pre-treatment color-coded airway segmentation indicates reduced airway size (red and black) and the location of the minimum cross-sectional area slightly below the level of the CV2 lower border. (**b**) The post-treatment segmentation shows an increasein the airway size (yellow, green, red) and the minimum cross-sectional area (red). The increase isnot as remarkable as in the Class II patient, but it is still evident

ment, and smaller minimum cross-sectional area. Also the OSA group showed elliptic shaped airway, while the non-OSA group showed round, or square airway [37].Recent study evaluated the upper airway dimensions of OSA and control subjects using CBCT. Results showed that OSA subjects had a significantly smaller average minimum cross-sectional area, average airway volume, total airway volume, and mean airway width. OSA subjects had a significantly larger airway length measurement [38].

5.5.1 Evaluation of OSA Treatment Approaches Using CBCT

5.5.1.1 Continuous Positive Airway Pressure (CPAP).

CPAP is the most effective method to manage OSA. It improves subjective and objective measures of sleepiness [39].The most significant effect is enlargement of the airway by dimensional changes of the lateral pharyngeal walls. A recent study evaluated OSA patients by taking CBCT scans during application of positive pressure to the respiratory system while awake and seated [40]. The scan was taken during a cycle of resting breathing. Another image was obtained when pressure was applied using a full facemask also in the seated posture during wakefulness. The mask was connected to a positive pressure source. Scan was taken while breathing on a mask pressure of +10 cm H_2O (Fig. 5.18). Positive pressure application of +10 cm H_2O showed significant airway volume increase in all regions (36%). The hypopharynx volume increased the most with 50%, followed by oropharynx with 23%, and the nasopharynx with 17.7%. The minimum cross-sectional area changed from 100.57 ± 38.74 mm^2 to 130.64 ± 64.01 mm^2.

5.5.1.2 Oral Appliances

An oral appliance is fitted to the upper and lower teeth and is designed to work by fixing and/or anterior positioning the mandible, preventing the collapse of the tongue and/or increasing the posterior oropharyngeal air-

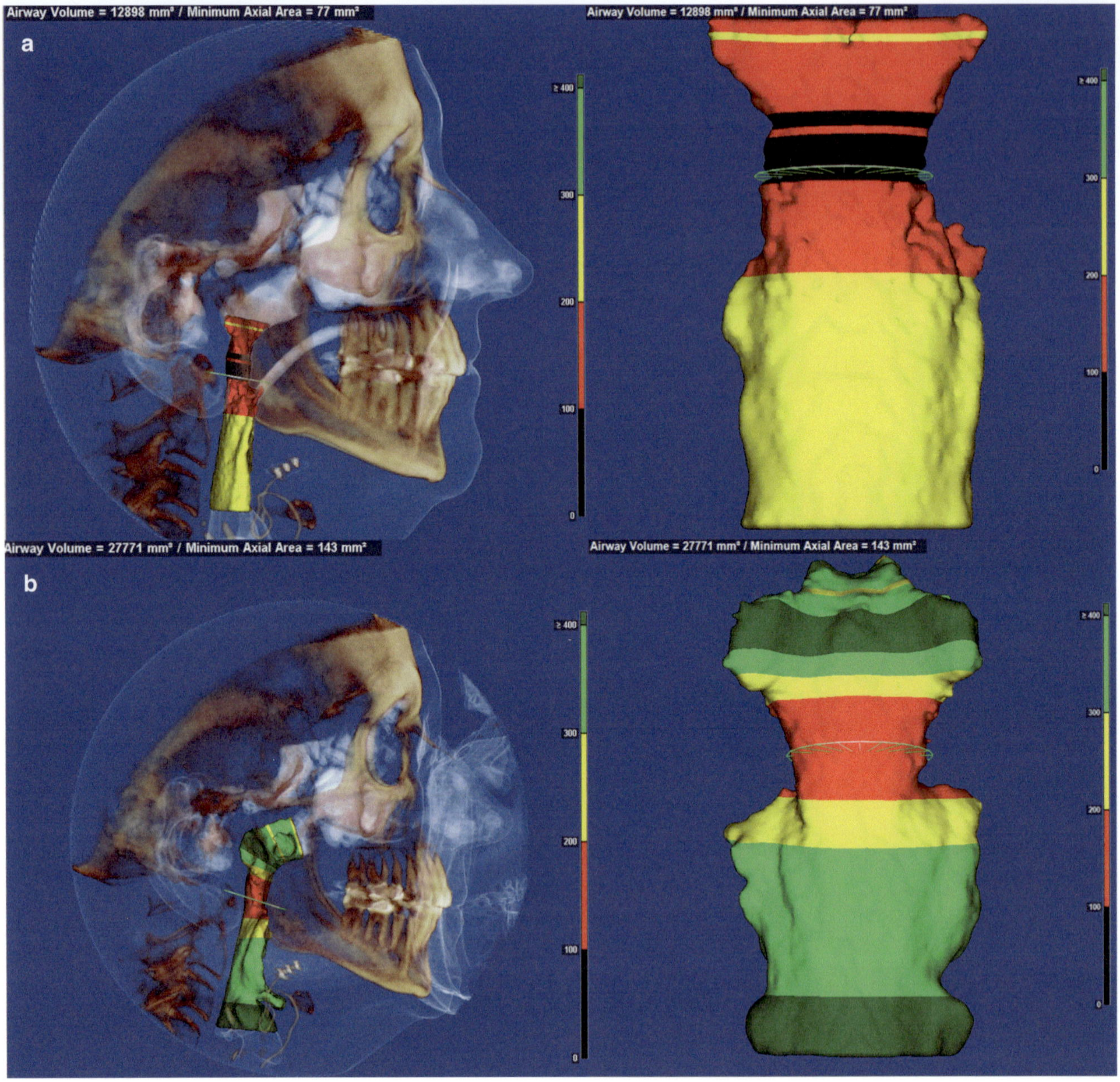

Fig. 5.18 Three-dimensional rendering images of the upper airway with cone beam computed tomography for one patient. (**a**) Resting Breathing: Sagittal view during a cycle of resting breathing showing the upper airway volume (**b**) Application of positive pressure (+10 cmH_2O) by facemask. Sagittal view during application of +10 cmH_2O with an increase in airway volume

way space, therefore reducing the collapse of the upper airway during sleep [41]. Oral appliances can be first-line therapy but are more commonly used for patients who are not compliant with CPAP and diagnosed with mild and moderate OSA; and oral appliance also treats simple snoring. Recently, the American Academy of Sleep Medicine recommended the oral appliances as a first line of therapy in patients with mild to moderate OSA. The most commonly used oral appliances are the mandibular advancement devices which reposition the mandible, tongue, and hyoid bone anteriorly to increase dimensions of the upper airway [42, 43]. Figure 5.19 shows airway volume changes for one patient with and without oral appliance.

5.5.1.3 Maxillomandibular Advancement

Maxillomandibular advancement (MMA) surgery is a well-established treatment of obstructive OSA [44]. The rationale for MMA is to increase the anteroposterior and the lateral dimensions at multi-levels of the upper airway [45].Also reducing upper airway collapsibility by the superior and anterior movement of the hyoid bone [46]. Schendel et al.

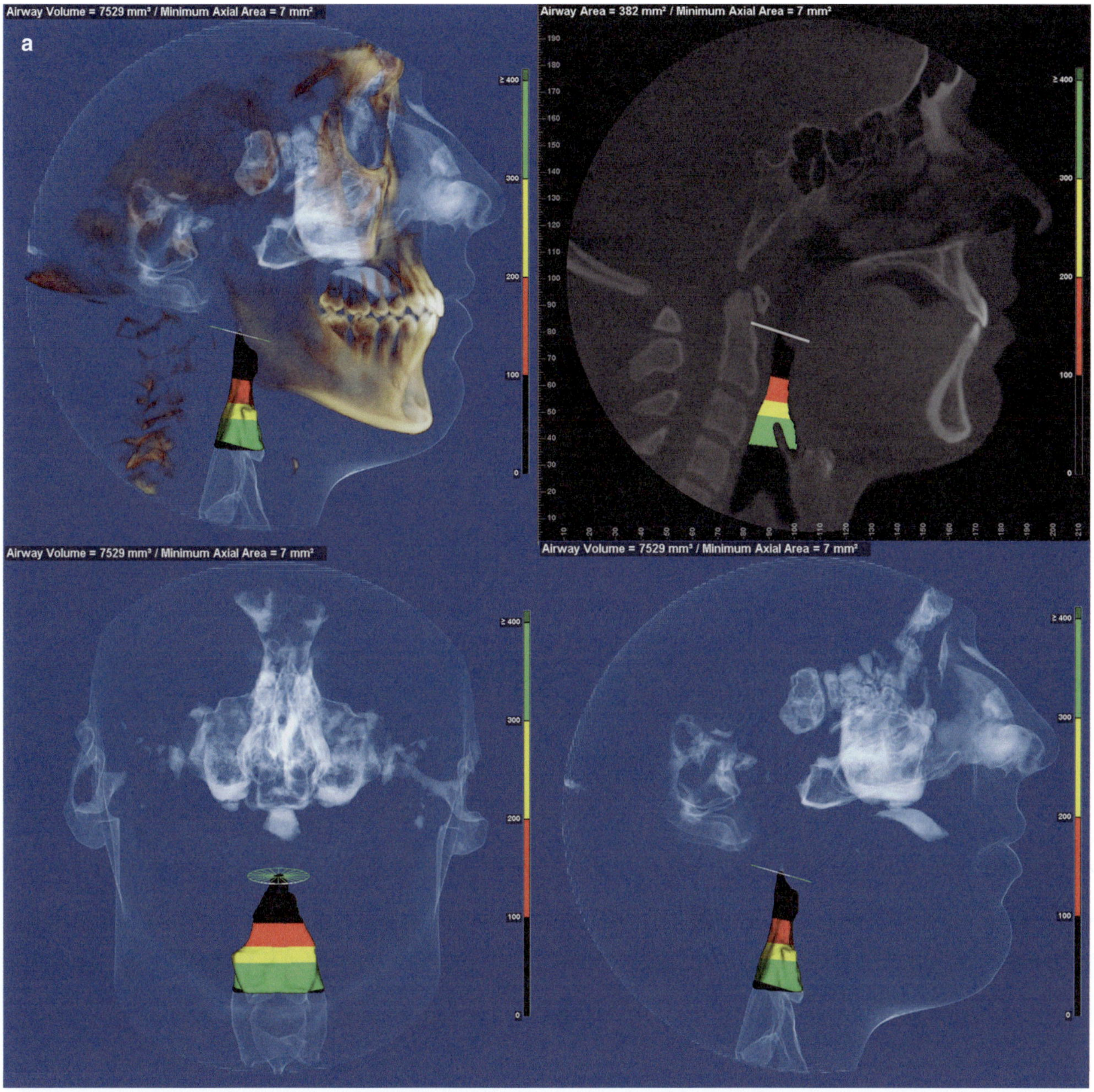

Fig. 5.19 Three-dimensional rendering images of the upper airway with cone beam computed tomography for one patient. (**a**) Resting Breathing: Sagittal view during a cycle of resting breathing showing the upper airway volume. (**b**) Same patient with oral appliance showing an increase in airway volume

evaluated ten patients with moderate or severe OSA who underwent MMA surgery by preoperative and postoperative cone beam computed tomography scans and polysomnograms. The volume of the UAS increased significantly by 237% as a result of the MMA. The retropalatal volume increased more than retroglossal volume, 361–165% [27]. Volumetric morphological changes of upper airway after MMA for OSA patients were assessed using CBCT. It was shown that MMA increased airway total volume (Fig. 5.20) [47].

5.5.1.4 Upper Airway Stimulation

A relatively novel and cutting edge treatment is upper airway electrical stimulation (UAS) therapy using a fully implanted system. The Inspire implant (Inspire Medical Systems, Inc., Maple Grove, MN and FDA approved in April 2014) is offered for the treatment of moderate-to-severe obstructive sleep apnea who cannot use CPAP therapy, and is known to decrease the severity and symptoms of OSA in selected patients [49–51]. The therapeutic approach, as initially described, is to deliver stimulation to the hypo-

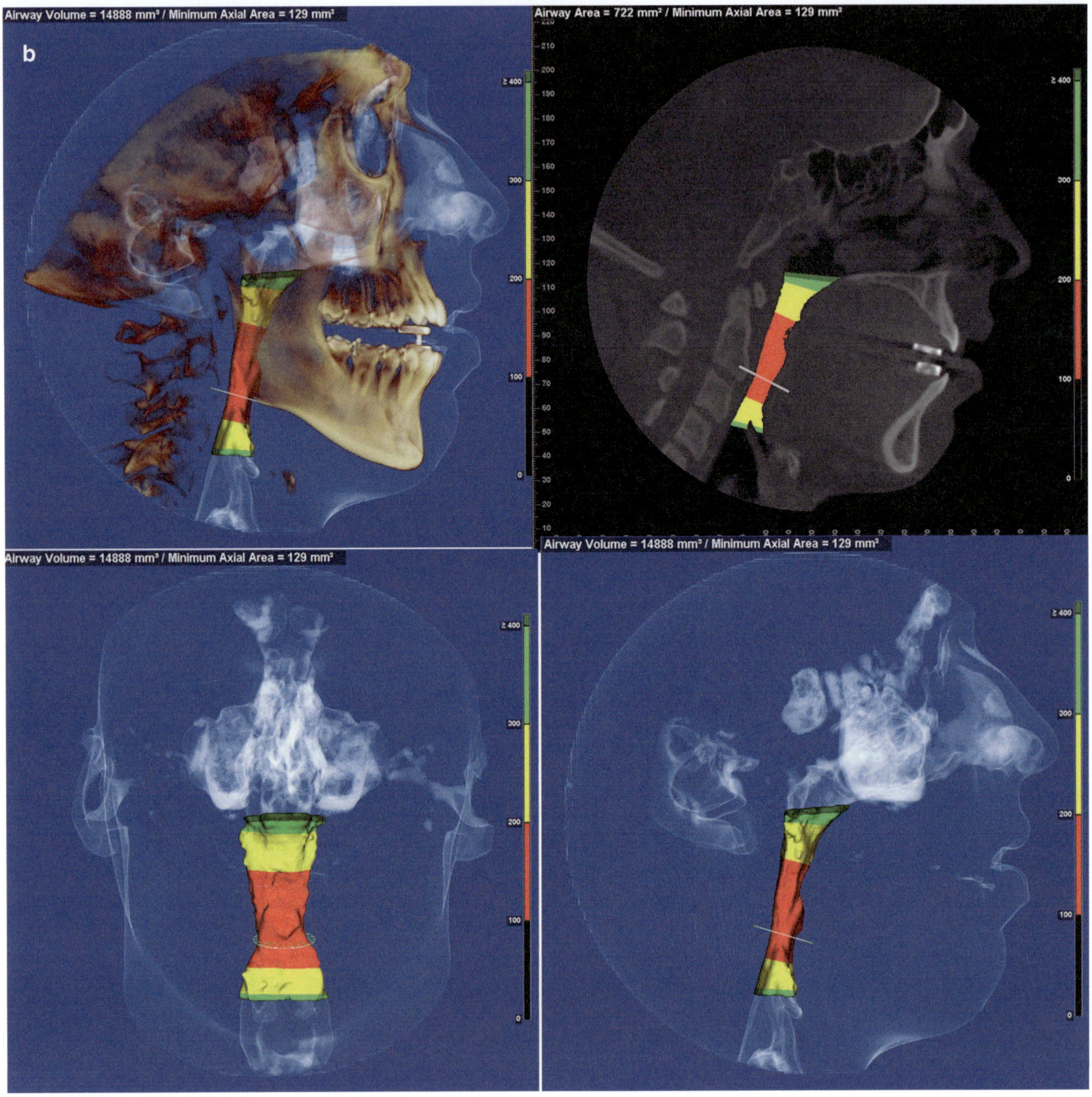

Fig. 5.19 (continued)

glossal nerve, synchronized with breathing efforts [45].The patient can turn the therapy on before bedtime, and off in the morning using a remote control. When the device is activated, it senses the person's breathing patterns, delivering mild stimulation in order to keep the airway open, acting in a similar way than a pacemaker. The level of stimulation can be custom to each patient depending on patient's unique BMI and AHI. A recent study evaluated seven patients who had previously undergone surgical implantation for UAS therapy at the University Hospitals Case Medical Center (Cleveland, OH); all were regularly using therapy. Subjects were evaluated by CBCT scans. The first scan was taken during a cycle of resting breathing. The second scan was taken during stimulation at voltage amplitude at or near that used therapeutically during sleep in that patient. The CBCT volumes taken under UAS of the hypoglossal nerve showed a significant increase along the upper airway (+48%). The hypopharynx increased 63%, followed by the oropharynx with 54%, and the nasopharynx with a 15% increase. The average minimum cross-

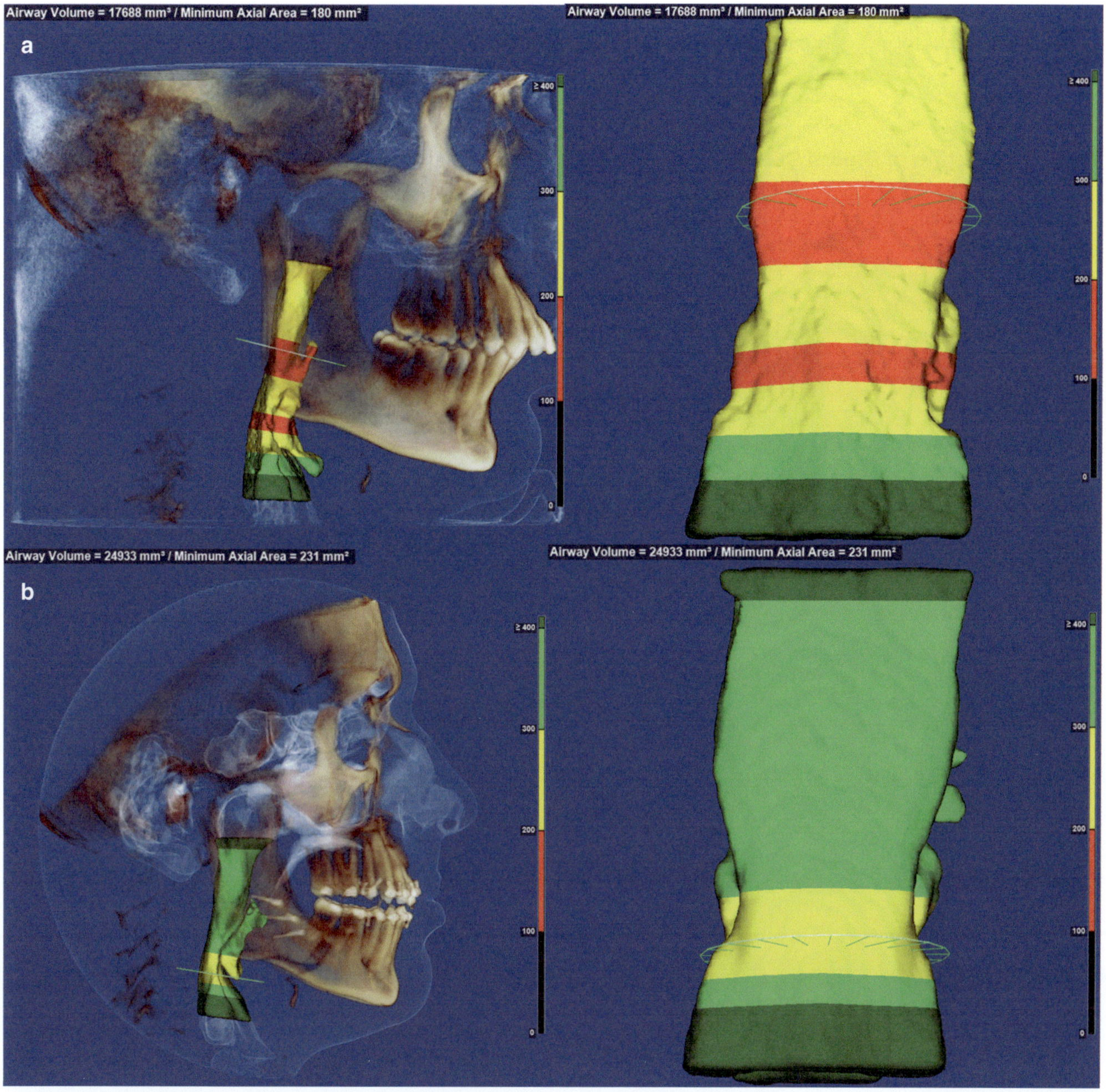

Fig. 5.20 Three-dimensional rendering images of the upper airway with cone beam computed tomography for one patient. (**a**) Resting Breathing: Sagittal view during a cycle of resting breathing showing the upper airway volume. (**b**) Same patient after MA showing increase in the airway volume

sectional area before stimulation was 100.5 mm^2 and after stimulation it was 139.2 mm^2 [40, 48].

5.6 The 3D Virtual Surgical Planning

For many years, clinicians relied on 2D cephalometrics, articulators, facebow transfer, dental casts, photos, and physical clinical examination for planning and fabricating guides for orthognathic surgery. The decision-making and planning process were mainly focusing on dental casts neglecting the anatomical information coming from the whole skull [52]. In today's practice, we are on the verge of a technology that allows the user to assess not only the occlusal relationships but also facial soft tissues and underlying hard tissues. To achieve these goals, the use of several VSP software along with powerful hardware is mandatory. Currently existing software show similarities to each other and mostly have a step by step interface guiding the user while planning the case. Therefore, the VSP procedure is not about learning the programs or which software to use, but more of transferring the clinician's knowledge and treatment philosophy using these software as a comprehensive tool in order to obtain desired results.

5.6.1 Collection of Digital Data

The digital data that is required for performing VSP for a specific patient are:

(a) Digital Photographs
  - Extraoral Photographs: Especially the frontal and profile photos help to identify asymmetry and sagittal/vertical discrepancies, respectively. Frontal smiling photos are used for evaluating the upper incisor exposure, upper and lower lip response while smiling and upper incisor midline shift with respect to facial midline. Additionally, in order to identify the midline shifts for both arches and canting of the occlusal plane, photos can be taken with cheek/lip retractors (Fig. 5.21a–d).
  - Intraoral Photographs: These photos are generally taken to check the accuracy of occlusal relationships after integrating the digital casts to CBCT data (Fig. 5.21e–i)

(b) CBCT
  - The reliability and sensitivity of CBCT has been demonstrated by several studies and it has been shown that the acquired 3D data is comparable to measurements obtained directly from dry skulls [53]. Therefore, this makes CBCT the most important digi-

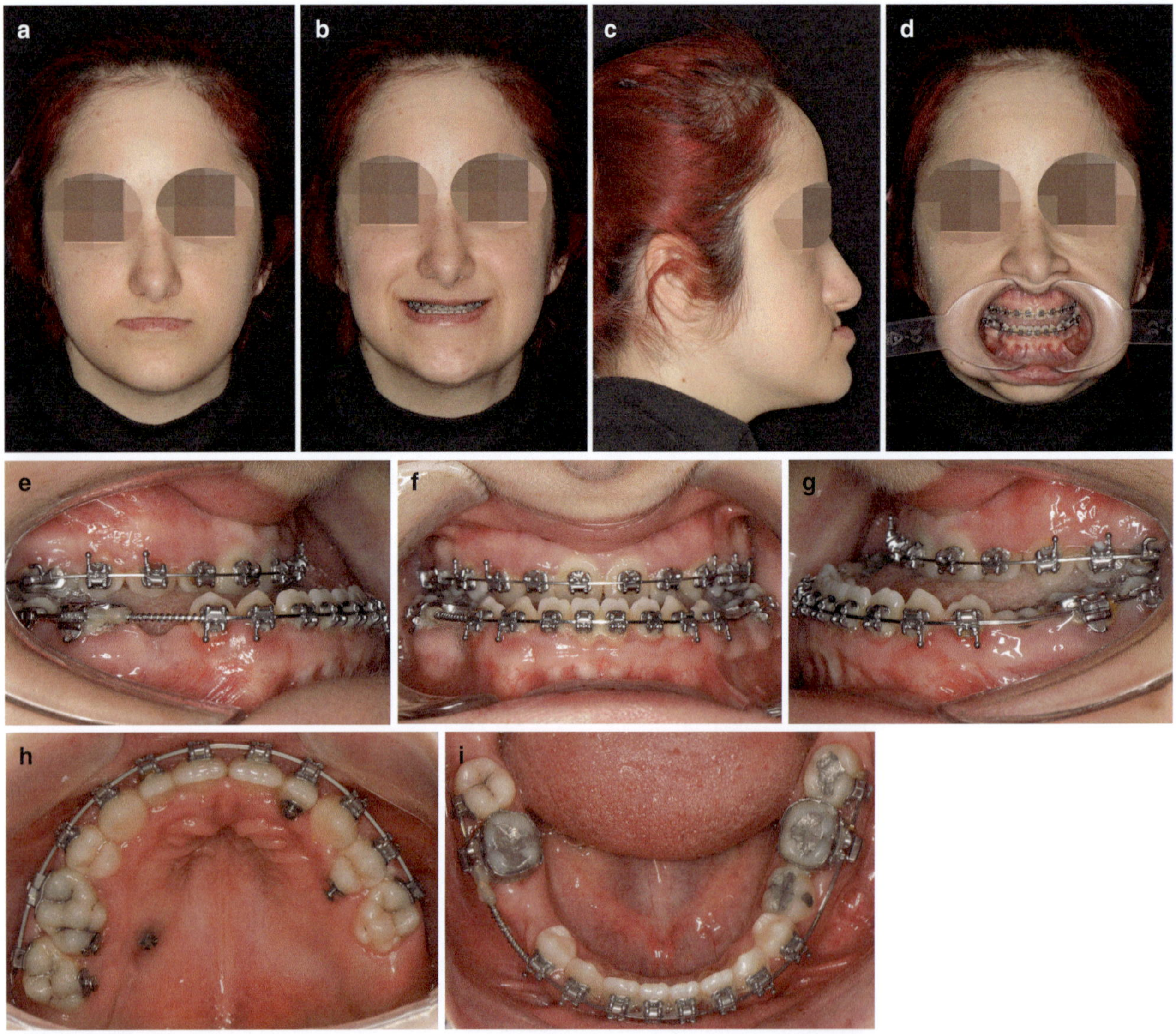

Fig. 5.21 Typical facial frontal (**a**), facial frontal smile (**b**), facial profile (**c**), and facial frontal retracted lips/open mouth (**d**) photographs taken prior to surgery for the purpose of VSP procedure. Intraoral photo series (**e–i**) do not contribute to planning phase as much as the extraoral photographs. The actual contribution in terms of intraoral dental relationships comes from the clinical analysis

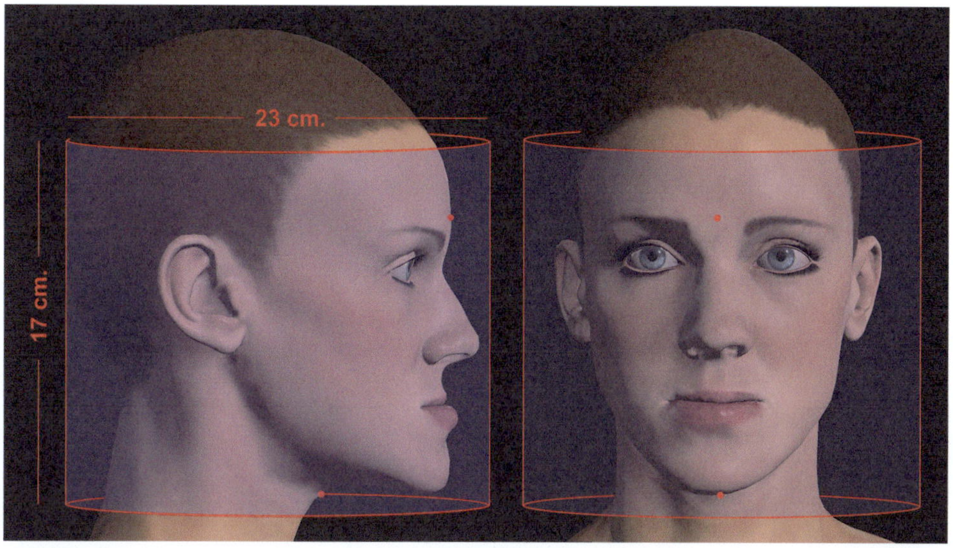

Fig. 5.22 CBCT devices with 23 × 17 cm FOV setting are generally able to capture all the vital information required for VSP. The upper and lower red dots represent the soft tissue glabella and neck-throat point, respectively

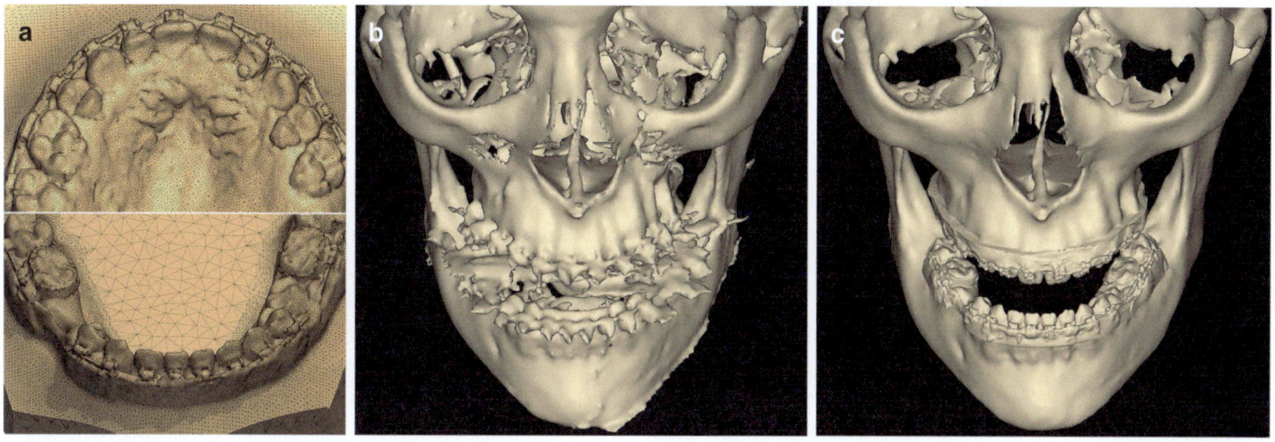

Fig. 5.23 Digital casts obtained from intraoral or desktop scanners provide accurate results. (**a**) Please note that the accuracy from the 3Shape Trios 3 scanner is approximately 6.9 ± 0.9 μm (high polygon density) compared to the surface of the model base formed automatically (low polygon density) by 3Shape OrthoAnalyzer software (3Shape A/S, Copenhagen, Denmark). (**b**) The raw CBCT data showing metal scatter artifacts at the occlusal level. (**c**) Digital casts integrated to the CBCT data

tal data of the whole planning procedure. For this purpose, a large Field of View (FOV) and related mA and kVp settings should be selected. The vertical height of the FOV should preferably be at least 15–17 cm. By this means, soft tissue glabella point for the superior limit and neck–throat junction for the inferior limit can be contained in the images even for patients with a dolichocephalic pattern (Fig. 5.22). Head orientation prior to image acquisition in the CBCT device is done using the laser/shading aligners [54]. Every effort should be made to adjust the head position with minimal stress on soft tissues or the bite. It should be noted that the final orientation of the head will be processed in the preferred VSP software.

(c) Digital Casts

- There are three main reasons for integrating digital casts to CBCT data:
  - The spatial resolution of digital casts scanned with intraoral and/or desktop scanners are better than CBCT images [55]. Replacing the dental region in the CBCT data with a high-quality dentoalveolar region scan allows preparation of an accurate surgical guide (Fig. 5.23a).
  - Considering that VSP procedure is often performed in patients during orthodontic treatment, CBCT provides insufficient visualization of the dental arches. The reason that the teeth are not accurately rendered is that CBCT scans are subject to metal scattering artifacts at the occlusal level [56] (Fig. 5.23b). Therefore, the first two matters are for fabrication purposes.
  - If a CBCT scan is acquired without any kind of registration wax bite and while the patient is in habitual biting position, the resultant dental region may seem somewhat "intertwined." This may result as the mis-

recognition of maxillary and mandibular regions by the software and end up with an error. In order to properly separate and create the regions including the dental area we have to show the limits of the maxilla and mandible to the software by integrating the digital casts (Fig. 5.23c). This is the technical reason for dental cast integration.

(d) 3D Photo
- Soft tissue skin can be obtained through CBCT or 3D photos. The construction of soft tissue skin is particularly useful to simulate the reflection of hard tissue movements to the face and measuring the soft tissue thicknesses in various regions to be able to predict the approximate response to hard tissue relocations. Currently, stereophotogrammetry, laser scanning, and structured light techniques are used to accurately and non-invasively capture the soft tissue skin of the facial region and the data retrieved from the capture is fully integratable with CBCT data thanks to VSP software [57] (Fig. 5.24).

5.6.1.1 Creation of the Virtual Patient

The VP is mainly made up of CBCT data. The soft tissue and hard tissue information can be separately processed using different threshold levels. Due to the reasons mentioned previously, digital cast integration to the CBCT volume is mandatory and is generally the first procedure to complete. Although there may be some differences, it is generally a straightforward procedure using a point to point registration algorithm such as Procrustes registration (Fig. 5.25). This step should be done with proper technique and diligence since improper registration may cause errors in the actual result and fabrication of surgical guides.

The next step is to extract the soft tissue skin from the CBCT volume using proper threshold values or to integrate the 3D soft tissue surface (3D photo). 3D photo can be integrated with similar methodology as the digital casts (Fig. 5.26). In order to extract the soft tissue from the CBCT volume, the threshold must be set to an extent where all soft tissue skin detail is captured.

There are also several other surfaces that can be added for a more detailed VP, such as the upper airway, right and left condyles, and inferior alveolar nerve (Fig. 5.27). Among these, the most important surface is the visualization and analysis of the upper airway. It is well documented that mandibular setback surgery has the potential of narrowing the oropharyngeal airway while maxillomandibular advancement surgeries tend to increase the airway space [58, 59]. Therefore, upper airway becomes an important factor that should be taken into consideration during VSP.

5.6.1.2 Head Orientation

Head orientation is the starting out point of the whole VSP procedure and thus can be considered as the most important step. Mostly used head orientation methods for VSP are:

- Frankfort horizontal (FH) plane orientation
- Natural head orientation

FH plane orientation has been a widely used orientation method for 2D cephalometric planning procedures. The main reason is that the facebow transfer also reflects the axio-orbital plane for positioning the models on the articulator. Therefore, all the records can be consistent with each other. However, for the 3D world it is not proper to use only a line passing from the orbitale and porion points because there are in fact two porion and two orbitale points. Thus, we

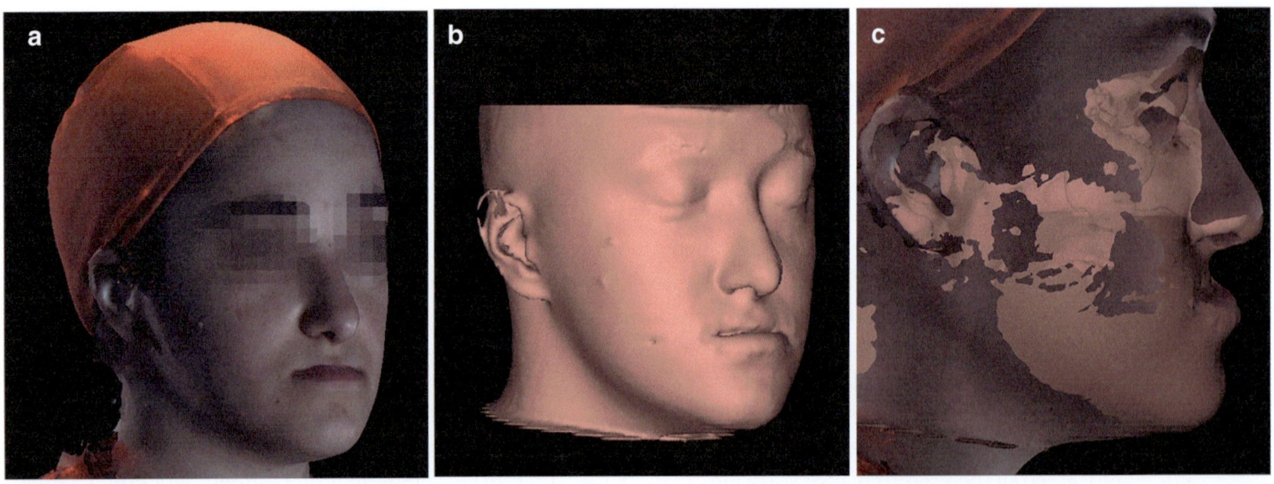

Fig. 5.24 (**a**) 3D soft tissue skin with true color depiction captured with 3dMd Face System (3dMD LLC, Atlanta, Georgia, USA). (**b**) Soft tissue skin obtained directly from the CBCT data using the relevant threshold values. (**c**) Precise integration of 3D photo to the soft tissue skin from the CBCT data is essential. If this is not the case, then use CBCT data is recommended

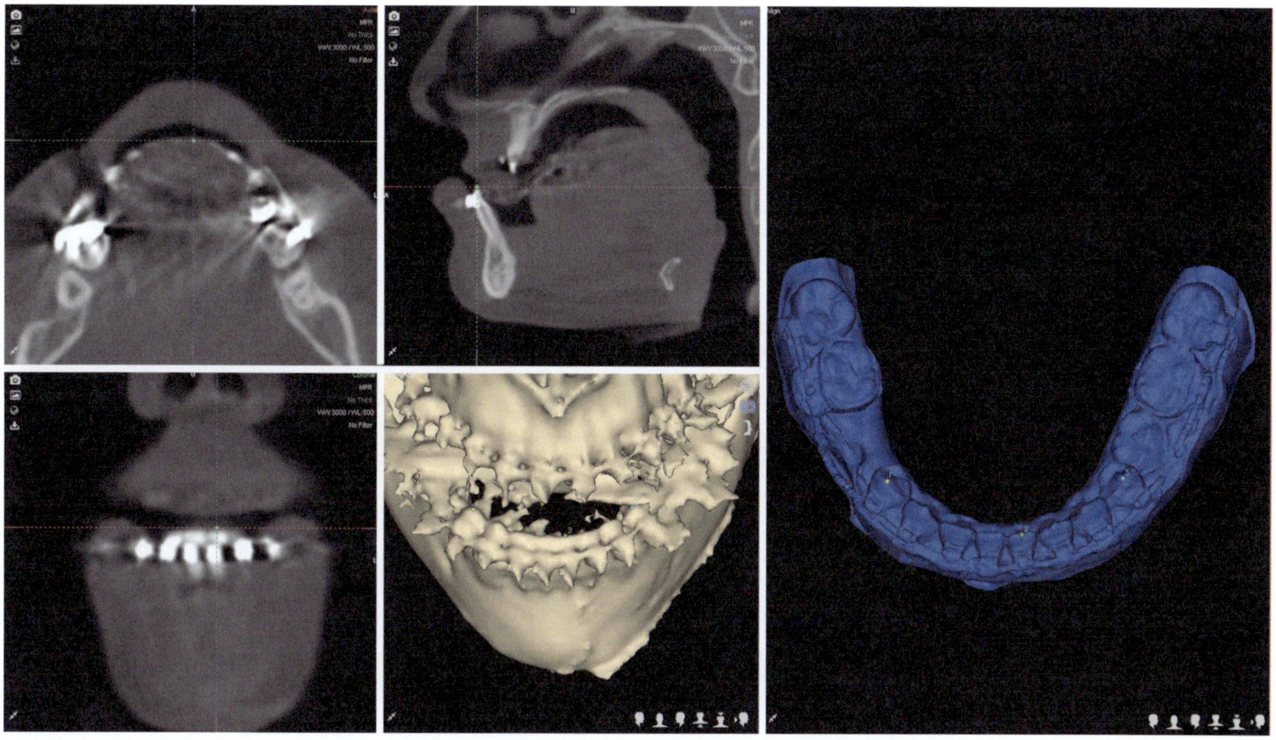

Fig. 5.25 Point to point registration is done by using three or more points. First, a point is placed on a well-defined surface on the volume render view of the CBCT data and fine-tuned using the MPR slices (axial, sagittal, and coronal). Then another point at the exact same location is marked on the digital cast. Finally, the integration is done by automatic and manual alignment

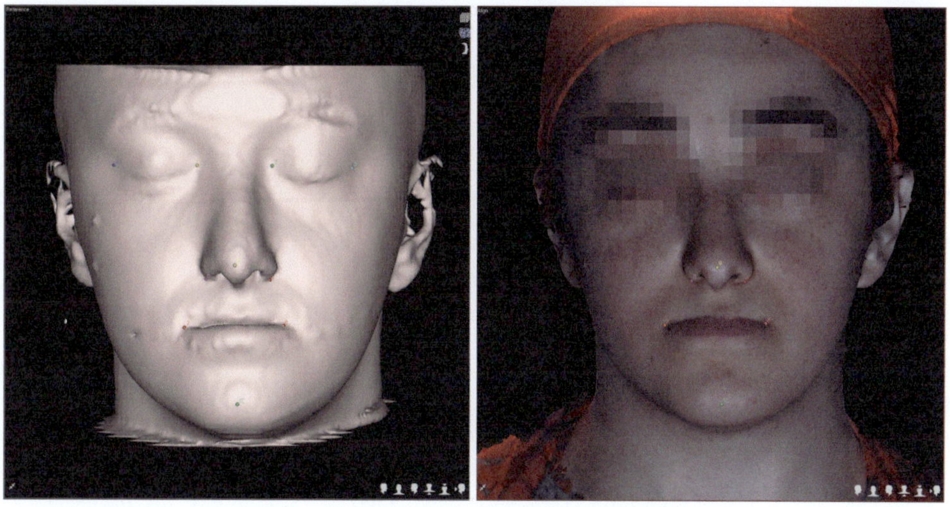

Fig. 5.26 Integration of the 3D photo to the soft tissue skin surface of the CBCT data is exactly the same as digital cast integration. Some typical landmarks that can be used for point to point registration is shown. Fiducial markers on the face also provides for a better and easier integration

have to form planes instead of lines and we have to perform this on three planes of space. For this purpose, FH, midsagittal and transporionic planes can be used as proposed [54]. This orientation method is also known to be closest to natural head position [60] (Fig. 5.28a).

Natural head position is considered as the most reproducible position and was suggested for use as a basis for cephalometric analysis [61]. It is also considered to be reproducible three-dimensionally [62]. Several methods have been proposed to register head position, such as laser light beams, mini-3D sensors, and gyroscope with fiducial landmarks [62–64]. Several software also let the user to trace orientation landmarks on the craniofacial skeleton and teeth along with data obtained from physical clinical analysis in order to automatically reproduce the natural head position. Furthermore, the head orientation can also be fine-tuned using the manual orientation tools such as yaw, roll and pitch rotational controls (Fig. 5.28b). The accuracy of the final orientation can be confirmed by comparisons with extraoral photographs taken using the true vertical line.

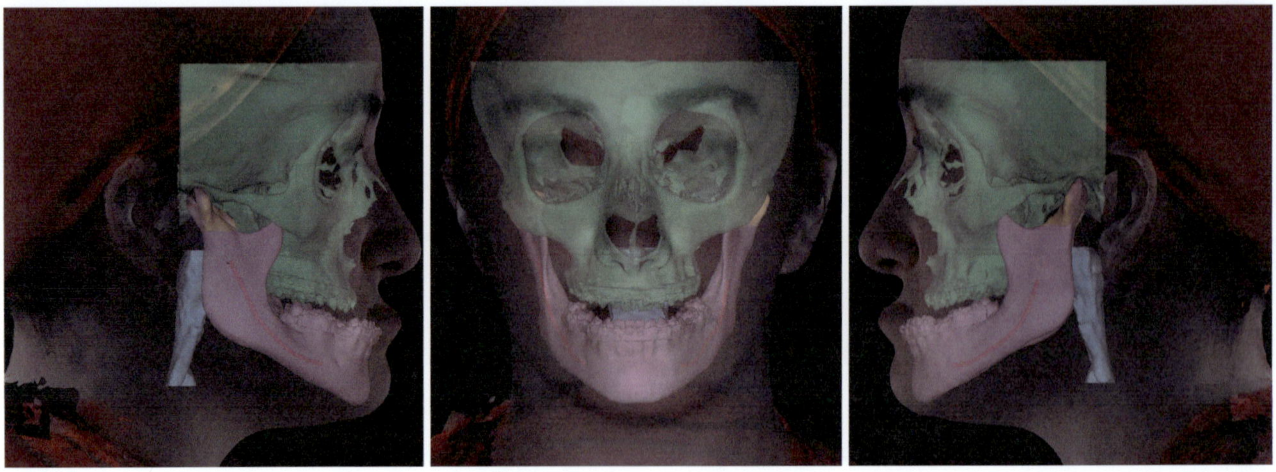

Fig. 5.27 The VP ready for VSP procedure. The meshes that are created using the NemoFAB 2019 software (Nemotec, Madrid, Spain) are maxilla attached to the cranial base (green), mandible (pink) with condyles (orange) reconstructed, inferior alveolar nerve (red), and the oropharyngeal airway (blue)

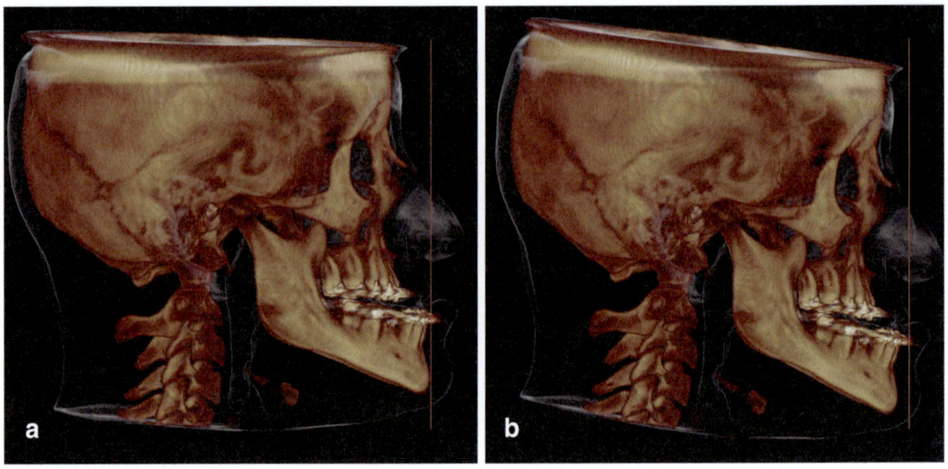

Fig. 5.28 (**a**) FH plane orientation vs. (**b**) natural head orientation using the Dolphin Imaging 11.95 software (Dolphin Imaging & Management Solutions, Chatsworth, CA, USA). Although there is a slight difference between two orientations, please note that how the perpendicular horizontal proximity of several landmarks change with respect to the true vertical line passing from the Subnasale point

5.6.1.3 Acquisition of 2D Radiographs and 2D Cephalometric Plan

2D conventional radiographs that can be obtained from CBCT data are: lateral, anteroposterior, submentovertex cephalograms, panoramic radiographs, and TMJ tomograms [54]. Generally, the most important 2D data to be extracted is the lateral cephalogram.

Lateral headfilms that are generated from CBCT are comparable with measurements obtained directly from dry skulls [65]. Thus, any 2D cephalometric analysis along with desired surgical movement simulation will reproduce true linear and angular measurements and can be reflected to the 3D environment (Fig. 5.29). However, it should be noted that only the changes in the vertical and sagittal directions of the required maxillary and mandibular movements can be transferred to the 3D plan. Transverse movements are determined according to the 3D cephalometric results.

5.6.1.4 Determination of Surgical Cuts

There are various types of cuts applied in orthognathic surgical procedures. The most common cut for the maxilla is LeFort I, for the mandible bilateral sagittal split osteotomy (BSSO) and for the chin genioplasty cuts. The osteotomy simulations are necessary to separate the segments that are going to be manipulated during the surgical planning procedure. Initially, the VP has two hard tissue meshes; maxilla attached to the cranial base and the mandible. After performing the standard osteotomies, there is one stable reference mesh; the cranial base and five movable meshes; maxilla, mandibular distal segment, two mandibular proximal segments, and the chin (Fig. 5.30).

5.6.1.5 Identification of 3D Landmarks

In this step all bony, dentoalveolar and soft tissue skin landmarks are identified one by one for the purpose of 3D cepha-

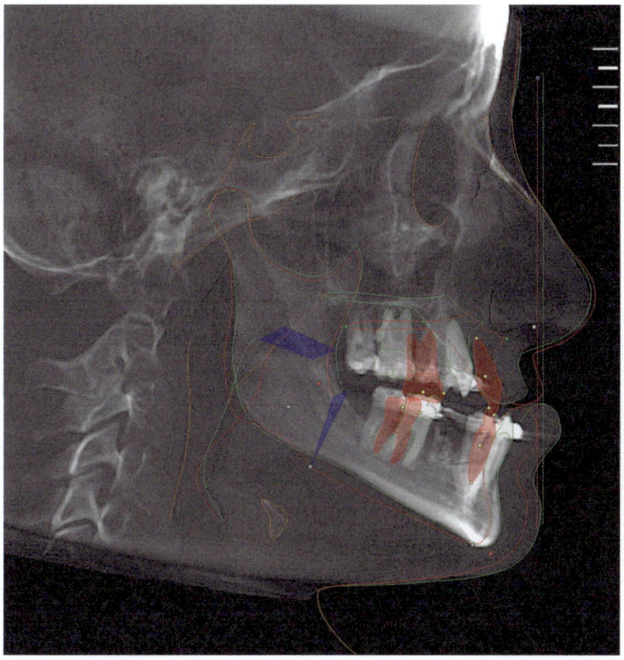

Fig. 5.29 The 2D cephalometric plan for the specific patient in order to reflect the vertical and sagittal positions of the maxillary and mandibular segments to the 3D plan. Here a 6.5 mm of maxillary advancement along with 4 mm of downgrafting and 3 mm of mandibular setback and a counterclockwise rotation of the whole complex was planned

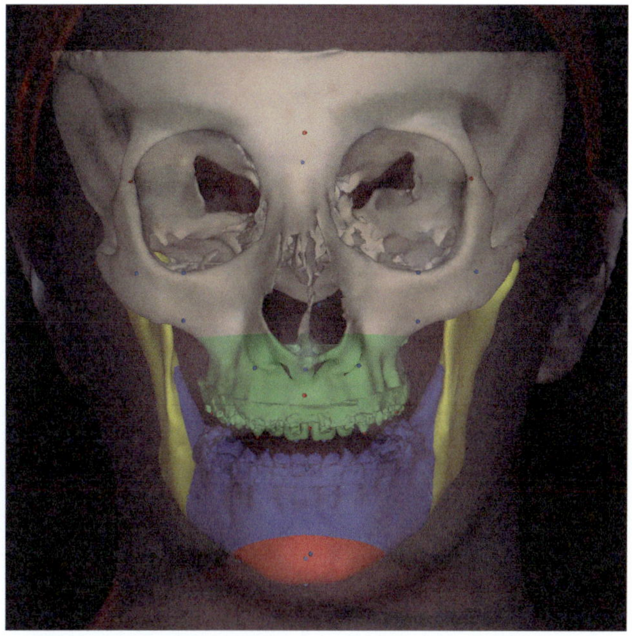

Fig. 5.31 Landmarks placed on the soft and hard tissues for a thorough 3D analysis and for the evaluation of 3D displacement of certain landmarks while planning the case

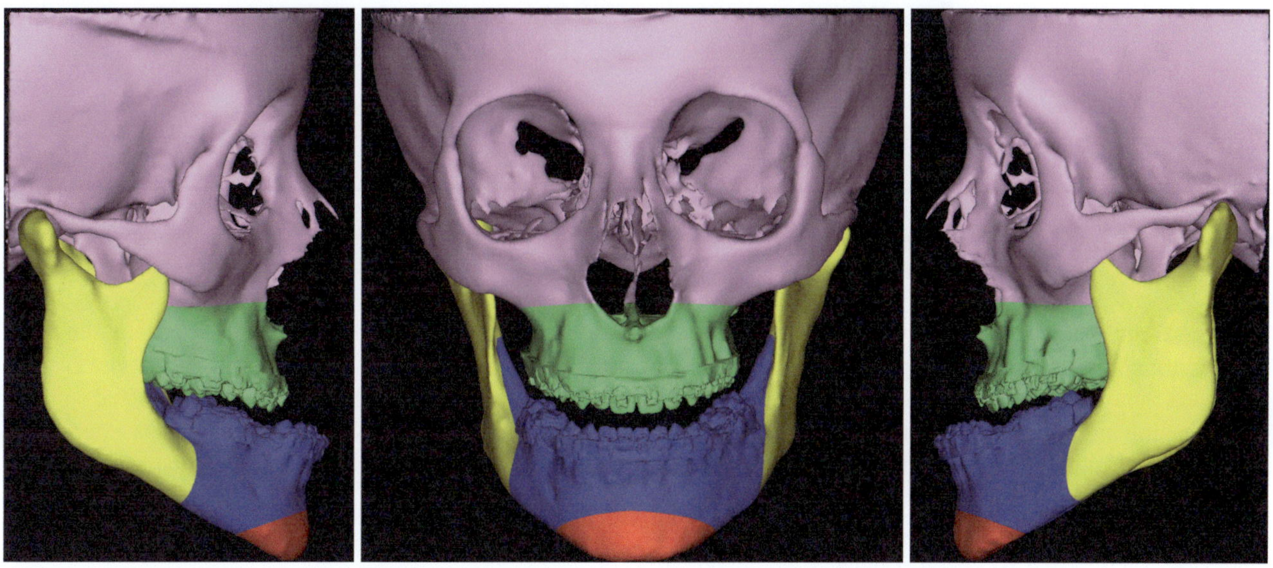

Fig. 5.30 Typical osteotomies (BSSO, LeFort I, and genioplasty) planned using the NemoFAB 2019 software

lometric evaluation (Fig. 5.31). These landmarks are also useful to compare the changes between the initial and final state of the repositioned segments. It is advisable to first determine the landmark points on the 3D volume render view and fine tune its position using the multiplanar reformatting (MPR) slices.

5.6.1.6 Surgical Simulation

Segments are first repositioned using the sagittal aspect of the volume render view as if doing a 2D cephalometric plan. At this stage, the data obtained from the 2D surgical plan is reflected to the 3D environment automatically or manually, depending on the software being used. These movements

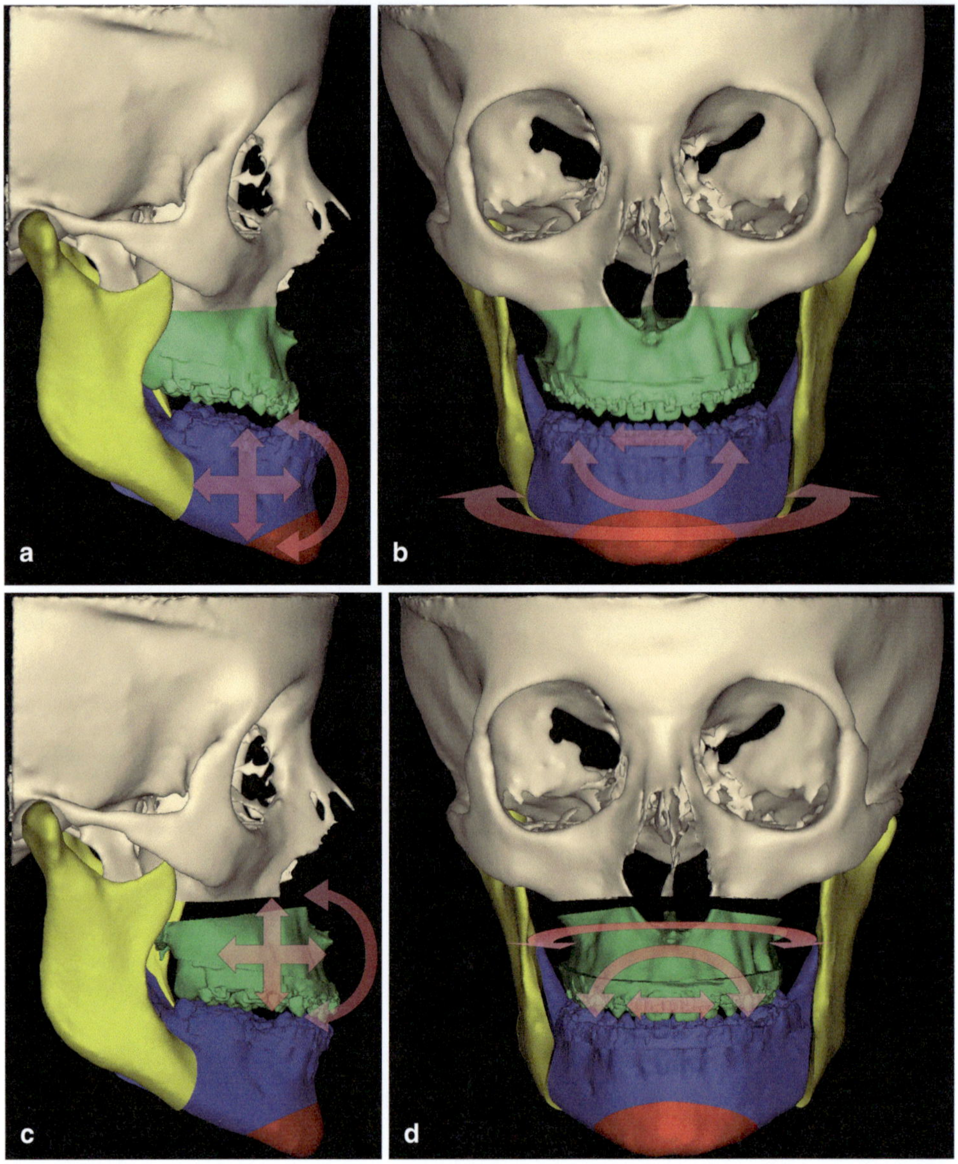

Fig. 5.32 Segments are positioned from the sagittal (**a** and **c**) and coronal (**b** and **d**) aspects, respectively. Anteroposterior and superoinferior linear movements and pitch type of rotations (clockwise or counterclockwise) are performed on the sagittal view. Mediolateral linear movements and roll and yaw type of rotations are performed on the coronal view

include advancement/setback (sagittal plane corrections) and downgrafting/impaction (vertical plane corrections) along with pitch type of rotations (clockwise or counterclockwise). Following this step, the 3D volume render is viewed from the coronal aspect in order to correct transverse discrepancies. For this purpose, several reference planes such as the midsagittal plane is used to determine the deviation of specific landmarks such as the pogonion. Deviated landmarks are aligned to the midsagittal plane in a linear fashion first and then yaw and roll type of rotations are applied if needed (Fig. 5.32).

5.6.1.7 Designing the Surgical Splints

When it is decided that all surgical movements are satisfactory, the final stage is to produce the digital splints. First of all, it should be determined which jaw is going to be osteotomized primarily. Then, by simply moving only the desired jaw and keeping the other in its original position, the intermediate splint is prepared. Subsequently, the previously passive jaw is placed in its final position and the final splint is arranged. The digital data can be exported to an external 3D printer software and the splints can be obtained physically (Figs. 5.33 and 5.34).

5.7 3D Superimposition Methods Using CBCT

In 1931 Birdsall Holly Broadbent published a technique for superimposition of successive cephalometric films to study the physical changes that occurred during facial growth with time [6]. This imaging approach also became a standard part of orthodontic records for confirming diagnosis and evaluating treatment outcomes. Several methods have been pro-

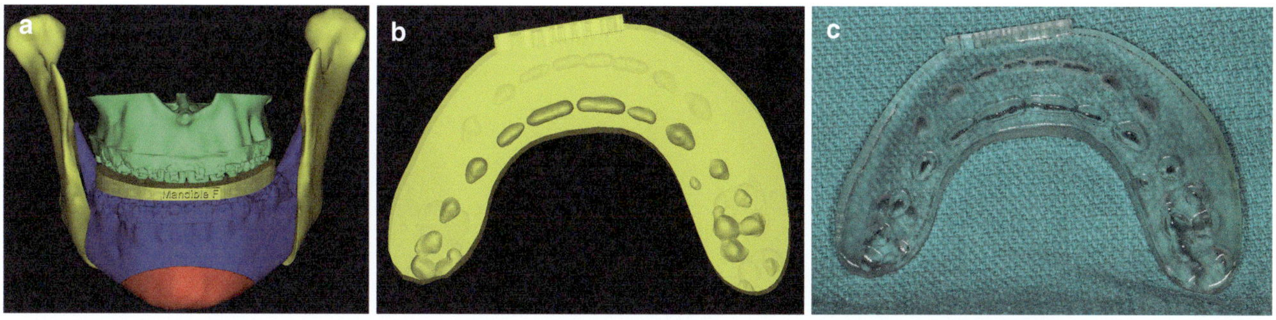

Fig. 5.33 Mandible was the first jaw to be operated for this specific patient. (**a**) Therefore, the intermediate splint was prepared while keeping the maxilla in its initial position and repositioning the mandible only. (**b**) The digital splint. (**c**) The 3D printed physical splint

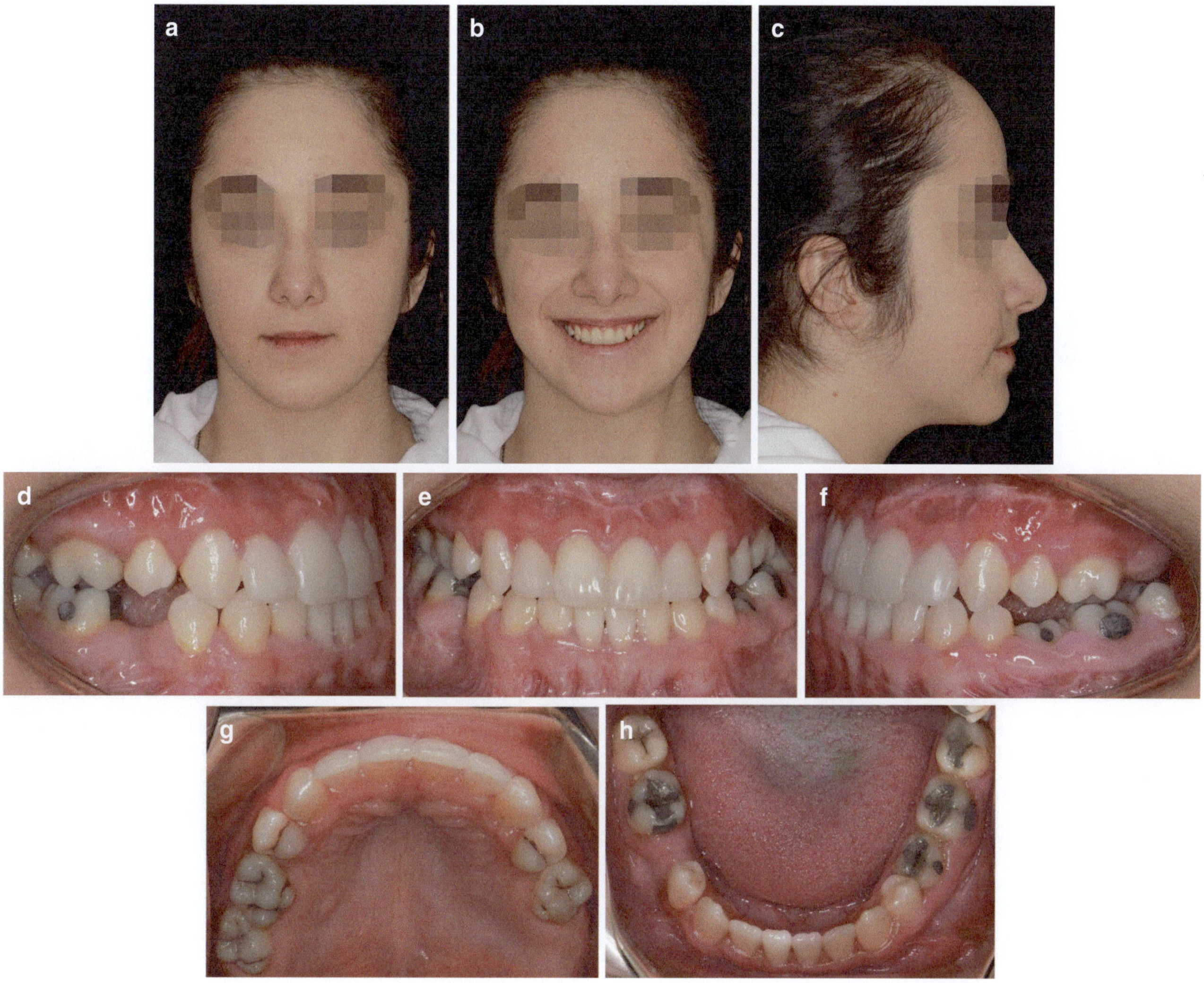

Fig. 5.34 The final extraoral (**a**–**c**) and intraoral (**d**–**h**) photos of the digitally planned case

posed for superimposing serial cephalograms in 2D [66, 67]. Cephalometric superimpositions allow clinicians to evaluate growth and treatment by evaluation of changes in the maxillary and mandibular displacement through a general superimposition on the cranial base, evaluation of changes in the maxillary dentoalveolar complex through local maxillary superimposition, and evaluation of dentoalveolar mandibular changes through local mandibular superimposition. However, cephalometrics was limited to viewing 3D craniofacial structures in only 2D.

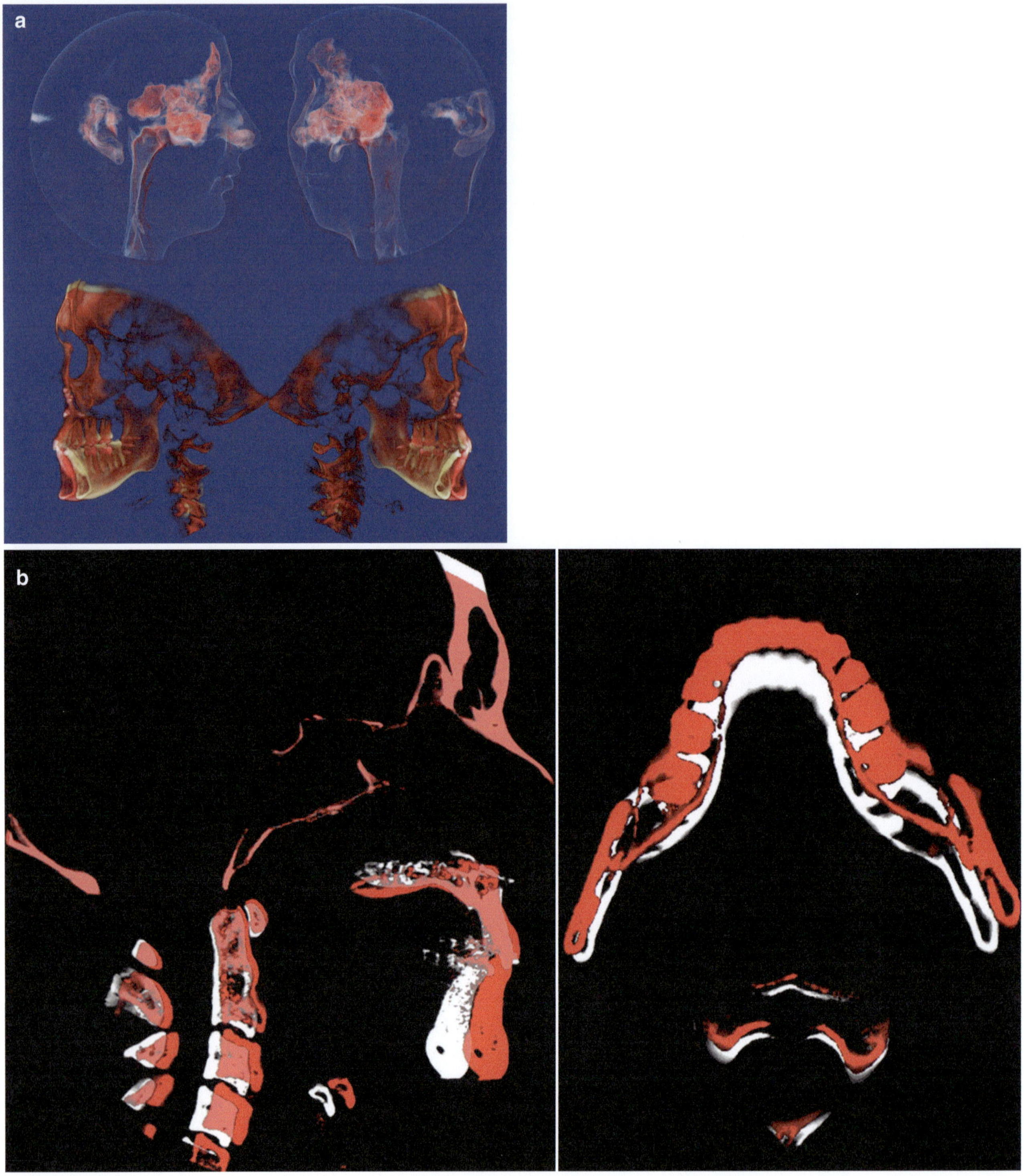

Fig. 5.35 Different views for superimpositions. 3D superimposition allows clinicians to assess the craniofacial structures in different views. a) shows 3D superimposed volume render of an orthognathic case (the red color represents the postsurgical volume) and b) shows the same superimposition from sagital and axial views

The importance of the third dimension for orthodontic and surgical purposes has been emphasized for decades, and several attempts have been made to be able to view the third dimension [33]. Recently, advancement of CBCT devices and abundant development of software packages has led not only to better diagnosis and treatment planning but also in evaluation of treatment outcomes in 3D (Fig. 5.35). The resolution of CBCT imaging is determined by the individual volume elements (voxels) produced from the volumetric dataset. The size of a voxel is defined by its height, width, and depth, and CBCT voxels are generally isotropic—equal in 3 dimensions [68].The voxel size of a 3D image is equivalent to the pixel resolution in 2D images, and each voxel contains an intensity or density of the grayscale level. This grayscale level can be analyzed to identify areas of stability within an image when comparing two images. The superimposition of CBCT volumes in 3D space after changes of the craniofacial structures over time due to growth or orthodontic/surgical treatment requires understanding different types of 3D superimpositions. With the development of software packages, different methods have been proposed for superimposition of volume images from a CBCT scan.

5.7.1 Landmark-Based Superimposition

Landmark-based superimposition requires accuracy in anatomical landmarks identification [69]. Landmark superimposition works by calculating the difference between selected anatomical landmarks on two CBCT images and accordingly the software overlays the two images. Most software programs provide superimposition tools for 3D images using anatomical landmarks [70].

5.7.1.1 Steps for Landmark Superimposition

The initial (T1) and the final (T2) CBCT images are uploaded to the software, and landmarks are placed on anatomically stable structures to serve as registration references. Each software program requires a different number of landmarks, varying between three and seven. Once the two images are overlaid, a position-refining tool can be used to manually refine the registration of the two images to reach the best fit or match of the cranial bases. Changes between two images can be evaluated through the rendered superimposed volumes or through superimposed slices. Landmark superimposition methods using Dolphin Imaging software version 11.9 (Dolphin Imaging & Management Solutions, Chatsworth, CA) are shown in Fig. 5.36, and the

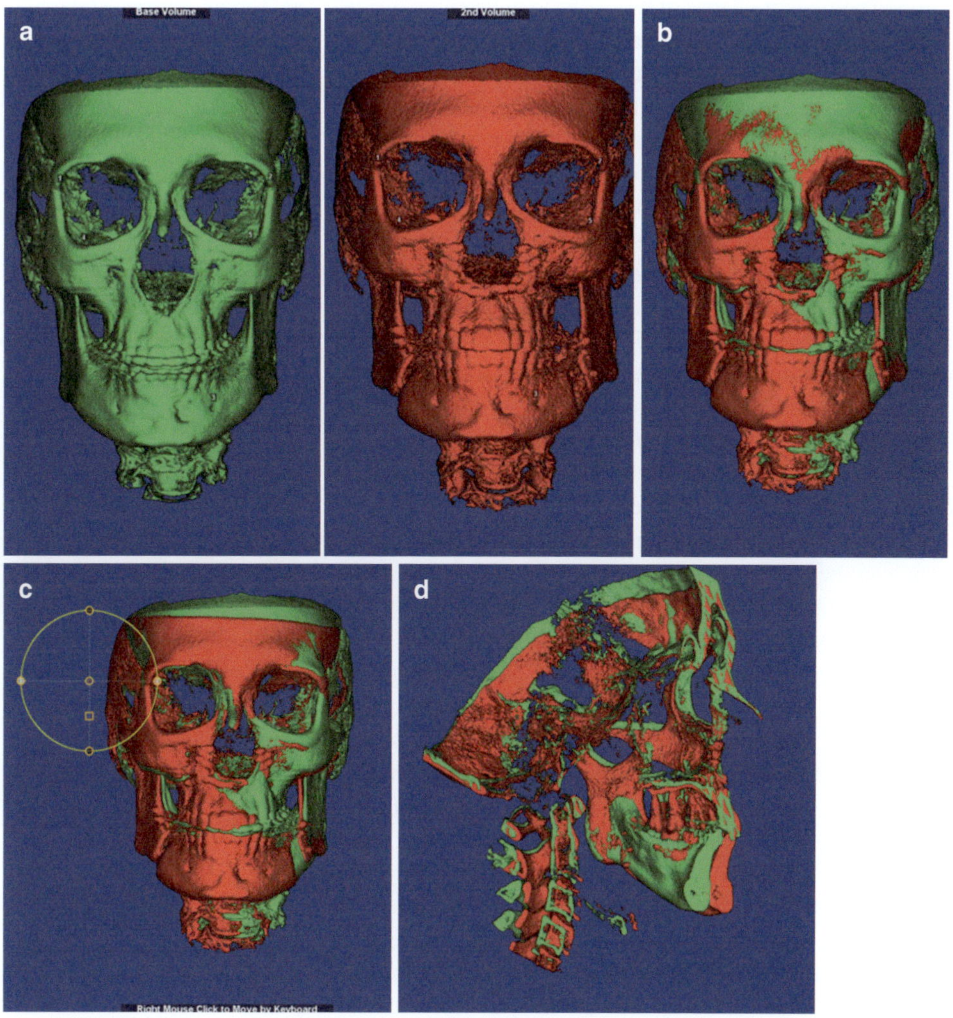

Fig. 5.36 Landmark-based superimposition using Dolphin 3D software. (**a**) Two CBCT images uploaded to the software. Same landmarks are placed on the two images as a registration reference. (**b**) The two images are overlaid together by the software after calculating the difference between the selected anatomical landmarks. (**c**) Manually refine the registration of the two images to reach the best fit or match of the cranial bases using the refining tool. (**d**) Final outcome after superimposition

one using InVivo version 5.1 (Anatomage, San Jose, CA) is shown in Fig. 5.37.

5.7.2 Surface-Based Superimposition

Surface-based registration implies separately selecting corresponding unchanged surfaces in two images. Once surfaces are selected, a manual approximation is performed by translating one of the two images to align the two surfaces. Finally, the software program performs a surface-to-surface registration to refine the initial manual registration.

5.7.3 Voxel-Based Superimposition

Cevidanes et al. introduced the voxel-based superimposition method to the dental field [71–75] It has been widely used previously in the medical field for superimposing CT, CBCT, and MRI images. Voxel-based registration method measures the unchanged grayscale intensity within each voxel in a defined volume of interest of two scans to register the images. This makes it a fully automated superimposition method, which can overcome the drawbacks of the previously described ones that mainly depend on accurate landmark identification. It can be performed using the Slicer open-source software (www.slicer.org), for which video tutorials are available at https://www.youtube.com/user/DCBIA/playlists [71–75]. The image analysis steps include: (1) 3D registration and construction of segmentations, (2) construction of surface models, and (3) quantification of changes. Initially, the major drawback is that it requires several steps performed using more than one software, which takes about 1 h for a well-trained user. Recently, commercial software packages started to offer a new tool for cranial base superimposition that is also voxel based and does not require the construction of surface models prior to superimposition. This tool is user-friendly in most of the software packages and superimposition can be performed in 30–40 s. Several studies have compared fast 3D voxel-based superimposition using commercial software programs with the Cevidanes method, which is considered the gold standard for voxel-based superimposition. Bazina et al. [76] compared the fast 3D voxel superimposition on the cranial base using Dolphin 3D software (version 11.9, Dolphin Imaging & Management Solutions, Chatsworth, CA) to the Cevidanes method using a sample of non-growing surgical patients to assess the accuracy of the software. No clinically significant differences were found between the two programs. Another study validated the method for fast 3D superimposition of CBCT images of growing patients and adults using commercial software (OnDemand3D; Cybermed, Seoul, Korea) and concluded it was reproducible in different clinical conditions and applicable for research and clinical practice [77]. After validation of commercial software packages against the gold standard method, Elshebiny et al. compared the fast commercial software packages. It was concluded that there were no clinically significant differences between the programs [78]. Eliliwi et al. [79] evaluated the effect of changing kVp, mA, and voxel size on the accuracy of voxel-based superimposition on the anterior cranial base to conclude that using different CBCT settings can affect the accuracy of the voxel-based superimposition method. Outcome can be changed when using low kVp values, while changes in mA or voxel sizes did not significantly interfere with the superimposition outcome.

5.7.4 Steps for Fast 3D Voxel-Based Superimposition on the Cranial Base

The base volume and the second volume CBCT images are uploaded to the software, and are approximated using at least three landmarks placed on each volume. Different software programs require different numbers of landmarks, usually a minimum of three and maximum of seven. After approximation, a position-refining tool is used to manually refine the registration of the two images to reach the best fit or match of the cranial bases. Anatomical structures of the anterior cranial base are then selected on different slice views of the used volumes by placing a size adjustable box on the area of interest. Next, the automated registration tool is performed to align the volumes using the unchanged voxels within superimposition box of the two CBCT volumes. Figure 5.38 shows the voxel-based superimposition method using Dolphin software program.

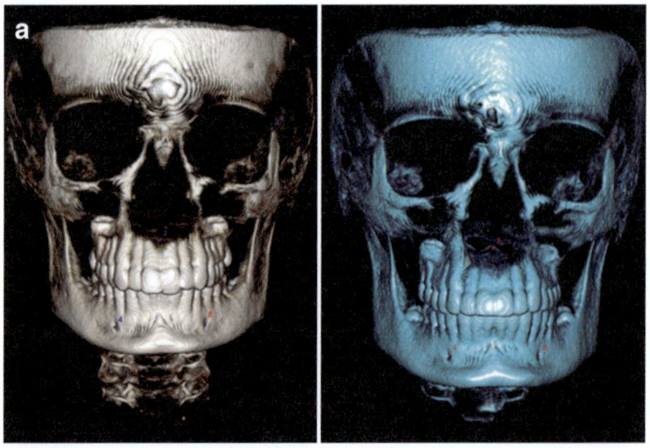

Fig. 5.37 (**a**) Two CBCT images uploaded to the software. Same landmarks are placed on the two images as a registration reference. (**b**)The two images are overlaid together by the software after calculating the difference between the selected anatomical landmarks. (**c**) Manually refine the registration of the two images to reach the best fit or match of the cranial bases using the refining tool

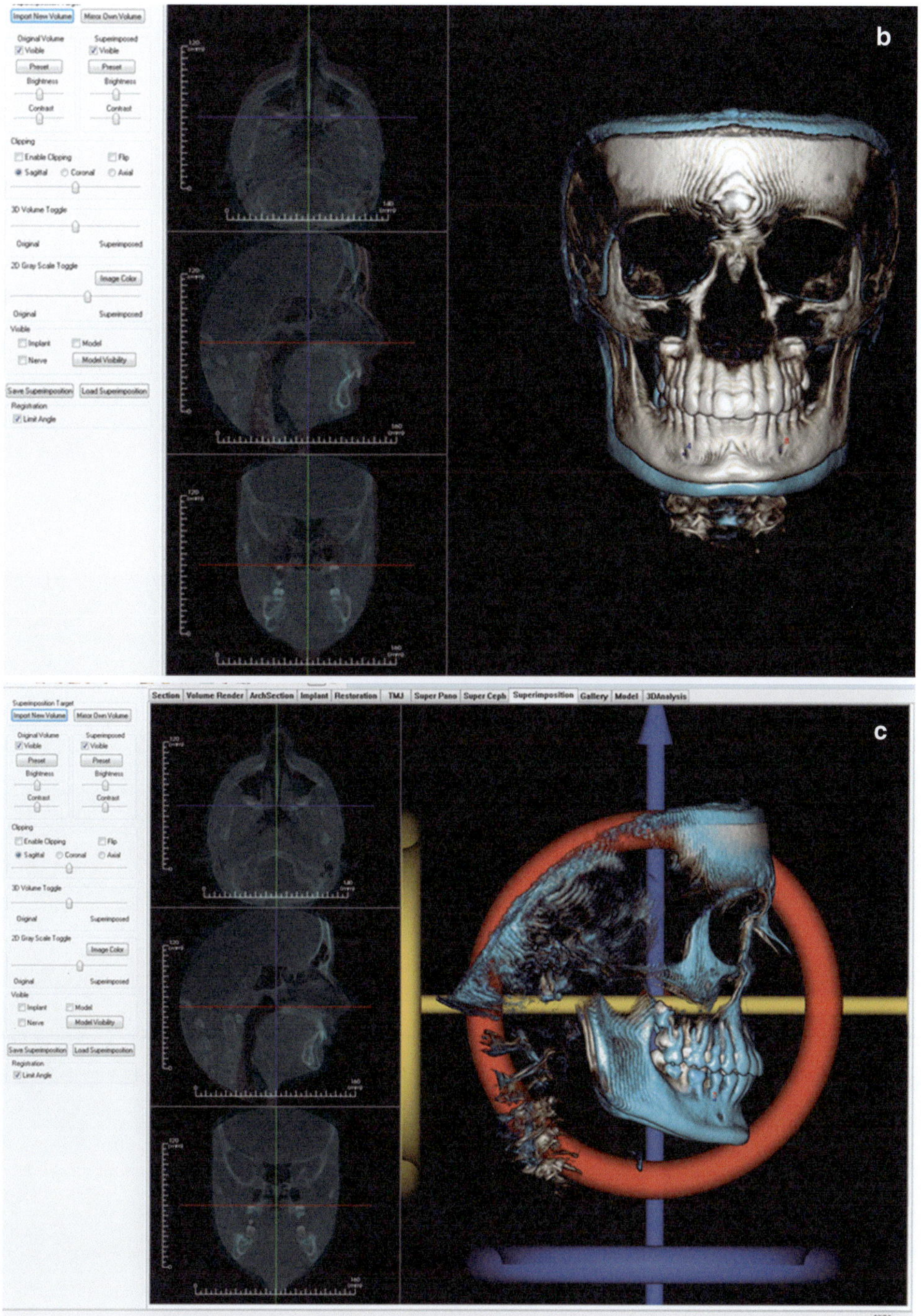

Fig. 5.37 (continued)

5.7.5 Superimposition Assessment

Color maps: After complete registration of the two volumes, the outcome can be assessed based on the absolute value of the maximum distance between surfaces, and then graphically displayed as color maps. Colored segments corresponding to the distance (mm) are used to highlight the differences between the two surfaces in the regions of interest (Fig. 5.39). Another method to assess the superimposition is by visualizing of the semitransparent surface models, axial, sagittal and coronal cross-sectional slices of the base and second volumes (Fig. 5.40). Figures 5.41 and 5.42 show different views of 3D superimposition that can be assessed in volume rendering and different slices to allow clinicians to evaluate and assess their treatment outcome.

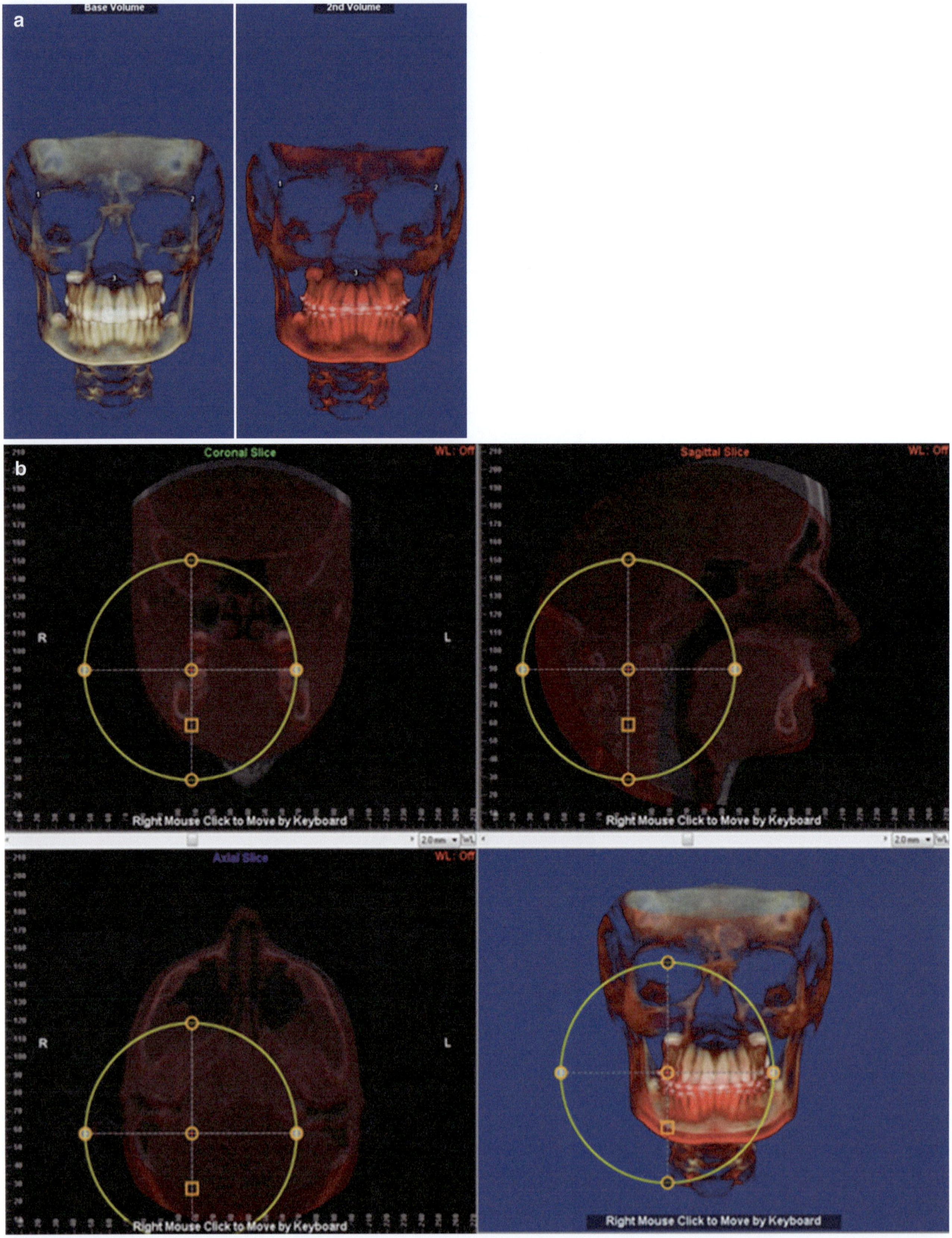

Fig. 5.38 Voxel-based superimposition. (**a**) Approximation of the two CBCT images using at landmarks placed on each volume. (**b**) Selection of the anterior cranial base on different slices views of the used volumes by placing a size adjustable box on the area of interest. (**c**) Final superimposition image after aligning the volumes using the unchanged voxels within superimposition box of the two CBCT volumes. (**d**) Final superimposition viewed in volumetric mode

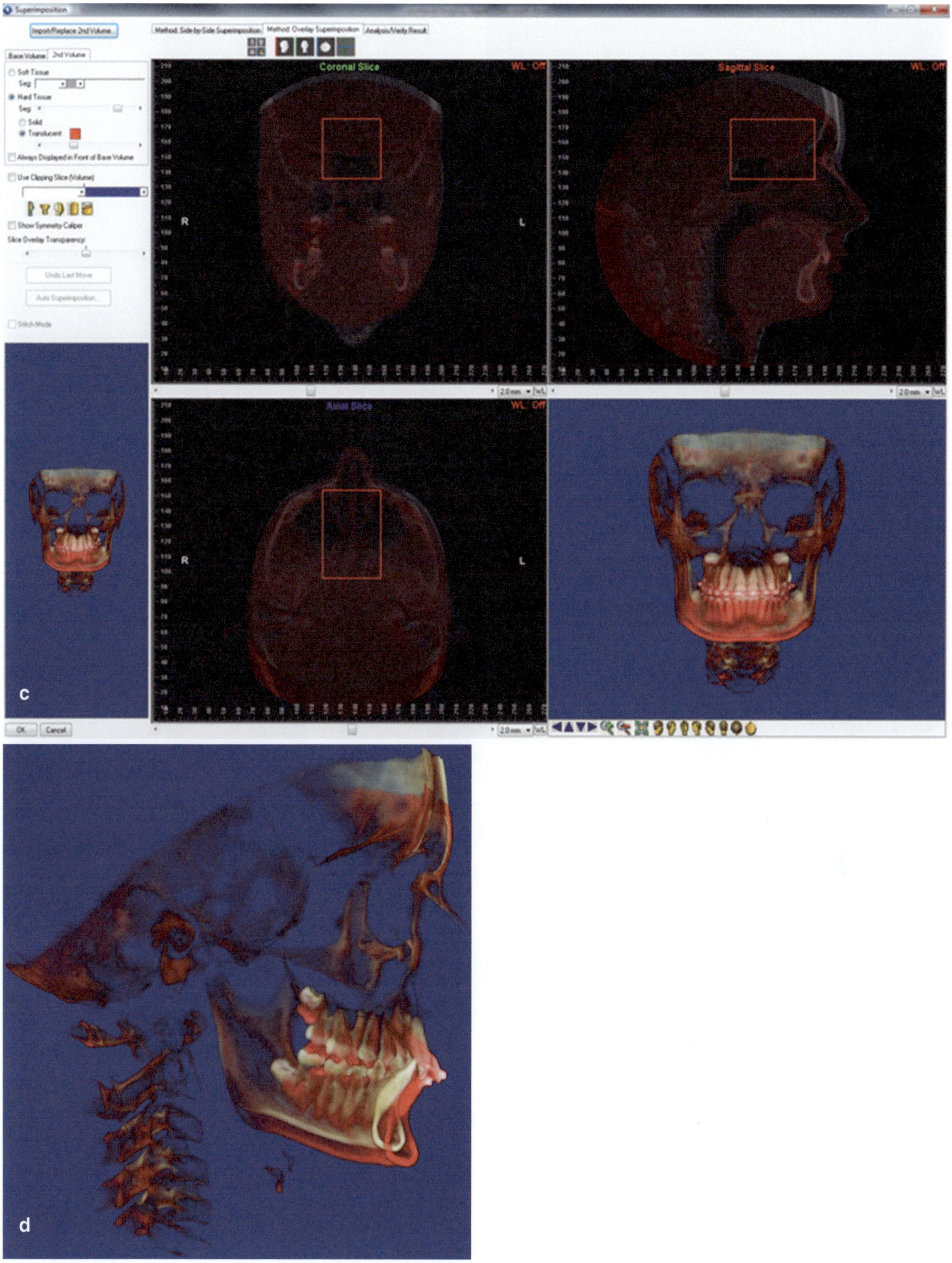

Fig. 5.38 (continued)

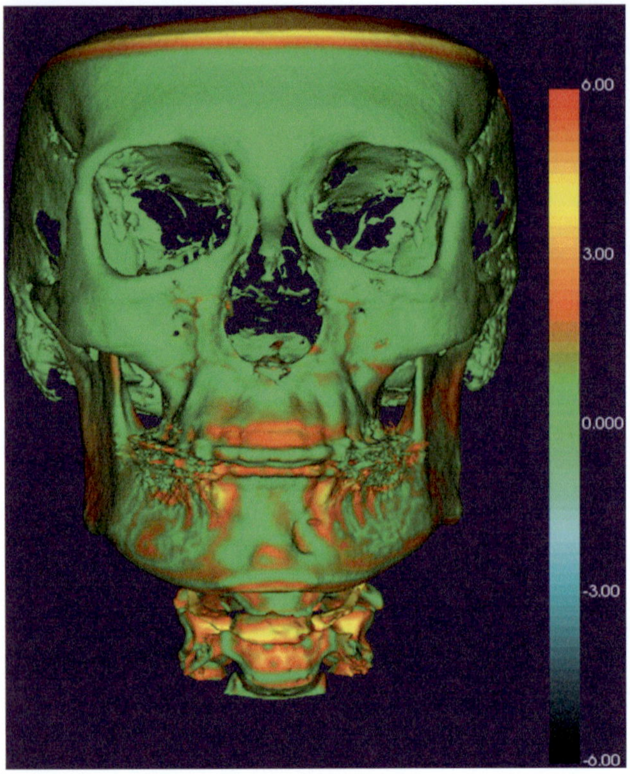

Fig. 5.39 Colormap showing the changes before and after surgery

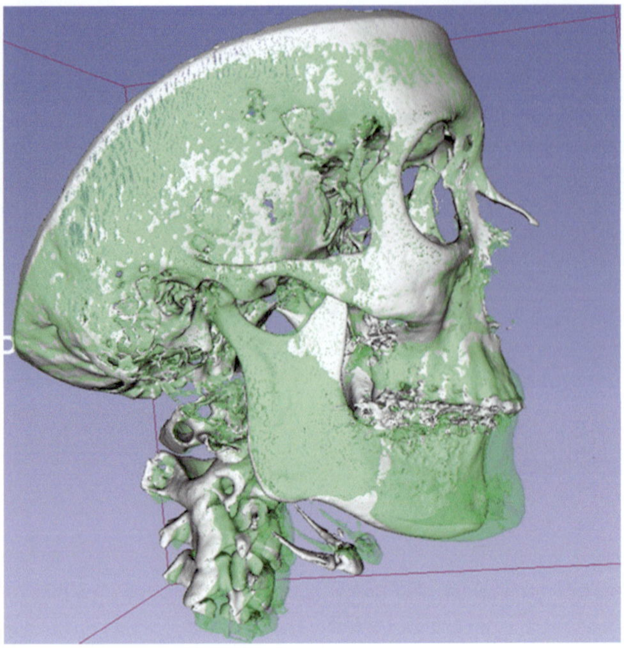

Fig. 5.40 CBCT superimposition of the same patient showing the presurgical surface in white and the postsurgical surface in semitransparent green color, showing the changes after mandibular advancement and maxillary rotation

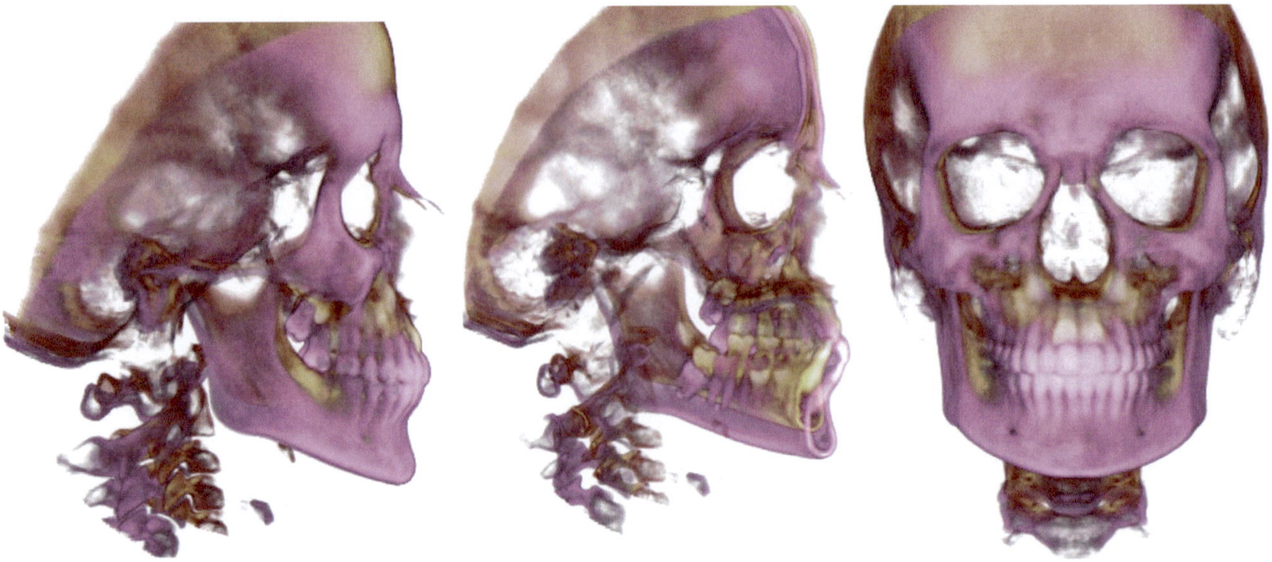

Fig. 5.41 3D superimposition allows clinicians to assess the craniofacial structures in different views. This figure shows 3D superimposed volume render of a growing patient (the purple color represents the second time point)

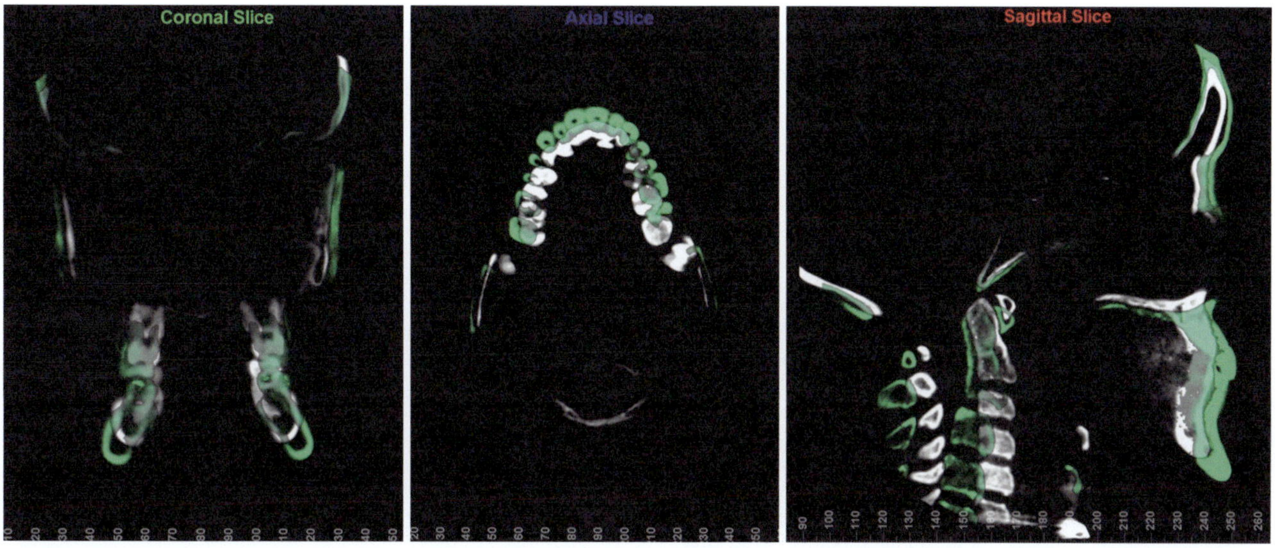

Fig. 5.42 3D superimposition of a growing patient (the green color represents the second time point) showing the changes in a sagittal view, coronal view, and an axial view

5.8 Conclusions

The introduction of the CBCT into everyday orthodontic practice made 3D cephalometry a reality. Landmarks can now be identified in the sagittal, vertical, and transverse dimension of the 3D image. This has significantly reduced errors in the lateral, but even more frontal cephalometric analyses, improving orthodontists' diagnostic ability and enhancing treatment planning. Moreover, it has become possible to analyze upper airway in all three planes of space, allowing clinicians to evaluate different OSA treatment modalities, like the CPAP machines, oral appliances, MMA surgery, or upper airway stimulation. Three-dimensional surgical planning which incorporates CBCT images, digital models, and photographs enables the creation of the virtual patient for which different surgical movements in the three planes of space can be planned and a surgical splint designed and exported for 3D printing. Finally, 3D images can be superimposed using different methods that are landmark, surface or voxel based, and analyzed numerically or graphically.

References

1. Broadbent BH. The face of the normal child. Angle Orthod. 1937;7:183–208.
2. Todd TW. The orthodontic value of research and observations in developmental growth of the face. Angle Orthod. 1931;1:67–9.
3. Todd TW, Broadbent BH, Turner OA. Growth of the pharyngeal tonsil. Anat Rec. 1934;58:41.
4. Broadbent BH. Measurement of dentofacial changes in relation to the cranium. In: Dewey M, Anderson GM, editors. Practical orthodontia. 5th ed. St Louis: C. V. Mosby; 1935. p. 184–204.
5. Broadbent BH. Investigations on the orbital plane. Dent Cosmos. 1927;69:797–805.
6. Broadbent BH. A new x-ray technique and its application to orthodontia. Angle Orthod. 1931;1:45–66.
7. Bourriau J, Bidange G, Foucart JM. Measurement errors in 2D cephalometrics. Orthod Fr. 2012;83:23–36.4.
8. Major PW, Johnson DE, Hesse KL, Glover KE. Landmark identification error in posterior anterior cephalometrics. Angle Orthod. 1994;64:447–54.
9. Zamora N, Llamas JM, Cibrian R, Gandia JL, Paredes V. Cephalometric measurements from 3D reconstructed images compared with conventional 2D images. Angle Orthod. 2011;81:856–64.
10. Lagravere MO, Gordon JM, Flores-Mir C, Carey J, Heo G, Major PW. Cranial base foramen location accuracy and reliability in cone-beam computerized tomography. Am J Orthod Dentofac Orthop. 2011;139:e203–10.
11. De Oliveira AE, Cevidanes LH, Phillips C, Motta A, Burke B, Tyndall D. Observer reliability of three-dimensional cephalometric landmark identification on cone-beam computerized tomography. Oral Surg Oral Med Oral Pathol Oral Radiol Endod. 2009;107:256–65.
12. Nur RB, Çakan DG, Arun T. Evaluation of facial hard and soft tissue asymmetry using cone-beam computed tomography. Am J Orthod Dentofac Orthop. 2016;149:225–37.
13. Park JU, Kook YA, Kim Y. Assessment of asymmetry in a normal occlusion sample and asymmetric patients with three-dimensional cone beam computed tomography: a study for a transverse reference plane. Angle Orthod. 2012;82:860–7.

14. Sievers MM, Larson BE, Gaillard PR, Wey A. Asymmetry assessment using cone beam CT. A Class I and Class II patient comparison. Angle Orthod. 2012;82:410–7.
15. Lee JK, Jung PK, Moon CH. Three-dimensional cone beam computed tomographic image reorientation using soft tissues as reference for facial asymmetry diagnosis. Angle Orthod. 2014;84:38–47.
16. De Moraes ME, Hollender LG, Chen CS, Moraes LC, Balducci L. Evaluating craniofacial asymmetry with digital cephalometric images and cone-beam computed tomography. Am J Orthod Dentofac Orthop. 2011;139:e523–31.
17. Damstra J, Oosterkamp BC, Jansma J, Ren Y. Combined 3-dimensional and mirror-image analysis for the diagnosis of asymmetry. Am J Orthod Dentofac Orthop. 2011;140:886–94.
18. Linder-Aronson S. Respiratory function in relation to facial morphology and the dentition. Br J Orthod. 1979;6(2):59–71.
19. McNamara JA. Influence of respiratory pattern on craniofacial growth. Angle Orthod. 1981;51(4):269–300.
20. Rubin RM. Mode of respiration and facial growth. Am J Orthod. 1980;78(5):504–10.
21. Subtelny JD. Oral respiration: facial maldevelopment and corrective dentofacial orthopedics. Angle Orthod. 1980;50(3):147–64.
22. El H, Palomo JM. Three-dimensional evaluation of upper airway following rapid maxillary expansion: a CBCT study. Angle Orthod. 2014;84(2):265–73.
23. Smith T, Ghoneima A, Stewart K, Liu S, Eckert G, Halum S, et al. Three-dimensional computed tomography analysis of airway volume changes after rapid maxillary expansion. Am J Orthod Dentofac Orthop. 2012;141(5):618–26.
24. Rizk S, Kulbersh VP, Al-Qawasmi R. Changes in the oropharyngeal airway of Class II patients treated with the mandibular anterior repositioning appliance. Angle Orthod. 2016;86(6):955–61.
25. Carvalho FR, Lentini-Oliveira DA, Prado LB, Prado GF, Carvalho LB. Oral appliances and functional orthopaedic appliances for obstructive sleep apnoea in children. Cochrane Database Syst Rev. 2016;10:CD005520.
26. Fairburn SC, Waite PD, Vilos G, Harding SM, Bernreuter W, Cure J, et al. Three-dimensional changes in upper airways of patients with obstructive sleep apnea following maxillomandibular advancement. J Oral Maxillofac Surg. 2007;65(1):6–12.
27. Schendel SA, Broujerdi JA, Jacobson RL. Three-dimensional upper-airway changes with maxillomandibular advancement for obstructive sleep apnea treatment. Am J Orthod Dentofac Orthop. 2014;146(3):385–93.
28. Eslami E, Katz ES, Baghdady M, Abramovitch K, Masoud MI. Are three-dimensional airway evaluations obtained through computed and cone-beam computed tomography scans predictable from lateral cephalograms? A systematic review of evidence. Angle Orthod. 2017;87(1):159–67.
29. Ghoneima A, Kula K. Accuracy and reliability of cone-beam computed tomography for airway volume analysis. Eur J Orthod. 2013;35(2):256–61.
30. Kuo GP, Torok CM, Aygun N, Zinreich SJ. Diagnostic imaging of the upper airway. Proc Am Thorac Soc. 2011;8(1):40–5.
31. Stuck BA, Maurer JT. Airway evaluation in obstructive sleep apnea. Sleep Med Rev. 2008;12(6):411–36.
32. Tsolakis IA, Venkat D, Hans MG, Alonso A, Palomo JM. When static meets dynamic: comparing cone-beam computed tomography and acoustic reflection for upper airway analysis. Am J Orthod Dentofac Orthop. 2016;150(4):643–50.
33. El H, Palomo JM. Measuring the airway in 3 dimensions: a reliability and accuracy study. Am J Orthod Dentofac Orthop. 2010;137(4 Suppl):S50.e51–9.
34. Weissheimer A, Menezes LM, Sameshima GT, Enciso R, Pham J, Grauer D. Imaging software accuracy for 3-dimensional analysis of the upper airway. Am J Orthod Dentofac Orthop. 2012;142(6):801–13.
35. Obelenis Ryan DP, Bianchi J, Ignacio J, Wolford LM, Goncalves JR. Cone-beam computed tomography airway measurements: can we trust them? Am J Orthod Dentofac Orthop. 2019;156(1):53–60.
36. Strohl KP, Redline S. Nasal CPAP therapy, upper airway muscle activation, and obstructive sleep apnea. Am Rev Respir Dis. 1986;134(3):555–8.
37. Ogawa T, et al. Evaluation of cross-section airway configuration of obstructive sleep apnea. Oral Surg Oral Med Oral Pathol Oral Radiol Endod. 2007;103(1):102–8.
38. Buchanan A, et al. Cone-beam CT analysis of patients with obstructive sleep apnea compared to normal controls. Imaging Sci Dent. 2016;46(1):9–16.
39. Patel SR, et al. Continuous positive airway pressure therapy for treating sleepiness in a diverse population with obstructive sleep apnea: results of a meta-analysis. Arch Intern Med. 2003;163(5):565.
40. ElShebiny T, Venkat D, Strohl K, Hans MG, Alonso A, Palomo JM. Hyoid arch displacement with hypoglossal nerve stimulation. Am J Respir Crit Care Med. 2017;196(6):790–2.
41. Ng AT, et al. Effect of oral appliance therapy on upper airway collapsibility in obstructive sleep apnea. Am J Respir Crit Care Med. 2003;168(2):238–41.
42. Kushida CA, et al. Practice parameters for the indications for polysomnography and related procedures: an update for 2005. Sleep. 2005;28(4):499–521.
43. Doff MH, et al. Oral appliance versus continuous positive airway pressure in obstructive sleep apnea syndrome: a 2-year follow-up. Sleep. 2013;36(9):1289–96.
44. Butterfield KJ, et al. Linear and volumetric airway changes after maxillomandibular advancement for obstructive sleep apnea. J Oral Maxillofac Surg. 2015;73(6):1133–42.
45. Fairburn SC, et al. Three-dimensional changes in upper airways of patients with obstructive sleep apnea following maxillomandibular advancement. J Oral Maxillofac Surg. 2007;65(1):6–12.
46. Gale A, Kilpelainen PV, Laine-Alava MT. Hyoid bone position after surgical mandibular advancement. Eur J Orthod. 2001;23(6):695–701.
47. El AS, et al. A 3-dimensional airway analysis of an obstructive sleep apnea surgical correction with cone beam computed tomography. J Oral Maxillofac Surg. 2011;69(9):2424–36.
48. Woodson BT, et al. Three-year outcomes of cranial nerve stimulation for obstructive sleep apnea: the STAR trial. Otolaryngol Head Neck Surg. 2016;154(1):181–8.
49. Woodson BT, et al. Randomized controlled withdrawal study of upper airway stimulation on OSA: short- and long-term effect. Otolaryngol Head Neck Surg. 2014;151(5):880–7.
50. Strollo PJ Jr, et al. Upper-airway stimulation for obstructive sleep apnea. N Engl J Med. 2014;370(2):139–49.
51. Soose RJ, et al. Upper airway stimulation for obstructive sleep apnea: self-reported outcomes at 24 months. J Clin Sleep Med. 2016;12(1):43–8.
52. Chin SJ, et al. Accuracy of virtual surgical planning of orthognathic surgery with aid of CAD/CAM fabricated surgical splint—a novel 3D analyzing algorithm. J Craniomaxillofac Surg. 2017;45(12):1962–70.
53. Ludlow JB, et al. Accuracy of measurements of mandibular anatomy in cone beam computed tomography images. Oral Surg Oral Med Oral Pathol Oral Radiol Endod. 2007;103(4):534–42.
54. Palomo JM, et al. Diagnostic value of 3D imaging in clinical orthodontics. In: Kadioglu O, Currier G, editors. Craniofacial 3D imaging: current concepts in orthodontics and oral and maxillofacial surgery. Berlin: Springer; 2018. p. 113–39.
55. Brullmann D, Schulze RK. Spatial resolution in CBCT machines for dental/maxillofacial applications-what do we know today? Dentomaxillofac Radiol. 2015;44(1):20140204.
56. Rangel FA, et al. Integration of digital dental casts in cone-beam computed tomography scans. ISRN Dent. 2012;2012:949086.

57. Kau CH, et al. Three-dimensional surface acquisition systems for the study of facial morphology and their application to maxillofacial surgery. Int J Med Robot. 2007;3(2):97–110.
58. Yajima Y, et al. Computational fluid dynamics study of the pharyngeal airway space before and after mandibular setback surgery in patients with mandibular prognathism. Int J Oral Maxillofac Surg. 2017;46(7):839–44.
59. Chang KK, et al. Fluid structure interaction simulations of the upper airway in obstructive sleep apnea patients before and after maxillomandibular advancement surgery. Am J Orthod Dentofac Orthop. 2018;153(6):895–904.
60. Ruellas AC, et al. Common 3-dimensional coordinate system for assessment of directional changes. Am J Orthod Dentofac Orthop. 2016;149(5):645–56.
61. Lundstrom F, Lundstrom A. Natural head position as a basis for cephalometric analysis. Am J Orthod Dentofac Orthop. 1992;101(3):244–7.
62. Weber DW, Fallis DW, Packer MD. Three-dimensional reproducibility of natural head position. Am J Orthod Dentofac Orthop. 2013;143(5):738–44.
63. Schatz EC, et al. Development of a technique for recording and transferring natural head position in 3 dimensions. J Craniofac Surg. 2010;21(5):1452–5.
64. de Paula LK, et al. Digital live-tracking 3-dimensional minisensors for recording head orientation during image acquisition. Am J Orthod Dentofac Orthop. 2012;141(1):116–23.
65. Kumar V, et al. In vivo comparison of conventional and cone beam CT synthesized cephalograms. Angle Orthod. 2008;78(5):873–9.
66. Tweed CH. Evolutionary trends in orthodontics, past, present, and future.pdf. Am J Orthod Dentofac Orthop. 1953;39:81–108.
67. Steiner CC. Cephalometrics in orthodontics.pdf. Angle Orthod. 1959;29:8–29.
68. Ballrick JW, et al. Image distortion and spatial resolution of a commercially available cone-beam computed tomography machine. Am J Orthod Dentofac Orthop. 2008;134(4):573–82.
69. van Vlijmen OJ, et al. Measurements on 3D models of human skulls derived from two different cone beam CT scanners. Clin Oral Investig. 2011;15(5):721–7.
70. Grauer D, Cevidanes LS, Proffit WR. Working with DICOM craniofacial images. Am J Orthod Dentofac Orthop. 2009;136(3):460–70.
71. Cevidanes LH, et al. Superimposition of 3D cone-beam CT models of orthognathic surgery patients. Dentomaxillofac Radiol. 2005;34(6):369–75.
72. Cevidanes LH, Styner MA, Proffit WR. Image analysis and superimposition of 3-dimensional cone-beam computed tomography models. Am J Orthod Dentofac Orthop. 2006;129(5):611–8.
73. Cevidanes LH, et al. Incorporating 3-dimensional models in online articles. Am J Orthod Dentofac Orthop. 2015;147(5 Suppl):S195–204.
74. Cevidanes LH, et al. Superimposition of 3-dimensional cone-beam computed tomography models of growing patients. Am J Orthod Dentofac Orthop. 2009;136(1):94–9.
75. Cevidanes LH, et al. Three-dimensional cone-beam computed tomography for assessment of mandibular changes after orthognathic surgery. Am J Orthod Dentofac Orthop. 2007;131(1):44–50.
76. Bazina M, Cevidanes L, Ruellas A, Valiathan M, Quereshy F, Syed A, Wu R, Palomo JM. Precision and reliability of Dolphin 3-dimensional voxel-based superimposition. Am J Orthod Dentofac Orthop. 2018;153(4):599–606.
77. Weissheimer A, et al. Fast three-dimensional superimposition of cone beam computed tomography for orthopaedics and orthognathic surgery evaluation. Int J Oral Maxillofac Surg. 2015;44(9):1188–96.
78. Elshebiny T, ElBarnashawy S, Bennasir E, Nadim M, Palomo JM. Comparison of two fast three dimensional voxel based superimposition software programs. JCO/Nov 2019.
79. Eliliwi M, Bazina M, Palomo JM. kVp, mA, and voxel size effect on 3D Voxel-based superimposition. Angle Orthod. 2019;90(2):269–77. https://doi.org/10.2319/012719-52.1.

6 Intraoral Scanning

Tarek Elshebiny, Fernando Pugliese, Neda Stefanovic, Manhal Eliliwi, and Juan Martin Palomo

6.1 Introduction

The practice of orthodontics has been revolutionized to adapt to the digital world. Recent developments in three-dimensional (3D) digital models, digital intraoral scanners, and 3D printing are at the forefront of these technological advances. Intraoral scanning technology is now being used by orthodontists for different applications. The aim of this chapter is to outline the use of intraoral digital scanners in an orthodontic office and its integration with other technologies.

6.2 Scanning Technology

Intraoral scanners are composed of a handheld camera, a computer, and software to collect the scan data in the patient's mouth. The way this technology works is through energy from light projected from the wand onto an object and reflected back to a sensor within the wand with tens or hundreds of thousands of measurements taken per inch resulting in a 3D representation of the object's shape [1]. The measurement speed, resolution, and accuracy of the scanner are determined by the technology used by the wand to capture surface data.

Four types of imaging technology are currently employed [1–3]:

1. Triangulation is based on a principle that the position of a point of a triangle can be calculated knowing the positions and angles of two points of view. As light reflects off the object, the system determines the angle of reflection, and therefore the distance from the laser source to the object's surface, according to the Pythagorean Theorem.
2. Confocal imaging is a technique based on acquisition of focused and defocused images from selected depths. Images are projected point-by-point, line-by-line, or multiple points at once and three-dimensionally reconstructed with a computer, rather than obtained through an eyepiece.
3. Accordion fringe interferometry (AFI) uses two light sources to project three patterns of light called "fringe patterns." AFI delivers the most precise laser fringe projection available which quickly digitizes the shapes of 3D objects with the highest accuracy of point cloud data.
4. Three-dimensional in-motion video uses an HD video camera with trinocular imaging to capture three precise views of an object.

6.3 Advantages of Intraoral Scanners

Although alginate and PVS impressions have been associated with almost every dental work for decades, taking impressions is not comfortable for some patients and it may trigger some patients' gag reflex. In addition to that, some lab work needed to pour up the impressions plus the need of shipping them to labs which consider time consuming.

Using intraoral scanner to obtain a digital scan has so many advantages such as: more comfortable to patients compared to conventional impressions [4], accurate which makes digital scans a helpful tool for orthodontic diagnosis and treatment planning [5], less time is needed to obtain digital scan copy and no need to do any lab work, provide a new tool to communicate with patients and make them more involved in treatment planning, easy to communicate with labs, improve workflow, no storage area required [1, 6, 7].

T. Elshebiny · F. Pugliese · M. Eliliwi · J. M. Palomo (✉)
School of Dental Medicine—Department of Orthodontics, Case Western Reserve University, Cleveland, OH, USA
e-mail: tme18@case.edu; fdp10@case.edu; mxe181@case.edu; jmp5@case.edu

N. Stefanovic
Faculty of Dental Medicine—Department of Orthodontics, University of Belgrade, Belgrade, Serbia

J.-M. Retrouvey, M.-N. Abdallah (eds.), *3D Diagnosis and Treatment Planning in Orthodontics*, https://doi.org/10.1007/978-3-030-57223-5_6

6.4 Scanners Available in the Orthodontic Market

Intraoral scanners intended for the use in orthodontics need to be capable of capturing complete dental arches. Almost 10 years before such scanners became available, Cadent (Carlstadt, NJ) came up with the OrthoCAD™ system for 3D digital models. This system implied scanning the patient's plaster models, and later PVS impressions, at the Cadent scanning center, where they were further processed into downloadable digital files. It was the same company that introduced the first intraoral scanner that could be used to generate 3D digital orthodontic study models—the iTero® digital impressions system. A few years later, they launched the iOC system™ that could be used by orthodontists for diagnosis and treatment planning. The company was then purchased by Align Technology and the direct 3D digital scan submission for Invisalign® was enabled [1].

6.4.1 iTero® (Align Technology Inc)

iTero remains one of the most popular and widespread intraoral scanners in orthodontic offices, especially in North America where it is the only intraoral scanner compatible with Invisalign® (Figs. 6.1 and 6.2). The scanning technology built into the iTero is the scan-in-motion video sequencing. There is no set scanning sequence since the software automatically identifies and moves the starting and final scanning points when the wand is relocated. The software processes the scan and automatically stitches the images and removes the soft tissue during the scanning procedure. Therefore, it takes around 60 s for a well-trained operator to complete the upper and the lower dental arch scan. The iTero® scanner also has an integrated color sensor and the dual-aperture lens system that simultaneously captures 2D color images and highly accurate 3D laser scans. The data is automatically saved to the system's hard disk every 2 s [8].

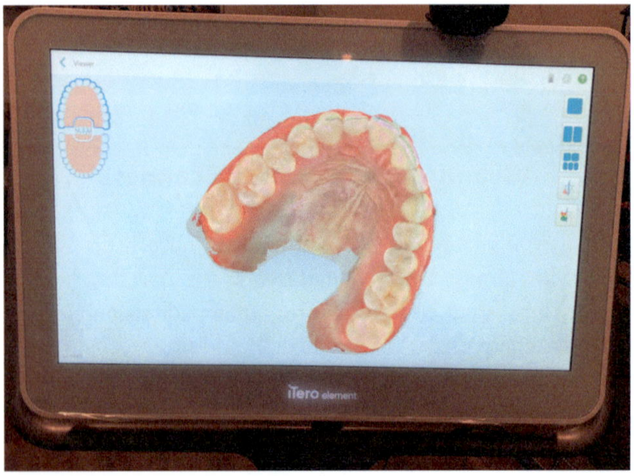

Fig. 6.1 iTero element scanner

6.4.2 3 Shape Trios 4

The latest 3Shape intraoral scanner, Trios 4, is a wireless scanner that uses the video sequencing TRIOS scanning technology and LED light source. There is no set scanning sequence, and software can easily identify and move scanning points. The artificial intelligence technology removes the excess soft tissue without any input from the operator, and the final high-quality scan features lifelike colors (Fig. 6.3). The integrated fluorescent technology enables surface caries identification, and the dedicated transillumination smart tip supports possible interproximal caries identification. Owing to the instant-heating smart tips, there is no need for pre-heating, and a well-trained operator can complete the upper and the lower dental arch scan in around 30 s [9].

6.4.3 Medit i500

Medit i500 is currently one of the most affordable intraoral scanners on the market. The scanning technology built into the Medit i500 is the 3D scan-in-motion video sequencing. Two high-speed cameras built into the scanner facilitate fast scanning, and there is no set scanning sequence. The final scan can be viewed in full color [10].

6.4.4 Dentsply Sirona Omnicam

Sirona introduced the first intraoral scanner to the dental market in 1987. In 2016 it merged with Dentsply, and today Dentsply Sirona offers two intraoral scanners Omnicam and Primescan. Omnicam is the preferred one for orthodontic purposes. Omnicam uses video sequencing data acquisition and the final scan can be viewed in natural color [11, 12].

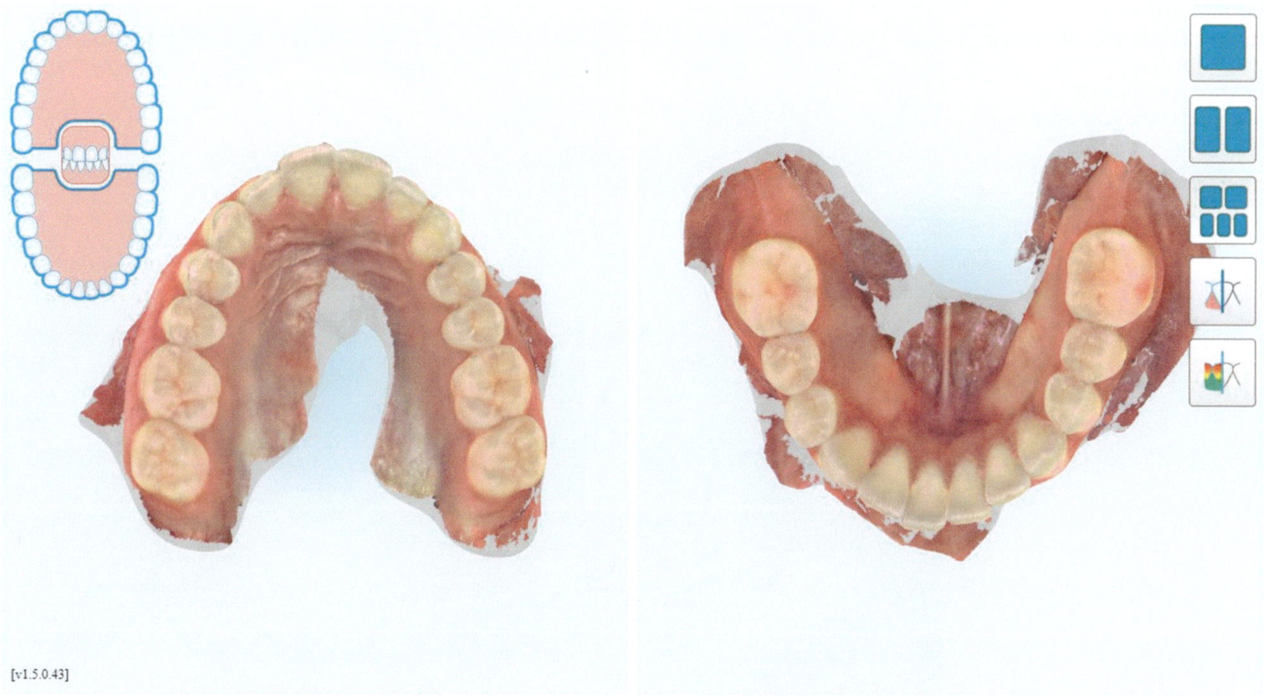

Fig. 6.2 A display of an intraoral scan using iTero scanner

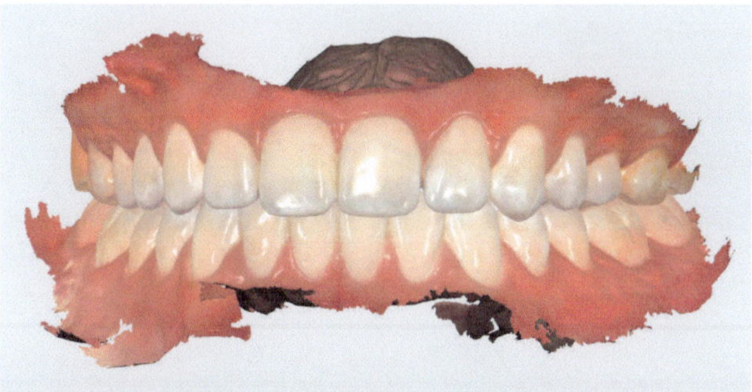

Fig. 6.3 A display of an intraoral scan using 3Shape scanner

6.5 Digital Models for Diagnosis and Treatment Planning

Orthodontic treatment planning is complex and requires the ability to simultaneously analyze multiple data obtained from different orthodontic diagnostic records. In this context, dental models are essential in providing a 3D record of a patient's occlusion [13].

The dental plaster model is the current gold-standard reference for 3D occlusal assessment in orthodontics [14]. Traditionally various measurements like tooth size, arch length, arch width, overjet, overbite, curve of Spee, Bolton discrepancy, and other different model analysis (Figs. 6.4, 6.5, and 6.6) can be performed on conventional plaster models using calipers or needle pointed dividers. In the new digital era, virtual models were developed as an alternative to the conventional plaster models. All software that provide 3D image virtual model systems are similar with respect to what assessments can be undertaken on them, bringing the ability to rotate, tilt and section models, and hold them in any position. OrthoCad (Cadent, Carlstadt, NJ) was the first software introduced to the orthodontic market in early 1999, followed by other software systems as DigiModel (OrthoProof, Nieuwegein, The Netherlands) and OrthoAnalyzer (3Shape, Copenhagen, Denmark).

Digital software systems have been carefully evaluated for accuracy and reproducibility. Scientific evidence consistently supports the validity of measurements from digital dental arch models [15]. Studies assessing the accuracy of measurements regarding tooth size, arch width and length, space analysis,

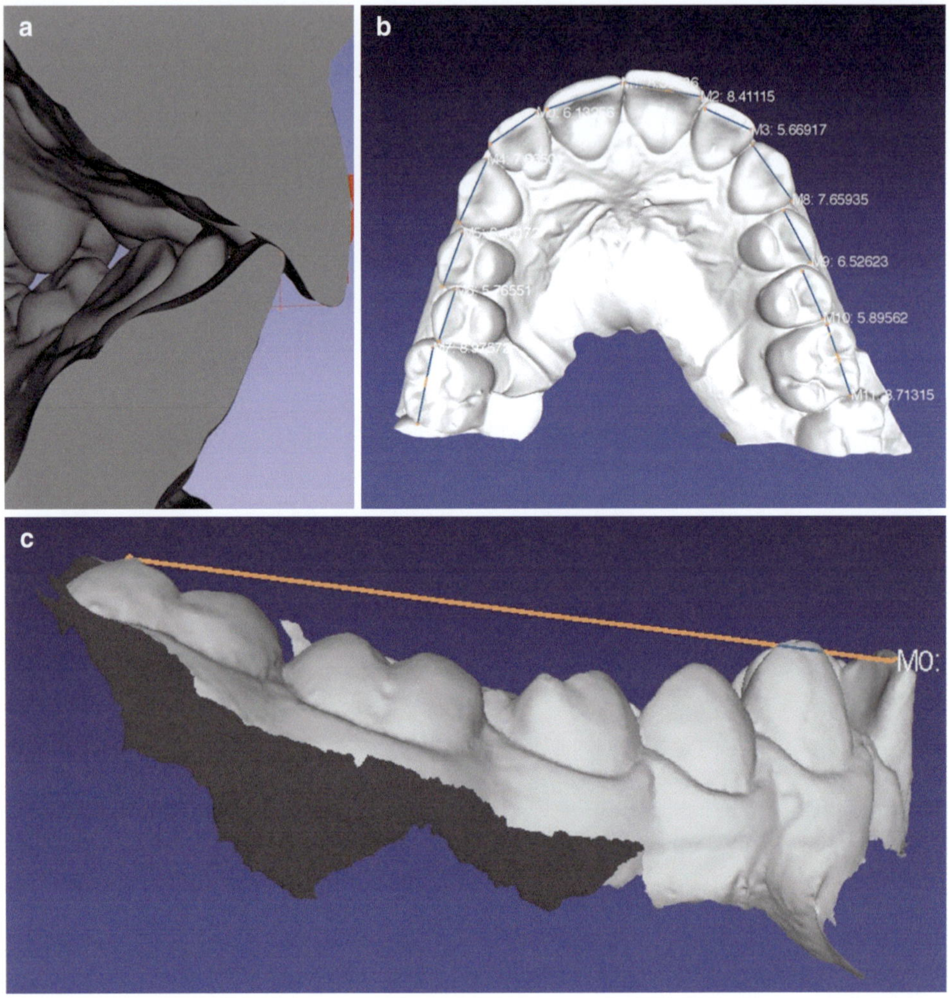

Fig. 6.4 (**a**) Overjet measurement on digital model. (**b**) Teeth size measurement for model analysis. (**c**) Curve of Spee assessment

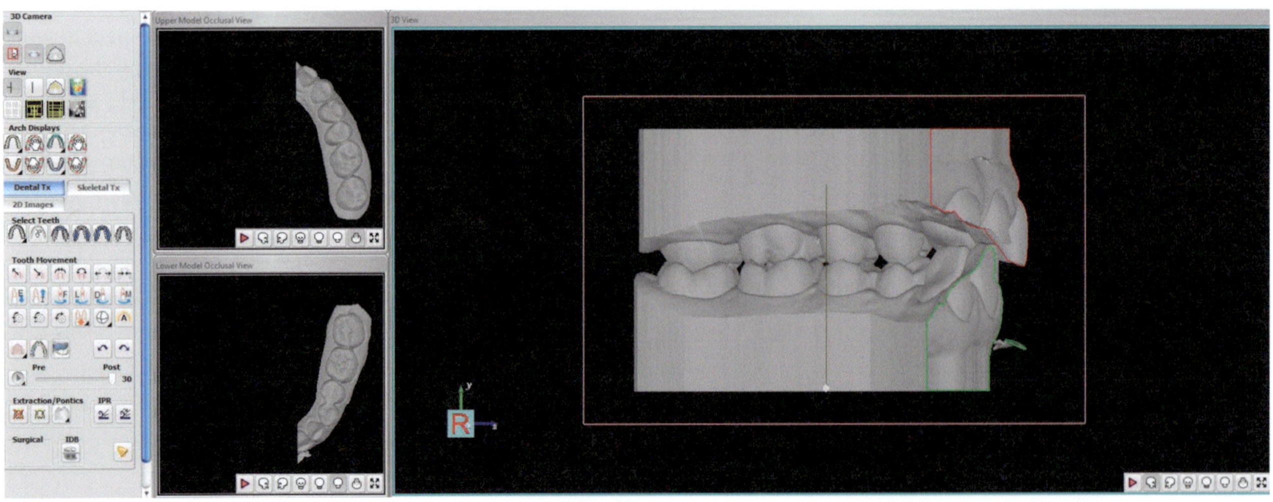

Fig. 6.5 Overjet measurement on digital model using Orthoinsight software

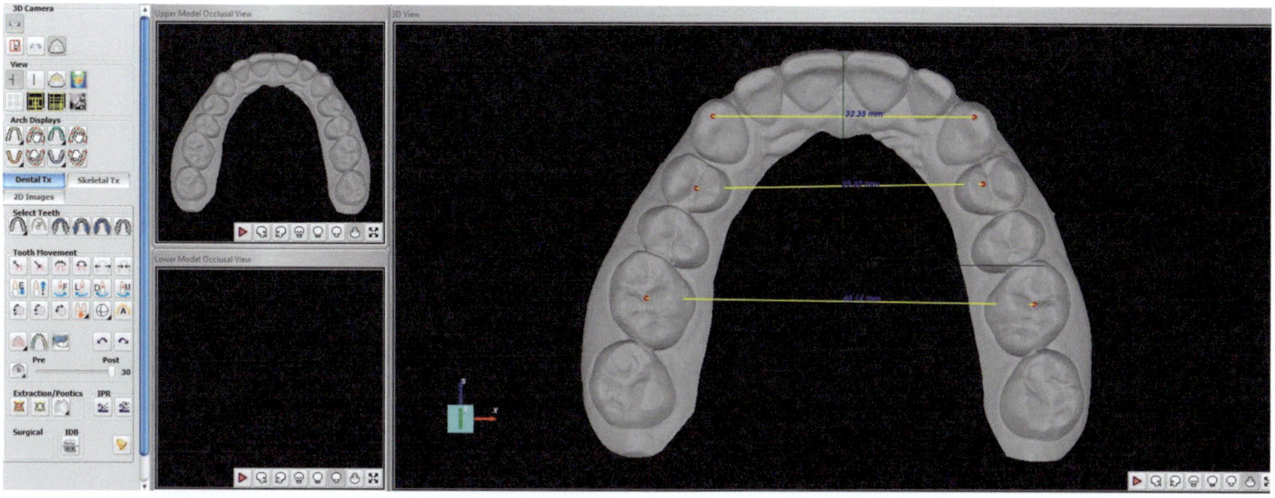

Fig. 6.6 Digital measurements of interarch width using orthoinsight software

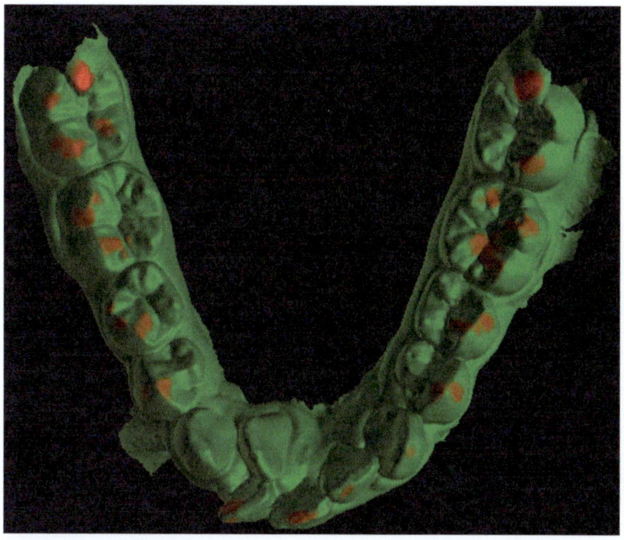

Fig. 6.7 Automatic occlusal contacts on red

reconstruction of the dental cast shape, and relationship between arches have shown that digital dental models are reliable and credible for clinicians [7]. Also, the use of digital models instead plaster models does not affect diagnostic and treatment planning decisions about different malocclusions [13].

New software features as digital diagnostic setup, automatic recognition of dental anatomic reference points, automatic recognition of occlusal contacts (Figs. 6.7 and 6.8), radiographic integration, simulation of proposed treatment planning and bracket positioning, help the orthodontist with an interactive diagnosis and treatment planning. A setup is a valuable diagnostic tool that can be used to confirm, modify, or reject a suggested treatment plan and can be particularly valuable in complex cases. The virtual setup is an alternative to the traditional setup (using a plaster model) and allows not only visualization of orthodontic treatment plans taking less time than making a conventional setup, but also can be used to make custom appliances based on the virtual setup, like the aligners (Fig. 6.9) [16].

6.6 Virtual Tooth Movement Software Programs for In-House Aligners

The goal of orthodontic treatment is to improve the malocclusion and to achieve as near perfect occlusion as possible. Orthodontic setup which was first introduced in 1946 [17] plays an important role in achieving predicted tooth movement. 3D virtual setup has become more popular in orthodontics with the introduction of intraoral scanners and diagnostic software programs [18]. 3D virtual setup can simulate the orthodontic treatment by segmenting each tooth as separate object and moving each individual tooth to its planned position. Virtual setup has been used to present different treatment options and can be useful when considering extractions, interproximal reduction (IPR), anchorage management, and pre-surgical orthodontics [19]. Virtual tooth movement had a great impact on the market of orthodontics by making the clear aligner therapy increasingly available as treatment tool not just to be used for minor tooth movement but also for comprehensive orthodontics for adults and teenager's population [20]. Align Technology which introduced Invisalign for orthodontic use in 1998 utilizes clinchek soft-

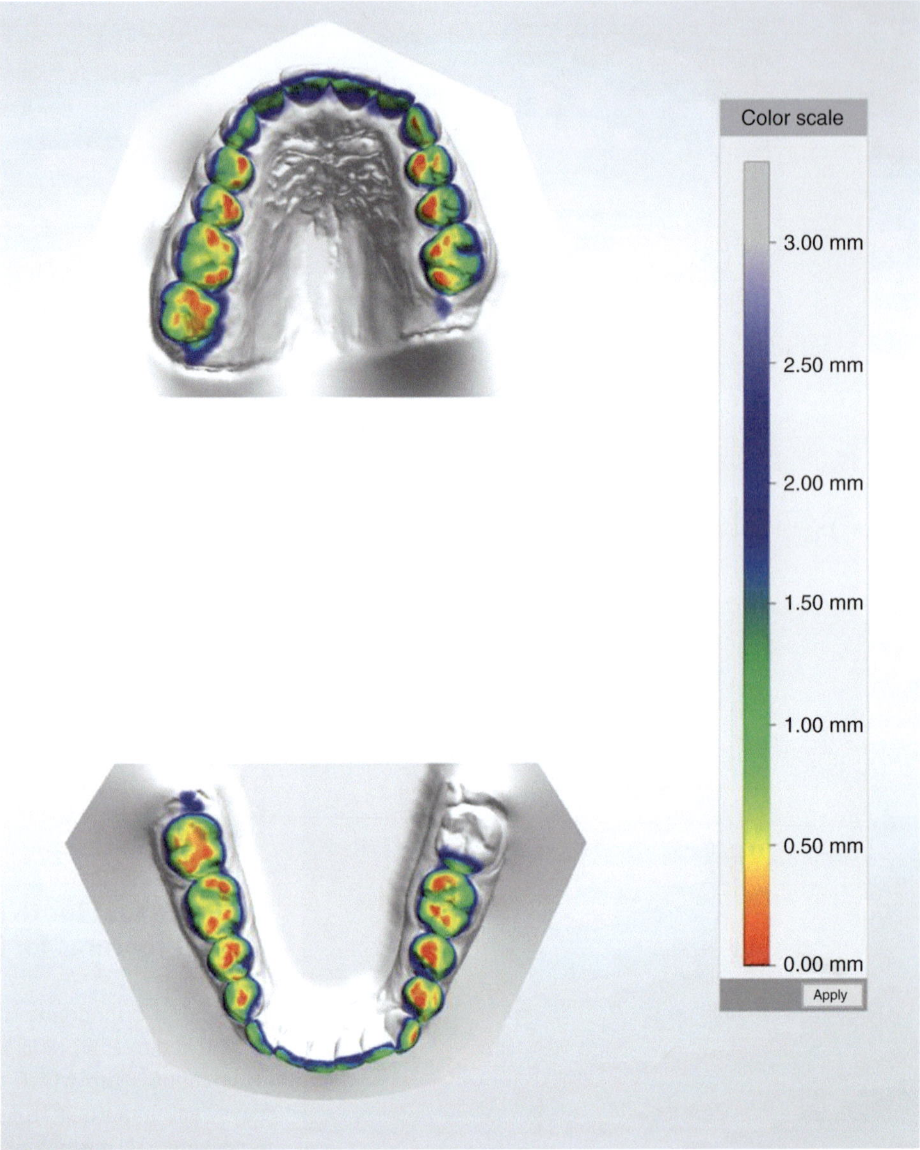

Fig. 6.8 Colormap for occlusal contacts using 3Shape software

ware program which presents stages of virtual tooth movements to achieve the desired tooth movements. Recently, 3D diagnostic software programs offered the virtual tooth movement feature which allowed orthodontists to produce clear aligners in-house via integration with 3D intraoral scanners and 3D printers. In this chapter, we will outline the steps involved in fabrication of in-house aligners using two different software programs.

6.7 Manual Segmentation Software

6.7.1 OrthoAnalyzer In-House Model Preparation and Teeth Segmentation

The first step using Clear Aligner studio in OrthoAnalyzer software is to prepare the model using the following steps.

1. Alignment of 3D Scan with CBCT image if present. The two files are aligned by placing three points around the first molars and one of the incisors (Fig. 6.10).
2. Setting up both occlusal and sagittal planes to orient the models and define references for different measurements.
3. Segmentation of upper and lower scans which allows separation of each individual tooth into a separate object to enable tooth movement in 3D directions. Segmentation works by virtually drawing lines between mesial and distal surfaces. The software will automatically outline the borders of each individual tooth, define the gingival margins and the rotation center of each tooth based on the user defined mesial-distal segmentation. Using the CBCT scan to define the teeth axes is highly recommended at this step (Fig. 6.11).
4. An optional step which allows the user to define an ideal arch that will act as a design guideline when the teeth are moved to the ideal setup.

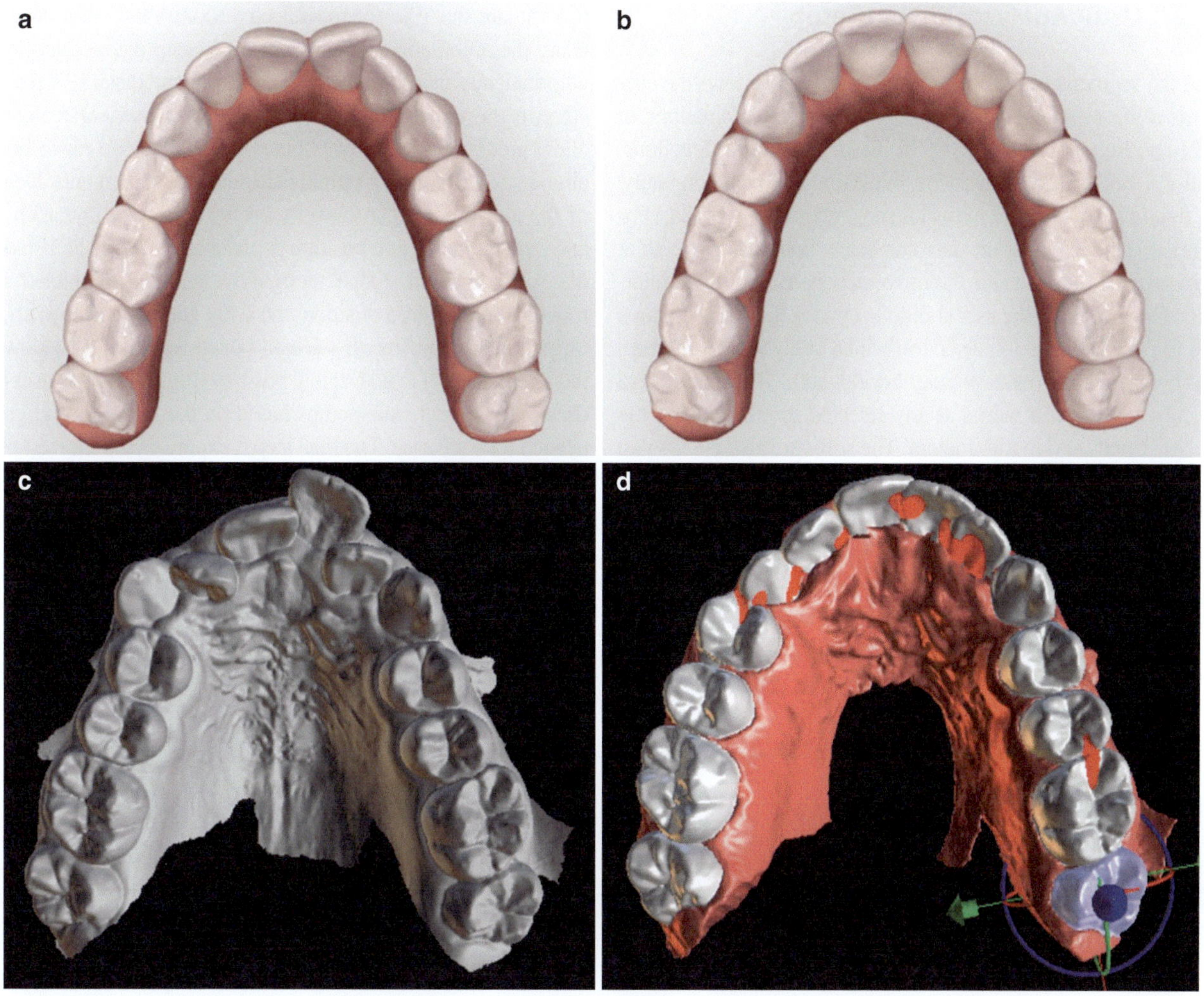

Fig. 6.9 (**a**) Initial digital model. (**b**) Virtual setup for custom aligners fabrication. (**c**) Initial digital model presenting negative model discrepancy. (**d**) Virtual setup showing interdental collisions and interproximal reduction necessity (red)

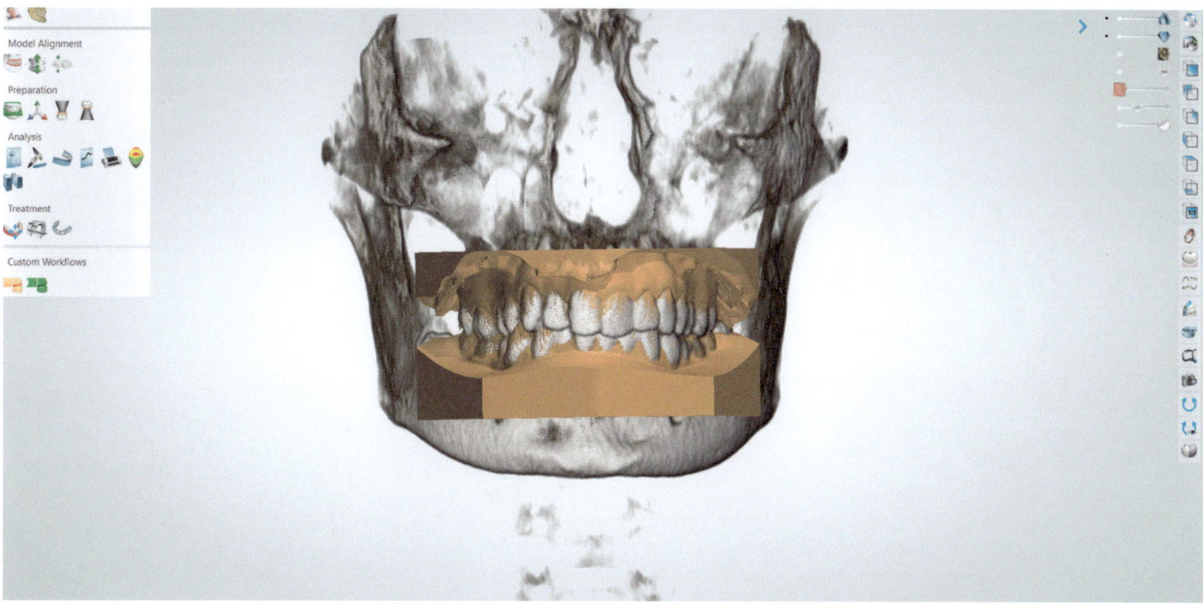

Fig. 6.10 Alignment of 3D scan with CBCT image if present. The two files are aligned by placing three points around the first molars and one of the incisors

6.7.2 OrthoAnalyzer Virtual Setup

Once the segmentation step is done, the software allows the user to move the segmented teeth in 3D to modify inclinations in labial and lingual directions, tip in mesial and distal directions, rotations, bodily movements mesiodistally and buccolingually, and finally extrusion and intrusion movements (Fig. 6.12a). For symmetric movements, the user can select contralateral teeth at the same time to make sure the movements are symmetric bilaterally. During setup, the user should keep in mind some features such as perform collision detection which analyzes the intersections between antagonists or neighboring teeth. This feature also provides intersection values at any selected tooth, showing the level of penetration in millimeters. The software also allows you to simulate the IPR for the selected tooth which can be done using the automatic stripping section to strip the selected tooth automatically or manually through mesial and distal IPR parameters in the corresponding fields. Another essential feature to allow predicted tooth movement with virtual setup for in-house aligners is the ability of virtual placement of attachments. Design of the attachments can be selected from an attachment library and then the shape and position of attachment can be adjusted on the selected tooth. Once tooth movement is completed and moved to the desired position, the setup can be viewed with the original position of teeth selected which recreates a shadow of the selected tooth in its original position (Fig. 6.13). The user can divide the setup to sub-setups based on the number of aligners needed for each case. The final step is exporting the sub-setups in STL format to be ready for in-house 3D printing.

Figures 6.14, 6.15, 6.16, 6.17, and 6.18 demonstrate the same concept of steps using Orthoinsight software.

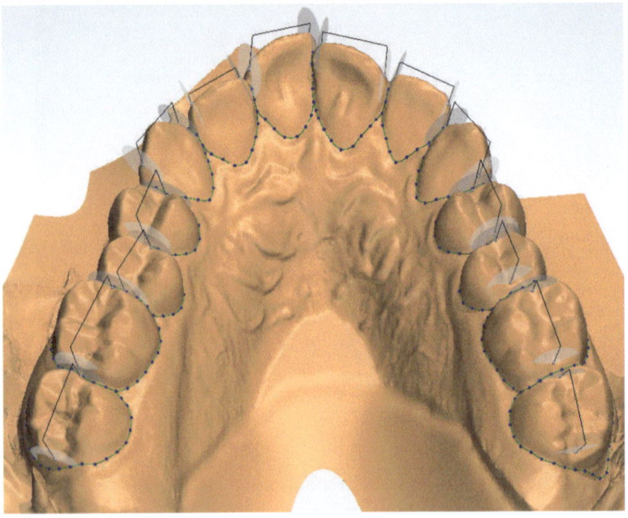

Fig. 6.11 Segmentation works by virtually drawing lines between mesial and distal surfaces. The software will automatically outline the borders of each individual tooth, define the gingival margins and the rotation center of each tooth based on the user defined mesial-distal segmentation

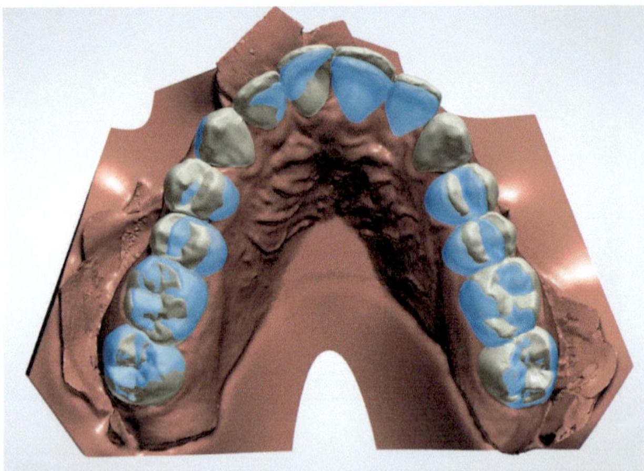

Fig. 6.13 The setup can be viewed with the original position of teeth selected which recreates a shadow of the selected tooth in its original position

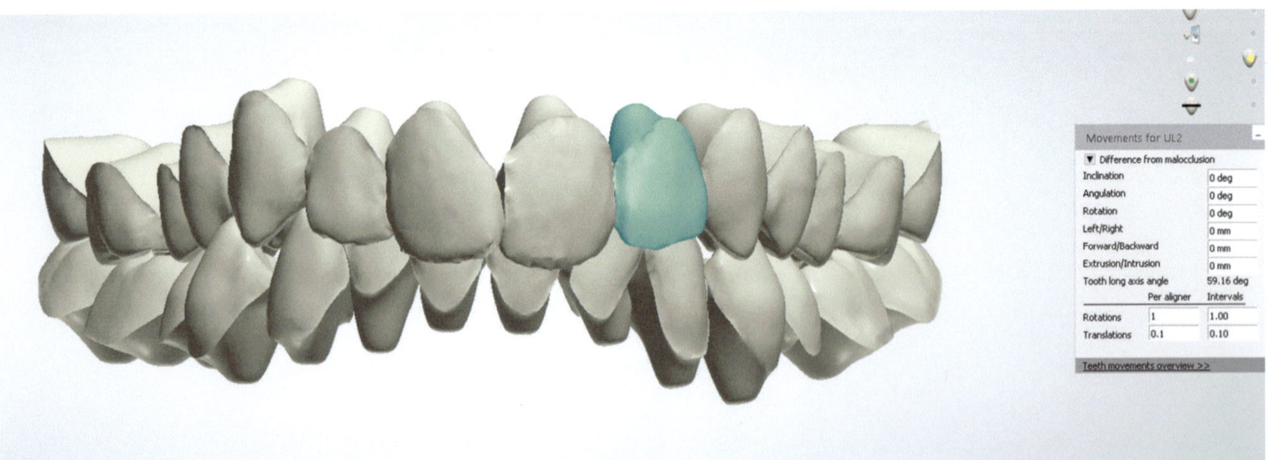

Fig. 6.12 The software allows the user to move the segmented teeth in 3D to modify inclinations in labial and lingual directions, tip in mesial and distal directions, rotations, bodily movements mesiodistally and buccolingually, and finally extrusion and intrusion movements

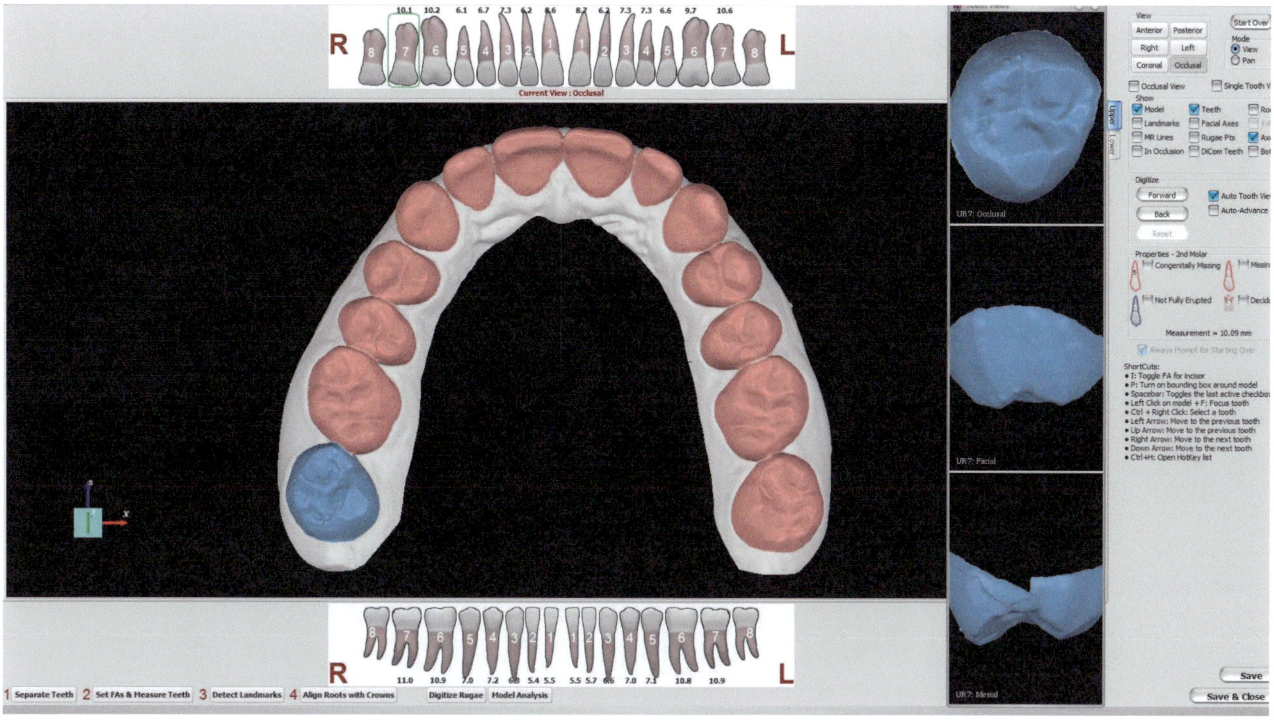

Fig. 6.14 Segmenting and digitizing the teeth to prepare for virtual tooth movement using Orthoinsight software

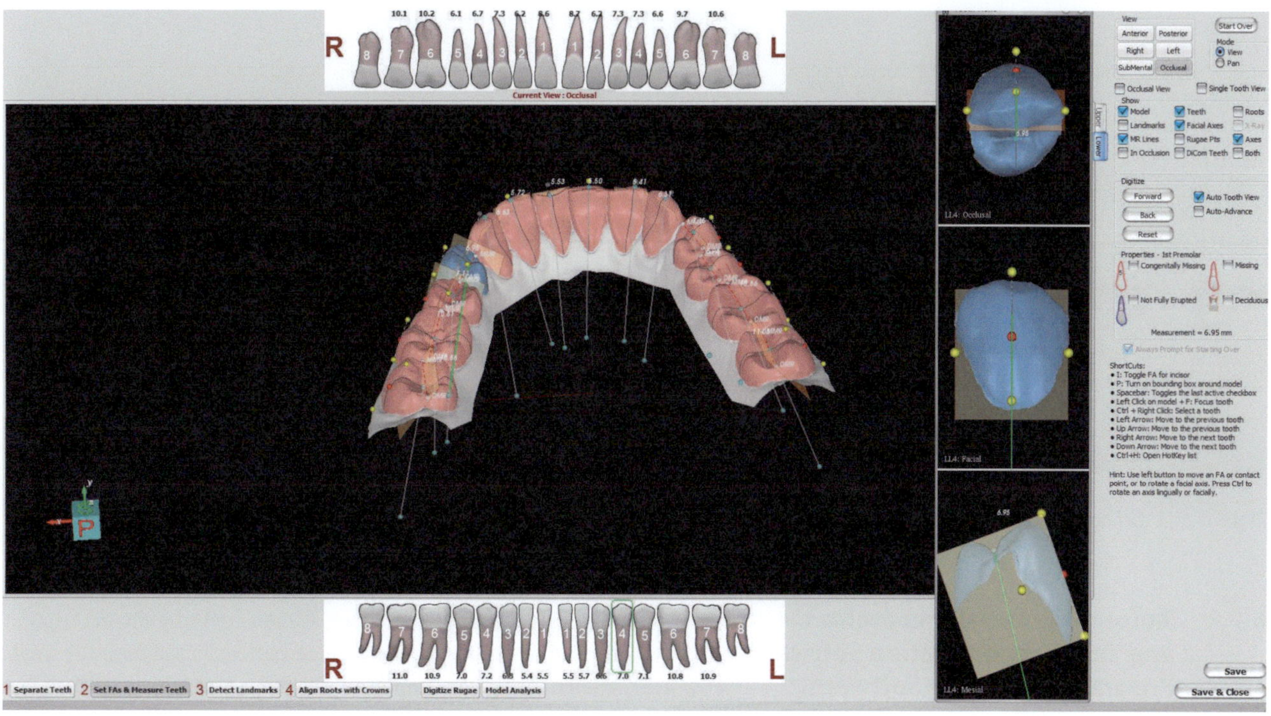

Fig. 6.15 Detecting landmarks to facilitate virtual setup

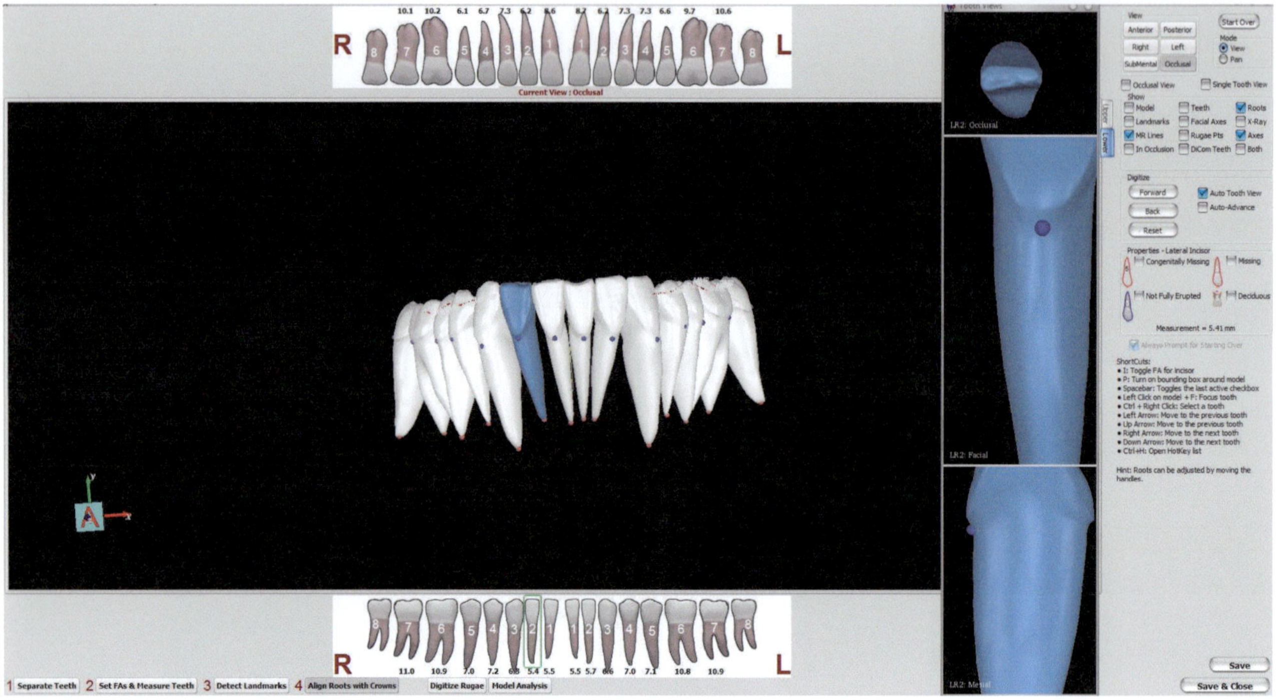

Fig. 6.16 Aligning the position of the crown with roots for proper virtual movement

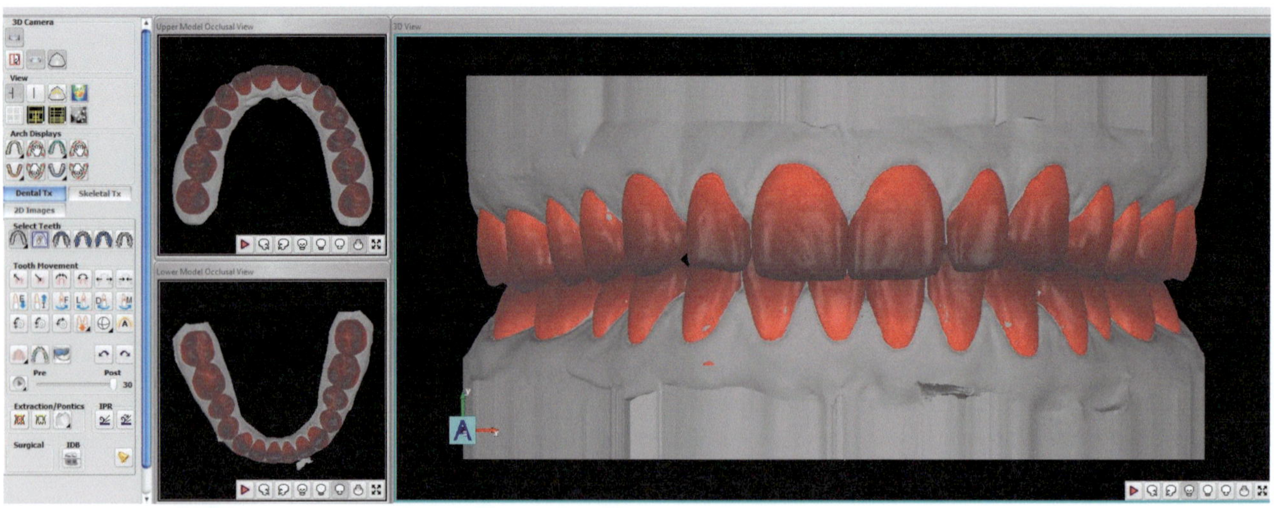

Fig. 6.17 A display of the selected teeth after digitization

6.7.3 Automatic Model Preparation and Teeth Segmentation Software Program (Suresmile Software)

The suresmile software for virtual tooth movements is cloud based which makes it an easy access to the user. Once the patient is created in the software, the user would choose from the options of doing it yourself aligner staging or full-service aligner staging. In this paper, we are covering the first option for the in-house aligners. Once patient is scanned for treatment, scans are imported to the software as STL files. Suresmile offers a paid service for the model preparation and teeth segmentation. Once this is completed, the user will have access to a prepared model with segmented teeth to be able to start the virtual setup (Fig. 6.19).

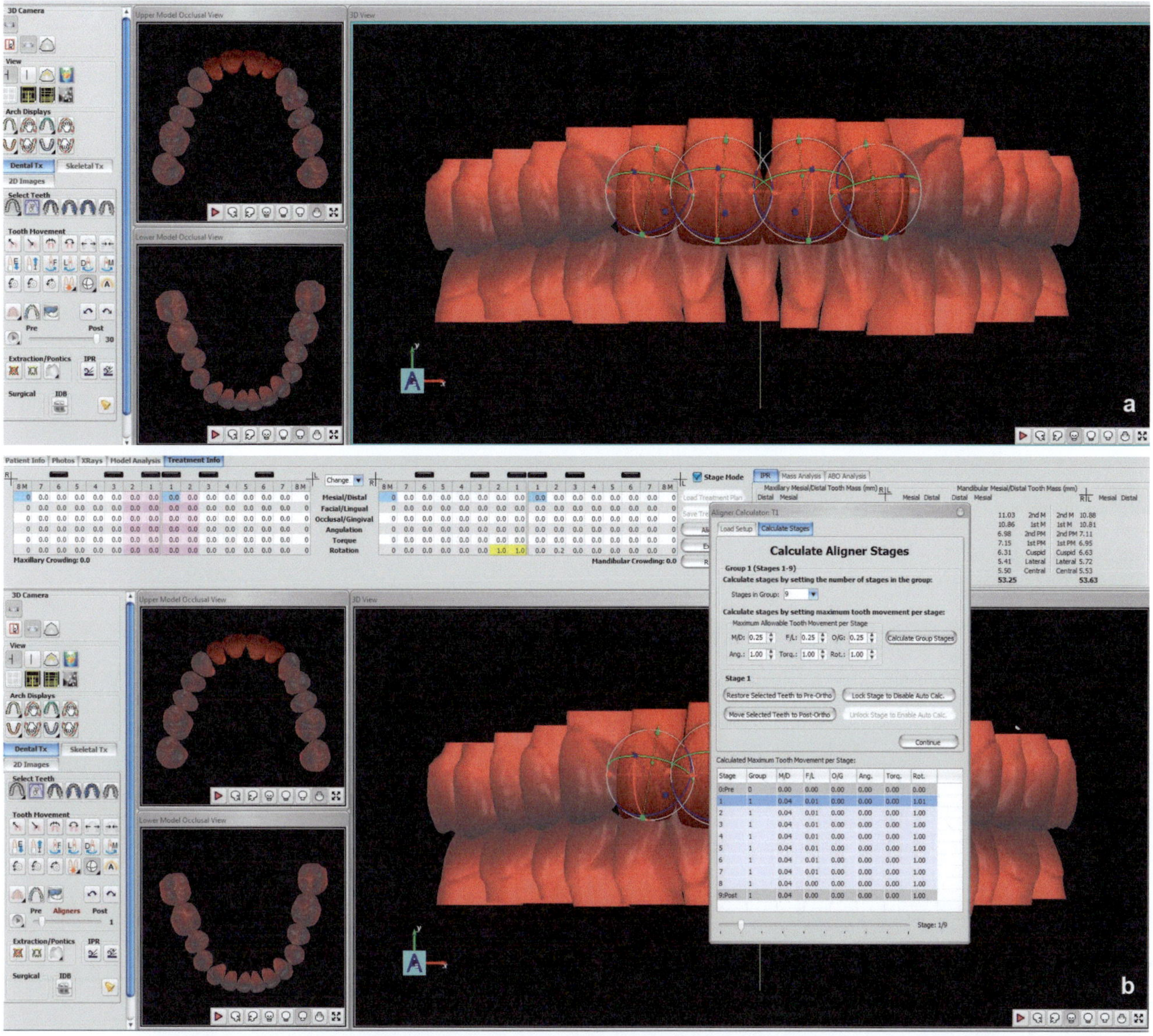

Fig. 6.18 (**a**) Circle tool to start the virtual tooth movement and saving the treatment plan. (**b**) Calculating number of aligners needed to achieve the desired tooth movement based on algorithms

6.7.4 Suresmile Virtual Setup

The software will display the prepared model with segmented teeth. The user can select the option to display only the segmented teeth without the gingiva and the option to select one arch at time. The software provides a table of displacements which represents in numbers the amount and direction of movement for each tooth separately. For virtual tooth movement, the user can use the arrows in the displacement table or the virtual box which appears on the selected tooth with different arrows for different 3D tooth movement (Fig. 6.20). Distal and mesial intersections tabs can be utilized to avoid any overlap with neighboring teeth. Now, setup is completed and the final tooth movements can be viewed with a reference of the original teeth position (Fig. 6.21). Once the user approves the setup, the software automatically calculates the stages of aligners and automatically places attachments on selected teeth for specific tooth movement (Fig. 6.22). Final step is exporting the staged models in STL format to be ready for in-house 3D printing (Fig. 6.23).

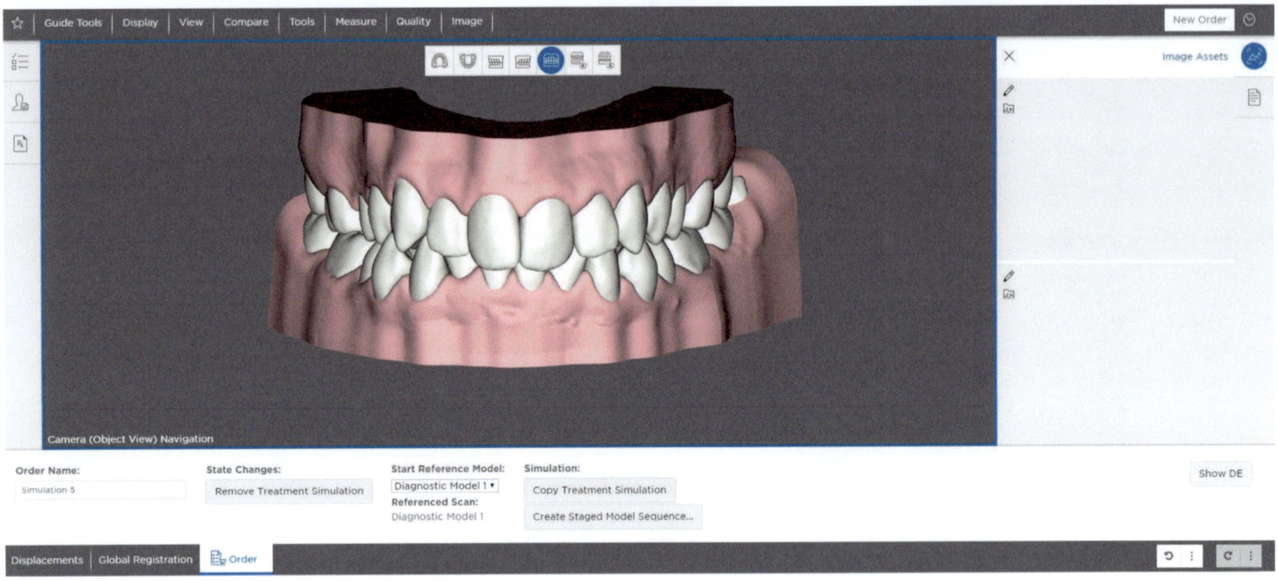

Fig. 6.19 A display of 3D models using Suresmile software

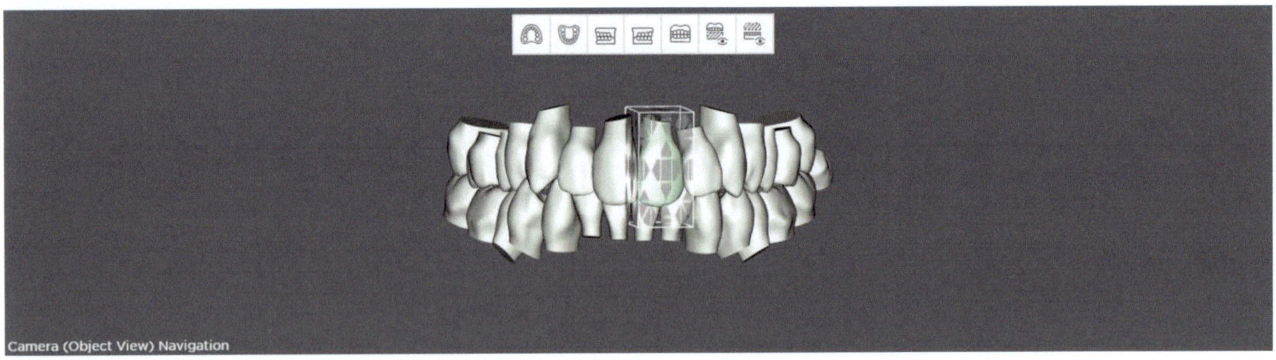

Fig. 6.20 Tool for virtual tooth movement using Suresmile Software

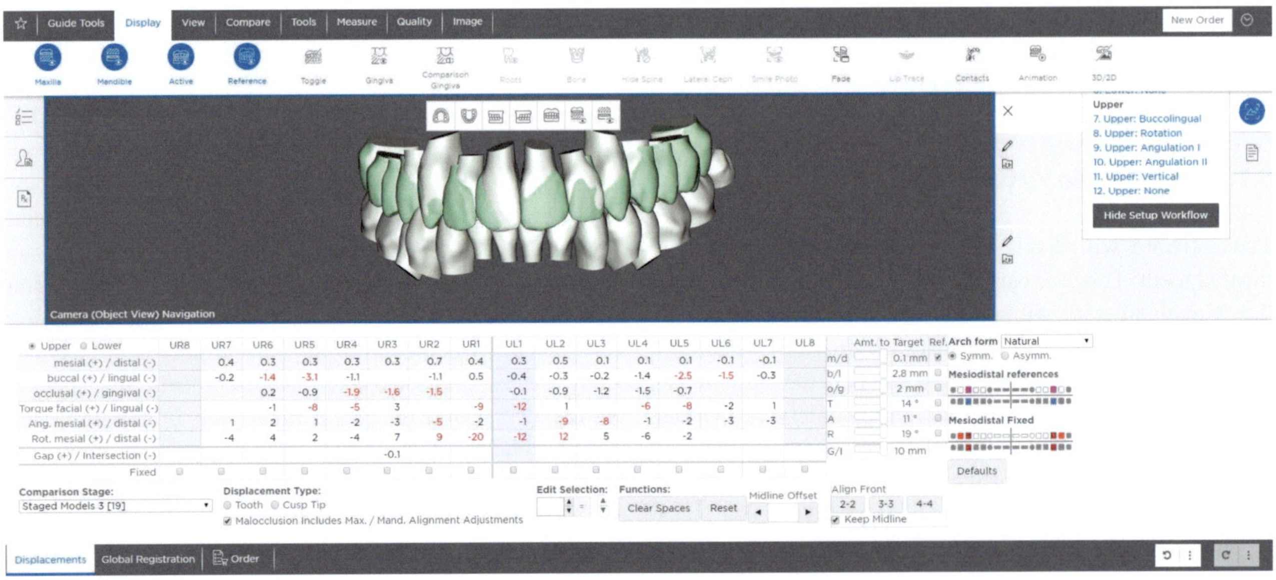

Fig. 6.21 Showing the number of stages to achieve the desired tooth movement using Suresmile software

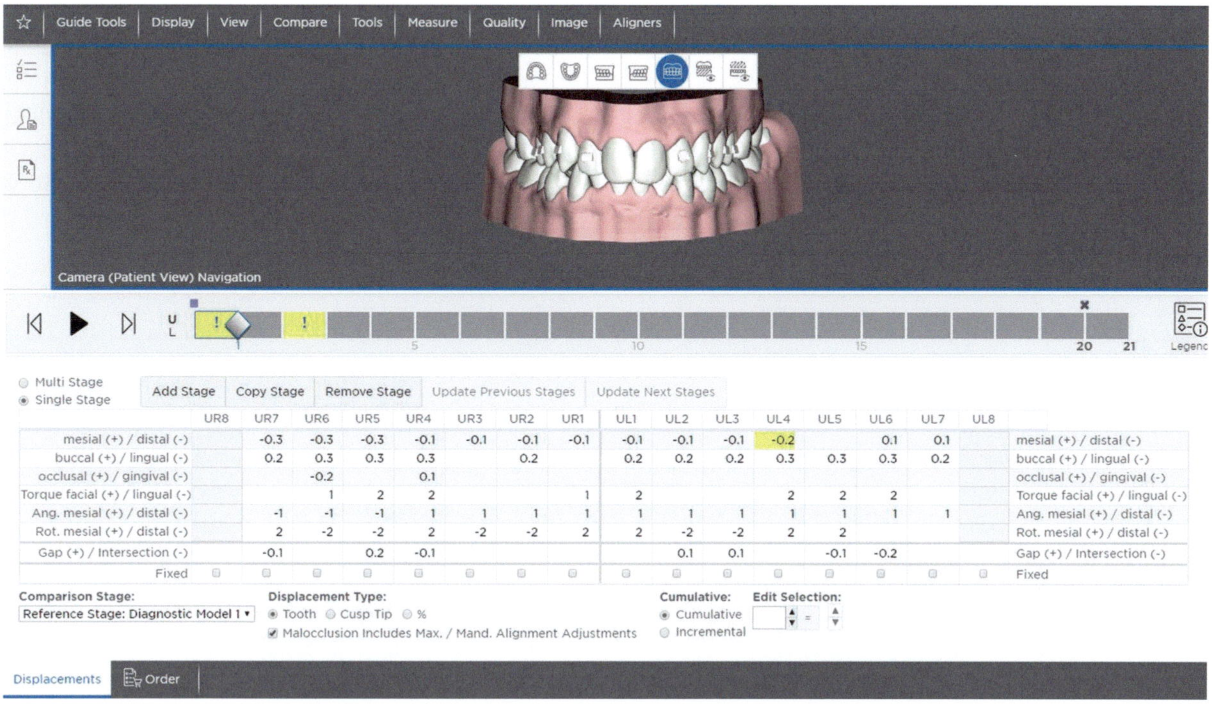

Fig. 6.22 The software automatically calculates the stages of aligners and automatically places attachments on selected teeth for specific tooth movement

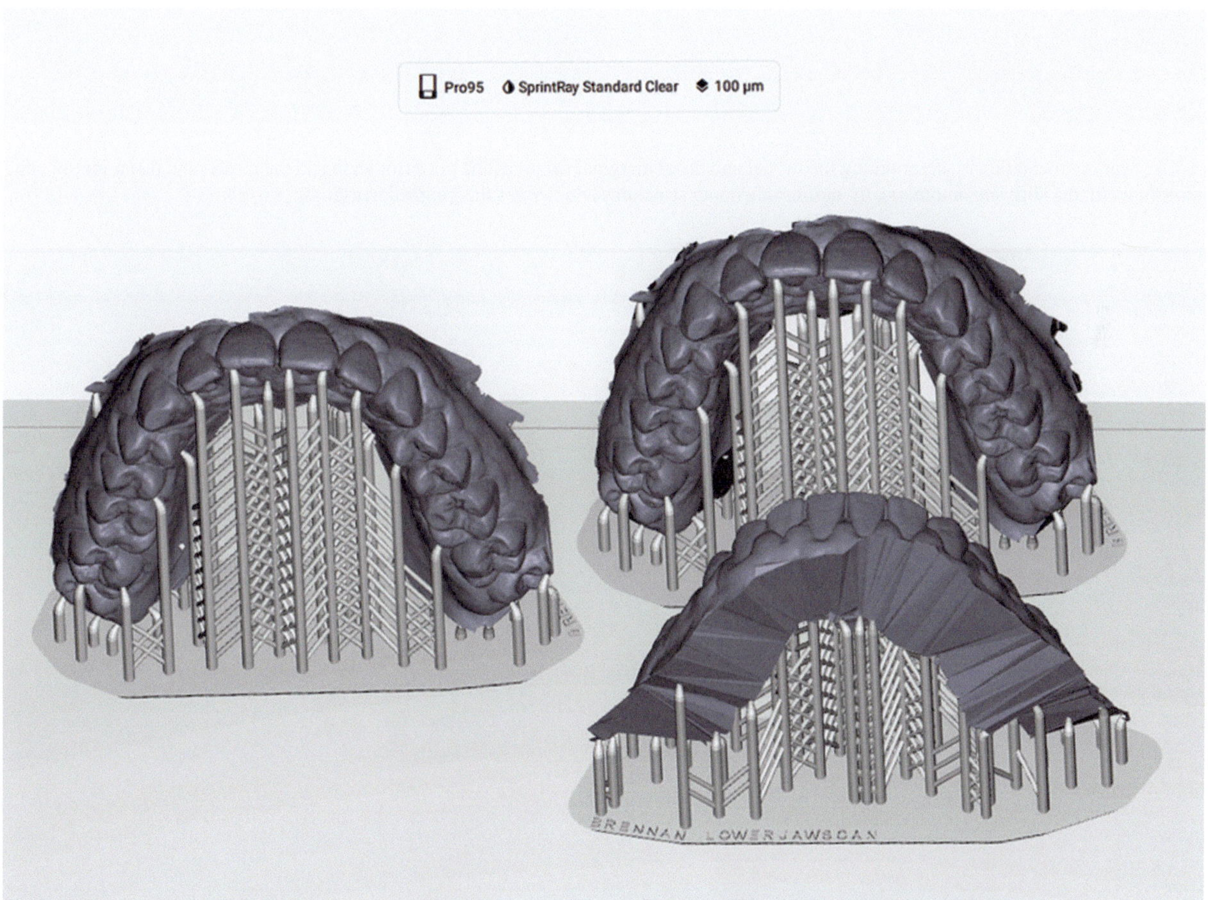

Fig. 6.23 The staged models in STL format to be ready for in-house 3D printing

6.8 Steps for 3D Virtual Indirect Bonding Using Orthoanalyzer Program

1. Scan segmentation by determining the mesial and distal marginal ridges of the posterior teeth and the mesial and distal incisal edges of the anterior teeth, the software automatically outlines the tooth structures and defines the gingival margins (Fig. 6.24).
2. Digitally place the brackets: Select the bracket icon to align the axis points along the clinical crown lines (Fig. 6.25).
3. Choose the brackets you use from the brackets library. The selected brackets will then populate on the model. A red dot indicates a bracket that can be moved to your desired position. Confirm the brackets position and save the file.

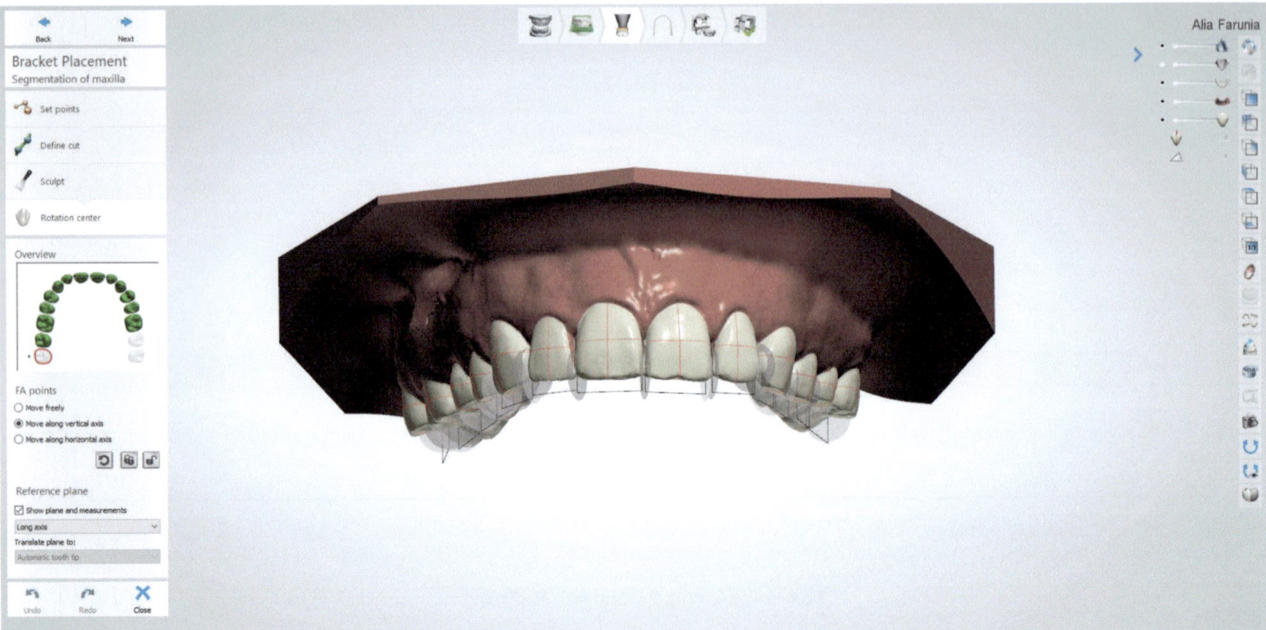

Fig. 6.24 Scan segmentation by determining the mesial and distal marginal ridges of the posterior teeth and the mesial and distal incisal edges of the anterior teeth, the software automatically outlines the tooth structures and defines the gingival margins

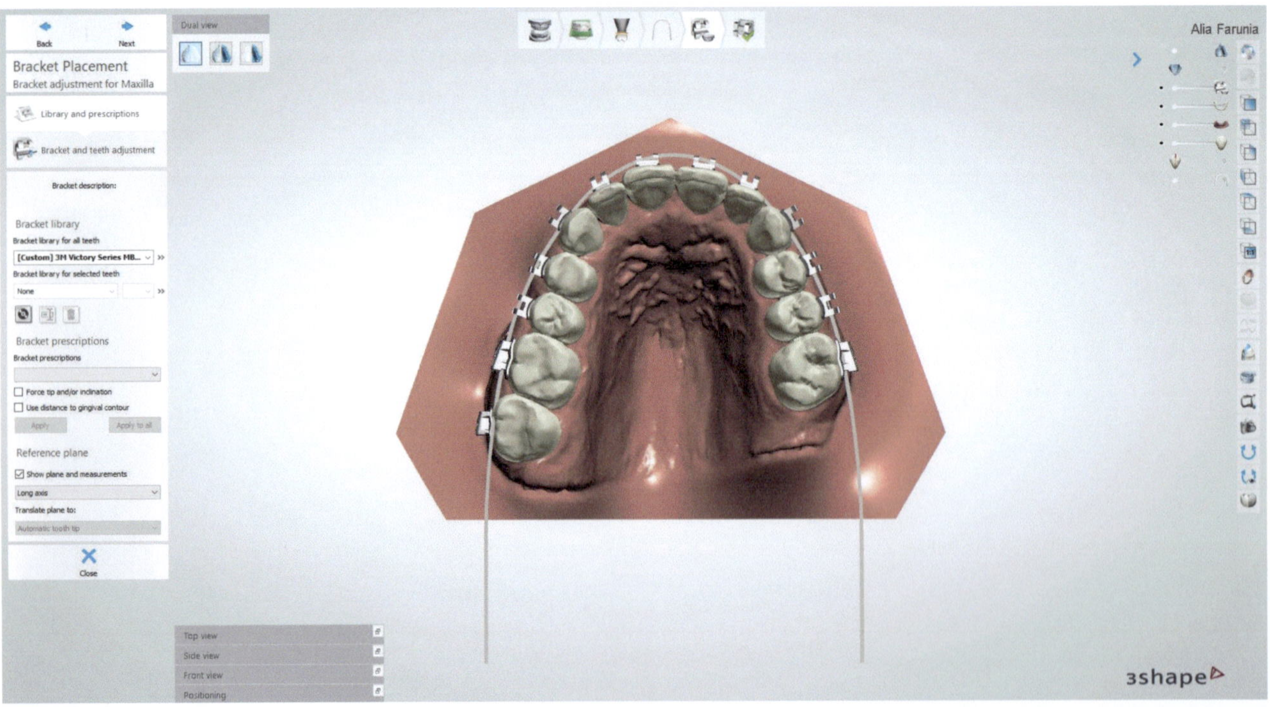

Fig. 6.25 Digitally placing brackets using 3Shape software

Figures 6.26, 6.27, and 6.28 demonstrate same concept of 3D virtual indirect bonding using Orthoinsight software programs.

Figures 6.29 and 6.30 demonstrate the steps of virtual debonding using Orthoanlyzer software.

6.8.1 3D Printing

Rapid prototyping is a generic name given to a range of related technologies that build models on a layer-by-layer basis. This technology offers the possibility to generate a physical orthodontic cast model from digital data in a fast and economic way [21].

6.8.1.1 Stereolithography (SLA)

SLA machine consists of: bath of photosensitive resin, model building platform, ultraviolet laser for curing the resin. SLA printing is a type of printing where an ultraviolet laser cures resin in a desired shape. During this process, the printing plate moves down in small increments, and the liquid polymer is exposed to an ultraviolet laser that cures a cross section layer by layer. This process is repeated until a printed model has been made.

6.8.1.2 Fused Deposition Modeling (FDM)

In order to produce the printed model, a part the material is supplied through a heated nozzle after a metal wire or a plastic filament wound in a coil are released. Instead of curing a liquid resin with projected light, an FDM printer extrudes a resin that has been heated just beyond its melting point, depositing it layer by layer. The heated material hardens immediately after being extruded.

6.8.1.3 Digital Light Processing (DLP)

DLP is identical to SLA except for the light source a projector is used to cure an entire layer at a time, similar to the difference between stamping and drawing an object. This

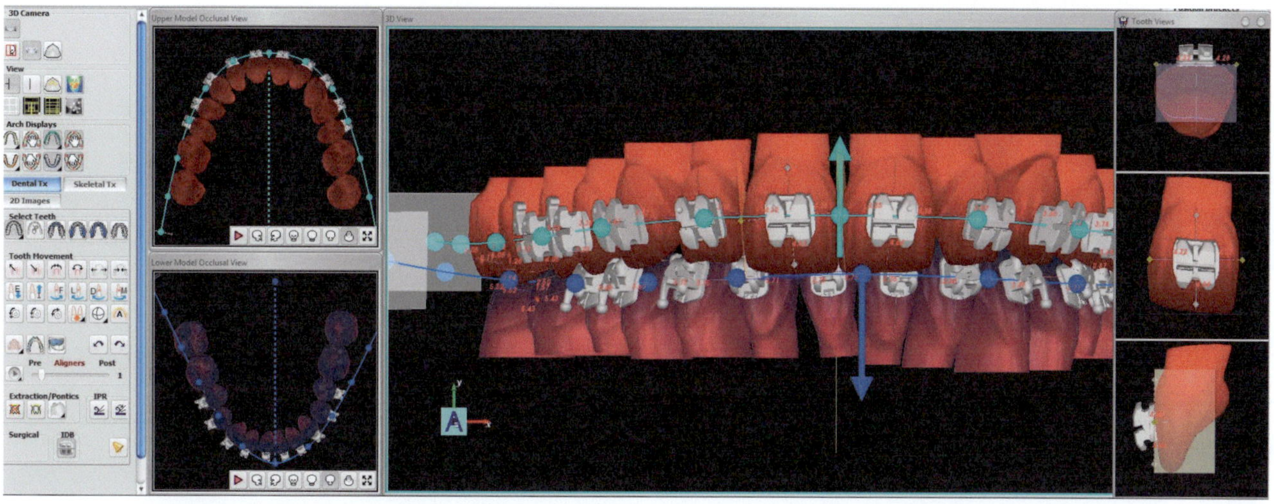

Fig. 6.26 Virtual bracket placement using Orthoinsight software

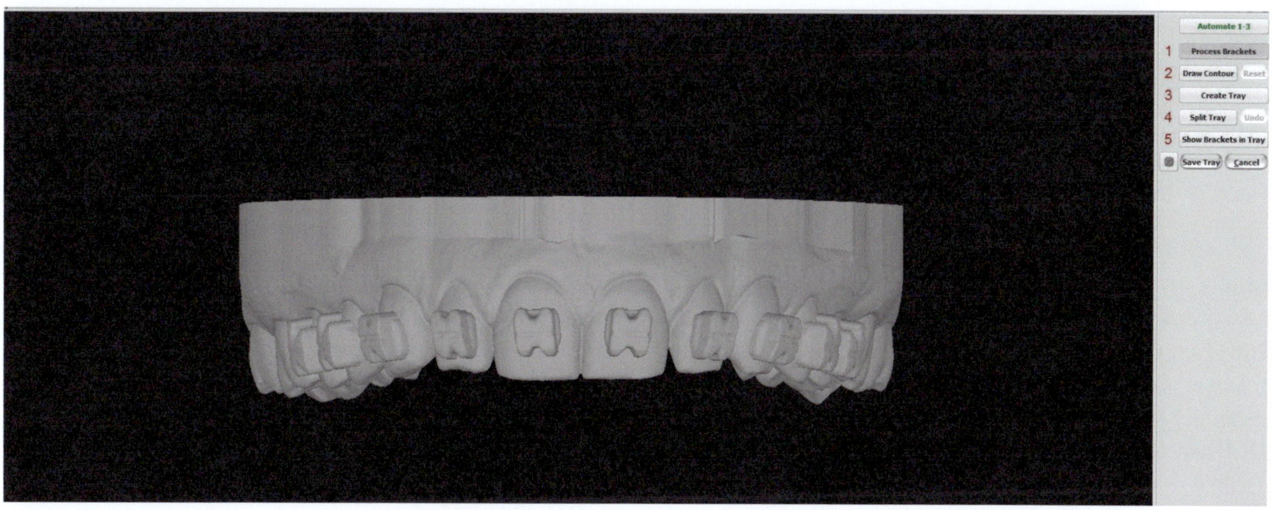

Fig. 6.27 3D model with brackets placed for indirect bonding tray fabrication

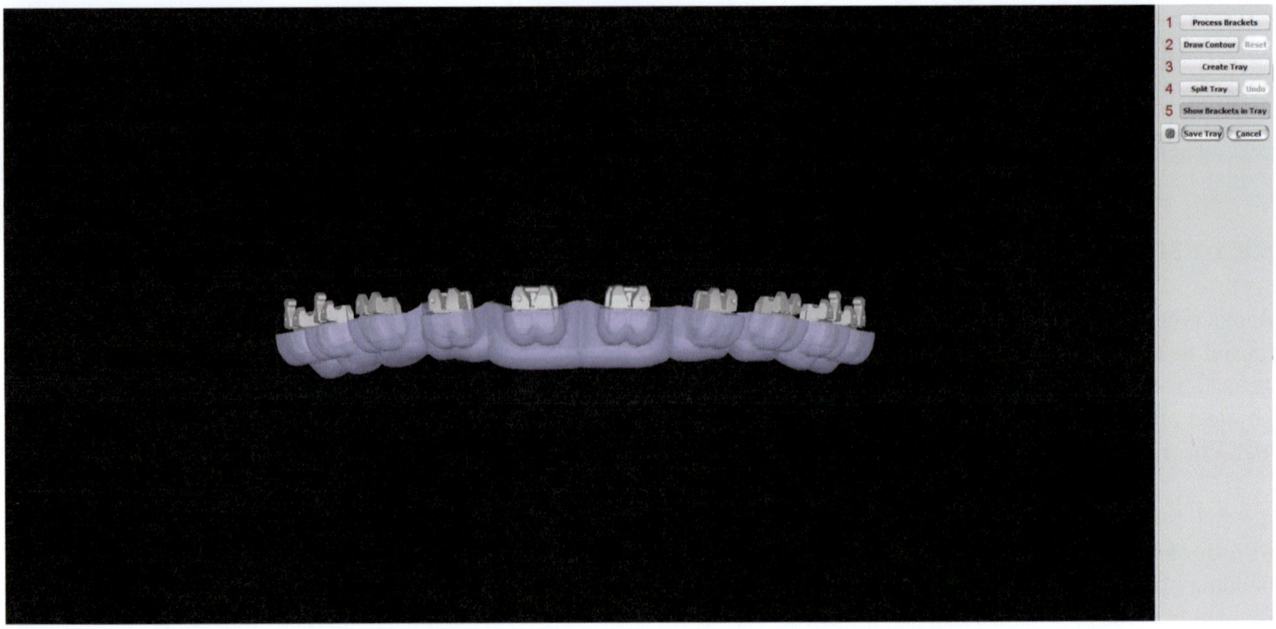

Fig. 6.28 Indirect bonding tray ready to be printed

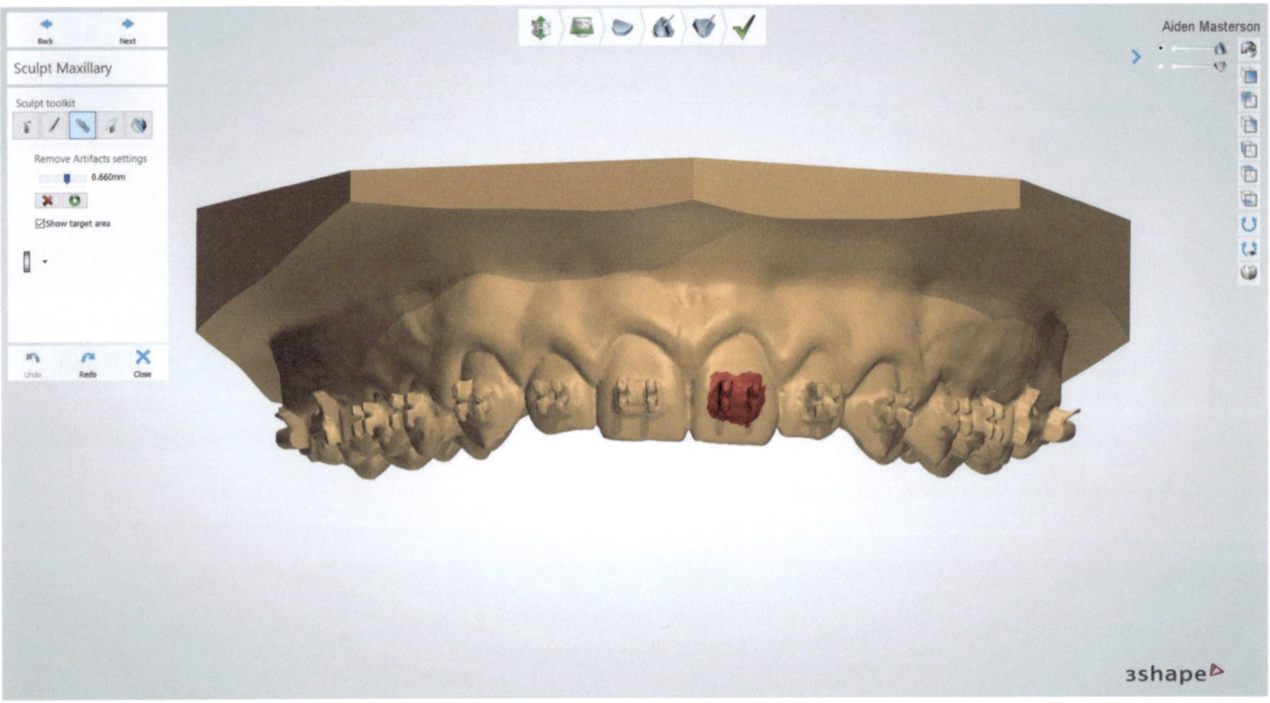

Fig. 6.29 Selecting a bracket for bracket removal

results in significantly faster print times. Like SLA, DLP also produces parts with high accuracy and high resolution. However, one advantage that DLP has over SLA is that it requires a shallow vat of resin to facilitate the process. This generally results in less waste and lower running costs. Also, DLP can be a faster process than SLA as the light source is applied to the whole surface of the vat of polymer resin at a single pass.

6.8.1.4 Polyjet Photopolymerization

Polyjet printing uses jet heads that spray or jet the resin in the desired areas. As the jet heads make subsequent passes, each sprayed layer is cured using an ultraviolet light source. A key element of the inkjet-based 3D printing process is the print head that sprays layers of photosensitive polymers, which precisely represent the cross-sectional profile of the model on the building platform.

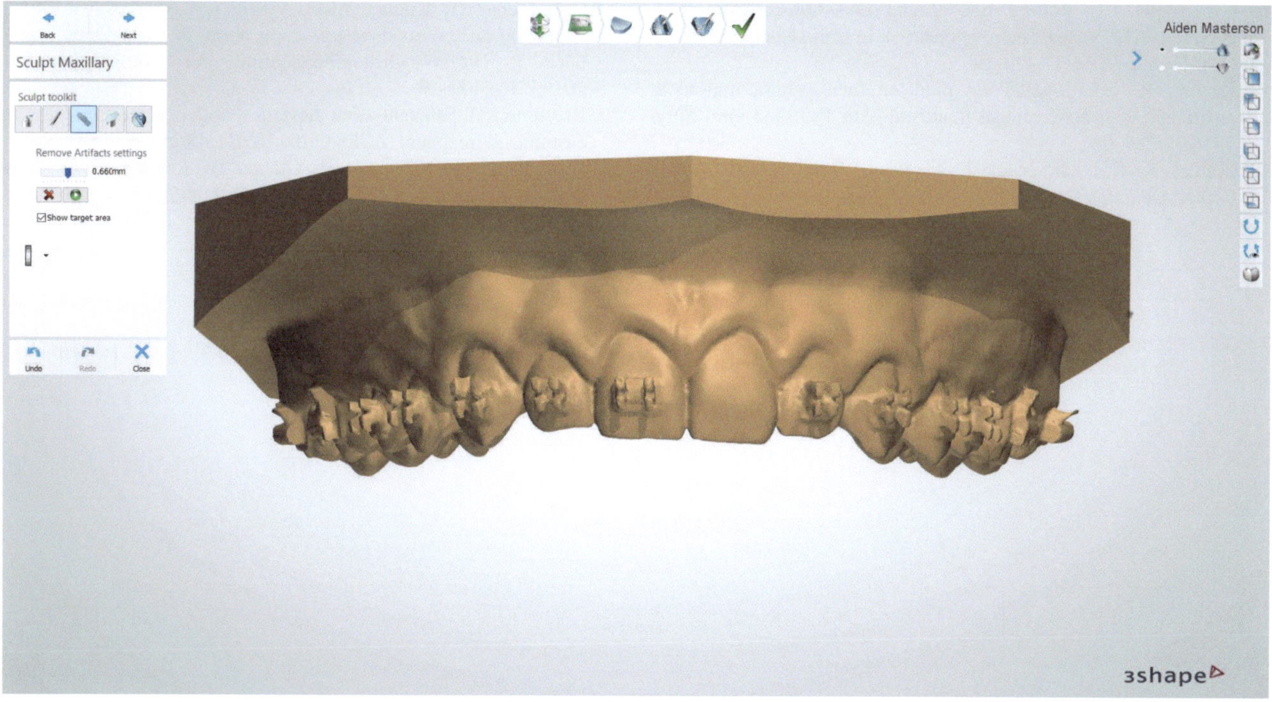

Fig. 6.30 Bracket removal using 3Shape software

6.9 Conclusions

1. Intraoral digital scanners are becoming integral to the modern orthodontic office.
2. Digital models can be used to replace plaster models for malocclusion diagnosis and treatment planning. Measurements can be made on digital models in an easy, accurate and sometimes, in an automatic way.
3. Virtual tooth movement for in-house aligners can be easily added to your workflow. This chapter demonstrated two different models for software programs for clinicians so each orthodontist can decide which model could be a better fit for their workflow in their practices.

References

1. Kravitz ND, Groth C, Jones PE, Graham JW, Redmond WR. Intraoral digital scanners. J Clin Orthod. 2014;48(6):337–47.
2. Logozzo S, Franceschini G, Kilpelä A, Governi L, Blois L. A comparative analysis of intraoral 3D digital scanners for restorative dentistry. Int J Med Technol. 2008;5.
3. Bloss R. Accordion fringe interferometry: a revolutionary new digital shape-scanning technology. Sensor Rev. 2008;28:22–6.
4. Yuzbasioglu E, Kurt H, Turunc R, Bilir H. Comparison of digital and conventional impression techniques: evaluation of patients' perception, treatment comfort, effectiveness and clinical outcomes. BMC Oral Health. 2014;14:10. https://doi.org/10.1186/1472-6831-14-10. Published 2014 Jan 30.
5. Akyalcin S, Cozad BE, English JD, Colville CD, Laman S. Diagnostic accuracy of impression-free digital models. Am J Orthod Dentofac Orthop. 2013;144(6):916–22. https://doi.org/10.1016/j.ajodo.2013.04.024.
6. Mangano F, Gandolfi A, Luongo G, Logozzo S. Intraoral scanners in dentistry: a review of the current literature. BMC Oral Health. 2017;17(1):149. https://doi.org/10.1186/s12903-017-0442-x. Published 2017 Dec 12.
7. Rossini G, Parrini S, Castroflorio T, Deregibus A, Debernardi CL. Diagnostic accuracy and measurement sensitivity of digital models for orthodontic purposes: a systematic review. Am J Orthod Dentofac Orthop. 2016;149(2):161–70. https://doi.org/10.1016/j.ajodo.2015.06.029.
8. Technology A. iTero. https://www.itero.com/en-us/products/itero_element. Accessed 31 Oct 2019.
9. 3Shape. Trios. https://www.3shape.com/en/scanners/trios. Accessed 31 Oct 2019.
10. Medit. i500. https://www.medit.com/dental-clinic. Accessed 1 Nov 2019.
11. DentsplySirona. Omnicam. https://www.dentsplysirona.com/en/explore/digital-impression/Omnicam.html. Accessed 1 Nov 2019.
12. Logozzo S, Zanetti EM, Franceschini G, Kilpelä A, Mäkynen A. Recent advances in dental optics—part I: 3D intraoral scanners for restorative dentistry. Opt Lasers Eng. 2014;54:203–21.
13. Rheude B, Sadowsky PL, Ferreira A, Jacobson A. Na evaluation of digital study models in orthodontic diagnosis and treatment planning. Angle Orthod. 2005;75:300–4.
14. Pacheco-Pereira C, De Luca Canto G, Flores-Mir C. Variation of orthodontic treatment decision-making based on dental model type: a systematic review. Angle Orthod. 2015;85:501–9.
15. Santoro M, Galkin S, Teredesai M, Nicolay OF, Cangialosi TJ. Comparison of measurements made on digital and plaster models. Am J Orthod Dentofac Orthop. 2003;124:101–5.

16. Camardella LT, Rothier EK, Vilella OV, Ongkosuwito EM, Breuning KH. Virtual setup: application in orthodontic practice. J Orof Orthop. 2016;77:409–19.
17. Kesling H. Coordinating the predetermined pattern and tooth positioner with conventional treatment. Am J Orthod Oral Surg. 1946;32:285–93.
18. Marcel T. Three-dimensional on-screen virtual models. Am J Orthod Dentofac Orthop. 2001;119:666–8.
19. Camardella LT, Rothier EKC, Vilella OV, Ongkosuwito EM, Breuning KH. Virtual setup: application in orthodontic practice. J Orofac Orthop/Fortschritte der Kieferorthopädie. 2016;77(6):409–19.
20. Breuning KH. Efficient tooth movement with new technologies for customized treatment. J Clin Orthod. 2011;45:257–62.
21. Groth C, Kravitz ND, Jones PE, Graham JW, Redmond WR. Three dimensional printing technology. J Clin Orthod. 2014;48(8):475–85.

7 TMD and Imaging Techniques Applied in Orthodontic Diagnosis

Juliana No-Cortes, Emad Eddin Alzoubi, Reinaldo Abdala-Junior, and Arthur Rodriguez Gonzalez Cortes

7.1 Anatomy

The temporomandibular joint (TMJ) is a synovial joint located between the condylar process of the mandible and the eminence of the temporal bone. The TMJ components are the condyle, glenoid cavity and articular tubercle, articular disc, retrodiscal tissue, synovial membrane, and joint capsule. The joint cavity is divided into an upper and a lower part by an intra-articular disc. This disc is predominantly a fibrous structure which acts as a cushion, to absorb shocks and stabilize the condyle while doing rotation and translation.

Disfunction in the TMJ system can cause a group of disorders and alterations known as temporomandibular disorders (TMD). Such disorders might present some signs and signals which may include myalgia, headache, pain in and around the ear, difficulty or even pain while chewing, and clicking sound or grating sensation when opening the mouth. It has been described that despite TMD etiology is not fully understood, there is involvement of multifactorial factors, including social, biologic, psychological, and environmental [1]. Some risk factors for TMD include various types of arthritis, jaw injury, stress, long-term parafunctional habits, postural condition, systemic predisposition, sleep disorders, and psychosocial alterations [2].

It is estimated that temporomandibular joint disorders (TMD) have a higher prevalence among female patients [3]. In addition, it has been described in the literature that approximately 30% of the population presents TMD in asymptomatic forms such as internal joint derangement, comprising disc dislocation and significant structural changes resulting from osteoarthritis and osteoarthrosis [4]. Among the important TMD alterations is the anterior displacement of articular disc, which can be verified with MRI. It is known that asymptomatic patients usually present approximately 30% of prevalence of TMJ disc anterior displacement. On the other hand, 85% of symptomatic patients present anterior displacement and related intracapsular disorders.

7.1.1 Relationship Between Orthodontic Treatments and TMJ Diagnosis

In the past, malocclusion was stated as the responsible factor for the TMD. For a long time, occlusion and temporomandibular disorders have been the subject of countless studies and forms of treatment. Rehabilitation, orthodontics, or occlusal adjustments were used trying to treat those disorders.

During the 1970s and 1980s, the belief that TMD was caused by dental malocclusion was evident. TMD should then disappear when malocclusion is eliminated, through orthodontic or prosthetic treatment (change of occlusal scheme). The scientific literature in the last decades, however, has shown that there is a very small relationship between TMD and orthodontic treatment [5]. On the other hand, another article in the literature suggests that orthodontic treatment could modify intracapsular dysfunctions and morphology [6]. Furthermore, there may be changes in

J. No-Cortes
Department of Restorative Dentistry, Faculty of Dental Surgery, University of Malta, Msida, Malta
e-mail: jcort02@um.edu.mt

E. E. Alzoubi
Department of Restorative Dentistry, Faculty of Dental Surgery, University of Malta, Msida, Malta

Department of Child Dental Health and Orthodontics, Faculty of Dental Surgery, University of Malta, Msida, Malta
e-mail: emad.alzoubi@um.edu.mt

R. Abdala-Junior
School of Dentistry, University of São Paulo, São Paulo, Brazil

Department of Radiology, UniFSP, Avaré, SP, Brazil

A. R. G. Cortes (✉)
Department of Dental Surgery, Faculty of Dental Surgery, University of Malta, Msida, Malta
e-mail: arthur.nogueira@um.edu.mt

J.-M. Retrouvey, M.-N. Abdallah (eds.), *3D Diagnosis and Treatment Planning in Orthodontics*,
https://doi.org/10.1007/978-3-030-57223-5_7

occlusal schemes occurring after the use of occlusal splints for stabilizing and reducing TMD symptoms of pain and clicking. Alterations of the facial muscles and intracapsular problems of the temporomandibular joint have also been the focus of discussions, but there is still a lack of conclusive individual findings reported by clinical studies. Studies have also shown that the correct occlusal relationship between the teeth did not cause a change in the physiological position of the condyles and articular discs in TMJ when MRI and CT were examined, whereas in cases of TMD, an improvement could be obtained as a result of orthodontic treatment [7, 8].

There is controversy in the literature regarding the association between the application of different orthodontic mechanics in Class II patients and incorrect articular disc–condyle relationship [9]. Existing articles present evidences that elastics mechanics, headgear, rapid maxillary expansion, Frankel functional appliance, Bionator, fixed functional orthopedic appliances, twin block, and functional mandibular advancement appliance do not cause physiological changes in the positioning of the condyle and articular disc. Implementation or not of extraction protocols do not seem to change such situation either. Several scientific studies also indicate that orthodontic treatment in the childhood does not increase the prevalence of signs and symptoms of TMD [10–12] and that orthodontic movement does not cause adverse effects to the TMJ [13].

Despite the above-mentioned evidences, some studies found changes in condylar position and in the volumes of the anterior and posterior joint spaces due to applied orthodontic mechanics [9]. The use of the chin-cup for class III patients, for instance, caused a morphological change in condylar growth, which may be associated with correction of skeletal malocclusion in conjunction with remodeling in the jaw [14].

There is also agreement among studies in the literature, suggesting stated that a prudent orthodontist, before starting orthodontic treatment, should identify and document any signs or symptoms of temporomandibular disorders, which could be treated so that the patient starts the orthodontic treatment with no pain or related TMD symptoms. If painful symptoms appear during treatment, therapy should be modified, heavy occlusal interference should be relieved, and forces intended to distalize teeth eliminated or altered. In other words, whenever pain and TMD symptoms arise, the orthodontic treatment should be suspended temporarily, in order to diagnose and perform conservative TMJ treatments until the patient feels no pain. Then, treatment planning should be re-evaluated accordingly, and the orthodontic treatment could be continued.

7.2 Diagnosis

Knowledge of several different 2D and 3D imaging tests, as well as their appropriate indications, is crucial to establish differential diagnosis of temporomandibular disorders, especially in patients with overlapping signs and symptoms. In this context, TMD diagnosis can usually be confirmed by evaluating medical history and by physical examination. Diagnostic TMJ imaging methods are mostly used to assess the integrity of its components and their functional association, to confirm the extent or progression of an existing disease, and to assess and document the effects of an already established treatment. In this context, imaging methods are essential for the assessment of cases of trauma, occlusal alterations, sudden limitation of mouth opening, presence of joint noises, systemic joint diseases, infection, and failure of conservative treatments.

To analyze TMD, complementary examinations are used such as radiographs (standard panoramic radiographs, TMJ X-rays), computed tomography, and MRI. The two latter, however, offer higher specificity and better visualization and are considered as gold standards for TMJ analyses.

7.2.1 Imaging Test Indication Criteria in the Diagnosis of TMD

One of the failures in diagnosis and treatment planning is an incorrect or unnecessary selection of unsuitable image-obtaining methods. This may occur due to a lack of knowledge from professionals regarding the adequate indications of the applicable tests. The correct indication of an image-obtaining method should be based on the patient's need for several aspects such as legal documentation, individual complaints, and identified clinical signs and symptoms during history-taking and physical examinations. Professionals should then still follow the basic principle that supplementary tests are only indicated whether clinical assessments are not sufficient to define the diagnosis and related treatment planning.

For TMD, measurement of occlusal movements, physical examinations of palpation, functional testing, and evaluation of joint noises are important procedures of diagnostic validity that should be performed by trained and experienced professionals. Nevertheless, overlapping of muscle and joint symptoms can prevent the achievement of an accurate diagnosis, since both the conditions show functional impairment. In such cases and those without specific symptoms (from, for example, inflammation, neoplasia, and trauma), complementary imaging tests are essential for diagnostic clarification and decision taking regarding an appropriate therapy.

Despite several imaging tests can be individually indicated for specific reasons in the diagnosis of TMD, there are factors that need to be assessed for the correct selection of TMJ imaging methods, including the following: the need to determine the presence of disease and its prognosis, amount of available clinical information, uncertainty of differential diagnosis, necessity of determining the stage of development of a disease, need for legal documentation, preoperative and follow-up assessments, as well as safety and accuracy of the proposed examination [2].

7.3 Characteristics and Drawbacks of Conventional 2D Radiographic Examinations

TMJ radiographs enable assessment of 2D morphological characteristics of bone components of the joint, including condyle, articular tubercle, and fossa, but are inefficient for assessing soft tissues. The 2D radiographic techniques that had been mostly used in the routine management of TMD were panoramic radiography, TMJ plain radiography, and transcranial radiography.

Radiographic visualization of TMJ in 2D was not always easy to acquire due to superposition of different structures on projections related to the TMJ. For this reason, a combined use of different techniques used to be necessary to locate and provide an accurate diagnosis of the alterations. The evaluation of the structures in different planes allowed for diagnosis of fracture extension, degenerative joint disease, postoperative status, ankylosis, neoplasms, acute fractures, dislocations, and severe degenerative articular disease. In this context, the main combined views are submental (or submento-vertex), reverse Towne, posterior-anterior, and lateral teleradiography. Lateral oblique, posteroanterior (Towne's), and caudocranial (Hertz) techniques were also commonly used.

Despite their lower sensitivity, 2D radiographic techniques have lower costs and employ lower radiation doses as compared to CT scans. Such conventional 2D methods can be indicated for the early assessment of less complex symptoms. In addition, they can help in the differential diagnosis between TMD and inflammatory dental-maxillofacial conditions.

The most commonly used method for dentists is the conventional or digital panoramic radiographs. Such radiographs provide a maxillary overview useful in the differential diagnosis of odontogenic alterations whose symptoms might overlap with TMD. It can reveal significant bone alterations in the condyle, such as erosions, osteophytes, asymmetries, fractures, changes in the morphology, degenerative and inflammatory processes, maxillary tumors, metastases, and ankylosis. Nevertheless, panoramic radiographs do not provide functional information on condylar excursion. In addition, some alterations in the articular tubercle morphology might be misdiagnosed because of superimpositions of anatomical structures from the skull base and zygomatic arches.

7.4 3D Radiographic Examinations

7.4.1 Computed Tomography

Computed tomography (CT) scans are images considered to be superior to 2D conventional examinations since it allows for assessments in multiplanar reconstructed images, which lead to accurate diagnosis of bone structures of the TMJ by means of images in the three orthogonal planes (i.e., sagittal, coronal, and axial), which can be assessed at the same time (Figs. 7.1, 7.2, and 7.3). It is also possible to have three-dimensional reconstructed models from the original Digital Communication in Medicine (DICOM) files of the CT scans by using DICOM viewer software. In CT scans, images in different planes with less than 1 mm of slice thickness can be assessed without distortions or overlap. For TMJ, CT is indicated for the diagnosis of bone abnormalities including fractures, dislocations, arthritis, ankylosis, and neoplasia. It is also used for assessing condyle implants, being adequate to detect erosion in the middle cranial fossa and ectopic bone growth.

Medical computed tomography uses sources of collimated X-rays, arranged in a fan shape to irradiate an anatomical region of interest. The patient is placed horizontally in a circular tunnel where there is a tube in which the rays are emitted on the one side and on the other they will be captured by a panel of receivers. Each receiver converts radiation into an electrical signal, which is sent and stored in a computer. In each scan, a two-dimensional matrix of pixels is produced with a calculated attenuation value, which results in the grayscale composing the image. Such grayscale, in turn, is dependent on the contrast resolution and the number of bits of the device and may be converted to different working scales such as the Hounsfield units (HU) which allows for bone density estimation, using a DICOM viewer software. In this context, a longer contrast scale depicts more details to differentiate pixel intensities within the tissues. For this reason, accuracy of medical CT is higher than conventional radiographs.

In contrast with medical CT, cone-beam computed tomography (CBCT) devices have been used for dental

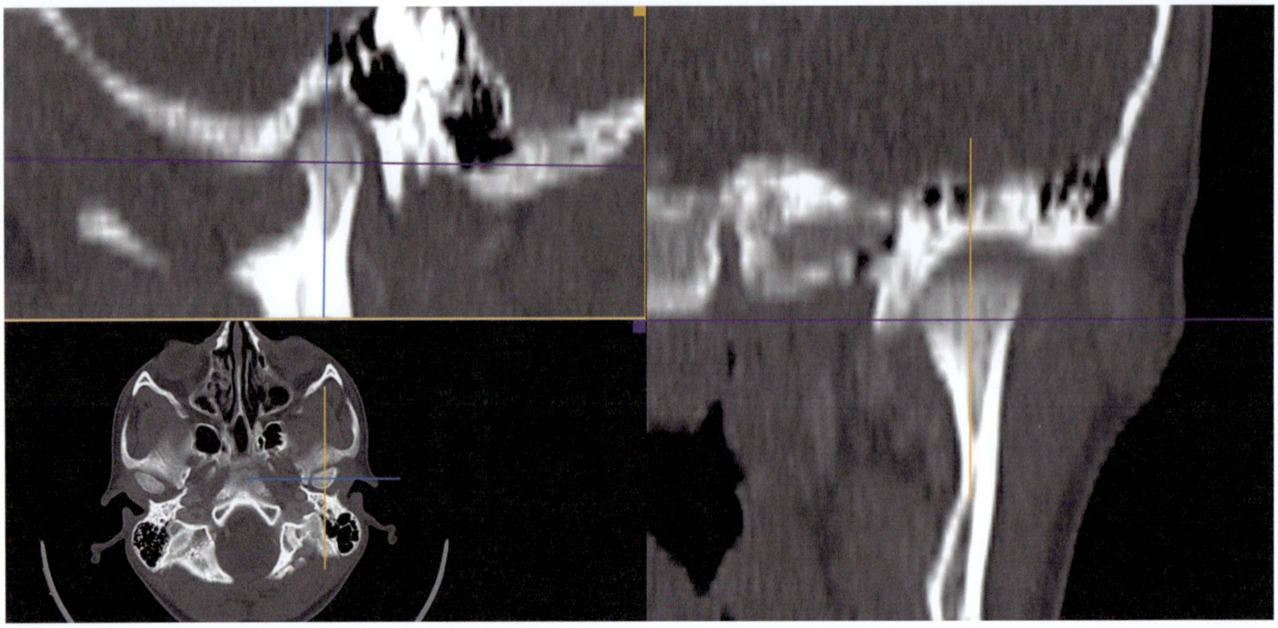

Fig. 7.1 Multi-planar reconstruction of a medical computed tomography showing bone components of the TMJ

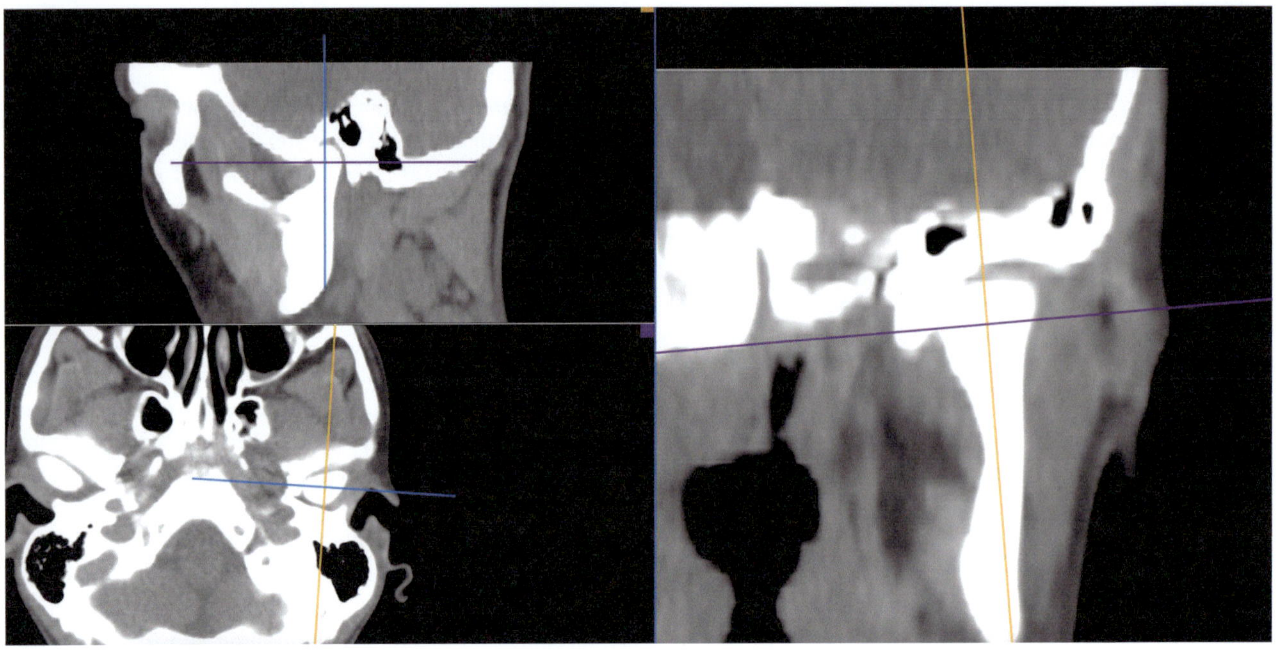

Fig. 7.2 Multi-planar reconstruction of a medical computed tomography showing soft tissue window images of the TMJ area

diagnosis due to its specific design for oral and maxillofacial regions. Important advantages of CBCT includes fast and easier imaging, as well as lower radiation doses as compared with medical CT. Despite having a shorter contrast scale, CBCT allows for observation of bone joint structures in the three planes: sagittal, coronal, and axial planes, as well as in 3D volumetric reconstructed models (Figs. 7.4, 7.5, 7.6, and 7.7).

The main indications of CBCT include structural assessment of bone components of the TMJ, which precisely determines the location and extent of boney alterations: fractures, neoplasms, and ankylosis; pseudocystic, erosive degenerative, and osteo-

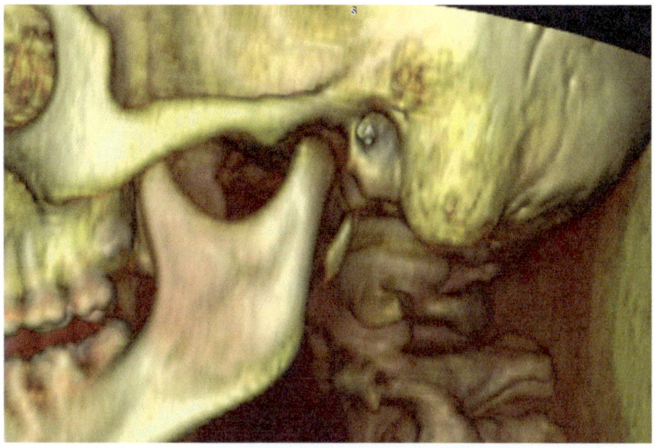

Fig. 7.3 3D reconstruction rendered from medical CT data

phytic alterations; presence of asymptomatic bone remodeling; evaluation of post-surgical conditions; morphologic alterations and hyperplasia of condylar, coronoid, and styloid processes; as well as intra-articular calcification derived from metabolic arthritis or synovial chondromatosis. Hard tissues, teeth, and bones are well demonstrated and measured in their real morphological condition, with minimal noise and artifacts [15].

On the other hand, due to its contrast resolution, CBCT is limited only to the evaluation of bone components of the TMJ. Therefore, when soft tissue imaging is required, such as in cases of injuries, the examination of choice should initially be MRI, to diagnose possible TMJ injuries, while CBCT will only be indicated when these alterations are involving TMJ bone components [16].

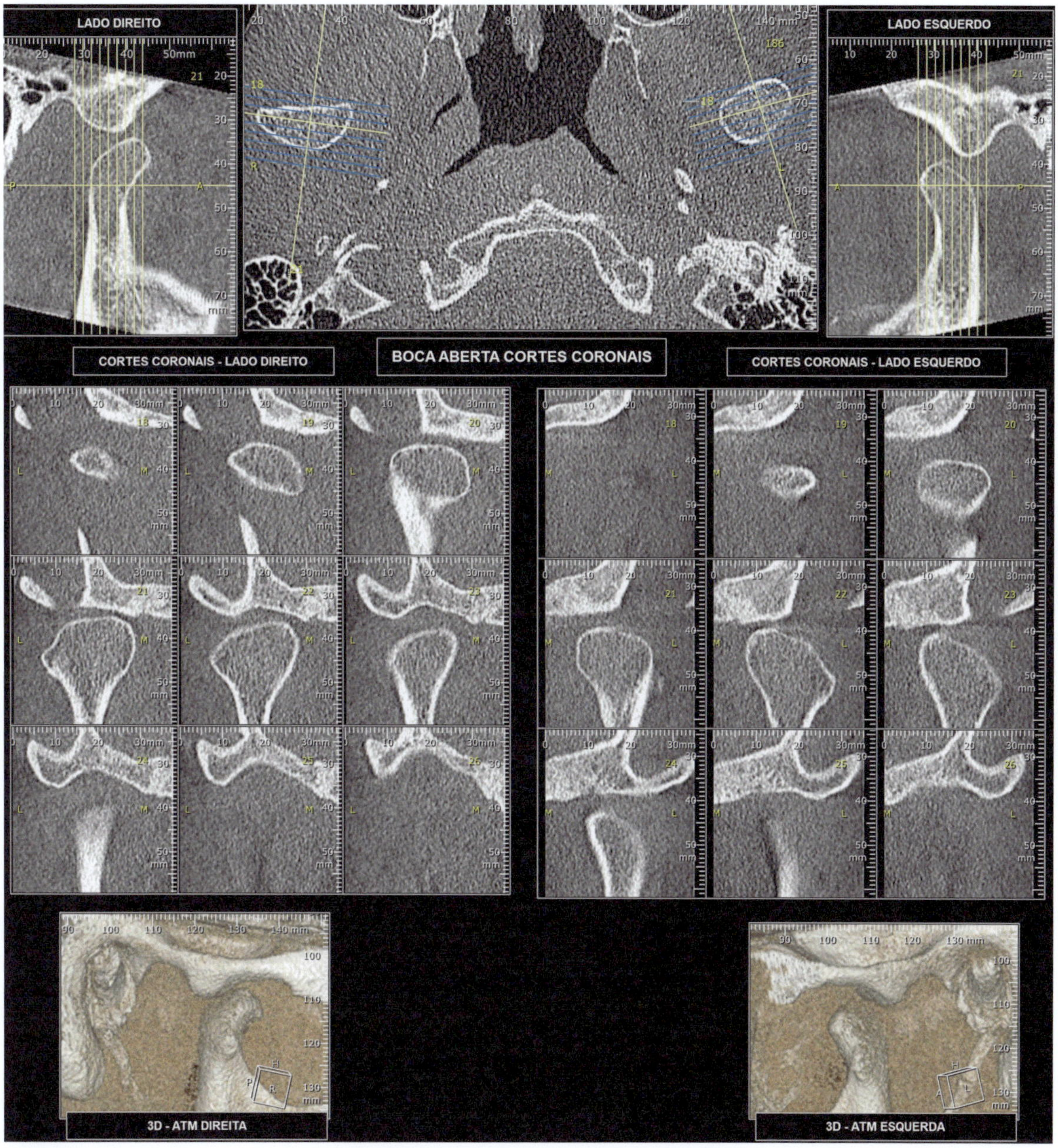

Fig. 7.4 Multiple coronal CBCT images showing the TMJ region of a patient with open mouth

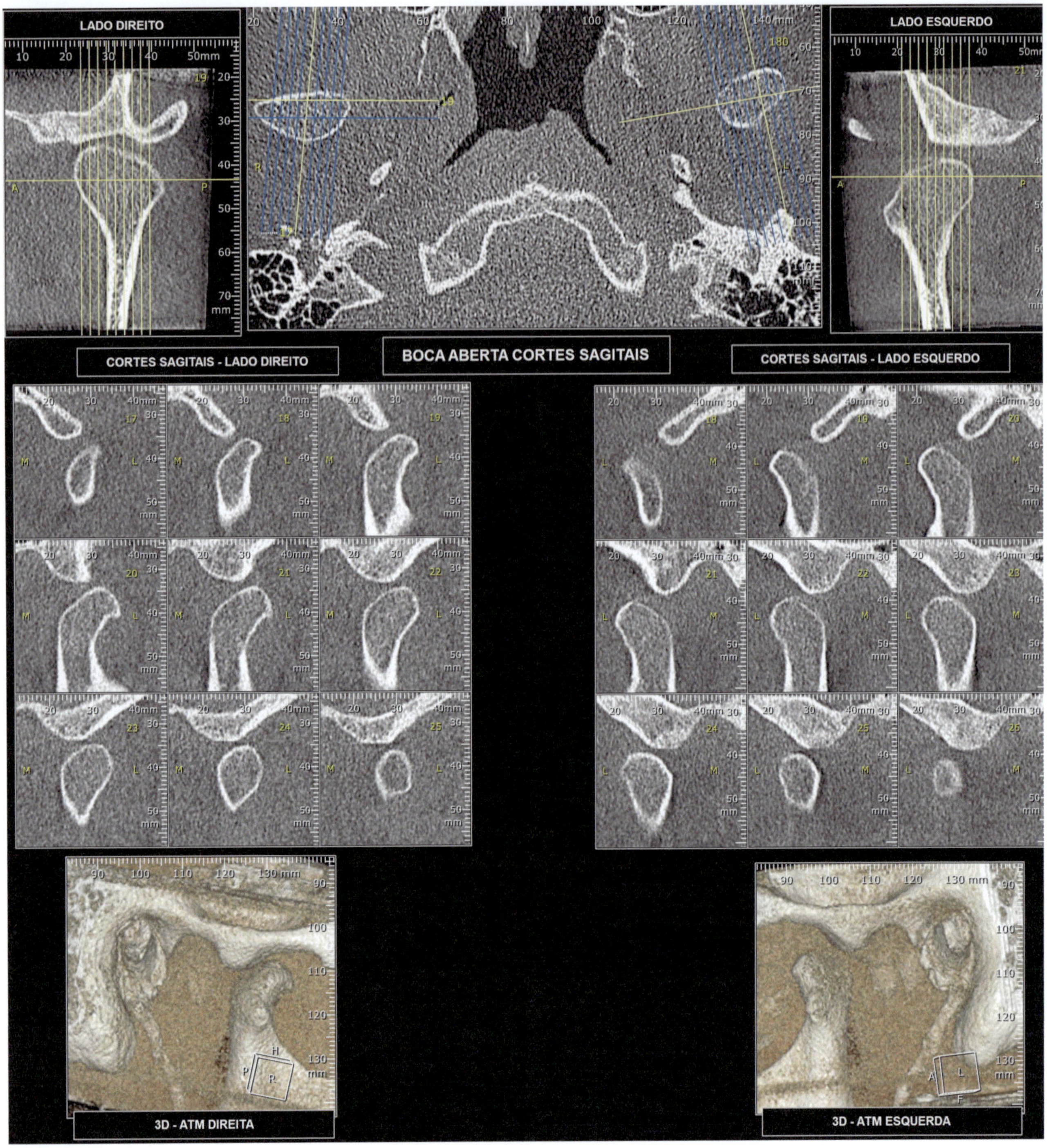

Fig. 7.5 Multiple sagittal CBCT images of a patient with open mouth, showing an osteophyte in the right condyle and excessive translation of both condyles

7.4.2 Magnetic Resonance Imaging

As mentioned briefly above, MRI has been considered the method of choice to study all alterations involving soft tissues and related TMJ components, such as the articular disc, ligaments, intracapsular synovial content, retrodiscal tissues, adjacent masticatory muscles, as well as cortical and trabecular integrity of bone component (Fig. 7.8).

In contrast with CT and other radiographic methods, MRI does not use ionizing radiation. Instead, it employs low-frequency radio waves that magnetize the protons of hydrogen atoms of the human organism. When such radiofrequency waves cease, the protons return to their original position, emitting other radio waves in the same frequency (frequency of resonance) which depends on the chemical and physical composition of each structure. Besides hydrogen, MRI sig-

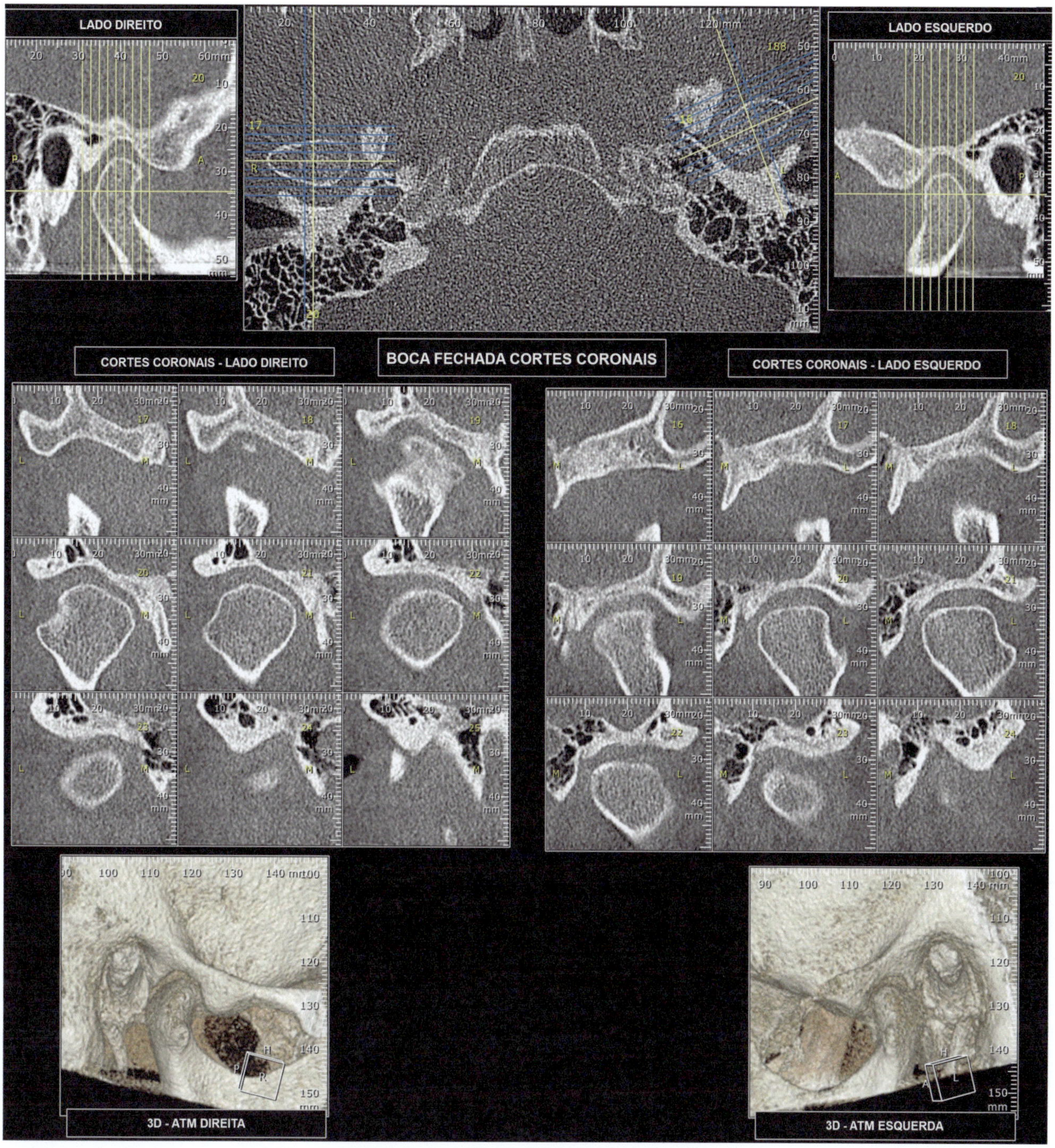

Fig. 7.6 Multiple coronal CBCT images showing the TMJ region of a patient with closed mouth

nals can be generated by other certain nuclei of atoms in tissues. By the image of the hydrogen density in the tissues, the density of the water can be measured. In this way, a structure rich in water (H_2O) or fat (which is basically composed by CH_2 molecules) emits a hypersignal, producing a clear image. The cortical bone, being avascular and therefore poor in water, emits a hyposignal, producing a dark image. The intermediate signals produce grayscale images. The TMJ is usually analyzed with the patient with the mouth closed, to detect the anterior displacement of the disc, and with the mouth open, to classify the abnormal joint in three categories: anterior displacement with reduction of the disc, anterior displacement without reduction of the disc, and anterior displacement without reduction associated with arthrosis.

Ferromagnetic materials move under the influence of the field on MRI. Therefore, the examination is contraindicated in patients with pacemakers and metallic implants in noble structures, such as large-caliber vessels, as they can displace.

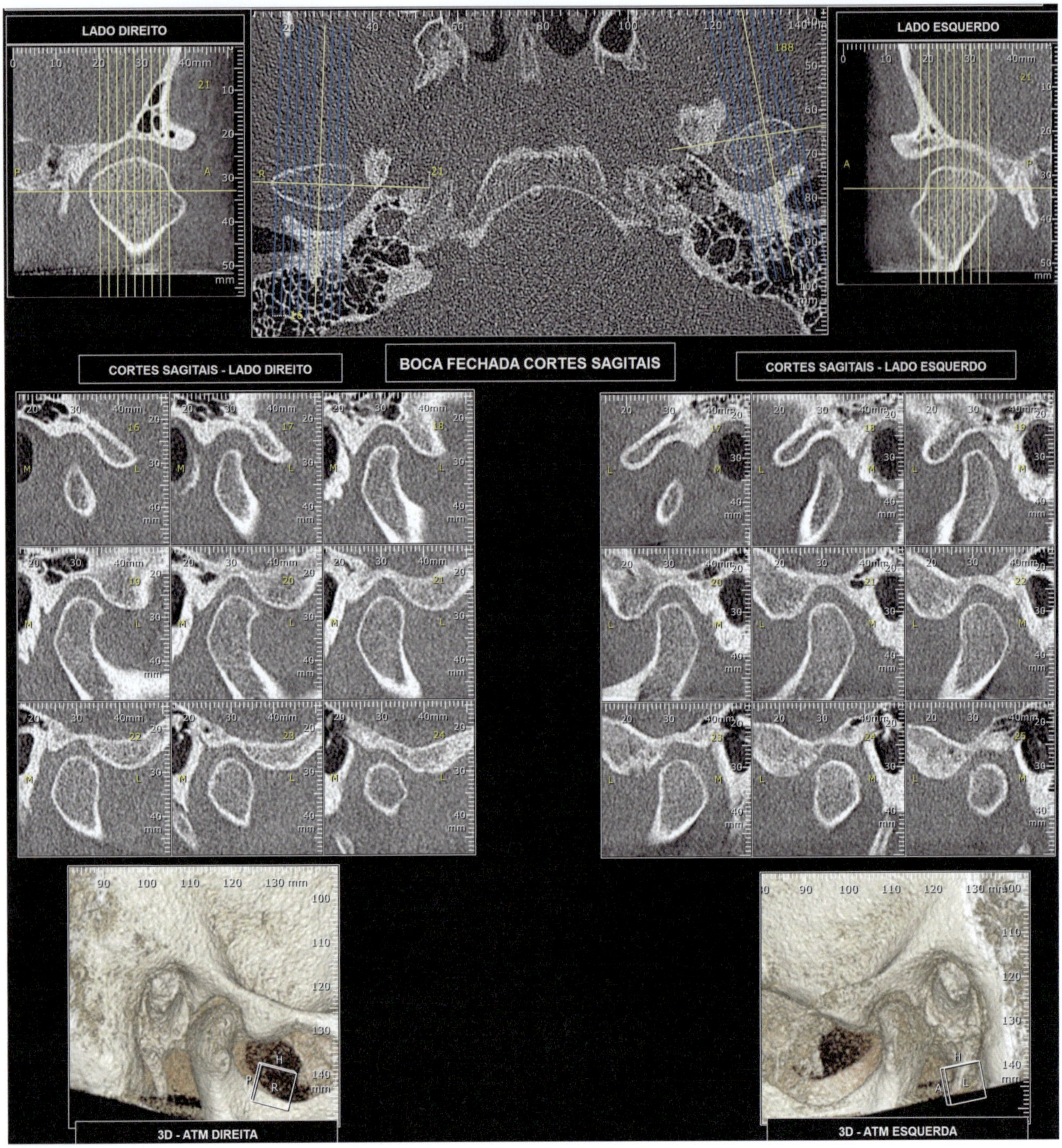

Fig. 7.7 Sagittal view of the CBCT imaging showing the TMJ region with closed mouth

Amalgam and gold restorations do not produce changes in the image; however, other metal alloys, such as those used in prostheses and orthodontic appliances, can produce artifacts that interfere in the interpretation of the image. The most apprehensive patients may need sedation, especially claustrophobic ones. Attempts should be made to minimize the time required for the examination by instructing the patient not to move.

Similar to CT scans, MRI also allows for three-dimensional analysis in the axial, coronal, and sagittal planes. It is considered the gold standard for assessing disc position and is highly accurate for intra-articular degenerative diseases. Common clinical conditions that require MRI scans include persistent symptoms of joint or pre-auricular pain, functional alterations such as lateral projections of the condyle during mouth opening, presence of clicking and

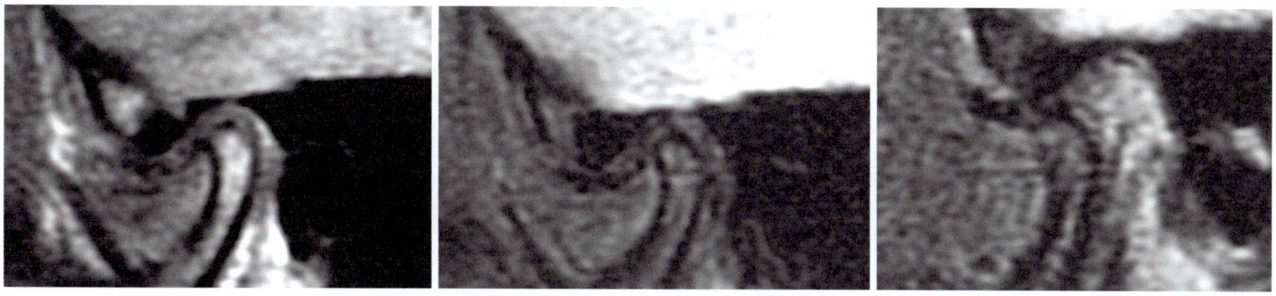

Fig. 7.8 (Left) Magnetic resonance imaging (MRI): T1-weighted image showing anteriorly disc displaced in a patient with closed mouth. (Middle) MRI, proton density (PD) image taken with closed mouth. (Right) MRI PD, image taken with open mouth showing an anteriorly disc displaced without reduction

crepitation noises, frequent subluxations and dislocations, limited mouth opening movement with terminal stiffness, and presence of osteoarthritic symptoms or asymptomatic osteoarthrosis [16].

The most common MRI protocols usually include scans in the MHI and MMO position, using weighted T1, T2, and proton density (PD), in the sagittal and coronal planes [2]. With T1-weighted images, it is possible to obtain satisfactory anatomic detail, while proton density results in satisfactory spatial resolution of joint disc injuries and is considered the best choice for the evaluation of medial and lateral disc displacements. On the other hand, T2-weighted images record the presence of joint effusion and medullary bone edema.

The main drawbacks of MRI are related to the high cost, the need for sophisticated facilities, and artifacts caused by metallic devices [17]. It is also contraindicated in patients with pacemakers and metallic heart valves, claustrophobic patients, ferromagnetic foreign bodies, and pregnant women.

7.4.3 Ultrasound

The US examination, especially by high-resolution imaging equipment, can be a useful option in the assessment of disc position in internal TMJ disorders. Despite its lack of resolution for assessing cortical and articular disc morphology, US allows for identifying effusion in patients with inflammatory conditions associated with pain, also diagnosed by MRI. Even with limitations, it can become a useful option for the initial study of the internal dysfunctions of the TMJ particularly in patients with contraindications to MRI. Moreover, it is less expensive, also without using ionizing radiation, being fast and comfortable. Another indication of the US assessment is the correct location of joint spaces for infiltrative therapies, arthrocentesis. The main advantage is dynamic visualization in real time of the location of joint components, providing adequate lubrication and washing, which are verified by the increase in joint space after treatment [18].

7.5 Conclusion

Diagnosis is most often based on history and physical examination. Diagnostic imaging may be beneficial when malocclusion or intra-articular abnormalities are suspected. The decision in choosing the examination must consider its influence on the proposed diagnosis and therapy. If the clinical indication is a conservative therapy that can control symptoms in the short term, image requests can be considered. Moreover, when conservative therapy has failed and an invasive therapy is indicated, highly sensitive diagnostic tests such as CT and MRI are selected.

Conflict of Interest and Source of Funding The authors do not have any financial interests, either directly or indirectly, to the products or information identified in the chapter.

References

1. Güler N, Uçkan S, Imirzalioğlu P, Açikgözoğlu S. Temporomandibular joint internal derangement: relationship between joint pain and MR grading of effusion and total protein concentration in the joint fluid. Dentomaxillofac Radiol. 2005;34:175–81.
2. Hunter A, Kalathingal S. Diagnostic imaging for temporomandibular disorders and orofacial pain. Dent Clin N Am. 2013;57:405–18.
3. Lai YC, Yap AU, Türp JC. Prevalence of temporomandibular disorders in patients seeking orthodontic treatment: a systematic review. J Oral Rehabil. 2020;47(2):270–80.
4. Fujiwara M, Honda K, Hasegawa Y, Hasegawa M, Urade M. Comparison of joint pain in patients diagnosed with and without articular disc displacement without reduction based on the research diagnostic criteria for temporomandibular disorders. Oral Surg Oral Med Oral Pathol Oral Radiol Endod. 2013;116:9–15.
5. Michelotti A, Iodice G. The role of orthodontics in temporomandibular disorders. J Oral Rehabil. 2010;37(6):411–29.
6. Sondhi A. Orthodontics and patients with temporomandibular disorders: inform before you perform. Am J Orthod Dentofac Orthop. 1999;115(5):551–2.

7. Kinzinger G, Roth A, Gulden N, Bucker A, Diedrich P. Effects of orthodontic treatment with fixed functional orthopaedic appliances on the condyle-fossa relationship in the temporomandibular joint: a magnetic resonance imaging study (part I). Dentomaxillofac Radiol. 2006;35(5 Pt 1):339–46.
8. Kinzinger G, Roth A, Gulden N, Bucker A, Diedrich P. Effects of orthodontic treatment with fixed functional orthopaedic appliances on the disc-condyle relationship in the temporomandibular joint: a magnetic resonance imaging study (part II). Dentomaxillofac Radiol. 2006;35(5 Pt 2):347–56.
9. Al-Saleh MA, Alsufyani N, Flores-Mir C, Nebbe B, Major PW. Changes in temporomandibular joint morphology in class II patients treated with fixed mandibular repositioning and evaluated through 3D imaging: a systematic review. Orthod Craniofac Res. 2015;18(4):185–201.
10. Egermark I, Magnusson T, Carlsson GE. A 20-year follow-up of signs and symptoms of temporomandibular disorders and malocclusions in subjects with and without orthodontic treatment in childhood. Angle Orthod. 2003;73(2):109–15.
11. Mohlin B, Axelsson S, Paulin G, Pietila T, Bondemark L, Brattstrom V, et al. TMD in relation to malocclusion and orthodontic treatment. Angle Orthod. 2007;77(3):542–8.
12. Kim MR, Graber TM, Viana MA. Orthodontics and temporomandibular disorder: a meta-analysis. Am J Orthod Dentofac Orthop. 2002;121(5):438–46.
13. Franco AA, Yamashita HK, Lederman HM, Cevidanes LH, Proffit WR, Vigorito JW. Fränkel appliance therapy and the temporomandibular disc: a prospective magnetic resonance imaging study. Am J Orthod Dentofac Orthop. 2002;121(5):447–57.
14. Zurfluh MA, Kloukos D, Patcas R, Eliades T. Effect of chin-cup treatment on the temporomandibular joint: a systematic review. Eur J Orthod. 2015;37(3):314–24.
15. Kim JH, Arita ES, Pinheiro LR, Yoshimoto M, Watanabe PCA, Cortes ARG. Computed tomographic artifacts in maxillofacial surgery. J Craniofac Surg. 2018;29(1):e78–80.
16. Al-Saleh MA, Alsufyani NA, Saltaji H, Jaremko JL, Major PWMRI. CBCT image registration of temporomandibular joint: a systematic review. J Otolaryngol Head Neck Surg. 2016; 45(1):30.
17. Cortes AR, Abdala-Junior R, Weber M, Arita ES, Ackerman JL. Influence of pulse sequence parameters at 1.5 T and 3.0 T on MRI artefacts produced by metal-ceramic restorations. Dentomaxillofac Radiol. 2015;44(8):20150136.
18. Almeida FT, Pacheco-Pereira C, Flores-Mir C, Le LH, Jaremko JL, Major PW. Diagnostic ultrasound assessment of temporomandibular joints: a systematic review and meta-analysis. Dentomaxillofac Radiol. 2019;48(2):20180144.

Part II

Indications, Applications, and Planning Based on Imaging Techniques

Potential and Applications of STL and DICOM Data Matching: MAPA Systems and F22 Aligners

8

Luca Lombardo, Mario Palone, Giuliano Bortolo Maino, Emanuele Paoletto, and Giuseppe Siciliani

8.1 Introduction

The relationship between dental, skeletal and soft tissues is three-dimensional [1], and the dentoskeletal apparatus is a complex system to investigate. Indeed, until recently, investigations were based on the 3D reconstruction of 2D radiographs, a difficult task that was heavily reliant on the analytical and technical skills of the operator [2]. Although the introduction of conventional computed tomography (CT) opened new horizons, especially in implantology, its application in orthodontics continued to be limited due to the large field of analysis and the relatively high levels of radiation exposure. However, with the introduction of cone-beam technology (Fig. 8.1), which features the emission of a conical rather than linear beam of X-rays, the quantity of ionising radiation emitted was drastically reduced, thereby paving the way to its routine use in orthodontics. This has also been facilitated by the high-performance detector systems available, and possibility of reducing the regions of interest (ROI) via modulation of the field of view (FOV) [3].

Volumetric datasets are acquired in DICOM format (Digital Imaging and Communications in Medicine), which can easily be opened using radiology software packages.

There are many advantages to the CBCT technique, notably:

- Ease of 3D rendering and 3D reconstruction (Fig. 8.1)
- Considerable reduction of radiations emitted with respect to conventional CT (426–1160 μSv) [4], thanks also to the introduction of image intensifiers
- The possibility to modulate the field of view (FOV), which enables focussing on the ROI, thereby reducing the extent of irradiated tissues (Fig. 8.2)
- Multiplanar reconstructions (MPRs) of acquired volumetric datasets (Fig. 8.3)
- The possibility of acquiring 2D images from the volumetric datasets such as panoramic radiograph, lateral head films and TMJ stratigraphy
- Lower cost than conventional CT
- The possibility of investigating even peripheral areas and therefore diagnosing occult pathologies [5]
- Clinical versatility and accurate matching between digital models in STL format and CBCT scans in DICOM format [6] (Fig. 8.4)

A recent meta-analysis conducted on 20 studies highlighted the considerable disparity in the amount of radiations emitted by CBCT scanners, with doses ranging from 5 to 1073 μSv in adults and from 7 to 769 μSv in children [7]. Therefore, the equivalent doses emitted by CBCT scanners are very difficult to generalise, depending on various factors including the size and shape (cylindrical or spherical) of the FOV (Fig. 8.2), the shape of the X-ray beam, the detector system technology (flat or rounded sensors), the exposure time and the resolution (voxel dimension), as well the amperage (mA) and voltage (kV) of the X-ray tube. Nonetheless, CBCT is able to provide precise, high-resolution radiographic images without any distortion, which can be used for multiplanar and volumetric reconstruction [8].

In a similar fashion, the introduction of digital technologies has made it possible to digitalise the dental arches. Dental analysis for orthodontic purposes has long been based on plaster casts, which, in addition to requiring laborious and time-consuming manual analysis, are bulky and difficult to store. Moreover, plaster models must be manually cast and

L. Lombardo (✉) · M. Palone · G. B. Maino · E. Paoletto
G. Siciliani
Ferrara University, Ferrara, Italy
e-mail: lab@orthomodul.it; sci@unife.it

J.-M. Retrouvey, M.-N. Abdallah (eds.), *3D Diagnosis and Treatment Planning in Orthodontics*,
https://doi.org/10.1007/978-3-030-57223-5_8

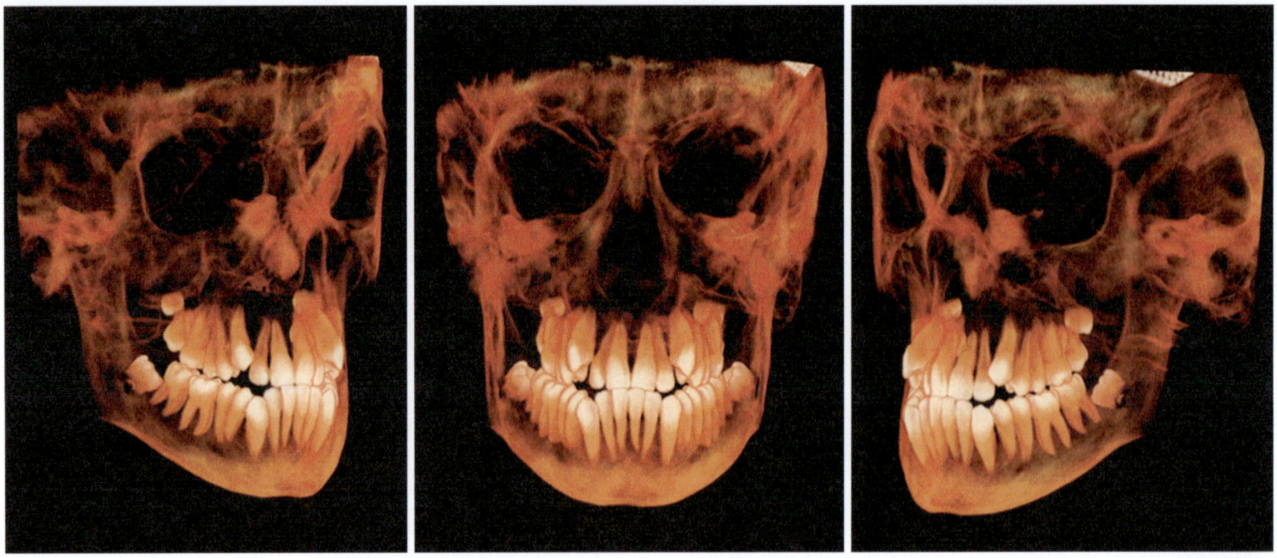

Fig. 8.1 Volumetric rendering images built from a dataset (DICOM data) obtained from a cone-beam computed tomography (CBCT) scan

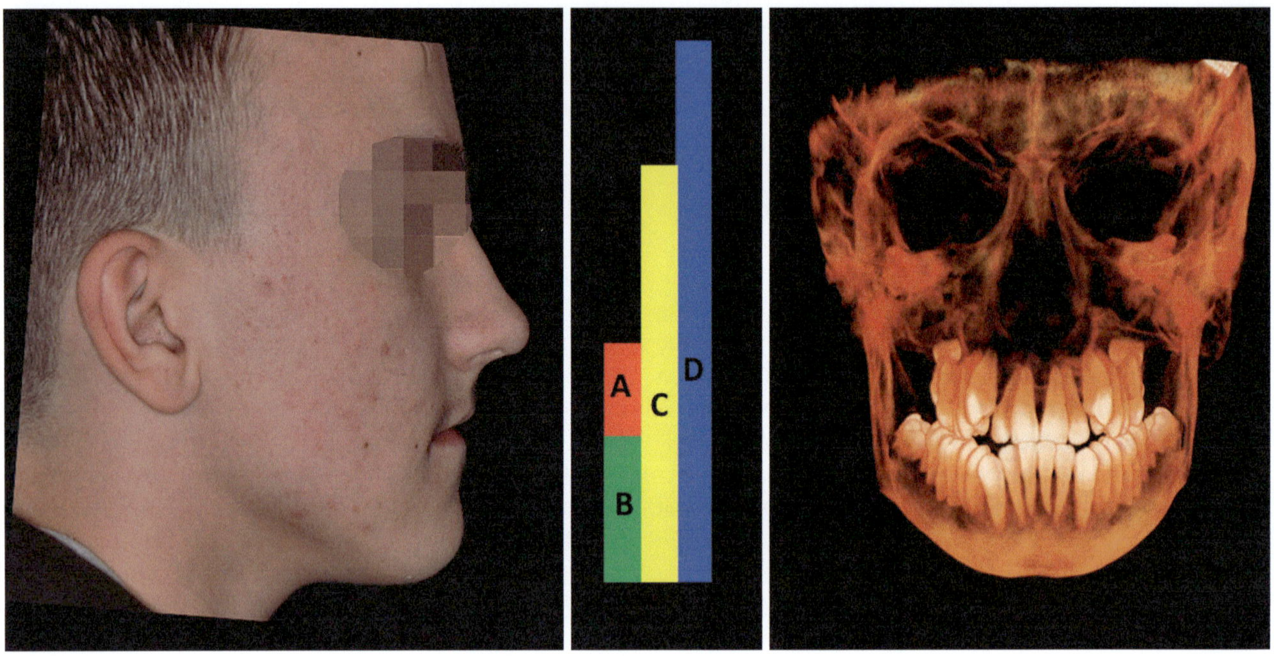

Fig. 8.2 Different sized fields of view (FOVs) that can be investigated using a CBCT examination (A = maxillary FOV, B = mandibular FOV, C = facial FOV, D = craniofacial FOV)

are therefore not immediately available for consultation. However, it is now possible to acquire digital models in STL format (standard triangulation language) immediately, which provides considerable versatility and ready clinical applications (Fig. 8.5).

Indeed, STL software enables the production of digital models composed of a polygonal mesh made up of contiguous triangles, each of which has points of known coordinates and a vector that identifies the normal to the surface (Fig. 8.6). The studies in the literature have provided irrefutable evidence that digital models, acquired directly or indirectly, can be routinely used for orthodontic purposes [9–11].

The advantages of using digital, as opposed to plaster, models, are as follows:

- No need for any physical storage space [12]
- The possibility of distance sharing via the internet [13, 14]
- Increased longevity with no risk of physical damage [15]

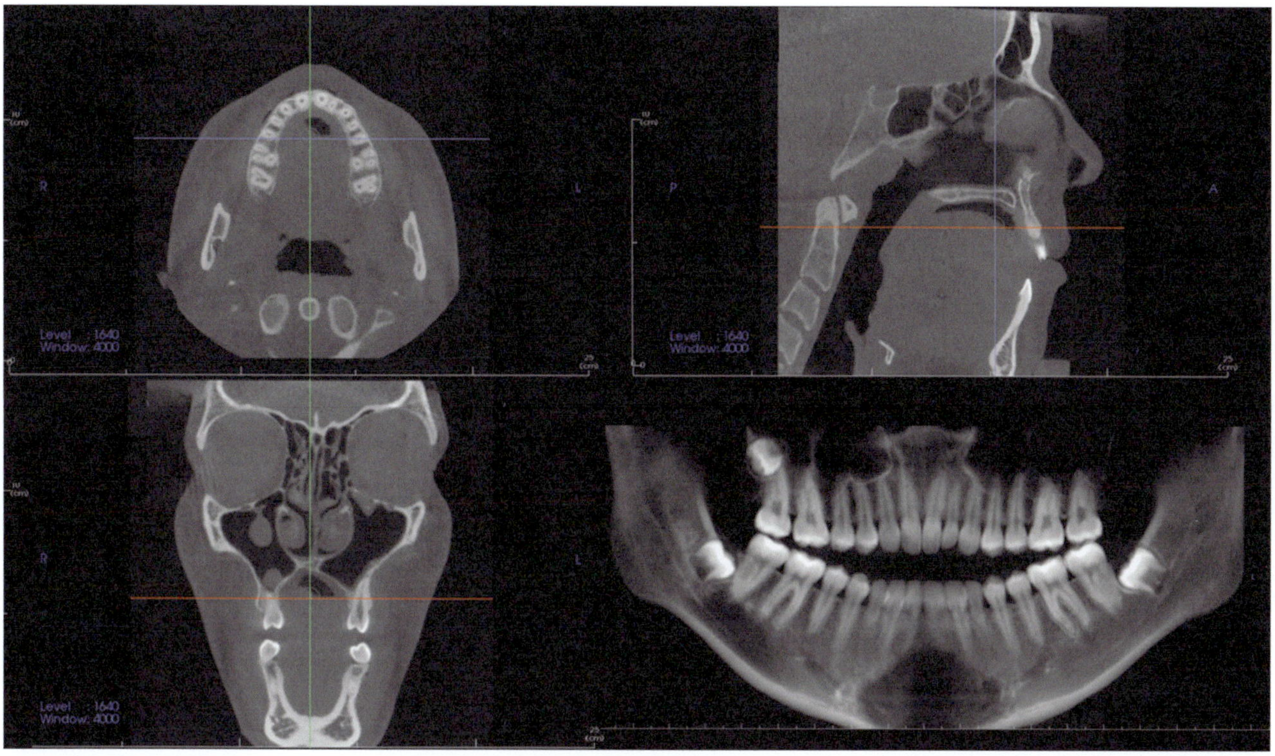

Fig. 8.3 Multiplanar reconstruction (MPR) of DICOM data obtained via CBCT

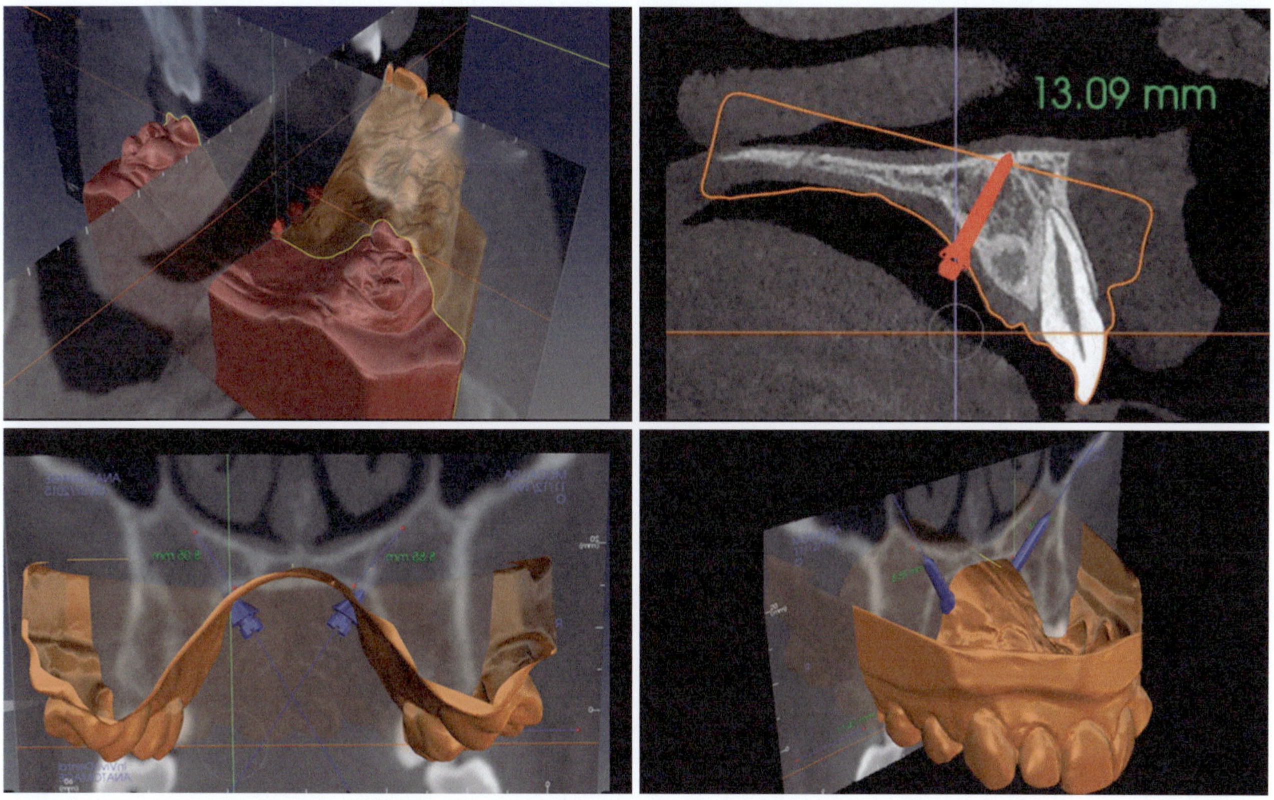

Fig. 8.4 Accurate 3D matching between DICOM data (CBCT) and STL file (digital cast)

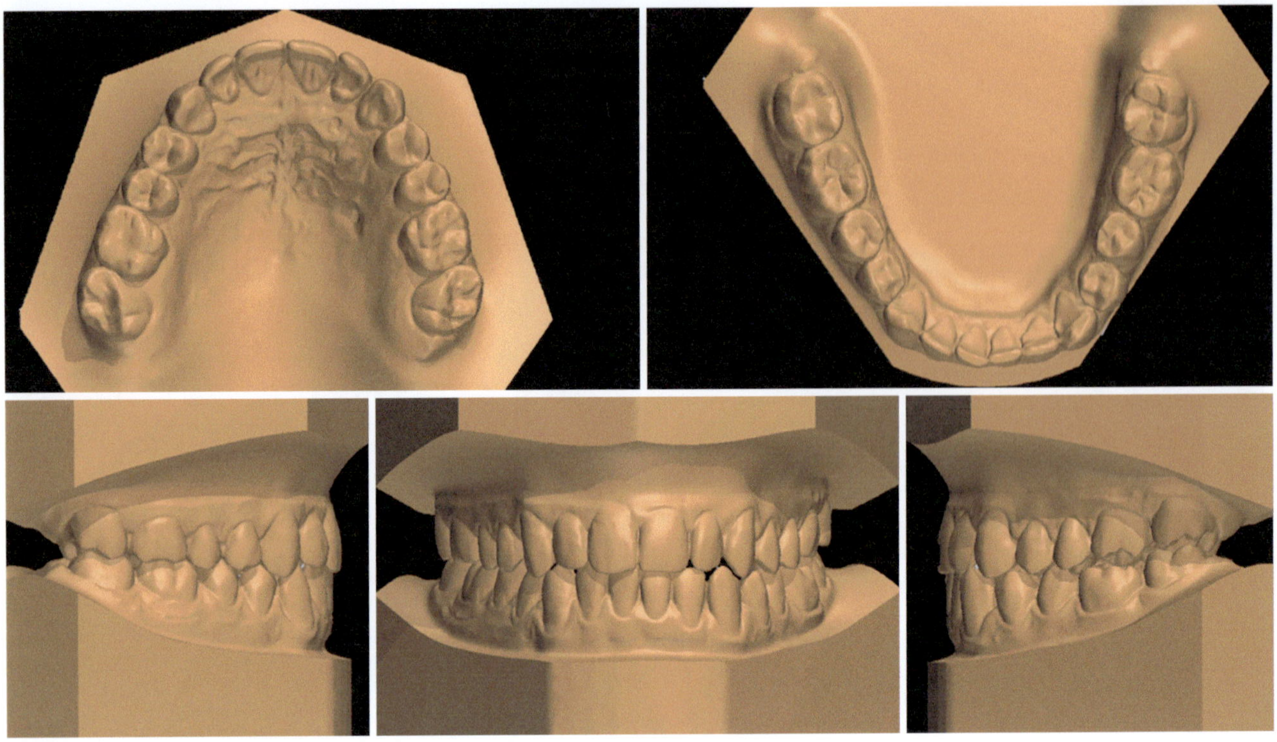

Fig. 8.5 Digital models in different views

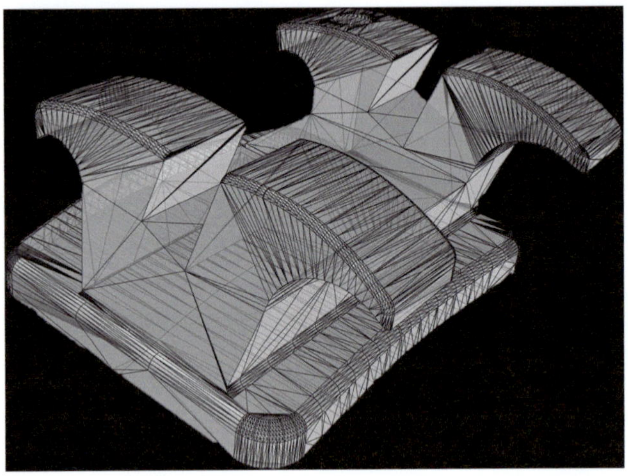

Fig. 8.6 Standard triangulation language (STL) file representing a bracket showing the polygonal (triangle) mesh used to map the object

- Extreme versatility, with applications that include diagnostic measurements (transverse diameters, arch length, total and anterior Bolton analysis, evaluation of molar and canine Class relationship, overjet and overbite analysis) with reduced handling times [16]; diagnostic set-ups [17] and working set-ups for the construction of orthodontic and other appliances using CAD/CAM technology, drastically reducing the time required for orthodontic set-up and laboratory costs [18]
- The possibility of measuring tooth position (tip, torque and in-out values) via the creation of virtual slices [9] or the use of reference point coordinates [19]
- The possibility of 3D printing models in the event that a tangible object is required for interaction with the patient, etc. [20]

8.2 Matching CBCT Scans (DICOM Data) and Digital Models (STL Files): Clinical Implications

As described in the previous chapter, the remarkable versatility of tomographic datasets enables 3D matching between them and digital models of dental arches acquired in STL format, obtaining a faithful reconstruction of the facial dentoskeletal apparatus. Together, this data enables the construction of surgical guides for assisted palatal orthodontic miniscrew insertion, ensuring that the miniscrews are of the correct length, providing bicortical or tricortical anchorage in a safe and a predictable manner.

8.2.1 Prerequisites for Adequate 3D Matching

In order to ensure an appropriate 3D matching between digital models and CBCT scans, the data acquired must have certain characteristics. As regards digital models, these must be accurate and precise, being free of distortion along the arch perimeter, and contain accurate and detailed renderings of all occlusal surfaces and the palatal vault.

As regards the CBCT scans, we must be sure that the scan is carried out with the patient's mouth open and the mandible stabilised by means of rolls of cotton placed between diatoric teeth during the examination. Moreover, the tongue should be positioned on the floor of the oral cavity, and this enables the dentition to be mapped in detail, without the mandibular arch overlapping, and the thickness of the palatal mucosa to be recorded, which would otherwise be indistinguishable from the tongue (Fig. 8.7).

8.2.2 Miniscrew-Assisted Palatal Application (MAPA System)

There are innumerable advantages to the construction of a surgical guide for orthodontic miniscrew insertion (Spider Screw K2 Regular Plus Konic, HDC, Thiene, Vicenza, Italy) in the palatal vault [6]. Surgical guides enable the degree of miniscrew parallelism to be selected, as well as the appropriate length for engaging the nasal cortical bone (bicortical anchorage). This provides excellent primary stability and enables the delivery of bone-borne appliances or tooth–bone-borne appliances, even in a single appointment [21, 22].

The literature reveals that the palatal vault is an ideal site for miniscrew insertion; indeed, it is of adequate thickness [23], features two cortical bone layers that can be easily engaged [24, 25], is free of important anatomical structures such as the tooth roots and has a thick, keratinised mucosa [26]. High survival rates have been consistently reported for miniscrews inserted into the palatal vault [27], and it is considered a safe site for miniscrew insertion [26].

However, the thickness of the palatal vault varies considerably between individuals, and therefore defies standardisation. Although Ardekian et al. reported no particular adverse effects in the event that the miniscrew perforates the nasal cavity floor by less than 2 mm, it is essential to avoid this in order to reduce patient discomfort [28].

After the 3D matching has been performed using eXam vision software (KaVo Dental GmbH, Biberach, Germany) integrated with Rhinoceros software (Robert McNeel & Associates, Seattle, WA, USA), miniscrews of the appropriate length and diameter can be selected from a large library. In this way, an adequate length for bicortical anchorage and safe insertion of miniscrews can be ensured (Fig. 8.8) and the MAPA surgical guide correctly designed. The K2 Regular Plus Konic miniscrews employed are self-drilling and have a diameter of 2 mm and a conical head which facilitates abutment connection with skeletal anchorage devices. Another advantageous feature of these miniscrews is that they have a port in the head of the mini-

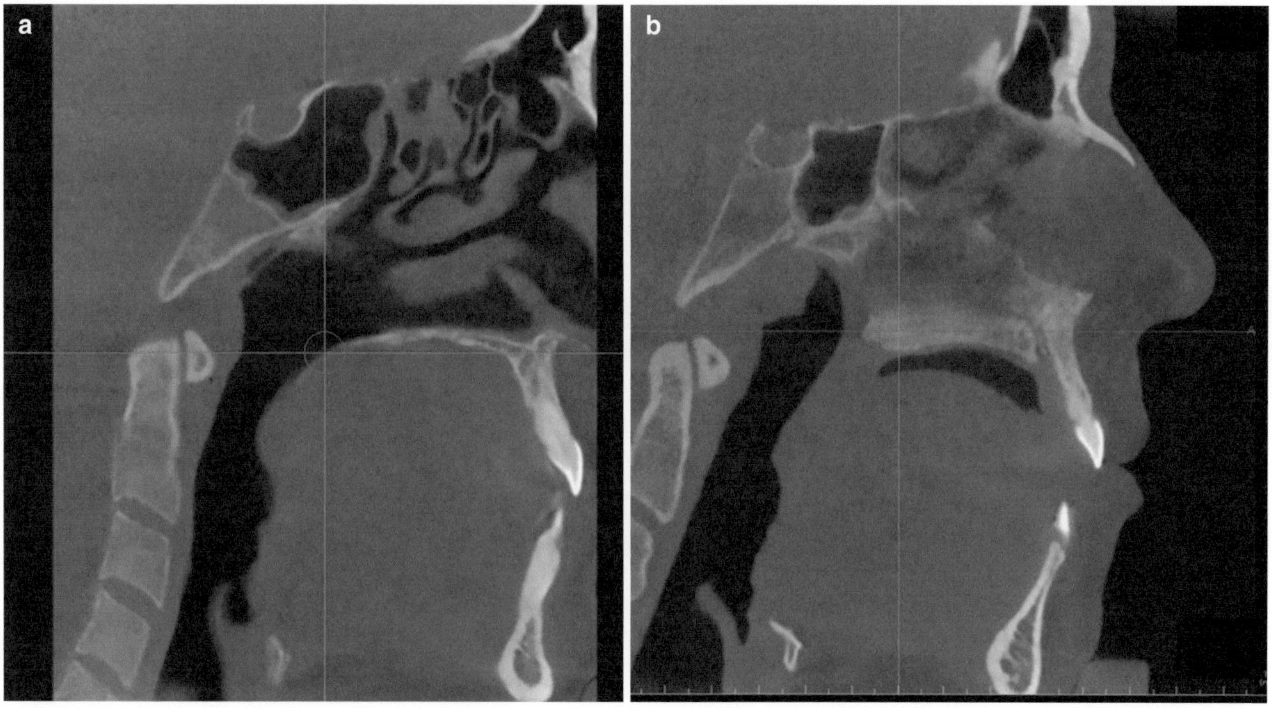

Fig. 8.7 Example of CBCT scans performed with the tongue in contact with the palatal mucosa (**a**), and on the floor of the mouth (**b**), the latter revealing the thickness of the palatal mucosa

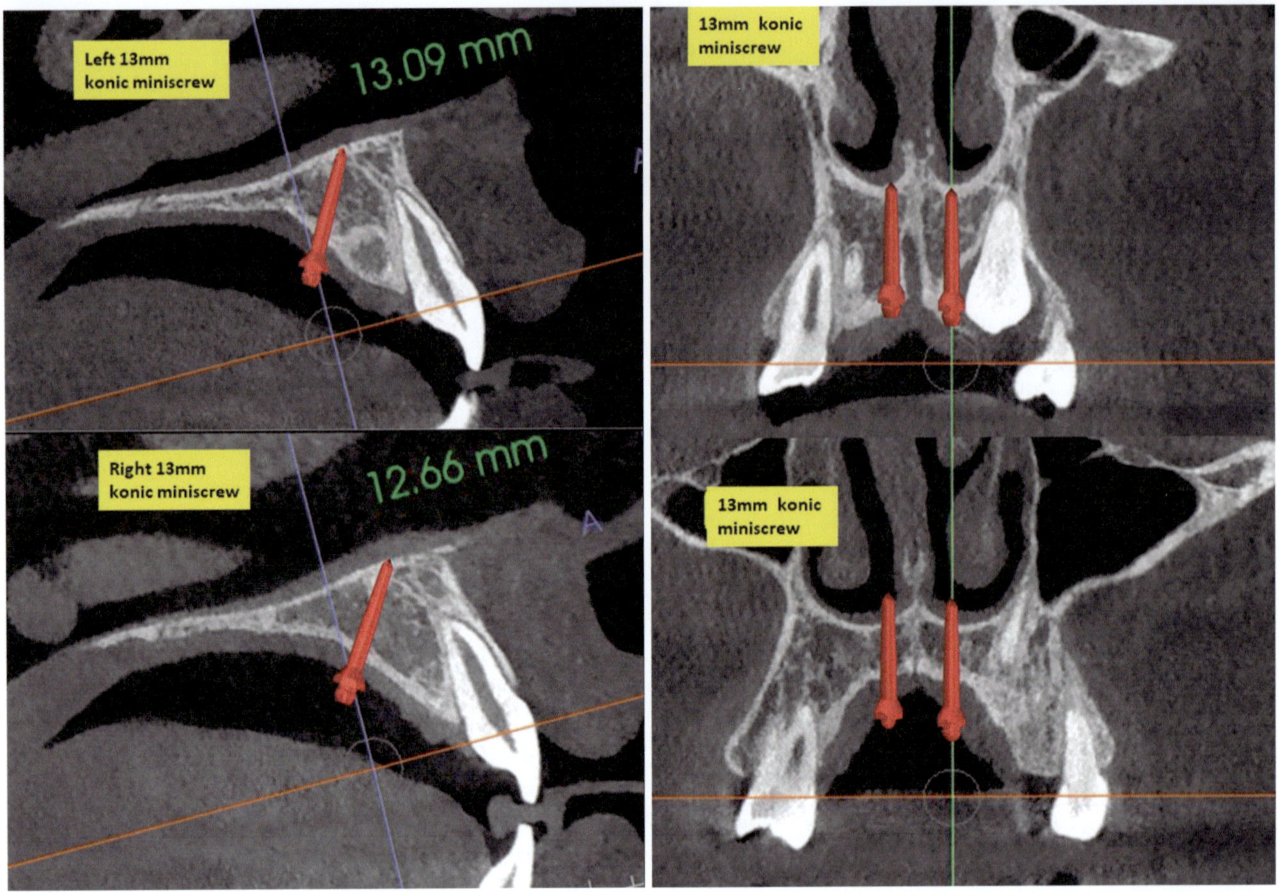

Fig. 8.8 After 3D matching between DICOM data and STL files, an accurate palatal miniscrew placement plan was devised in different views, selecting from a miniscrew library

screw that enables the insertion of a fixing screw to stabilise the abutment or device (Fig. 8.9).

8.2.2.1 MAPA Surgical Guide Design

After having identified the most favourable location, length and insertion axis for orthodontic miniscrew position, the MAPA surgical guide is then designed using Rhinoceros software (Robert McNeel & Associates, Seattle, WA, USA).

The MAPA surgical guide is composed of a main body, which is designed to fit precisely over the palatal and occlusal surfaces with the purpose of ensuring its stability during miniscrew insertion. Its original design included cylindrical sheaths that were designed to guide the accurate insertion of miniscrews into the palatal vault and resin 'bridges' that could be cut after miniscrew insertion to enable removal of the surgical guide (Fig. 8.10).

The latest design, however, features the addition of cylindrical metal rings, directly inserted into the main body of the guide (Fig. 8.11), of a size appropriate for housing both the

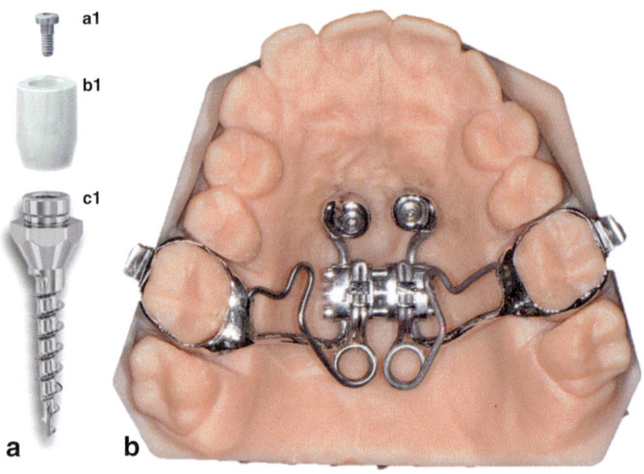

Fig. 8.9 Components of the Spider Screw system (**a**): the fixing screw (**a1**), the abutement (**b1**) and the Spider Screw Regular Plus Konic miniscrew (**c1**). An example of a tooth bone-borne appliance with all components represented (**b**)

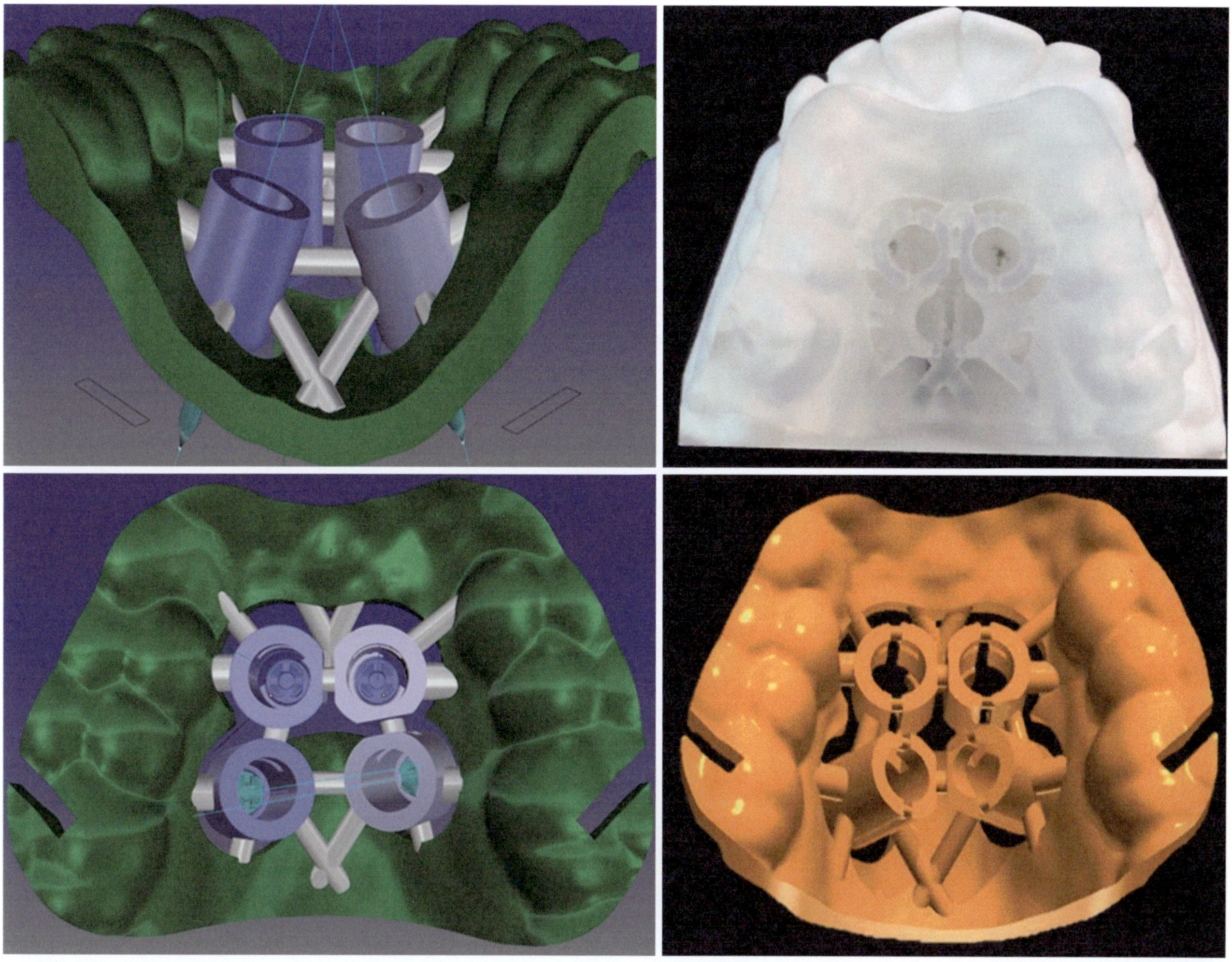

Fig. 8.10 First-generation miniscrew-assisted palatal appliance (MAPA) surgical guide, composed of main body (green), resin bridges (grey) and cylindrical sheaths (blue)

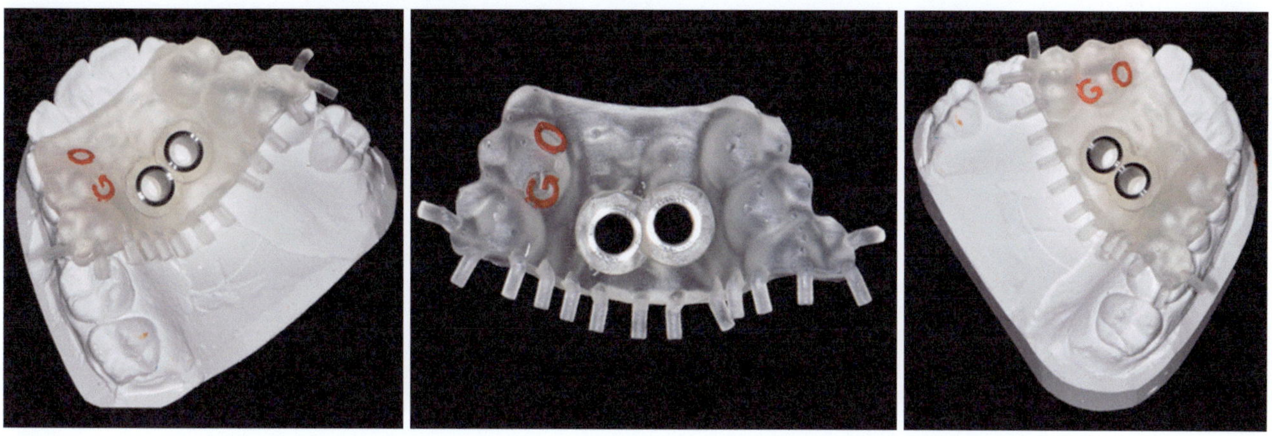

Fig. 8.11 Second-generation MAPA surgical guide showing the cylindrical metal rings embedded in the main body

pilot drill and the pick-up driver during the miniscrew insertion procedure; the rings are also designed as a drilling guide, ensuring that the miniscrews are not inserted beyond the pre-determined depth. In addition, the latest MAPA guide is designed with rear extensions to house a rubber dam, in order to prevent accidental ingestion of miniscrews or other dental equipment components.

8.2.2.2 Miniscrew Insertion Protocol

After performing local anaesthesia in situ (2% lidocaine or 3% mepivacaine), first the stability of the MAPA guide in the patient's mouth is verified, and then a low-viscosity light-cured composite (Optiband Ultra, Ormco, Glendora, CA, USA) is used to fix the surgical guide to the occlusal surfaces of the posterior teeth (Fig. 8.12). Then, a pilot drill is mounted on a dedicated implantation device or low-speed contra-angle handpiece. The pilot hole should be drilled at a speed of 60–80 rpm and have a diameter of roughly 80% of the diameter of the selected miniscrew; it will not only guide the miniscrew insertion but also reduce mechanical stress and the risk of accidental fracture.

Next, the pick-up driver is mounted on the low-speed contra-angle handpiece, and the miniscrew is inserted at a speed of roughly 25–30 rpm with 15–20 Ncm of torque value, until the stop on the pick-up driver comes into contact with the metal ring inserted in the MAPA guide

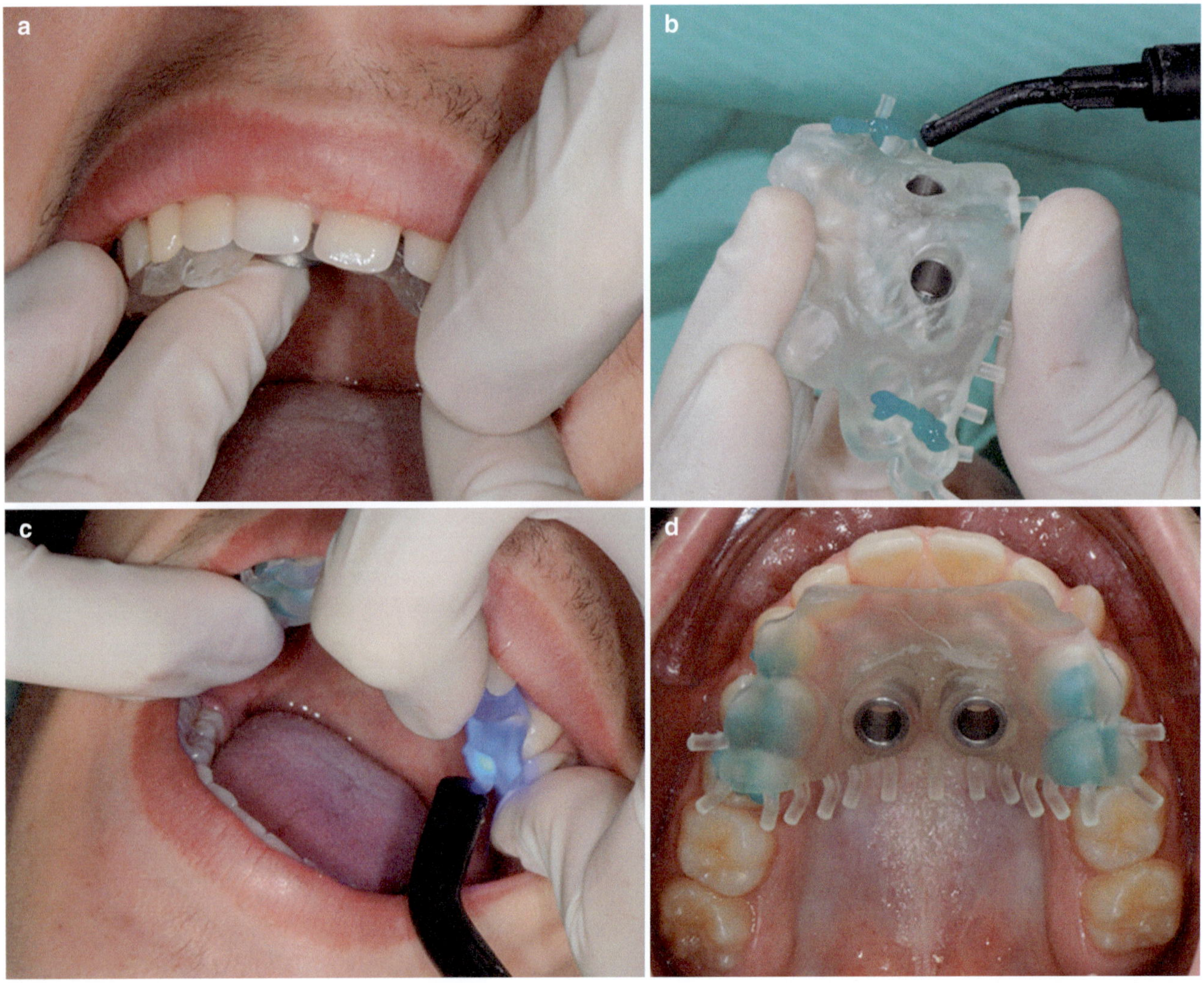

Fig. 8.12 Clinical phases of intraoral MAPA positioning: stability test (**a**), placing composite on the occlusal surfaces of the MAPA surgical guide (**b**), light-curing the resin in order to stabilise the MAPA surgical guide (**c**); occlusal view of the MAPA surgical guide in situ (**d**)

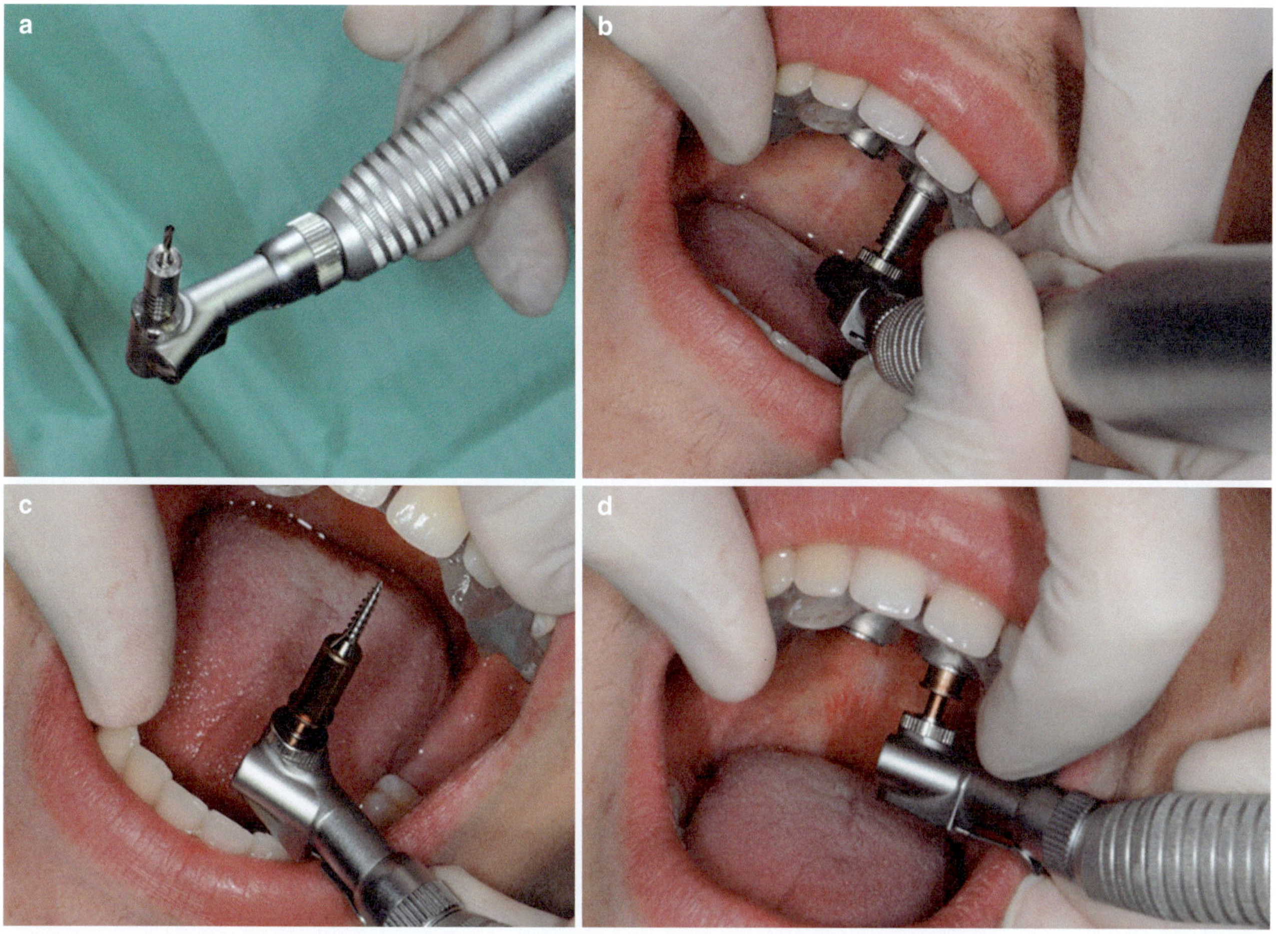

Fig. 8.13 Clinical phases of palatal miniscrew insertion: mounting the pilot drill on the low-speed (60/80 rpm) contra-angle handpiece (**a**), drilling the pilot hole (**b**), mounting the palatal miniscrew with the pick-up driver in the low-speed contra-angle hand-piece (**c**) and clinical placement of the palatal miniscrew (**d**). In the latter photo, the stop on the pick-up driver is visible

(Fig. 8.13). After the requisite number of miniscrews have been inserted, the guide is removed and the bone-borne appliance can be immediately fitted by connecting its abutments to the miniscrew necks, fixing them in place using screws and a manual screwdriver (Fig. 8.14). As shown in Fig. 8.15, a surgical guide enables palatal miniscrews to be inserted as programmed digitally (Fig. 8.15).

8.3 Clinical Case Reports: MAPA System and F22 Aligner

In this section we illustrate two clinical cases exploiting the full potential of the MAPA protocol and the F22 aligner system (Sweden & Martina, Due Carrare, Padua, Italy).

8.3.1 MAPA and F22 Aligners: An Adolescent Case

A 13-year-old female patient presented, along with her parents, complaining of excessive mandibular protrusion and an irregular smile. Extraoral examination revealed a symmetrical oval face with a predominant lower facial third; the mandibular prognathism was evident in profile, and buccal corridors were visible upon smiling (Fig. 8.16). Intraoral analysis revealed 3 mm-molar Class III on the right but molar Class I on the left, and bilateral canine Class I, with a tendency towards a Class II head to head relationship in the right side. Both overjet and overbite were reduced, and bilateral open-bite was present in the canine–premolar region (Fig. 8.17). In order to obtain all radio-

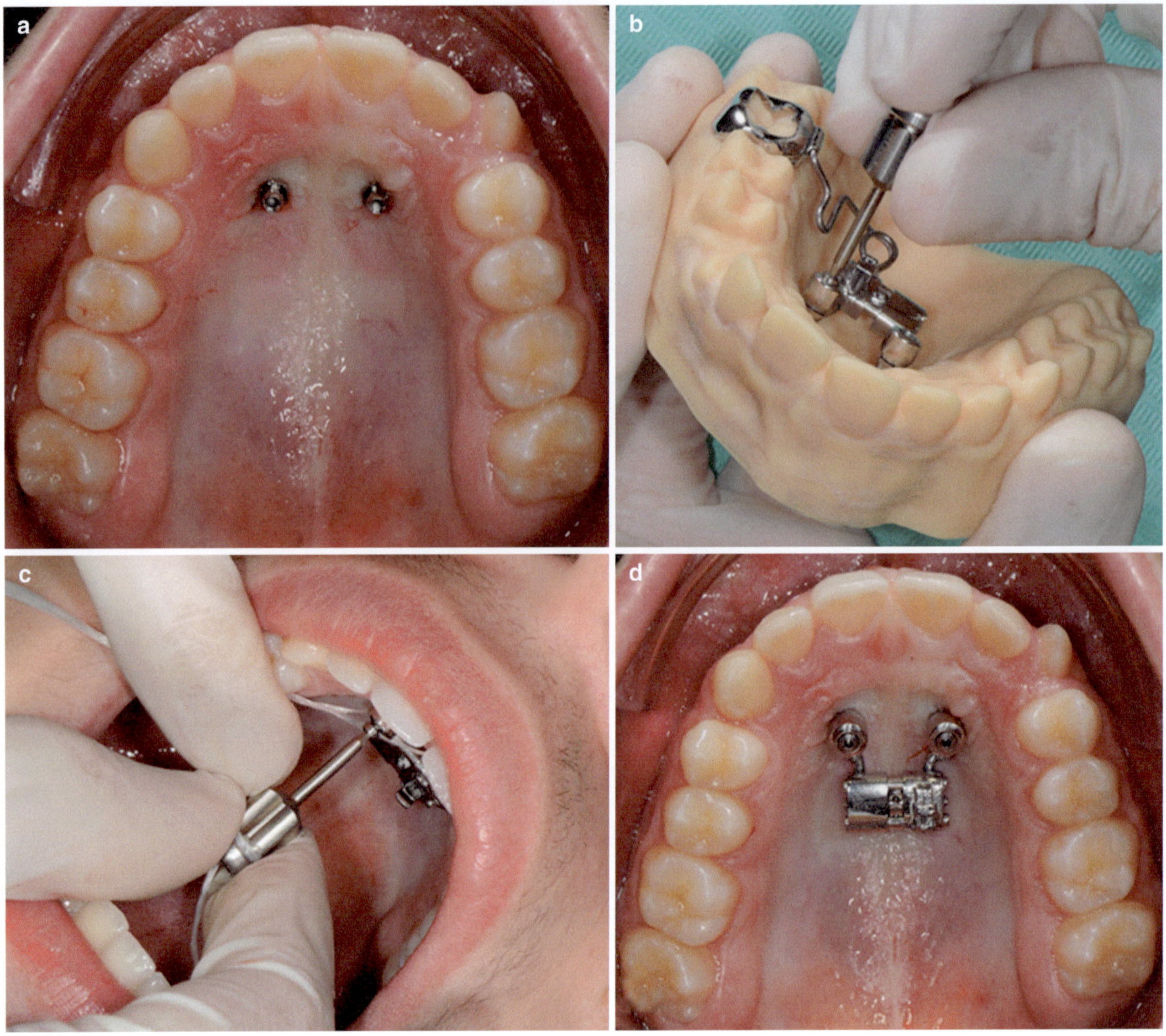

Fig. 8.14 Clinical phases of bone-borne appliance fitting: occlusal view with the palatal miniscrews inserted (**a**), disassembly of the bone-borne appliance on the working resin cast using manual screwdriver (**b**), fixing the bone-borne appliance onto the miniscrew heads (**c**) and clinical occlusal view of the bone-borne appliance

graphic records, a cranio-facial CBCT examination has been performed from which both panoramic and cephalometric radiographs should have been extrapolated through a professional analysing software (Invivo 6, Anatomage, San Jose, CA, USA). Unfortunately, this examination has been executed with mouth in a slight opened position (Fig. 8.18), but authors preferred to not repeat examination keeping in mind both the 'as low as reasonably achievable' (ALARA) principles, gender and early age of patient [3]; moreover, the entity of mouth opening during examinations was not considered so excessive to invalidate orthodontic measurements or to influence negatively orthodontic treatment planning.

Cephalometric radiograph showed a tendency towards skeletal Class III (ANB = 0.3°; Wits = −0.1 mm) and a normodivergent facial type (FMA = 25.6°). The upper incisors were proclined (123°), while the lower incisors had normal inclination (IMPA = 90.1°) (Table 8.1). The upper jaw was

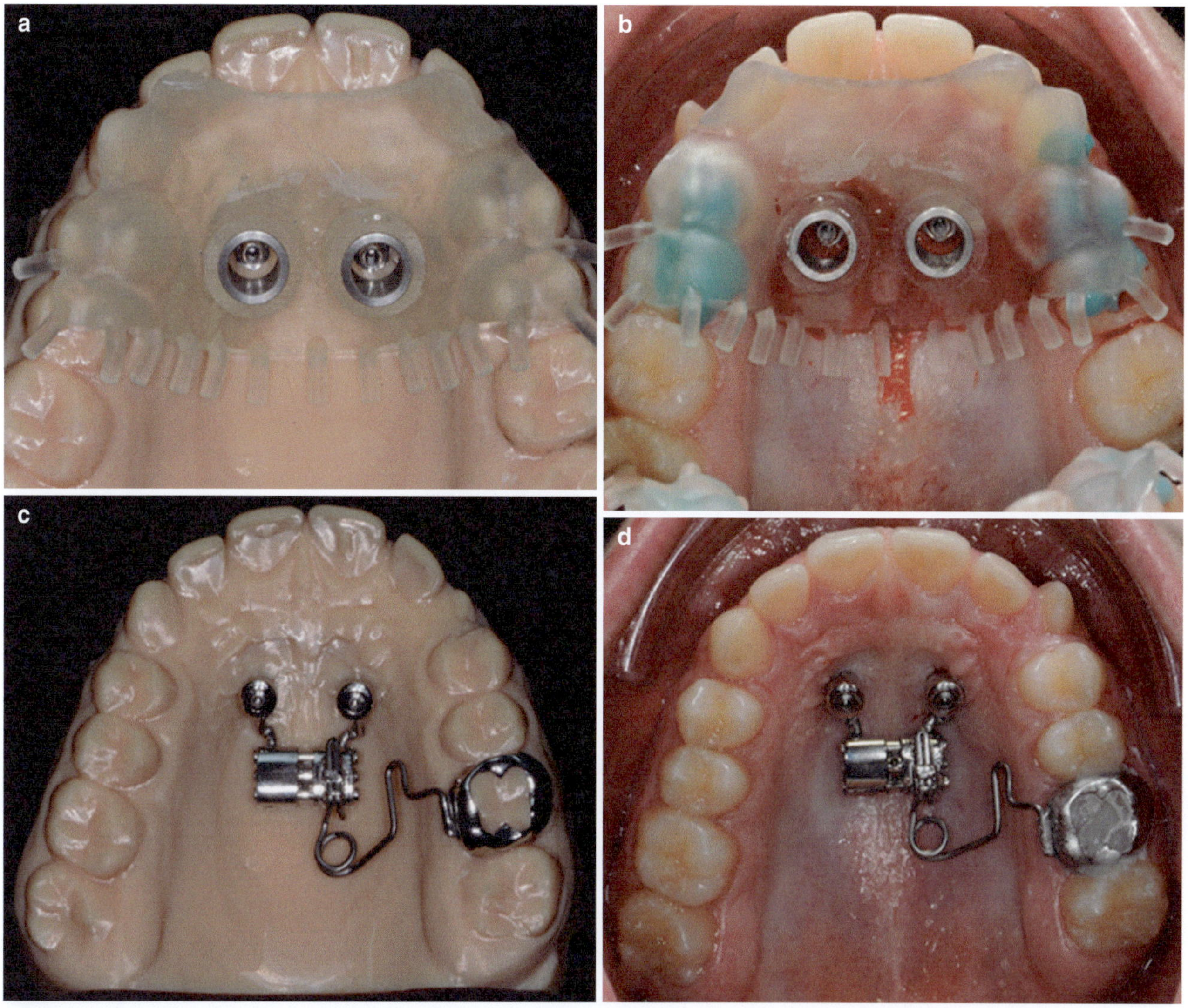

Fig. 8.15 Location of the palatal miniscrews in the working plaster cast and in the maxillary palatal vault (**a**, **b**). Bone-borne unilateral distalising appliance on the working resin cast (**c**) and its in vivo placement (**d**)

V-shaped, with reduced transverse diameters especially in the anterior sector.

In order to maximise skeletal results while minimising dental compensation such as mesialisation of first molars and flaring of upper incisors [29], we decided to use a hybrid-anchorage (skeletal and dental) expansion device and facemask to improve the skeletal relationship between upper and lower arches [30, 31]. Hence, after matching the CBCT scans with the patient's dentition (Fig. 8.19), the MAPA protocol was used to construct a surgical guide for palatal miniscrew insertion (Fig. 8.20). The expansion device used was a SKAR III (Skeletal Alt-RAMEC for Class II), which relies on hybrid anchorage and features welded vestibular arms for securing the facemask.

After miniscrew insertion and SKAR III appliance delivery in a single appointment, the ALT-RAMEC (Alternate Rapid Maxillary Expansion and Constriction) protocol was applied in order to achieve good mobilisation of the upper jaw and to increase response to the orthopaedic forces. This protocol consists of alternating weeks of 1 mm/die expansion and constriction for 4 weeks, followed by successive activations of the rapid maxillary expander from the fifth week onwards until the transverse deficit had been corrected [32] (Fig. 8.21). Once this had been achieved, a Petit face-

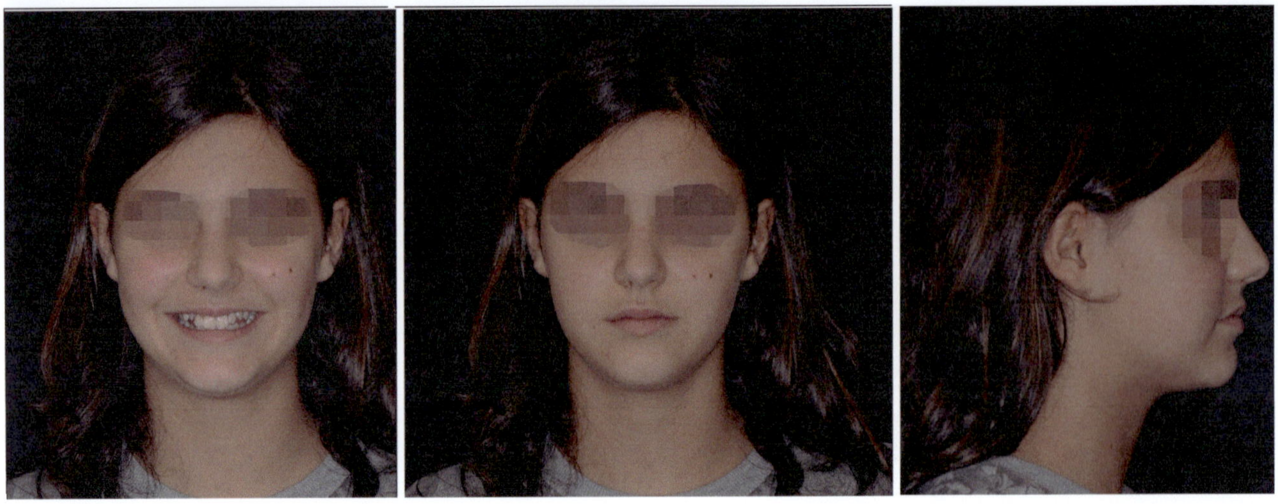

Fig. 8.16 Pre-treatment extraoral photographs

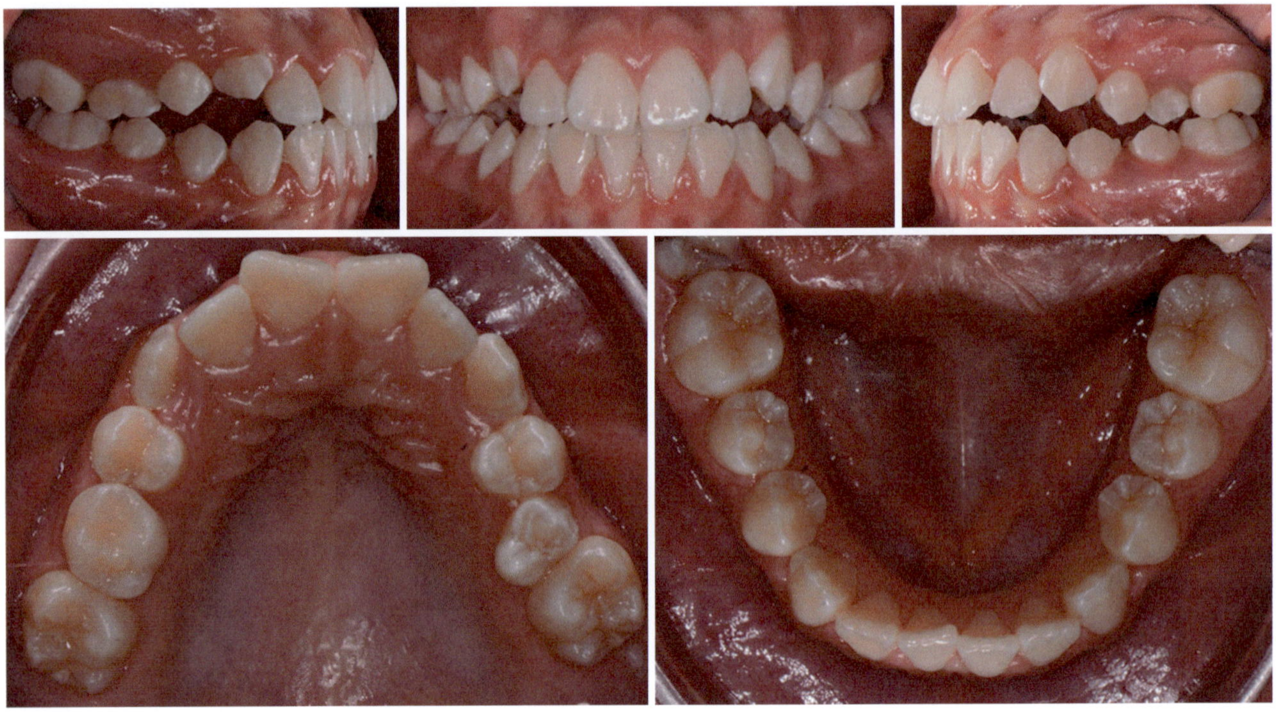

Fig. 8.17 Pre-treatment intraoral photographs

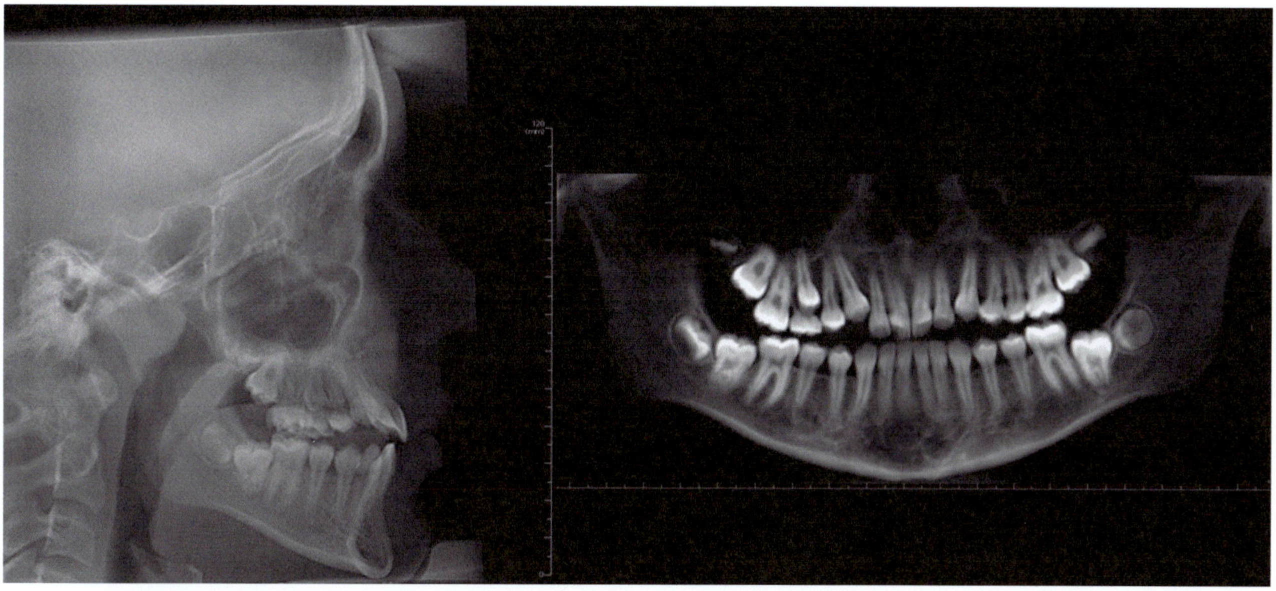

Fig. 8.18 Pre-treatment radiographs

Table 8.1 Pre-, post-SKAR III and post-treatment cephalometric values of case 1

Measurements	Pre-treatment cephalometric values	Post-SKAR III cephalometric values	Post-treatment cephalometric values	Normal values
Horizontal skeletal				
SNA (°)	75.8°	77.5°	76.5°	82.0°
SNB (°)	75.5°	75.8°	75.9°	80.0°
ANB (°)	0.3°	1.7°	0.6°	2.0°
Maxillary skeletal (A-Na Perp) (mm)	−0.4 mm	−0.1 mm	−0.3 mm	0.0 mm
Mandibular skeletal (Pg-Na Perp)	−0.6 mm	−0.4 mm	−0.2 mm	−4.0 mm
Witts appraisal (mm)	−0.1 mm	−0.2 mm	−0.2 mm	0.0 mm
Vertical skeletal				
FMA (MP-FH) (°)	25.6°	24.4°	23.7°	26.0°
MP-SN (°)	35.4°	34.8°	33.7°	33.0°
Palatal mandibular angle (°)	23.4°	22.5°	21.0°	28.0°
Palatal occlusal plane (PP-OP)	4.8°	5.0°	6.0°	10.0°
Mandibular plane to occlusal plane	18.7°	17.1°	15.0°	17.4°
Anterior dental				
U: Incisor protrusion (U1-APo) (mm)	0.5 mm	3.2 mm	2.6 mm	6.0 mm
L1: Protrusion (L1-APo) (mm)	0.1 mm	−0.3 mm	0.0 mm	2.0 mm
U1: Palatal plane (°)	123.0°	117.6°	115.2°	110.0°
U1: Occlusal plane (°)	52.3°	57.4°	58.8°	57.5°
L1: Occlusal plane (°)	71.2°	73.0°	75.5	72.0°
IMPA	90.5°	89.9°	89.5°	95.0°

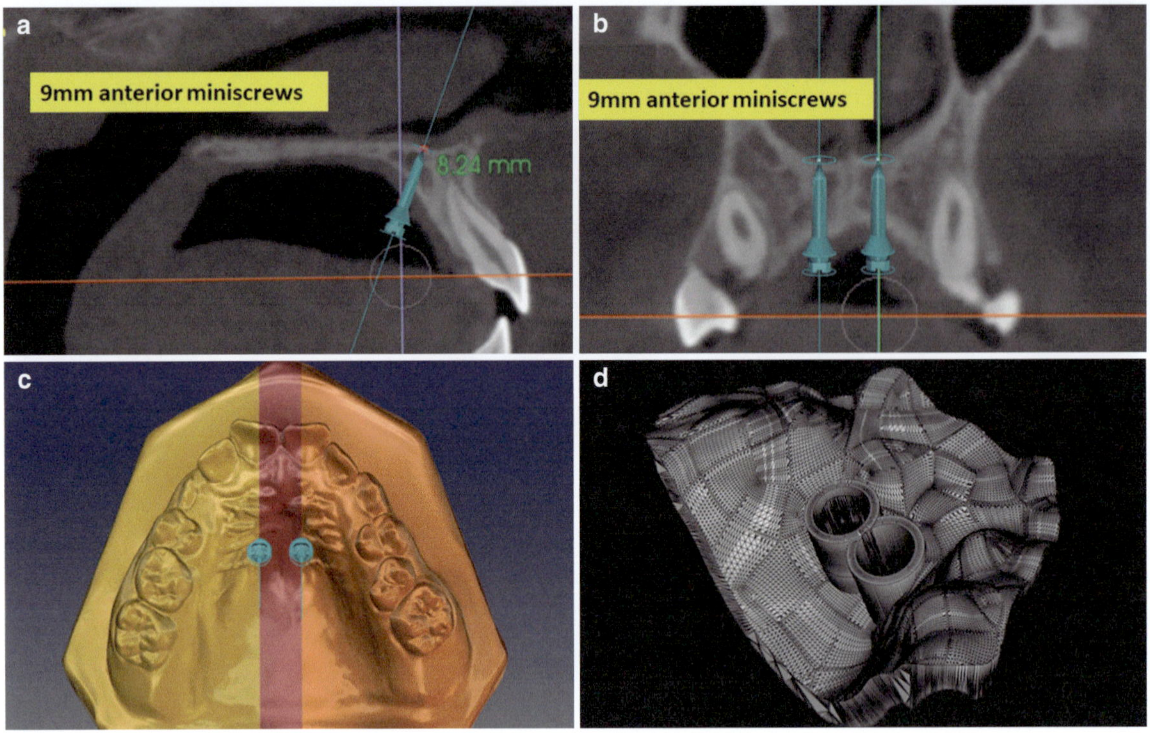

Fig. 8.19 Planning palatal miniscrew insertion after accurate matching between DICOM data and STL files in different views (**a**–**c**). Digital design of MAPA surgical guide (**d**)

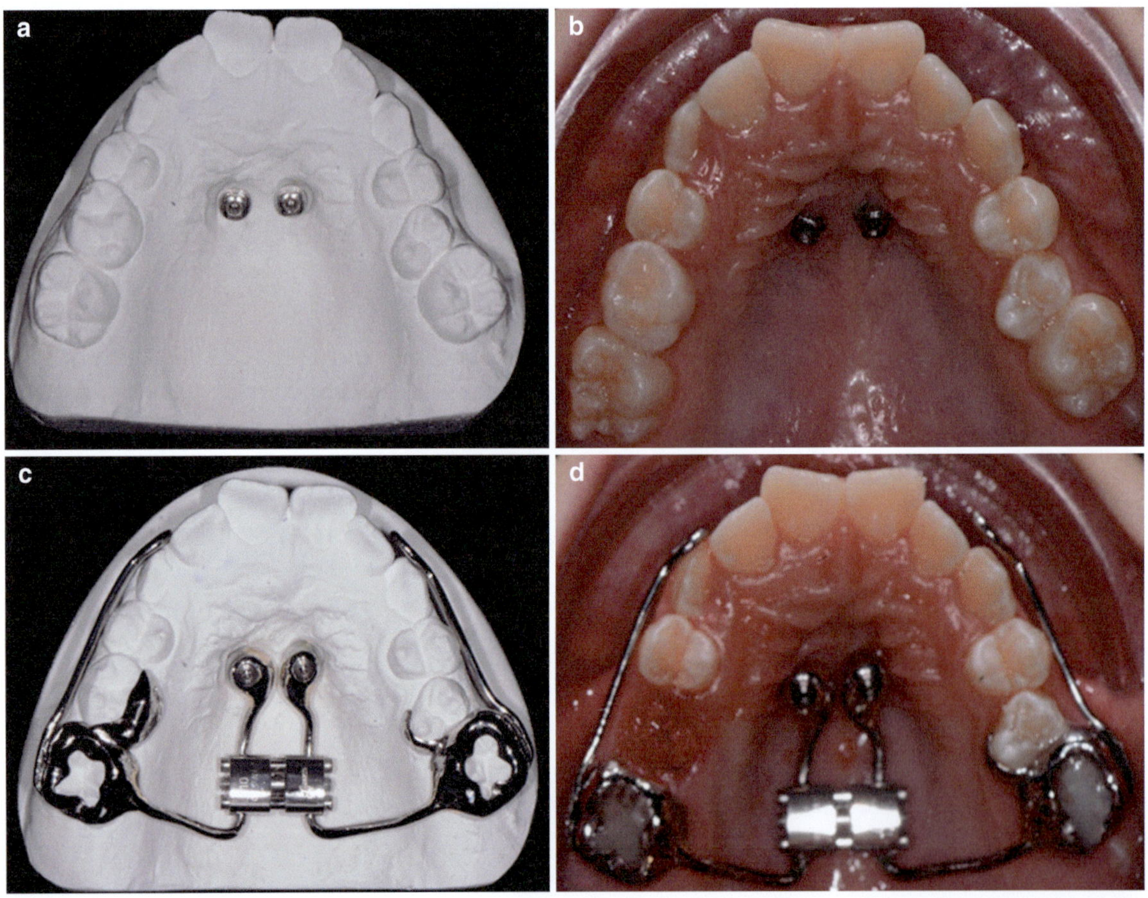

Fig. 8.20 Location of the two palatal miniscrews in the working plaster cast (**a**) and positioning of the two palatal miniscrews in the palatal vault (**b**). SKAR appliance positioned on the working plaster cast (**c**) and in the palatal vault (**d**)

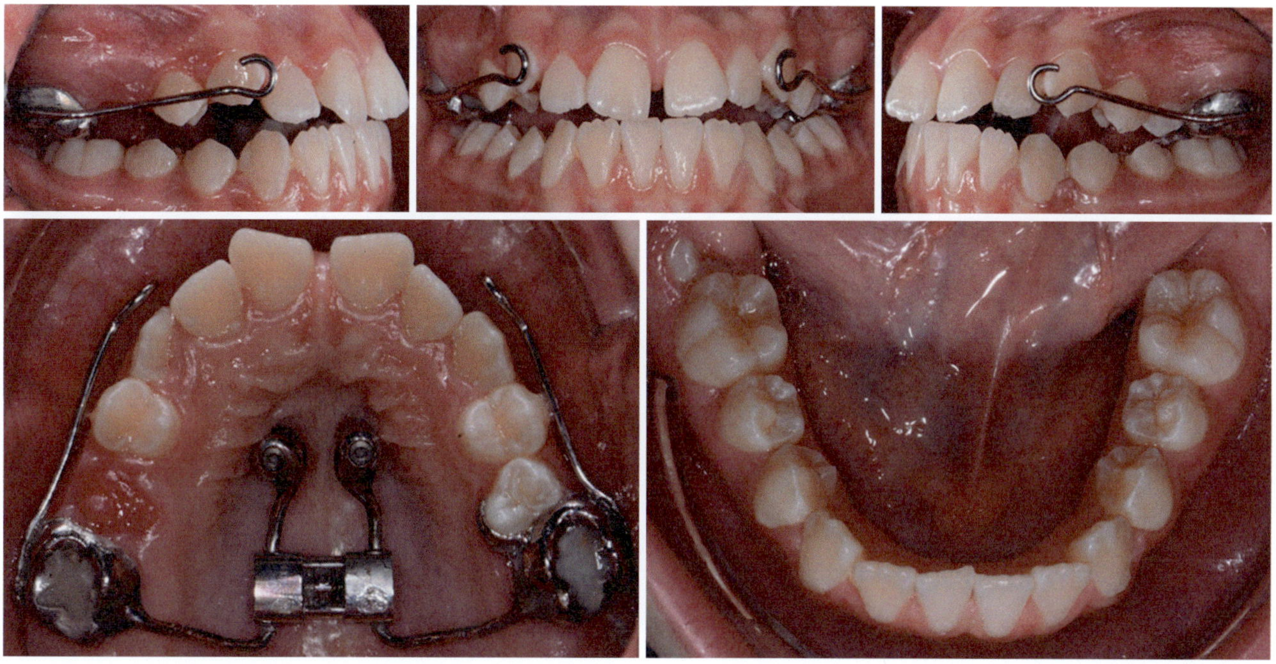

Fig. 8.21 Post-expansion intraoral photographs

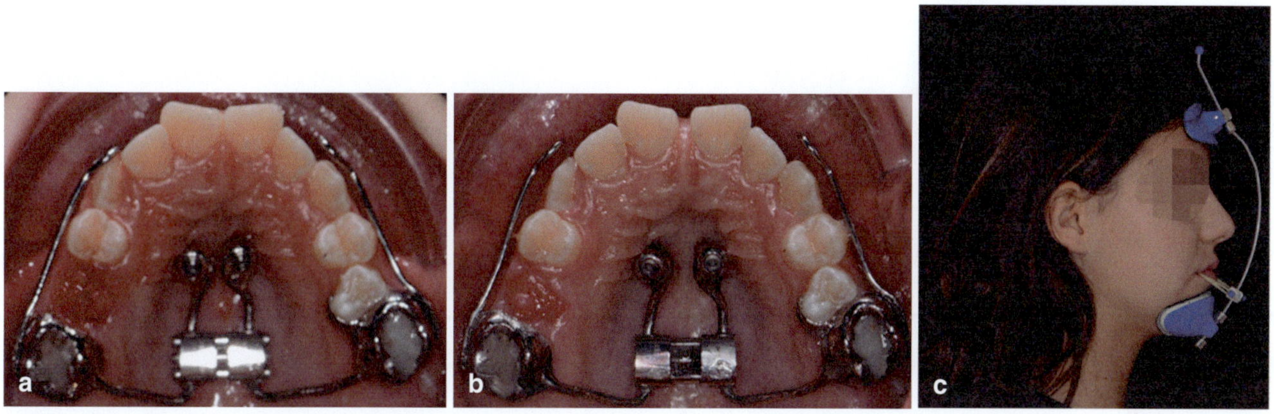

Fig. 8.22 Comparison between pre- and post-expansion photographs in the occlusal view (**a**, **b**) and fitting the facemask to the patient (**c**)

mask (Ormco, Glendora, CA, USA) (Fig. 8.22) was fitted and worn for 14 h per day until the sagittal dental relationships had been corrected and the overjet improved.

These objectives were achieved in 4 months of therapy, with a marked improvement in the patient's profile (Fig. 8.23) and in the cephalometric values (Table 8.1). As a matter of fact, skeletal relationship between arches has been improved with an augmentation of SNA values (1.5°) and a spontaneous retroclination of upper incisors (5.4°) probably caused by transverse augmentation of maxillary apical base and by the augmented upper lip pressure as a consequence of forward displacement of upper arch. Moreover, post-SKAR III extraoral investigation revealed an increased smile display, no longer featuring buccal corridors (Fig. 8.24) and increased transverse diameters in the anterior sector of the upper arch upon smiling. Also, the skeletal relationship was remarkably improved. In order to finish the occlusion (Figs. 8.25 and 8.26), a second phase of treatment using both F22 Aligners and a partial lingual fixed appliance in the area encompassing 2.4, 2.5 and 2.6 was planned (Sweden & Martina, Due Carrare, Padua, Italy).

This hybrid approach (fixed and removable appliances used synergistically) was adopted in order to satisfy both the request of the patient for a comfortable and aesthetic orthodontic treatment [33] and at the same time to increase the predictability of the treatment. Indeed, the orthodontic movement analysis revealed a roughly 29° rotation of tooth 2.5, a movement that would be poorly predictable if attempted using aligners alone, due to both the type and degree of the movement required and the conical crown of the premolars [34, 35].

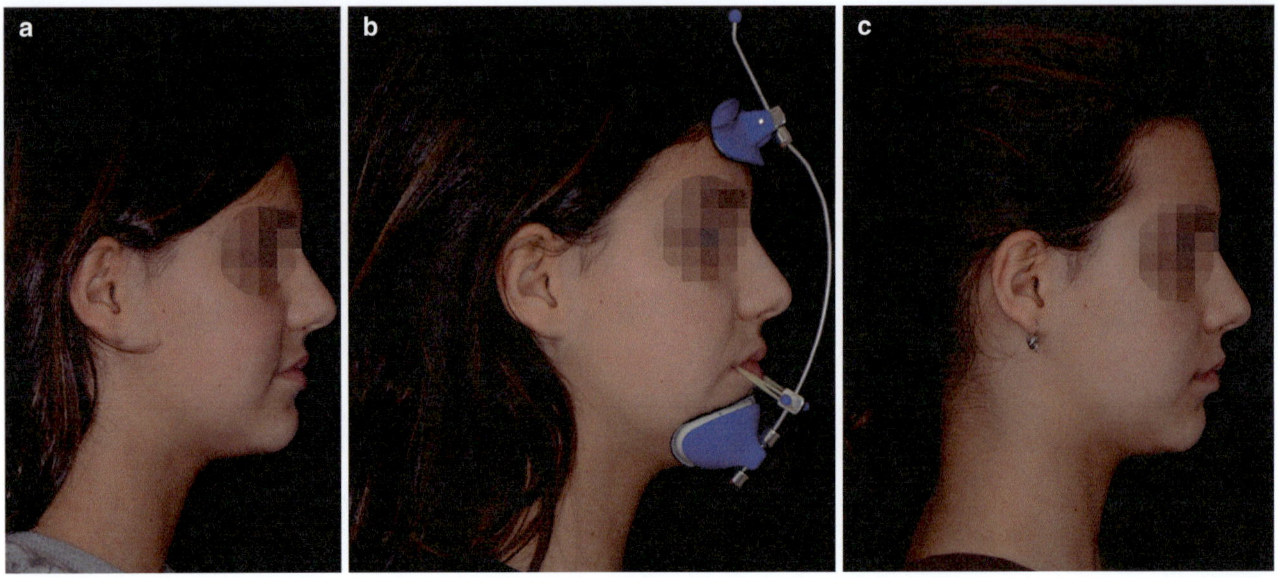

Fig. 8.23 Pre-facemask treatment (**a**), delivery of facemask (**b**) and post-facemask treatment (**c**)

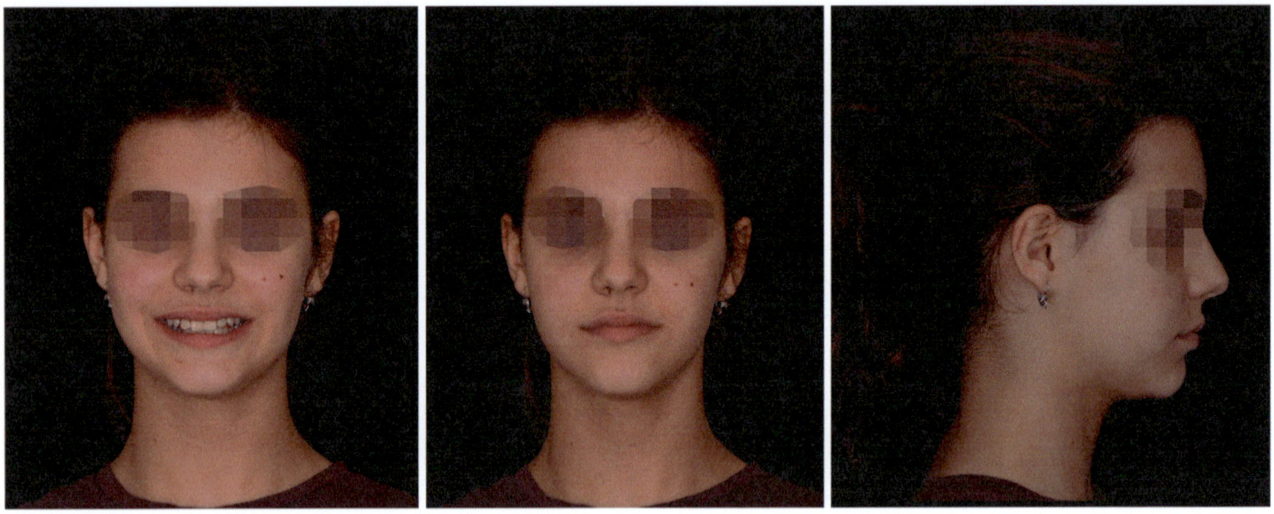

Fig. 8.24 Post-SKAR III extraoral photographs

Hence, in order to perform the most efficient treatment possible, three lingual brackets (Stb, Ormco, Glendora, CA, USA) were positioned on teeth 2.4, 2.5 and 2.6, and the arches were then scanned and digitalised, simulating a digital archwire passing through them (Fig. 8.27). The aligner treatment prescribed involved a series of 10 upper and lower F22 aligners with grip points positioned on teeth 1.6, 1.3, 2.3, 2.6, 3.3, 3.5, 4.4 and 4.6, in addition to slight IPR (0.2 mm) from the mesial side of the 2.6 to the mesial side of 1.2 in the upper jaw and from the mesial 3.4 to the mesial 4.6 in the lower.

A 0.013-inch NiTi archwire (Copper NiTi, Ormco, Glendora, CA, USA) was engaged in the lingual brackets, and F22 aligners were delivered immediately afterwards

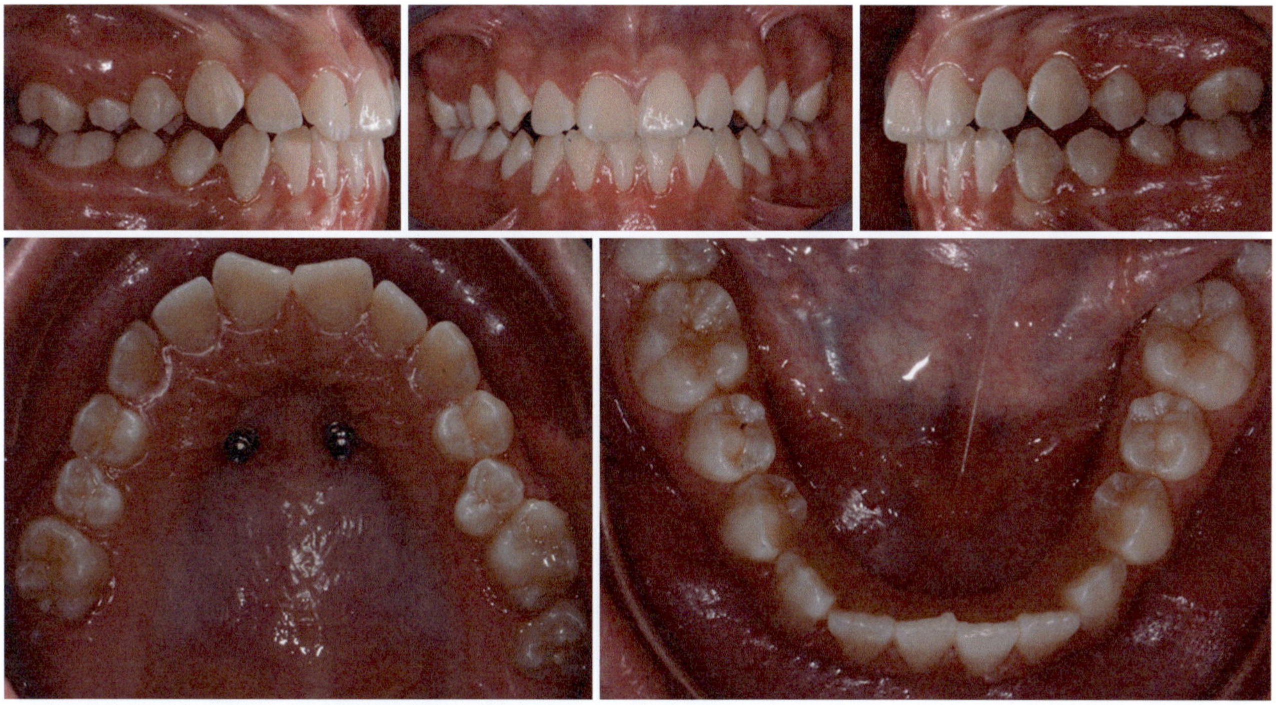

Fig. 8.25 Post-SKAR III intraoral photographs with palatal miniscrews inserted

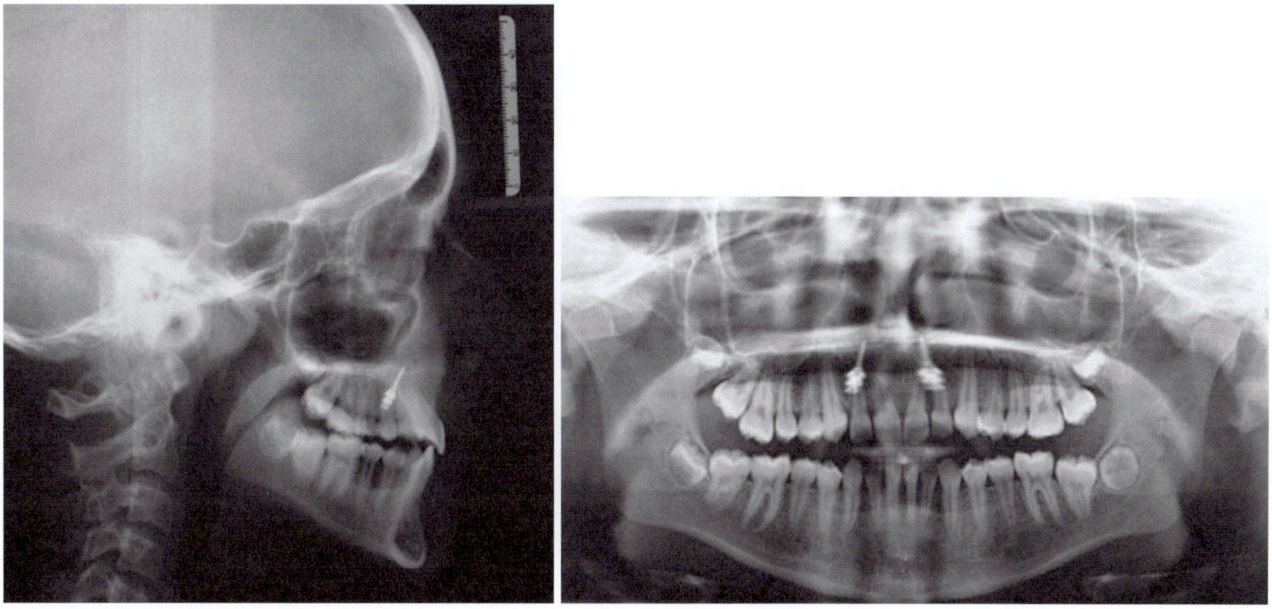

Fig. 8.26 Post-SKAR III radiographs

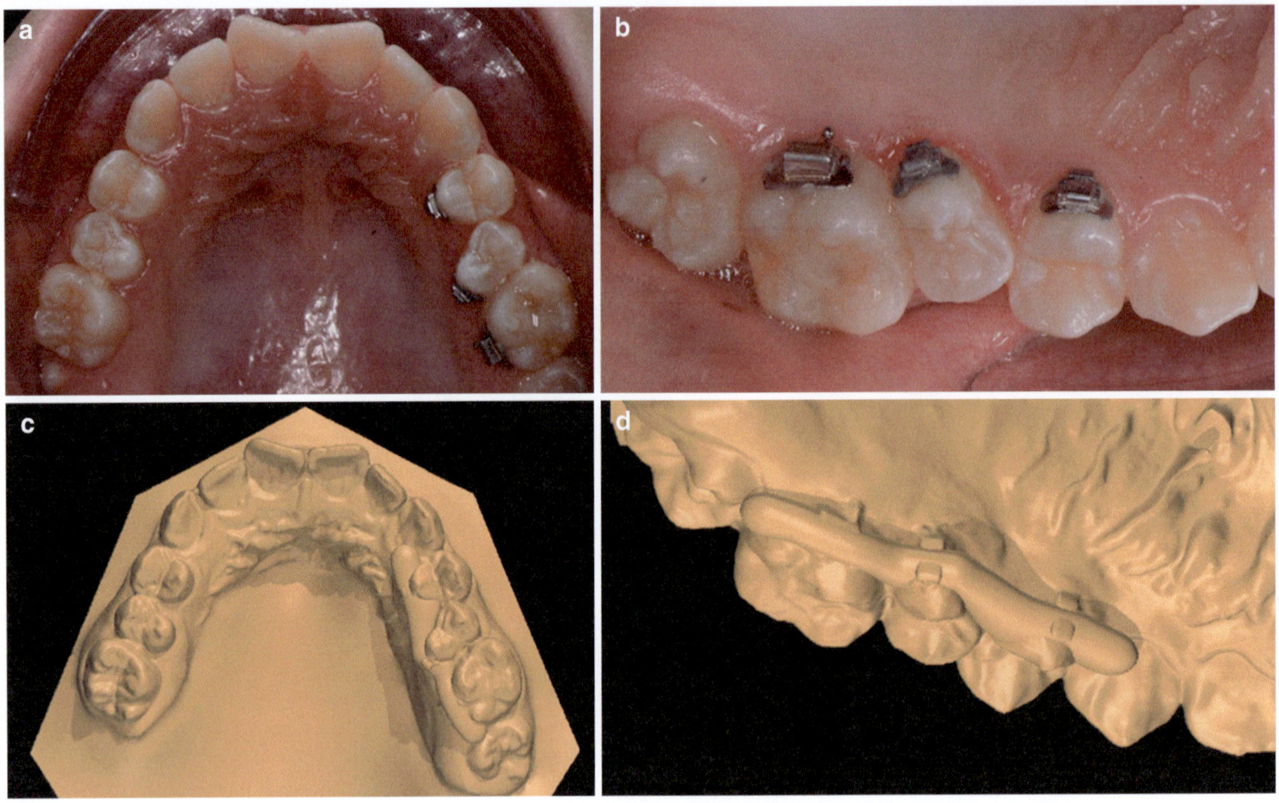

Fig. 8.27 Positioning of the lingual braces (**a**, **b**). Digital cast with digital lingual archwire (**c**, **d**)

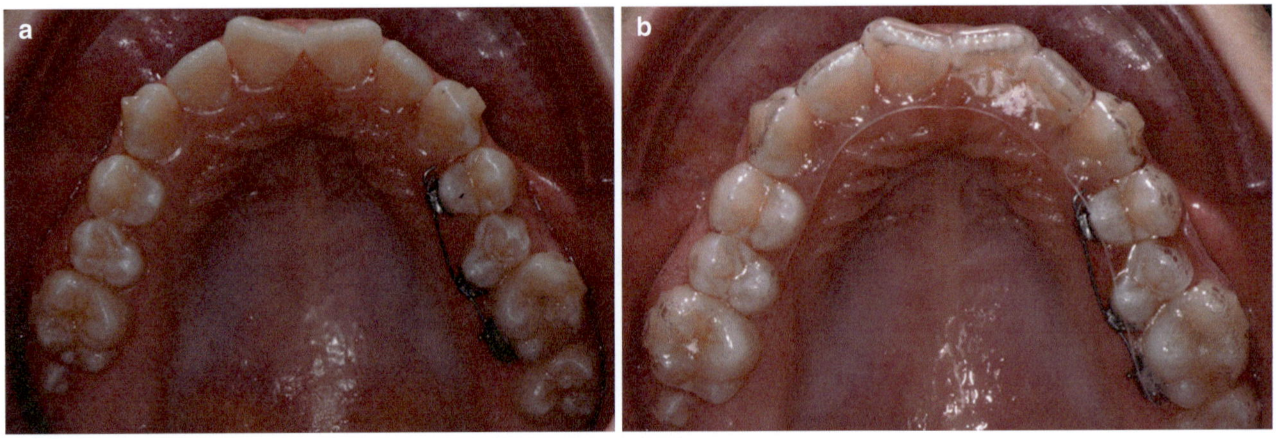

Fig. 8.28 Positioning of the 0.016-inch NiTi lingual archwire (**a**) and delivery of F22 aligners (**b**)

(Fig. 8.28). The patient was instructed to swap aligners every 10 days, and the archwire was replaced with a 0.016 NiTi after a month of aligner treatment.

This finishing phase lasted a total of 3 months and 10 days (Figs. 8.29 and 8.30), and the post-treatment extraoral photos confirm that a balanced profile with increased incisor display and a consonant smile arc was achieved (Fig. 8.31). Intraorally, despite occlusal contacts in the premolar area and centring of midlines should have been little improved, a good bilateral molar and canine Class I had been achieved and overbite and overjet were good (Fig. 8.32). The alignment of marginal ridges is acceptable (Fig. 8.33), and radiography revealed good root parallelism (Fig. 8.34) and improved dental and skeletal relationships (Table 8.1).

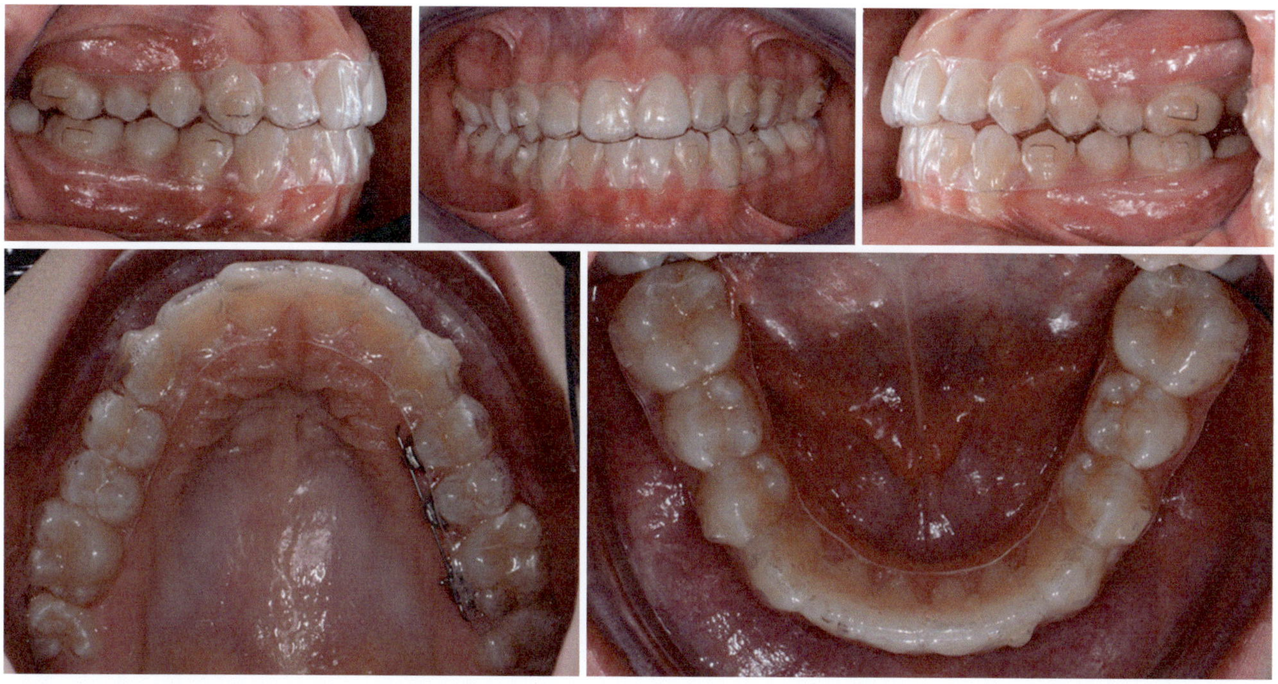

Fig. 8.29 Intraoral views of F22 aligners

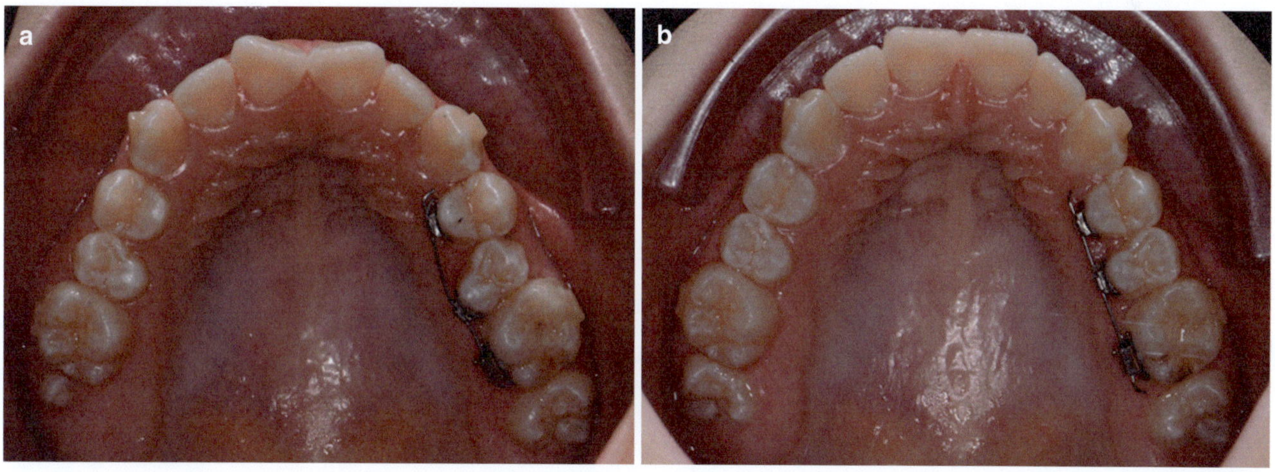

Fig. 8.30 Occlusal view of pre-F22 aligner treatment (**a**) and post-treatment outcome (**b**)

Cephalometric measurements show an advancement of both the maxilla (SNA = 76.5°), induced by SKAR III treatment, and mandible (SNB = 75.9°) that seems to be the expression of the mandibular growth. A mandibular counterclockwise rotation has been recorded with a subsequent reduction of facial divergency (FMA = 23.7°), but this effect could be explained by the slight opened position of the mouth during pre-treatment CBCT examination and only partially by improvement of occlusal contact in the posterior area, especially in the right side, and by the use of the hybrid anchorage used in the facemask therapy, avoiding the extrusion of upper molars. An overall improvement of intermaxillary relationship has been registered (ANB = 0.6°). As regards dental cephalometric measurements, a retroclination of upper incisors (115.2°) has been recorded, while lower incisors remain almost stable (IMPA = 89.5°) (Table 8.1).

Superimposition of pre-, post-SKAR III and post-treatment lateral cephalograms showed the skeletal and the dental effects of the treatment (Fig. 8.35). SKAR III protocol caused a forward displacement of maxilla (1.7°) and a spon-

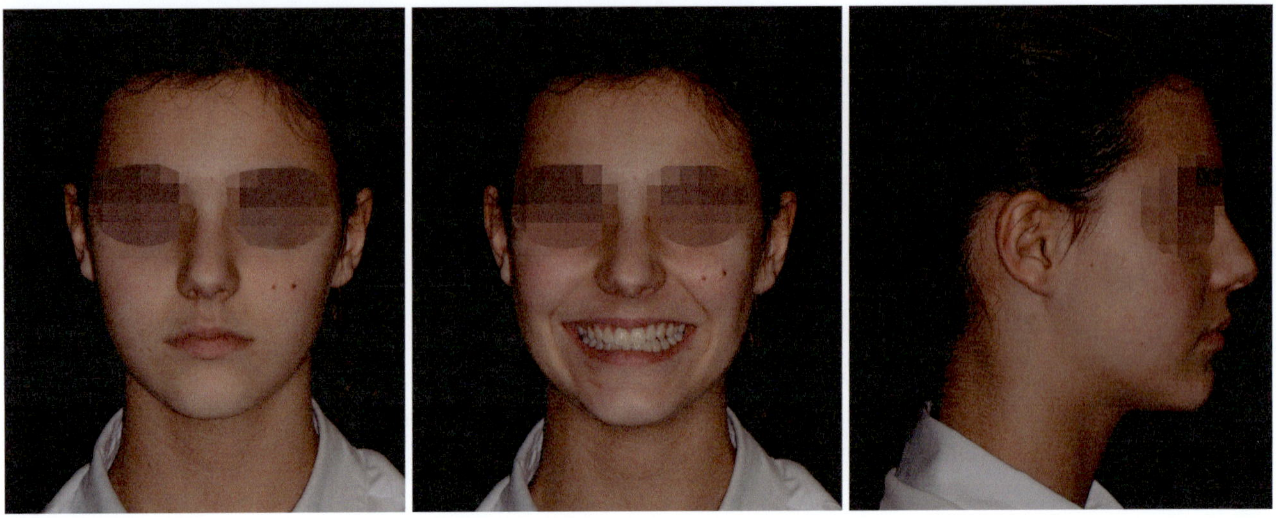

Fig. 8.31 Post-treatment extraoral photographs

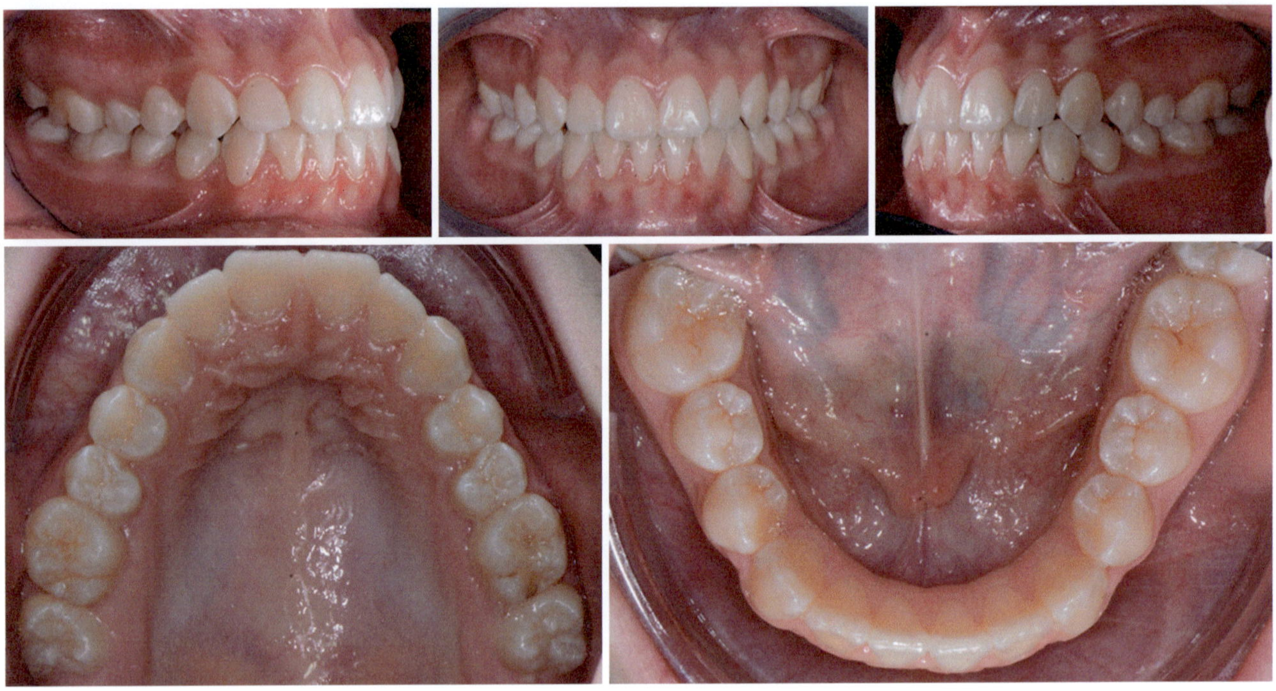

Fig. 8.32 Post-treatment intraoral photographs

taneous retroclination of upper incisors (5.4°). Skeletal anchorage provided a good control of the unwanted dental effects with good sagittal stability of upper molars with no mesialisation of these teeth detectable. As regarding the end results, despite a mesial movement of upper molars has been detected during the orthodontic therapy with F22 aligners, the upper incisors remain almost stable in their antero-posterior position, registering however an uprighting due to controlled palatal crown tipping. It could be due to the fact that space gained through skeletal expansion by SKAR III device has been filled up totally by the mesial movement of the upper molars and that widening of maxillary base allowed this retraction.

Figure 8.36 shows the situation before and after SKAR III treatment, and after aligner finishing, highlighting the good intra- and extraoral outcomes.

8.3.2 MAPA and F22 Aligners: An Adult Case

A 23-year-old female presented with the chief complaint of her front teeth 'sticking out' and the fact that her upper

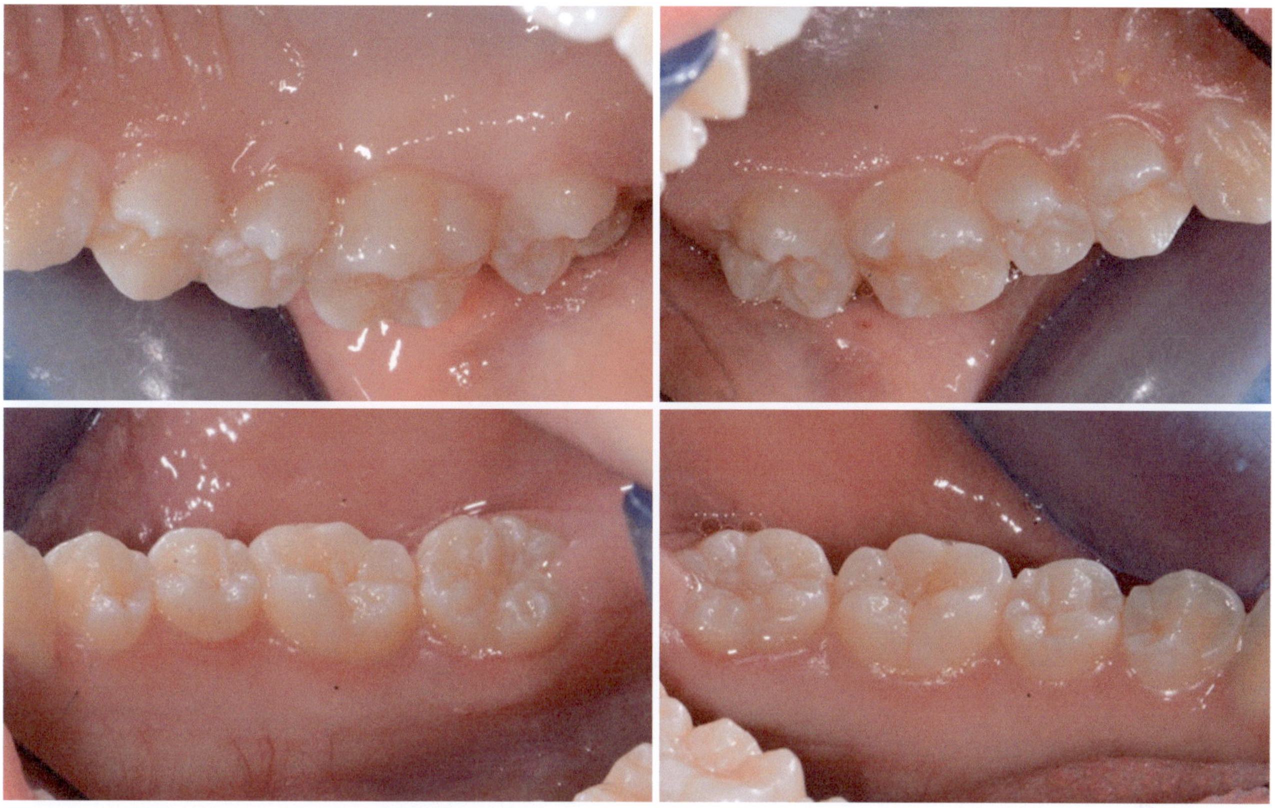

Fig. 8.33 Alignment of posterior marginal ridges

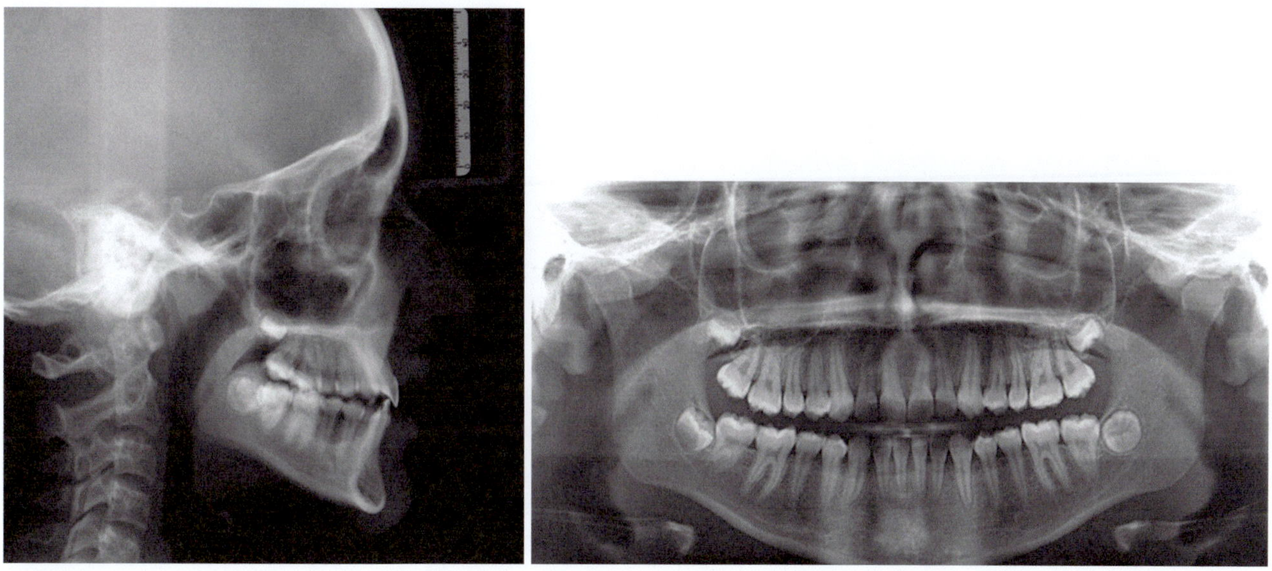

Fig. 8.34 Post-treatment radiographs

back teeth were 'inside' the lower. Extraoral assessment revealed mandibular asymmetry, with a deviation of the lower jaw towards the left, and a flat profile with steep mandibular plane. Upon smiling, there were wide buccal corridors, and an unsightly display of the anterior teeth (Fig. 8.37). Intraoral examination revealed bilateral 2 mm Class III molar and canine Class I and normal overjet, but reduced overbite (Fig. 8.38). Bilateral cross-bite was present, and the gingival biotype was thin, and several areas of gingival recession were present. Radiographic analysis showed the presence of all teeth, including the upper third molars (Fig. 8.39). Cephalometric analysis revealed skel-

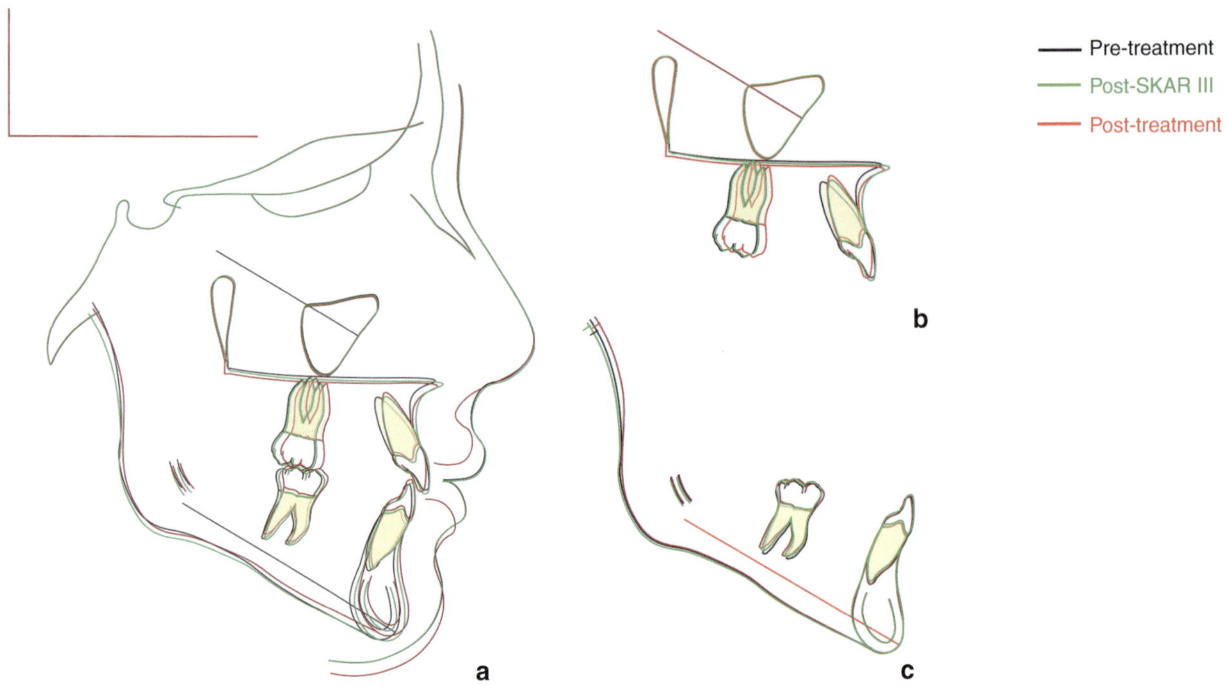

Fig. 8.35 Superimposed pre-, post-SKAR III and post-treatment tracings: superimposition on the cranial base (**a**), maxillary superimposition (**b**) and mandibular superimposition (**c**)

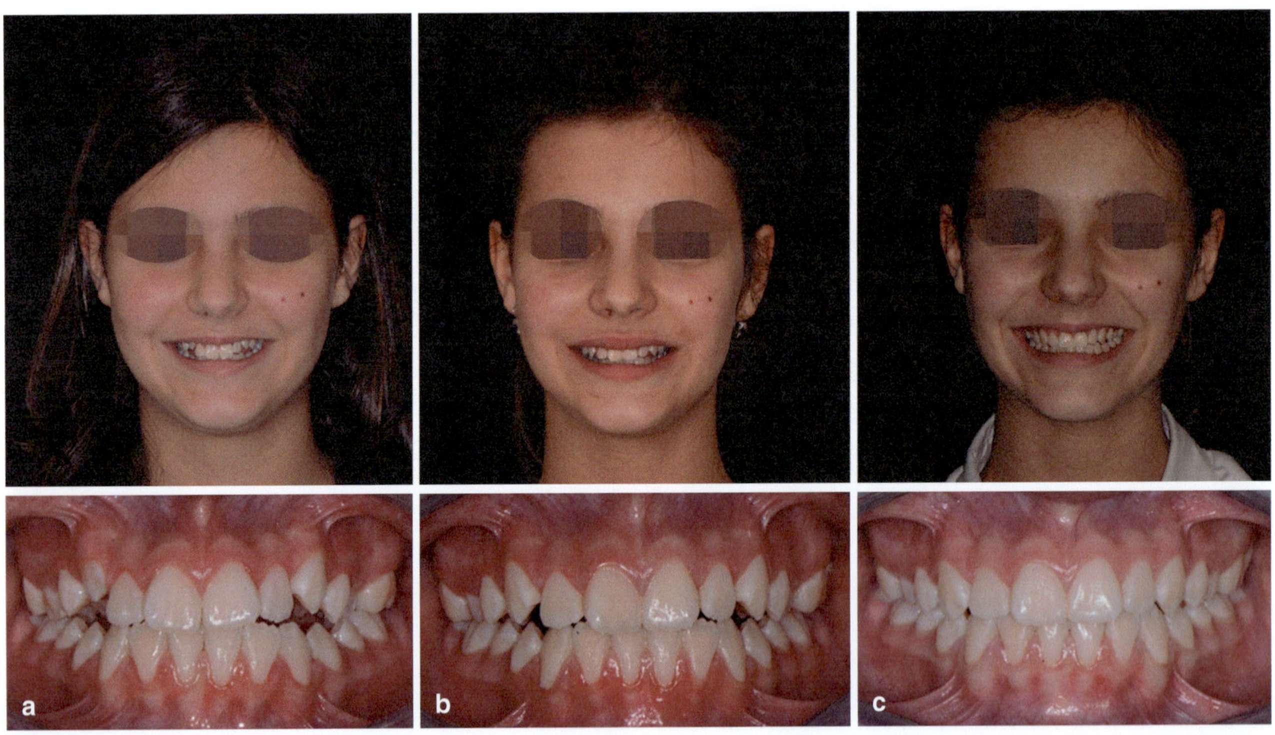

Fig. 8.36 Pre-SKAR (**a**), post-SKAR (**b**) and post-treatment results (**c**)

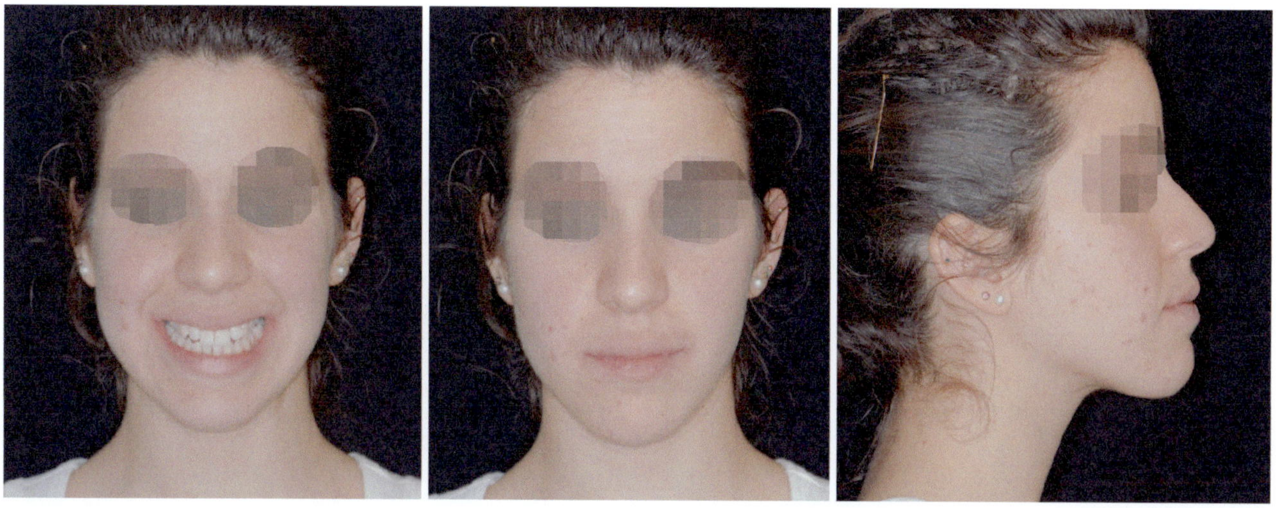

Fig. 8.37 Pre-treatment extraoral photographs

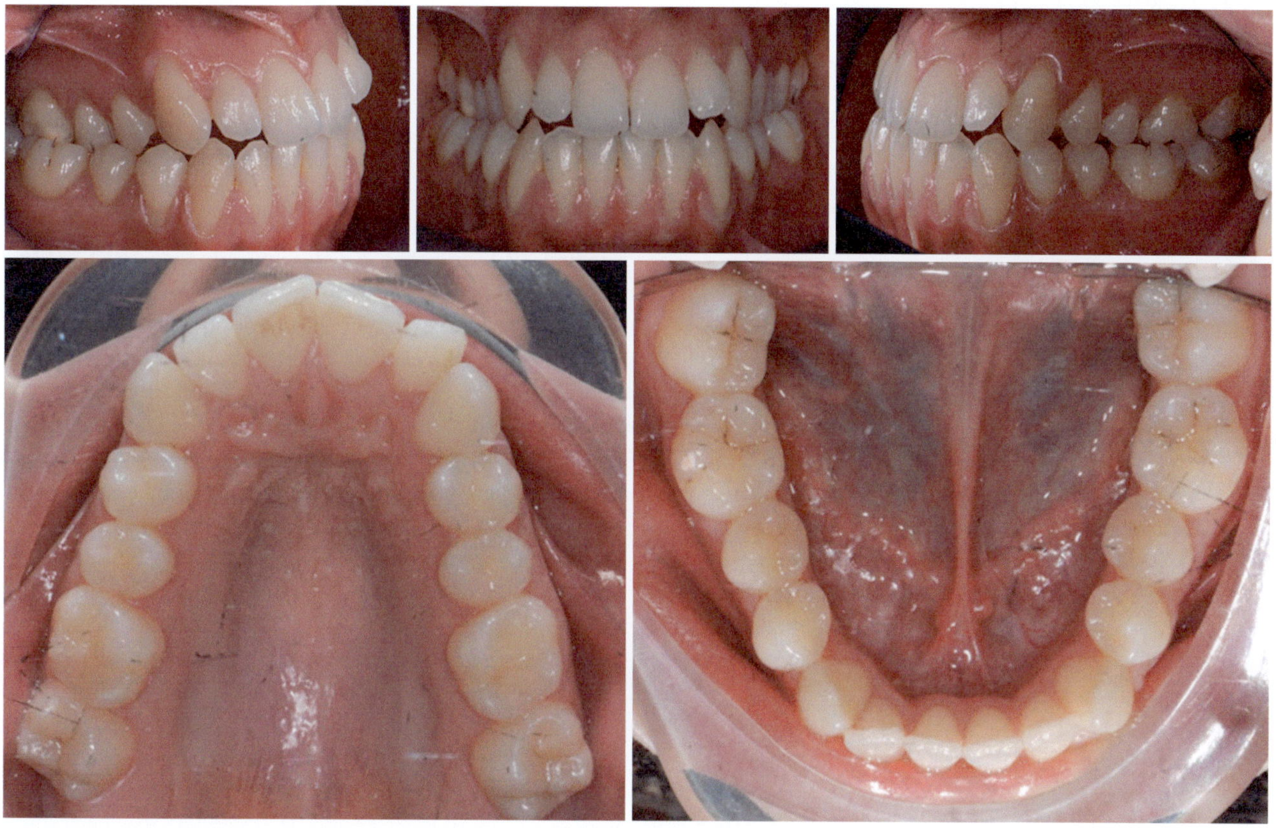

Fig. 8.38 Pre-treatment intraoral photographs

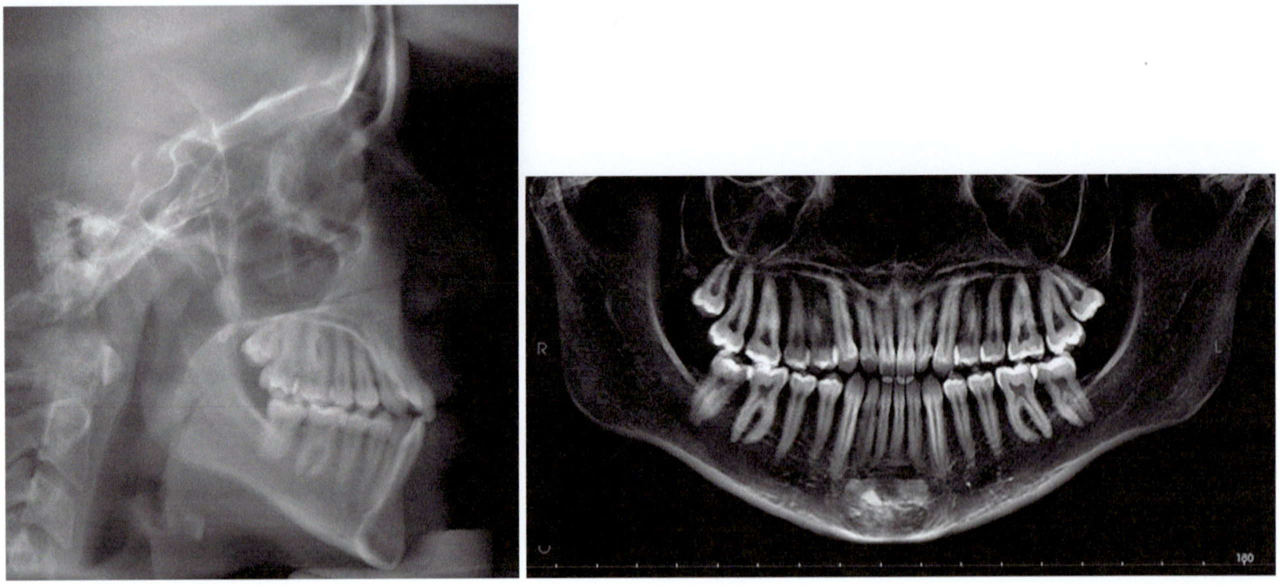

Fig. 8.39 Pre-treatment radiographs

Table 8.2 Pre-treatment, post-treatment and difference of bucco-palatal angulation measurements of teeth on CBCT coronal slice is reported

Measurements	Pre-treatement	Post-treatement	Differences
16 angulation	99.1°	99.7°	+0.6°
26 angulation	99.1°	99.2°	+0.1°
15 angulation	92.2°	92.2°	0.0°
25 angulation	90.6°	92.0°	+1.4°
13 angulation	102.2°	100.0°	−2.2°
23 angulation	104.2°	101.0°	−3.2°

Positive values state for vestibular crown tipping, while negative values for palatal crown tipping

etal Class III (ANB = 0°; Wits = −5 mm) with a hyperdivergent facial pattern (FMA = 30.8°). The upper incisors were proclined (117°), while the lower incisors were retroclined (IMPA = 82°), in an attempt at dental compensation (Table 8.2). Analysis of the CBCT scan highlighted thin supporting vestibular alveolar bone in the posterior sectors of the upper jaw, which limited the possibility of resolving the cross-bite using dental expansion (Fig. 8.40).

The patient refused orthognathic surgery, and in order to respect the patient's wishes, we therefore proposed an initial phase of non-surgical skeletal expansion of the upper jaw using a bone-borne appliance, with a subsequent phase of F22 aligners to detail the occlusion. This treatment plan was designed with the patient's periodontal issues [36, 37] and age [38] in mind; indeed, in order to expand the upper jaw without worsening the periodontal situation [39, 40], it would be necessary to rely on pure skeletal anchorage.

After the accurate matching of CBCT scans and digital models, optimum miniscrew insertion sites and adequate lengths (2 × 9 mm in the anterior palate and 2 × 11 mm in the posterior palate, each 2 mm in diameter) were identified, and the MAPA surgical guide was planned (Fig. 8.41). This was used for the correct insertion of the four miniscrews (Spider Screw K2 Regular Plus, HdC, Thiene, Vicenza, Italy) into the palate after local anaesthesia (mepivacaine 3%), and then a polyvinyl siloxane (PVS) (Elite HD+ Regular and Light Body, Badia Polesine, Rovigo, Italy) impression of the upper dentition was taken. In this way, a bone-borne expansion device was designed and was delivered at the subsequent appointment (Fig. 8.42). An activation protocol of two turns per day for a total of 24 days (48 activations) was performed until the mid-palatal suture opened (Fig. 8.43) and the bilateral cross-bite had been resolved. With 9 mm of appliance expansion, 7 mm of expansion was obtained at the upper first molars and 4 mm at the upper canines. Due to early contact between the upper and lower second molars, the open bite was increased, and the device was left in situ for 2 months to stabilise the expansion (Fig. 8.44).

Post-expansion intraoral scans were taken and used to plan the second phase with F22 aligner therapy (Sweden & Martina, Due Carrare, Padua, Italy). In this phase, interproximal reduction of teeth 13 and 22, 35 and 43 was performed to create space and facilitate the derotation movements. Then, 20 individualised upper and lower aligners were delivered to the patient after composite grip points had been attached to the buccal surfaces of teeth 1.3, 2.2, 2.3, 3.5, 4.4 and 4.5 and the lingual surfaces of teeth 1.2, 1.1 and 2.1 and from 3.1 to 4.2, as prescribed by the digital set-up (Fig. 8.45). Each aligner was worn for 7 days and, after this series, five upper and lower refinement aligners were prescribed in order to detail the occlusion (Fig. 8.46).

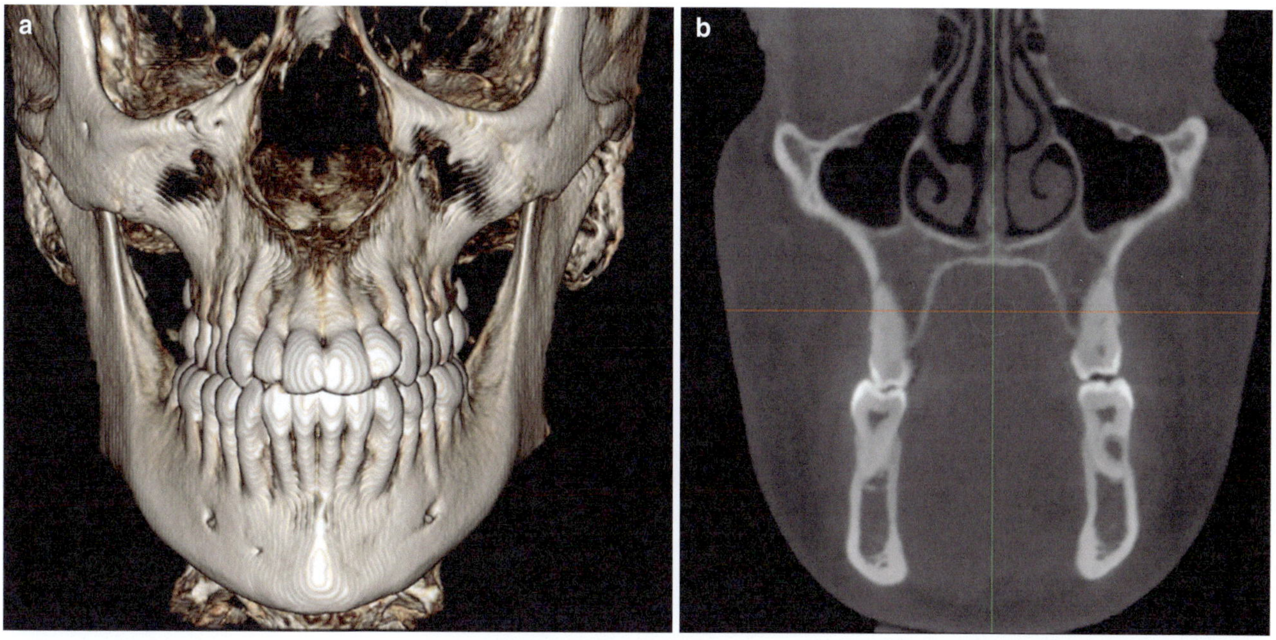

Fig. 8.40 CBCT volumetric rendering of the skeletal structure in frontal view (**a**). Coronal slices of the CBCT view investigating the vestibular bone thickness of the maxilla (**b**)

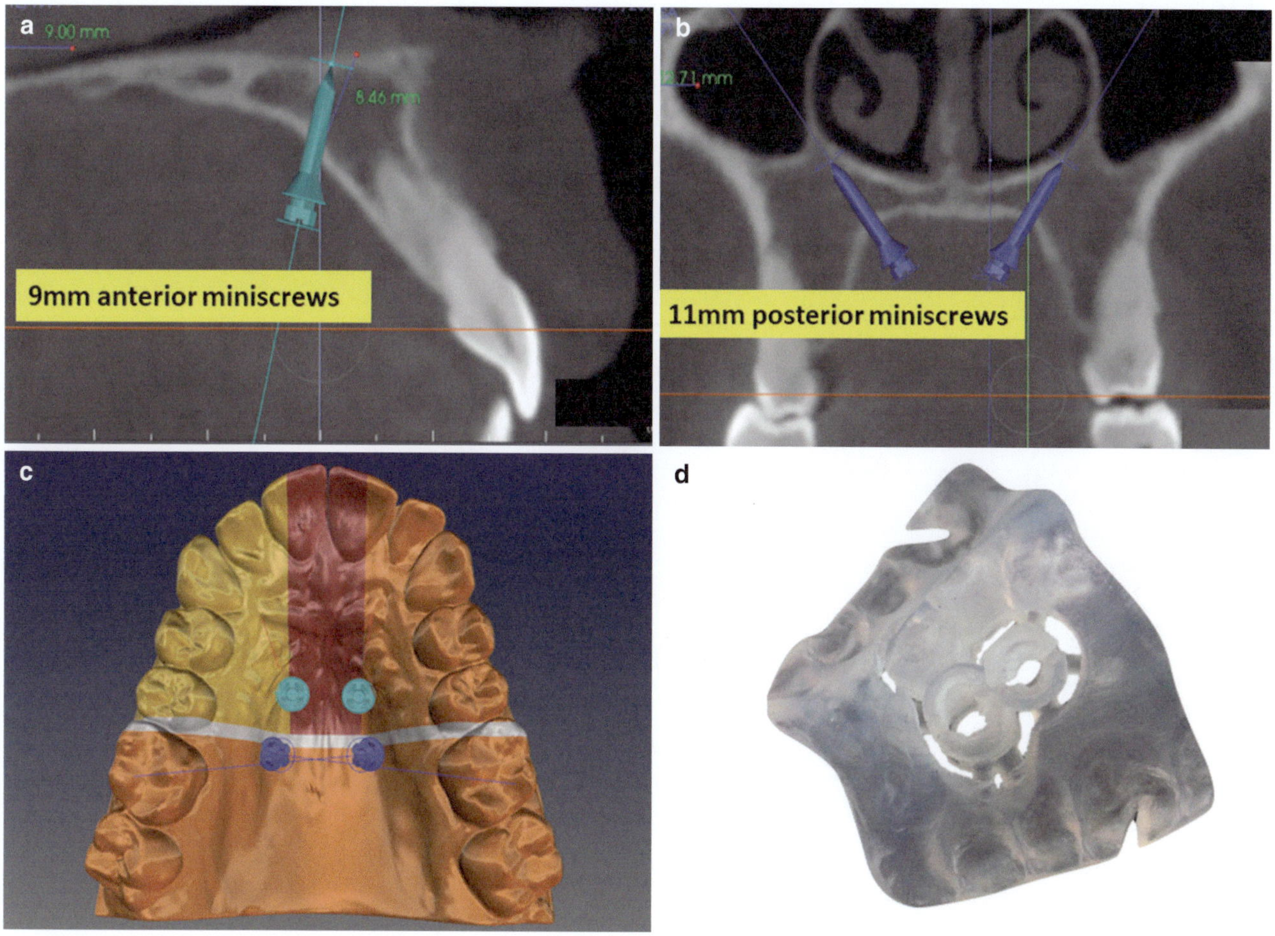

Fig. 8.41 Planning palatal miniscrew insertion: anterior (**a**) and posterior miniscrews (**b**). Digital occlusal view of the location of the miniscrew heads (**c**). MAPA surgical guide (**d**)

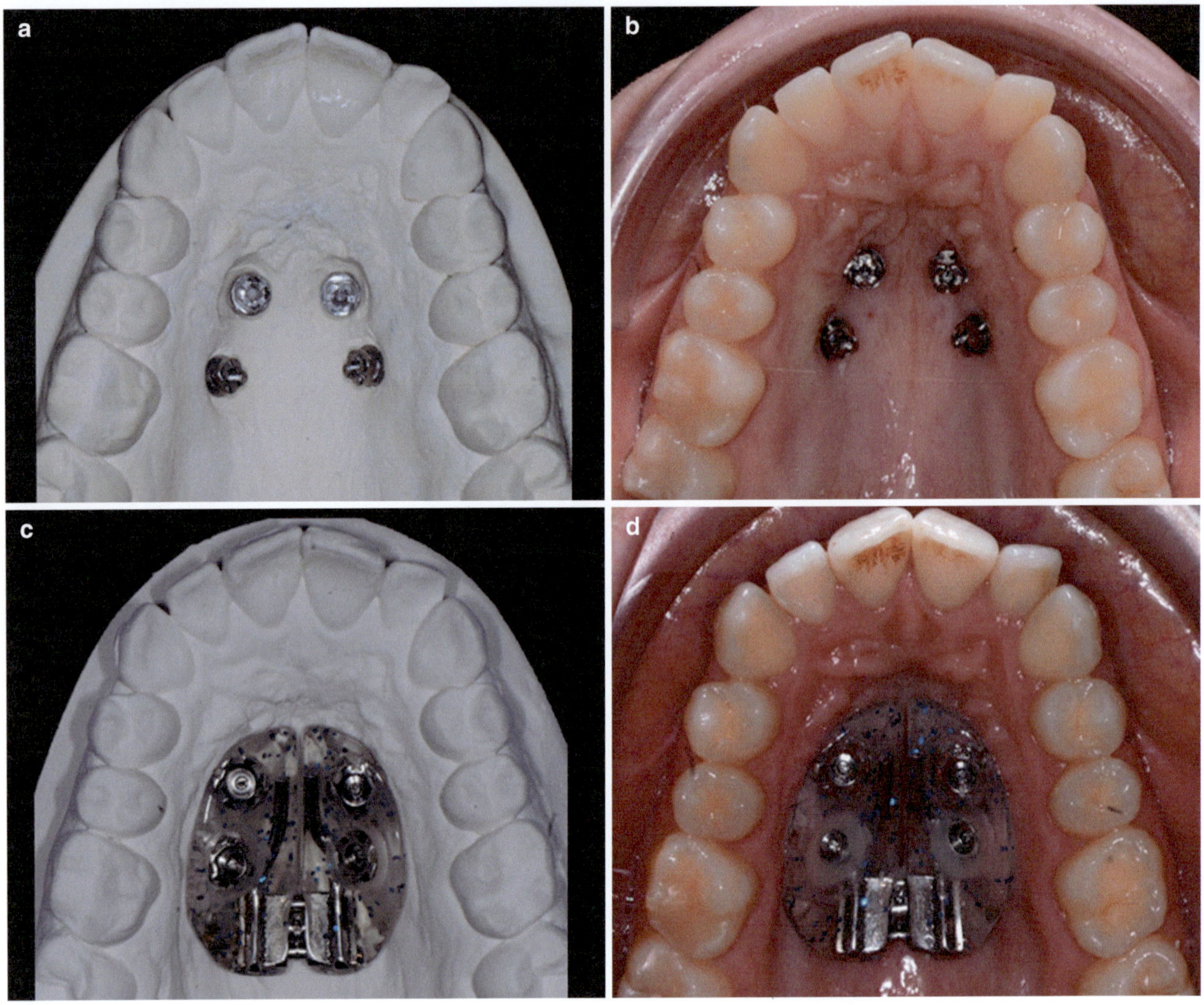

Fig. 8.42 Application of the four palatal miniscrews (**a**). Comparison of palatal miniscrew placement and bone-borne appliance placement in the working resin cast (**a**, **c**) and the palatal vault (**b**, **d**)

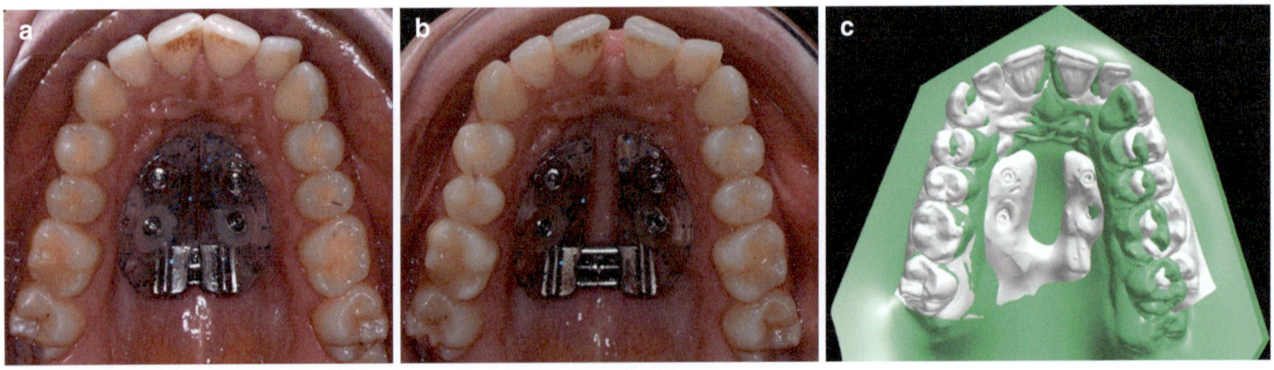

Fig. 8.43 Active phase of skeletal expansion. Placement of the bone-borne appliance (**a**), occlusal post-expansion photo (**b**) and digital superimposition of pre- and post-expansion digital casts (**c**)

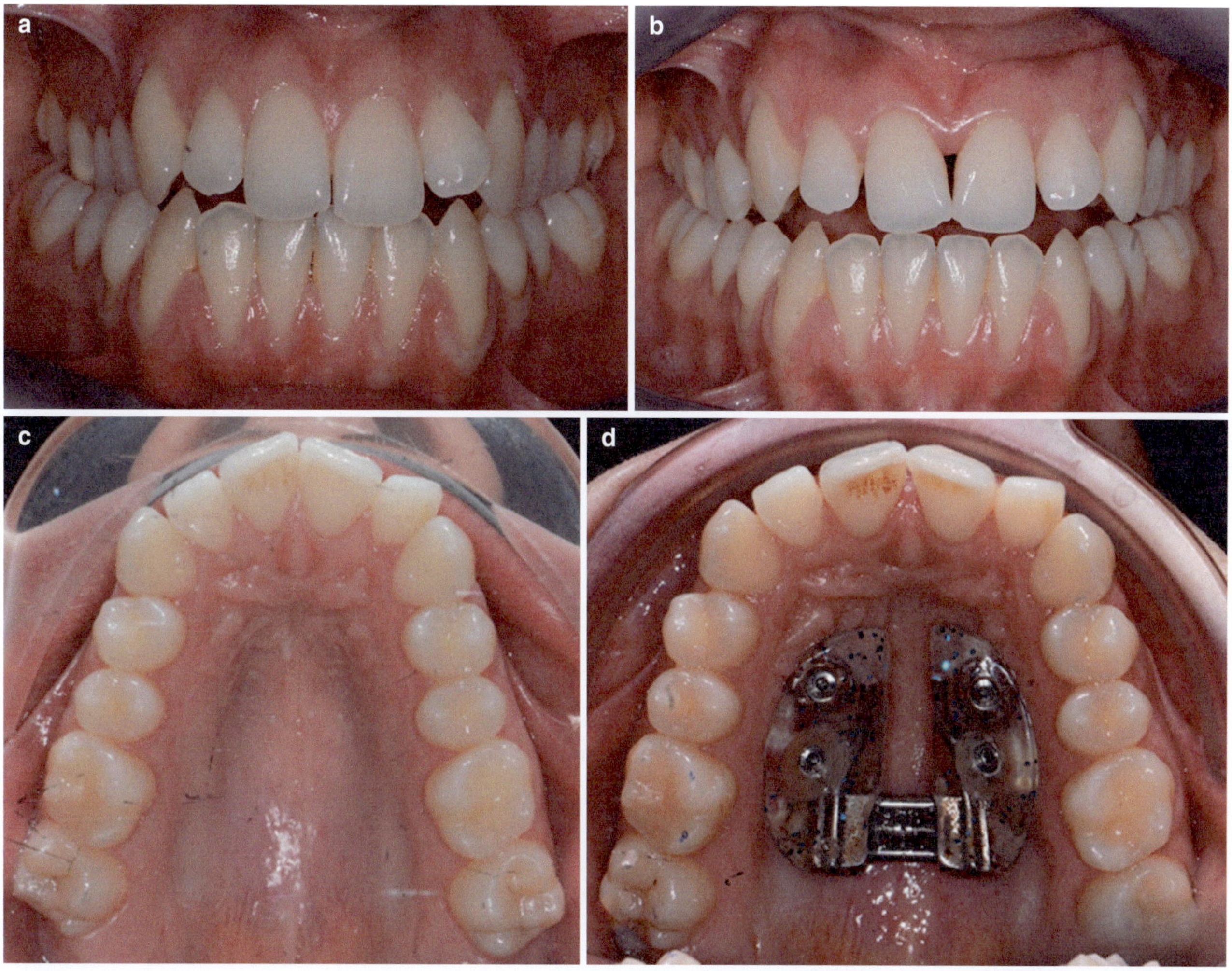

Fig. 8.44 Pre- (**a**, **c**) and post-expansion photos (**b**, **d**). The post-expansion photographs show resolution of posterior cross-bites without unwanted dental effects

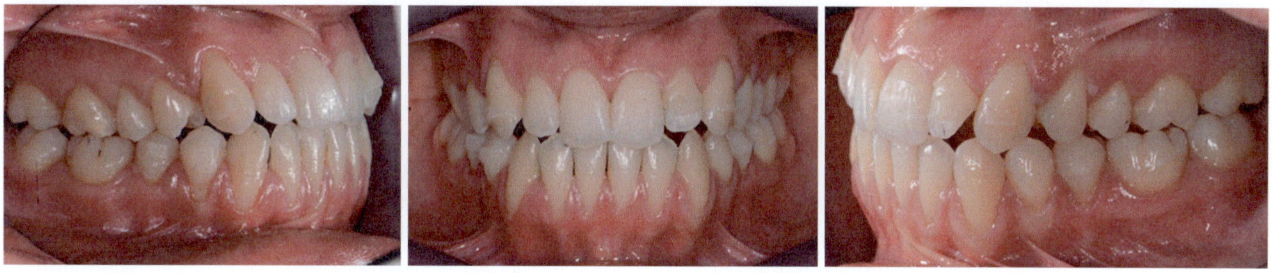

Fig. 8.45 Application of grip points and execution of IPR before the second phase of therapy with F22 aligners

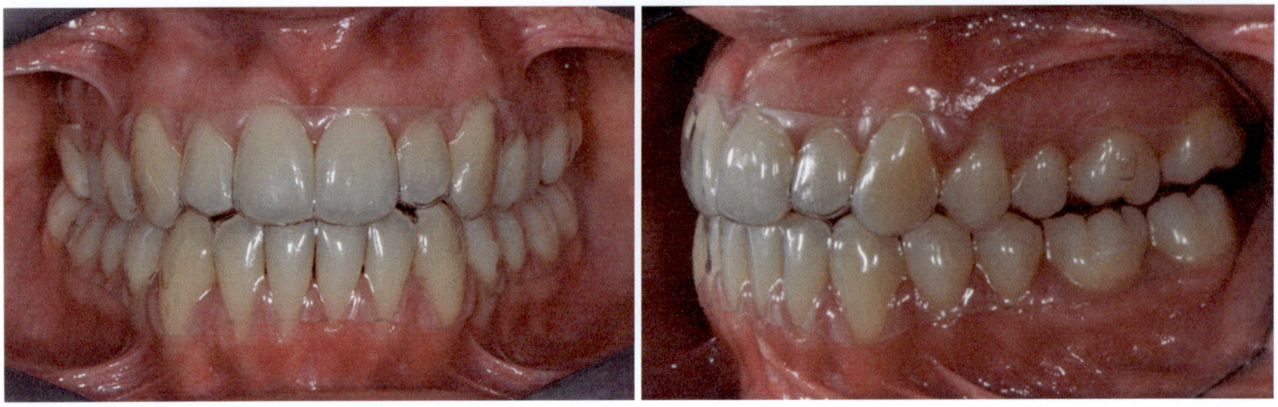

Fig. 8.46 Intraoral photos of F22 aligner treatment

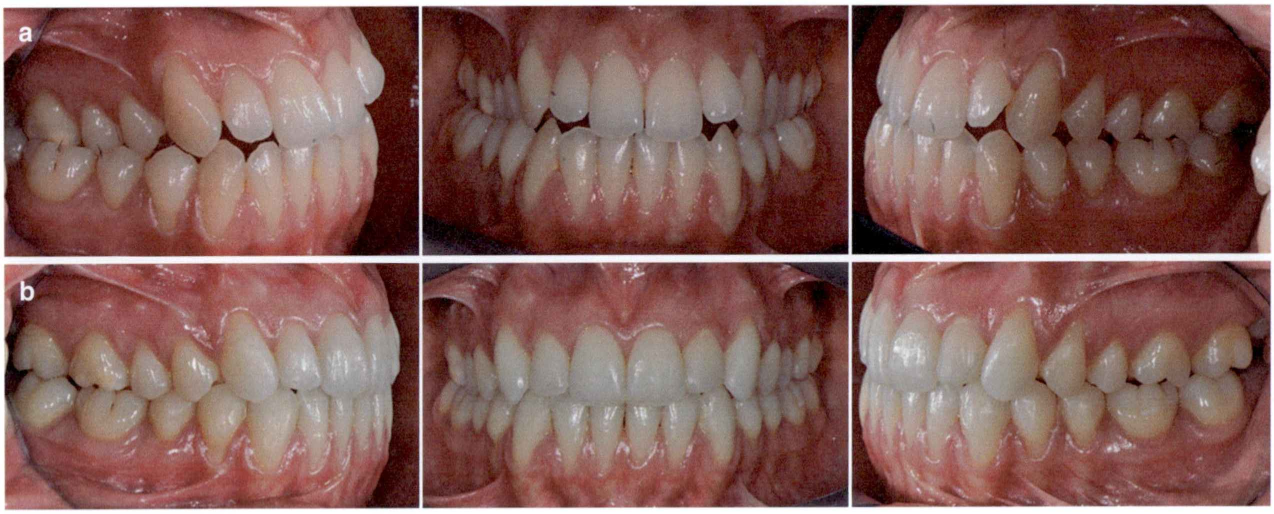

Fig. 8.47 Pre- (a) and post-treatment photos (b)

The treatment was completed in a total of 10 months. Thanks to the bone-borne expander, the transverse hypoplasia of the maxilla and the bilateral posterior cross-bite were resolved without any unwanted effect on posterior teeth that is well documented in literature when a dental-borne RPE was used [39]; this type of appliance-enabled maximisation of the skeletal results with no effect in the upper posterior sectors which could easily have worsened the patient's bone status and periodontal health (Fig. 8.47). As reported in Table 8.2, teeth angulation measured in CBCT axial slices (Fig. 8.48) revealed that they remained fairly stable during orthodontic treatment and that the slight differences between pre- and post-treatment tooth angulation values are due to the effect of clear aligners rather than first phase of orthopaedic expansion.

Extraoral analysis revealed an improvement in incisor display during smile, a significant reduction in buccal black corridors, and a balanced smile (Fig. 8.49). Intraoral examination showed bilateral molar Class I with a residual tendency towards Class III relationship and bilateral canine Class I with ideal overjet and overbite. The midlines were both coincident with the sagittal midline of the face (Fig. 8.50), and the marginal crests were well levelled (Fig. 8.51). Radiography revealed good root parallelism, although tooth 3.2 shows a slight distal inclination in the intraoral photos, with no evident signs of root resorption (Fig. 8.52), and cephalometric analy-

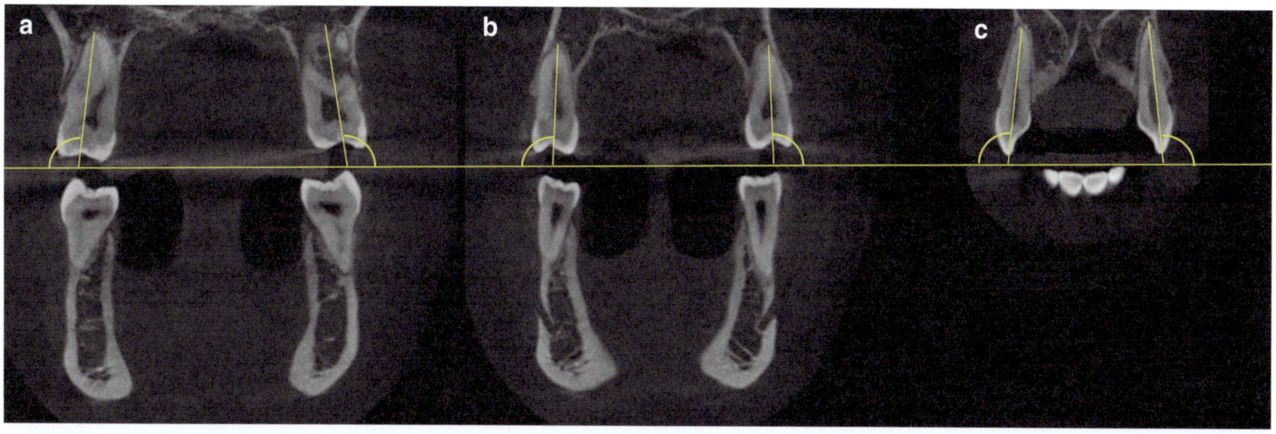

Fig. 8.48 Axial coronal slices of post-treatment CBCT examination, on which tooth angulation measurements have been performed in molar (**a**), premolar (**b**) and canine (**c**) regions. Results are summarised up in Table 8.2

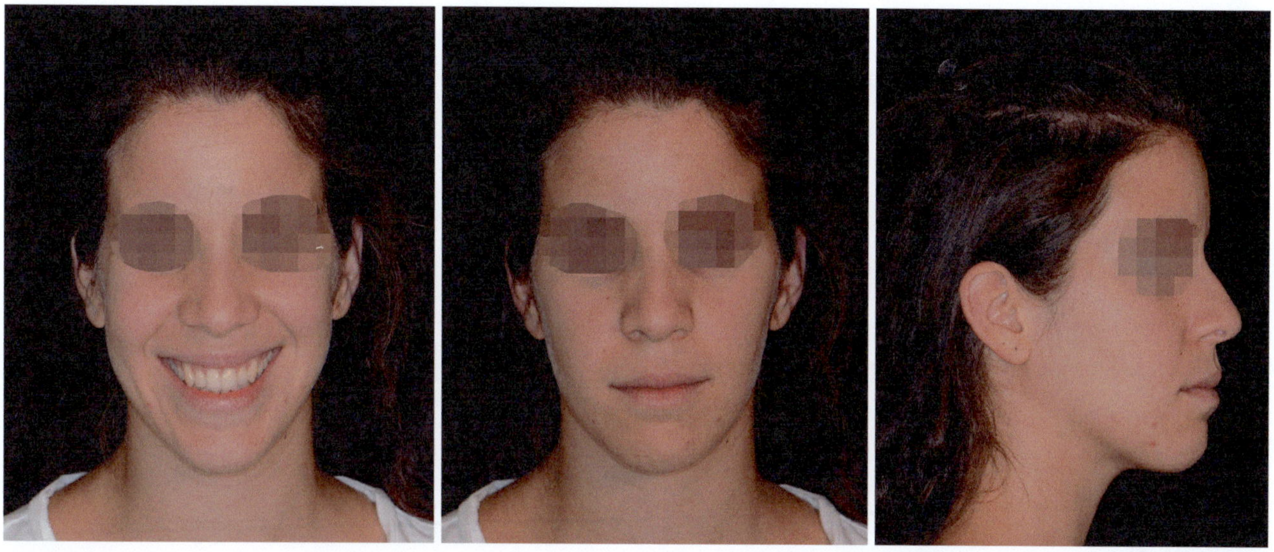

Fig. 8.49 Post-treatment extraoral photographs

sis highlighted slight retrusion of point B with a reduction of SNB value (0.6°) and an increase in ANB value (1°). On the vertical plane, there were no differences in the upper jaw, but the lower jaw was slightly post-rotated with an increase in FMA (31.7°), that could explain the slight retrusion of point B and the reduction of SNB value (0.6°). As regards the dental measurements, the upper incisors had been extruded and uprighted (107°), while the lower incisors had been slightly retroclined (IMPA = 81°) (Table 8.3).

Analysis of the superimpositions clearly shows the effects of the orthodontic treatment with a slight post-rotation of the mandible, retroclination of lower teeth and extrusion and uprighting of upper incisors (Fig. 8.53). Figures 8.54 and 8.55 confirm the excellent dental and skeletal stability at the 18-month check-up, and Fig. 8.56 shows the situation after periodontal surgery, with connective tissue graft, performed 2 months after completion of the orthodontic treatment.

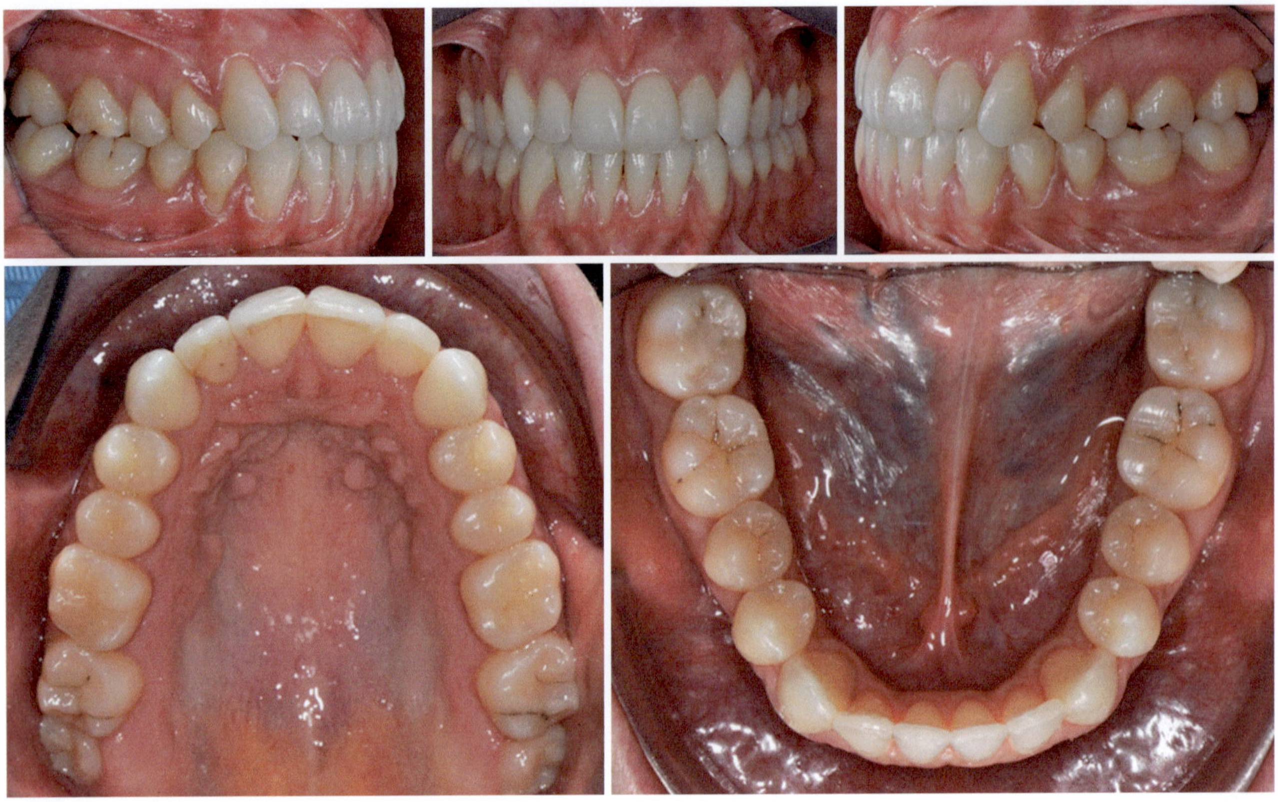

Fig. 8.50 Post-treatment intraoral photographs

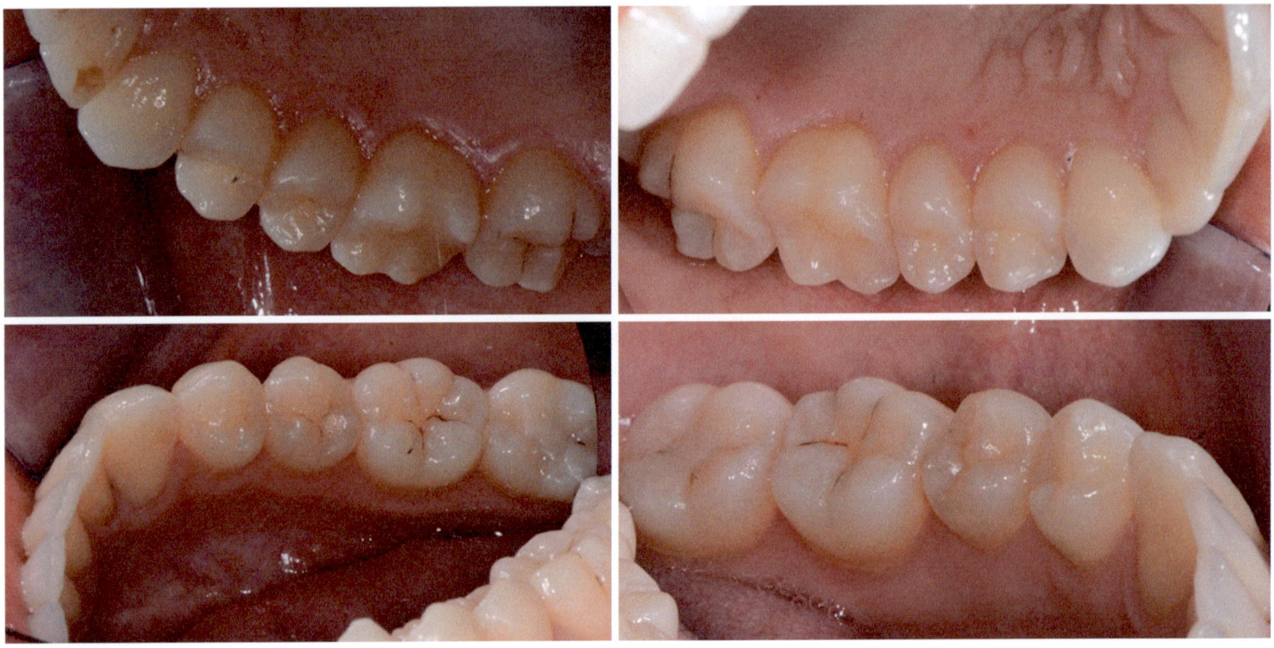

Fig. 8.51 Alignment of posterior marginal ridges

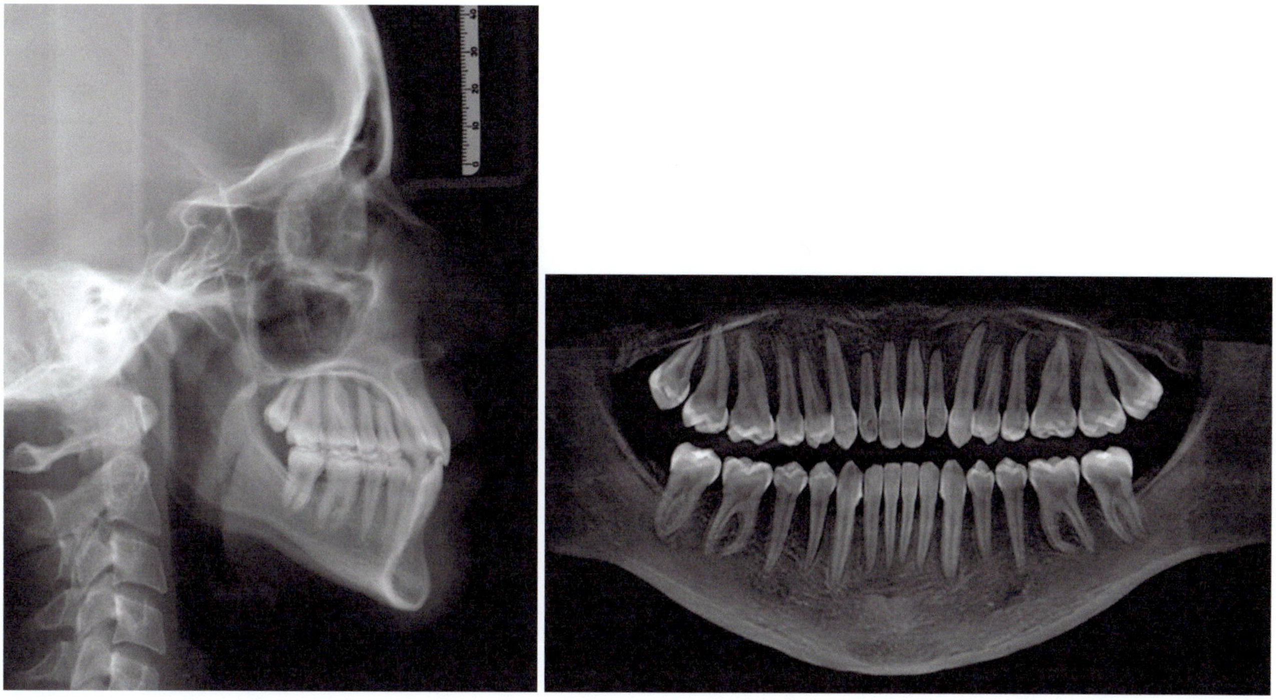

Fig. 8.52 Post-treatment radiographs

Table 8.3 Pre- and post-treatment cephalometric values of case 2

Measurements	Pre-treatment cephalometric values	Post-treatment cephalometric values	Normal values
Horizontal skeletal			
SNA (°)	82.0°	83.0°	82.0°
SNB (°)	82.0°	81.4°	80.0°
ANB (°)	0.0°	1.0°	2.0°
Maxillary skeletal (A-Na Perp) (mm)	−0.8 mm	−0.8 mm	0.0 mm
Mandibular skeletal (Pg-Na Perp)	−3.5 mm	0.8 mm	−4.0 mm
Witts appraisal (mm)	−5 mm	−5.0 mm	0.0 mm
Vertical skeletal			
FMA (MP-FH) (°)	30.8°	31.7°	26.0°
MP-SN (°)	40.0°	41.0°	33.0°
Palatal mandibular angle (°)	32.7°	30.9°	28.0°
Palatal occlusal plane (PP-OP)	12.1°	7.4°	10.0°
Mandibular plane to occlusal plane	20.6°	23.5°	17.4°
Anterior dental			
U: Incisor protrusion (U1-APo) (mm)	7.4 mm	6.5 mm	6.0 mm
L1: Protrusion (L1-APo) (mm)	5.3 mm	4.4 mm	2.0 mm
U1: Palatal plane (°)	117.0°	107.0°	110.0°
U1: Occlusal plane (°)	51.0°	64.4°	57.5°
L1: Occlusal plane (°)	73.9°	72.6°	72.0°
IMPA	82.0°	81.0°	95.0°

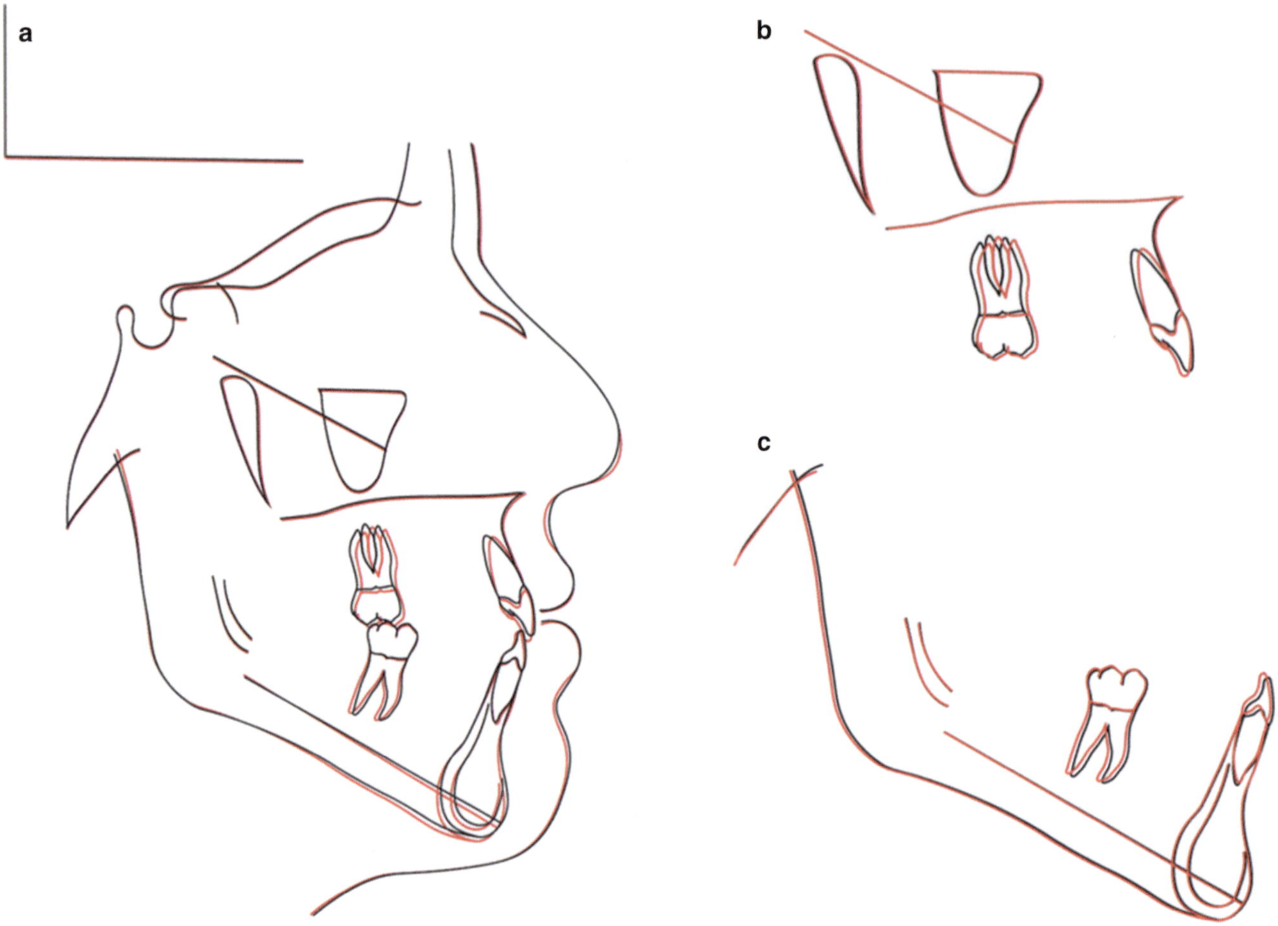

Fig. 8.53 Superimposed tracings: superimposition on the cranial base (**a**), maxillary superimposition (**b**) and mandibular superimposition (**c**)

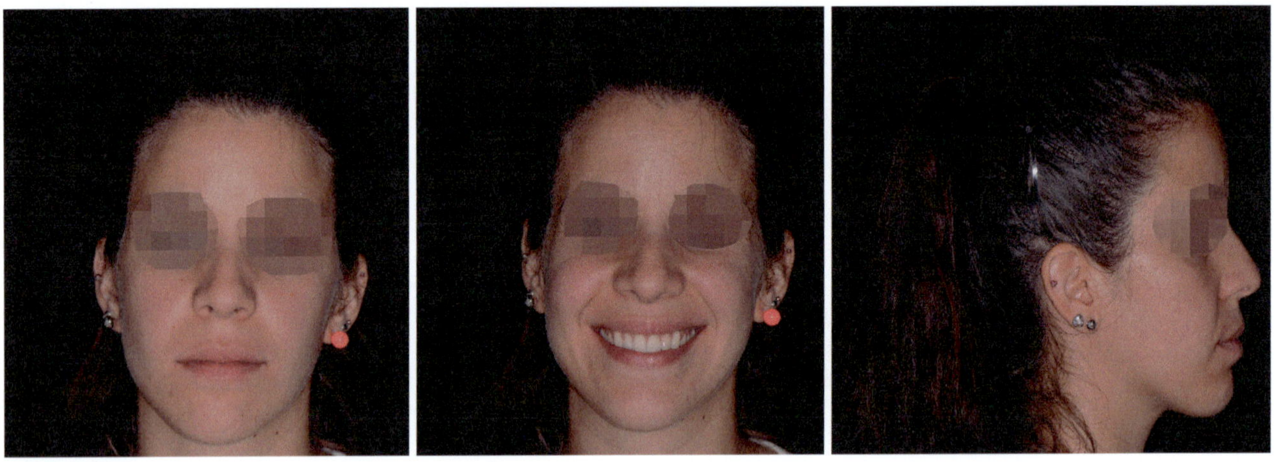

Fig. 8.54 Eighteen-month post-retention extraoral photos

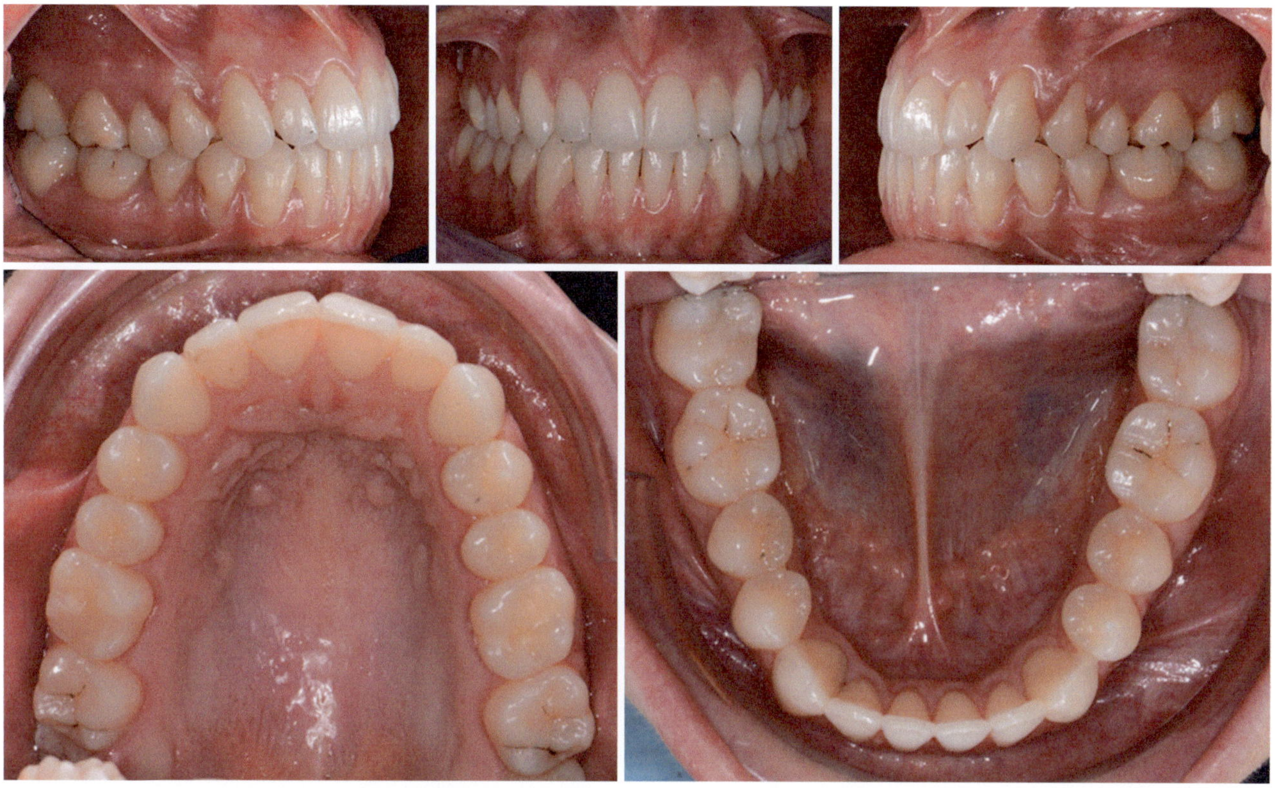

Fig. 8.55 Eighteen-month post-retention intraoral photos

Fig. 8.56 Intraoral photos after connective tissue graft (CTG)

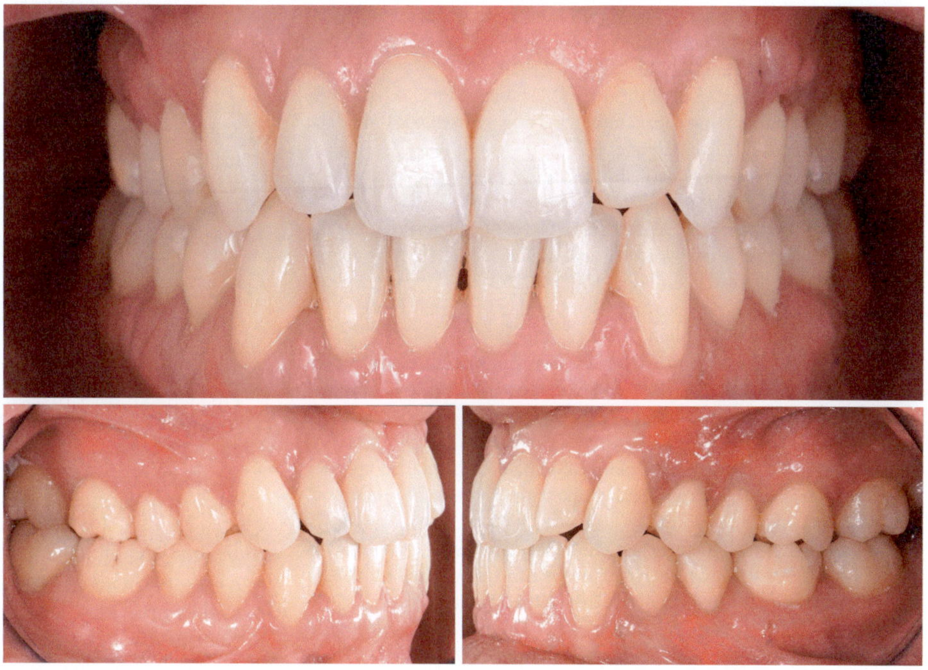

References

1. Graber LW, Vanarsdall RL, Katherine WLV, Huang GJ. Orthodontics. In: Current principles and techniques. 6th ed. St. Louis: Elsevier; 2017.
2. Gracco A, Lombardo L, Guarneri MP. La tomografia volumetrica in ortodonzia. Collana di Ortodonzia diretta dal prof. Damaso Caprioglio. Bologna: Edizioni Martina SRL; 2012.
3. SEDENTEXCT Guideline Development Panel. Radiation protection no 172. Cone beam CT for dental and maxillofacial radiology. Evidence based guidelines. Luxembourg: European Commission Directorate-General for Energy; 2012.
4. Garib DG, Calil LR, Leal CR, Janson G. Is there a consensus for CBCT use in orthodontics? Dent Press J Orthod. 2014;19(5):136–49.
5. Lombardo L, Arreghini A, Guarneri MP, Lauritano D, Nardone M, Siciliani G. Unexpected artefacts and occult pathologies under CBCT. Oral Implantol. 2017;10(2):97–104.
6. Maino G, Paoletto E, Lombardo L, Siciliani G. MAPA: a new high-precision 3D method of palatal miniscrew placement. EJCO. 2015.
7. Ludlow JB, Timothy R, Walker C, Hunter R, Benavides E, Samuelson DB, Scheske MJ. Effective dose of dental CBCT—a meta-analysis of published data and additional data for nine CBCT units. Dentomaxillofac Radiol. 2015;44(1):20140197.
8. Lamichane M, Anderson NK, Rigali PH, Seldin EB, Will LA. Accuracy of reconstructed images from cone-beam computed tomography scans. Am J Orthod Dentofac Orthop. 2009;136(2):156.e1–6; discussion 156–7.
9. Rossini G, Parrini S, Castroflorio T, Deregibus A, Debernardi CL. Diagnostic accuracy and measurement sensitivity of digital models for orthodontic purposes: a systematic review. Am J Orthod Dentofac Orthop. 2016;149(2):161–70.
10. Fleming PS, Marinho V, Johal A. Orthodontic measurements on digital study models compared with plaster models: a systematic review. Orthod Craniofac Res. 2011;14:1–16.
11. Luu NS, Nikolcheva LG, Retrouvey JM, Flores-Mir C, El-Bialy T, Carey JP, et al. Linear measurements using virtual study models. Angle Orthod. 2012;82:1098–106.
12. Marcel T. Three-dimensional on-screen virtual models. Am J Orthod Dentofac Orthop. 2001;119:666–8.
13. Sousa MV, Vasconcelos EC, Janson G, Garib D, Pinzan A. Accuracy and reproducibility of 3-dimensional digital model measurements. Am J Orthod Dentofac Orthop. 2012;142:269–73.
14. Peluso MJ, Josell SD, Levine SW, Lorei BJ. Digital models: an introduction. Semin Orthod. 2004;10:226–38.
15. Hazeveld A, Huddleston Slater JJ, Ren Y. Accuracy and reproducibility of dental replica models reconstructed by different rapid prototyping techniques. Am J Orthod Dentofac Orthop. 2014;145(1):108–15.
16. Gracco A, Buranello M, Cozzani M, Siciliani G. Digital and plaster models: a comparison of measurements and times. Prog Orthod. 2007;8(2):252–9.
17. Hajeer MY. Assessment of dental arches in patients with Class II division 1 and division 2 malocclusions using 3D digital models in a Syrian sample. Eur J Paediatr Dent. 2014;15:151–7.
18. Kravitz ND, Groth C, Jones PE, Graham JW, Redmond WR. Intraoral digital scanners. J Clin Orthod. 2014;48:337–47.
19. Huanca Ghislanzoni LT, Lineberger M, Cevidanes LHS, Mapelli A, Sforza C, McNamara JA. Evaluation of tip and torque on virtual study models: a validation study. Prog Orthod. 2013;14:19.
20. Azari A, Nikzad S. The evolution of rapid prototyping in dentistry: a review. Rapid Prototyping J. 2009;15:216–25.
21. Maino BG, Paoletto E, Lombardo L III, Siciliani G. A three-dimensional digital insertion guide for palatal miniscrew placement. J Clin Orthod. 2016;50(1):12–22.
22. Maino BG, Paoletto E, Lombardo L, Siciiani G. From planning to delivery of a bone-borne rapid maxillary expander in one visit. J Clin Orthod. 2017;51(4):198–207.
23. Gracco A, Lombardo L, Cozzani M, Siciliani G. Quantitative cone-beam computed tomography evaluation of palatal bone thickness for orthodontic miniscrew placement. Am J Orthod Dentofac Orthop. 2008;134(3):361–9.
24. Lombardo L, Gracco A, Zampini F, Stefanoni F, Mollica F. Optimal palatal configuration for miniscrew applications. Angle Orthod. 2010;80(1):145–52.
25. Lee RJ, Moon W, Hong C. Effects of monocortical and bicortical mini-implant anchorage on bone-borne palatal expansion using finite element analysis. Am J Orthod Dentofac Orthop. 2017;151(5):887–97.
26. Kim YH, Yang SM, Kim S, Lee JY, Kim KE, Gianelly AA, Kyung SH. Midpalatal miniscrews for orthodontic anchorage: factors affecting clinical success. Am J Orthod Dentofac Orthop. 2010;137(1):66–72.
27. Mohammed H, Wafaie K, Rizk MZ, Almuzian M, Sosly R, Bearn DR. Role of anatomical sites and correlated risk factors on the survival of orthodontic miniscrew implants: a systematic review and meta-analysis. Prog Orthod. 2018;19(1):36.
28. Ardekian L, Oved-Peleg E, Mactei EE, Peled M. The clinical significance of sinus membrane perforation during augmentation of the maxillary sinus. J Oral Maxillofac Surg. 2006;64:277–82.
29. Cordasco G, Matarese G, Rustico L, Fastuca S, Caprioglio A, Lindauer SJ. Efficacy of orthopedic treatment with protraction facemask on skeletal Class III malocclusion: a systematic review and meta-analysis. Orthod Craniofac Res. 2014;17:133–43.
30. Maino G, Turci Y, Arreghini A, Paoletto E, Siciliani G, Lombardo L. Skeletal and dentoalveolar effects of hybrid rapid palatal expansion and facemask treatment in growing skeletal Class III patients. Am J Orthod Dentofac Orthop. 2018;153(2):262–8.
31. Nienkemper M, Wilmes B, Franchi L, Drescher D. Effectiveness of maxillary protraction using a hybrid hyrax-facemask combination: a controlled clinical study. Angle Orthod. 2015;85(5):764–70.
32. Liou EJ, Tsai WC. A new protocol for maxillary protraction in cleft patients: repetitive weekly protocol of alternate rapid maxillary expansions and constrictions. Cleft Palate Craniofac J. 2005;42(2):121–7.
33. Lombardo L, Arreghini A, Maccarrone R, Bianchi A, Scalia S, Siciliani G. Optical properties of orthodontic aligners-spectrophotometry analysis of three types before and after aging. Prog Orthod. 2015;16:41.
34. Rossini G, Parrini S, Castroflorio T, Deregibus A, Debernardi CL. Efficacy of clear aligners in controlling orthodontic tooth movement: a systematic review. Angle Orthod. 2015;85(5):881–9.
35. Papadimitriou A, Mousoulea S, Gkantidis N, Kloukos D. Clinical effectiveness of Invisalign® orthodontic treatment: a systematic review. Prog Orthod. 2018;19(1):37.
36. Karkhanechi M, Chow D, Sipkin J, Sherman D, Boylan RJ, Norman RG, Craig RG, Cisneros GJ. Periodontal status of adult patients treated with fixed buccal appliances and removable aligners over one year of active orthodontic therapy. Angle Orthod. 2013;83(1):146–51.

37. Rossini G, Parrini S, Castroflorio T, Deregibus A, Debernardi CL. Periodontal health during clear aligners treatment: a systematic review. Eur J Orthod. 2015;37(5):539–43.
38. Melsen B. Palatal growth studied on human autopsy material. A histologic microradiographic study. Am J Orthod. 1975;68(1):42–54.
39. Baysal A, Uysala T, Velia I, et al. Evaluation of alveolar bone loss following rapid maxillary expansion using conebeam computed tomography. Korean J Orthod. 2013;43:83–95.
40. Lo Giudice A, Barbato E, Cosentino L, Ferraro CM, Leonardi R. Alveolar bone changes after rapid maxillary expansion with tooth-born appliances: a systematic review. Eur J Orthod. 2018;40(3):296–303.

9 Visualizing Treatment Objectives and Treatment Planning Using 2D and 3D Occlusograms

Franklin She Tsang Tsang, Asta Abunevičiūtė, and Giorgio Fiorelli

9.1 Conventional Approach of Treatment Planning

A major part of orthodontic diagnosis and treatment planning is done by studying the relationship of dentition, dental alveolar process, and the basal bones of maxilla and mandible with each other and to the skull and overlying soft tissues through clinical, radiographic, and dental model examinations [1]. By comparing the records to the subjective esthetic and functional goals, cephalometric norms and Andrew's six keys of normal occlusion [2], as well as considering the patient's chief complaint, a problem list can be formulated [1]. It leads to the setting of treatment objectives and treatment options with the involvement of the patient which is called shared decision-making [3].

Conventionally, there was a great emphasis on space analysis of dental models, and the Royal London Space Analysis is probably the most commonly taught procedure for undergraduate and postgraduate training worldwide [4, 5].

The analysis is done by filling in a form with a list of factors which affects the space condition of the dental arch. Some factors relate to the existing condition of the patient, e.g., arch length discrepancy to align the overlapped and rotated teeth. There are other factors which relate to the effect of the planned treatment, e.g., extraction and overjet correction. Their implications on space condition are recorded to the nearest millimeter and are positive when space is present or is created (e.g., by proclination of incisors) and is negative when there is crowding or space is required (e.g., for retraction of incisors). In theory, after the form is completed, the residual space requirement for each arch should sum to zero. Otherwise, it indicates that the treatment plan must be modified as the result does not conform to the Andrew's six keys of normal occlusion [2].

F. She Tsang Tsang (✉)
Orthodontics, Faculty of Dentistry, The University of Hong Kong, Hong Kong, China

BIOMEDE (International Association for Development and Spread of Orthodontic Biomechanics Knowledge), Lugano, Switzerland
e-mail: she@smileclinic.com.hk

A. Abunevičiūtė
BIOMEDE (International Association for Development and Spread of Orthodontic Biomechanics Knowledge), Lugano, Switzerland

Private Practice, Vilnius, Lithuania

G. Fiorelli
BIOMEDE (International Association for Development and Spread of Orthodontic Biomechanics Knowledge), Lugano, Switzerland

Orthodontic Department, University of Siena, Siena, Italy

9.2 Limitations of the Conventional Approach and the Need for Tools to Visualize Treatment Objectives and Plan Treatment

Although the teaching of the Royal London Space Analysis provides orthodontic students a very good foundation on understanding how a treatment can potentially affect the space condition of the arches, it is not used routinely for most clinicians after a few attempts due to its limitations such as measurement accuracy, space analysis on dental asymmetry, and definition of the anchorage needs for extraction [6].

While some of these limitations can be overcome by taking measurements on virtual dental models [7] and the use of custom-made orthodontic treatment planning software [8], these analyses generate only numbers relating to two-dimensional tooth movements (Figs. 9.1, 9.2, and 9.3). Therefore, it is very difficult to relate to the three-dimensional change in a real patient situation especially for difficult cases. As such, we need a system to visualize the change of jaw relationship and occlusion three dimensionally which is based on the proposed treatment objectives, and both the VTO and the occlusogram are the solutions [9].

J.-M. Retrouvey, M.-N. Abdallah (eds.), *3D Diagnosis and Treatment Planning in Orthodontics*,
https://doi.org/10.1007/978-3-030-57223-5_9

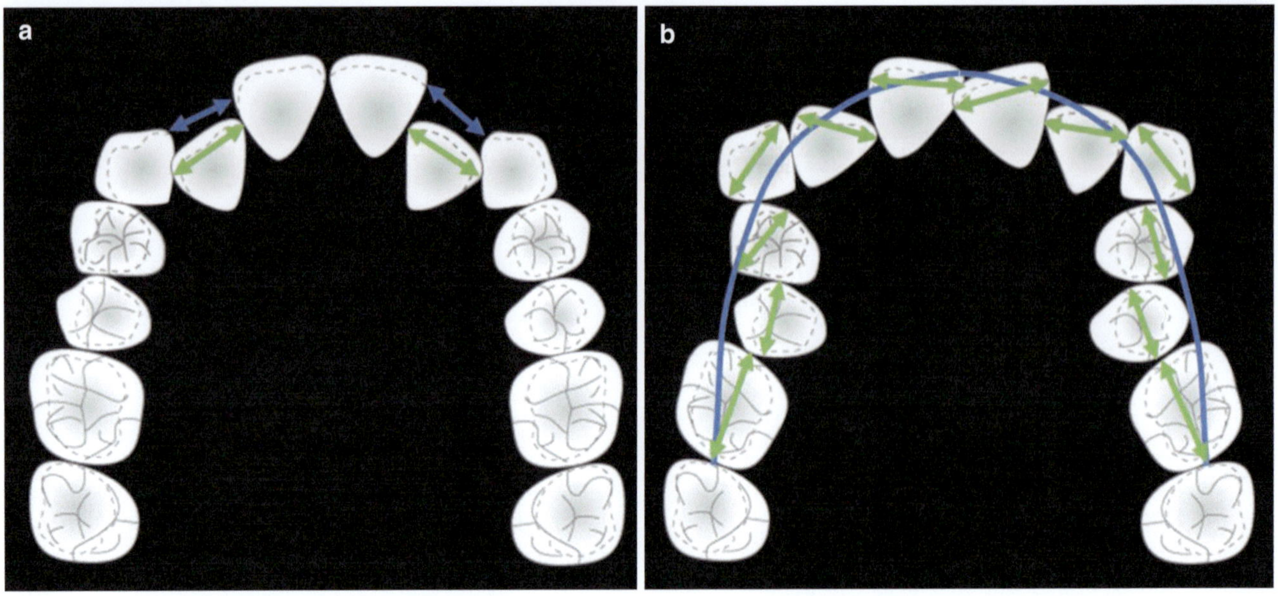

Fig. 9.1 Limitation of conventional approach. Scenario 1. (**a**) Both arches A and B were developed from the same well-aligned arch. However, space analysis can be done more accurately for case A as only four measurements are required as highlighted by the blue and green arrows. For case B, since all the teeth except 17 and 27 are displaced from the ideal arch form, the width of every tooth has to be measured (green arrows) and subtracted to the arch length (blue line), the crowding is often over-estimated as each measurement is rounded up to the nearest millimeter. The accumulated errors can be enormous which lead to extraction therapy if the buccal occlusion and profile are not considered

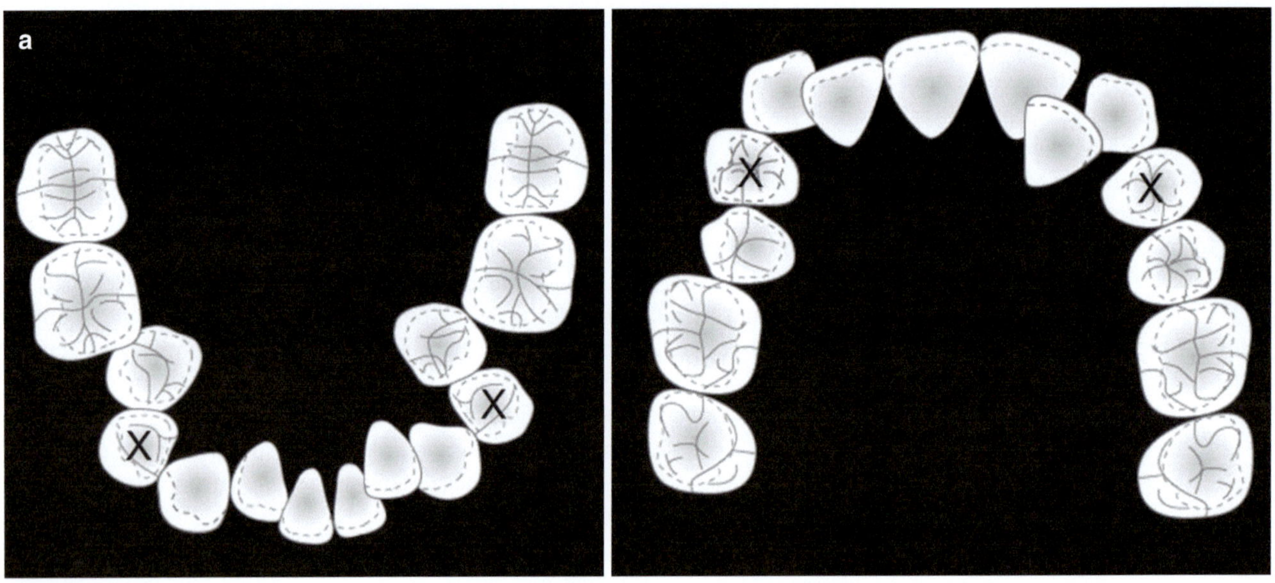

Fig. 9.2 Limitation of conventional approach. Scenario 2. (**a**) Midline of both lower and upper arches are shifted to left 2 mm, and there is crowding of 12 mm on each arch. There is 2 mm extra space left after extracting two 7 mm premolars (14, 24, 34 and 44) on each arch. (**b**) It would be difficult to determine the anchorage need by only referring to the space analysis form as it does not separate the space condition on each quadrant. More information is needed to formulate a treatment plan. (**c**) Extra information for treatment planning. Dental arch midlines (blue) are added to illustrate the shift of anterior midline. The perpendicular lines (red) to the dental arch midlines (blue) which are flushed on the mesial contacts of 26 and 36 show that 16 and 36 are shifted 2 mm mesial. (**d**) Extra information for treatment planning. Since molar relationships are class I on both sides and canine relationship is more class II on the right than the left side, 26 and 36 can move forward 2 mm. Therefore, after extraction, absolute anchorage need is required at quadrants 1 and 4, and maximum anchorage need is required on quadrants 2 and 3

b **Modified Royal London Space analysis form**

	Lower	Upper
Lower arch	+/-mm	+/-mm
Crowding/spacing	-12	-12
Level curve of Spee		
Arch width change		
Incisor AP change		
Tip/torque change		
Tooth reduction/Enlargement		
Extractions	+14	+14
Space opening for replacement		
Molar distalization		
Molar mesialization	-2	-2
TOTAL (should = 0)	0	0

+ = Space available or gained
- = Space required or lost
Overjet - lower incisor AP change/2 - 2 = Overjet to be corrected
Overjet to be correct × -2 = upper incisor AP change

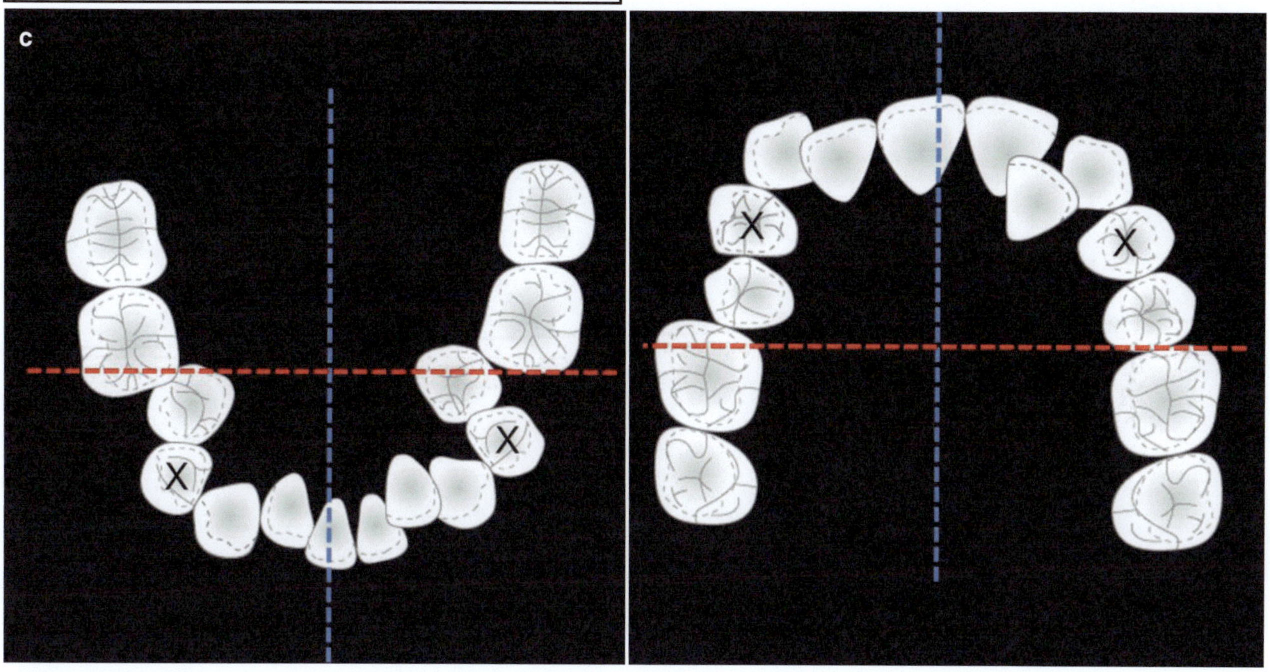

Fig. 9.2 (continued)

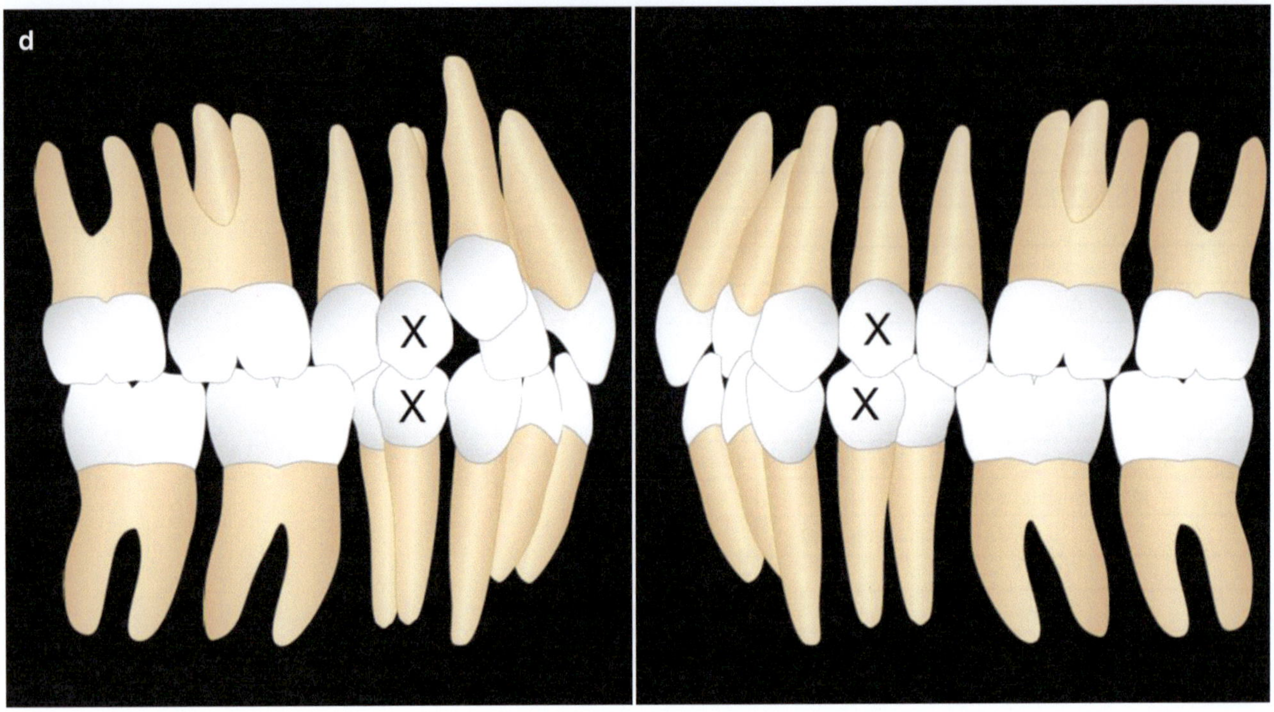

Fig. 9.2 (continued)

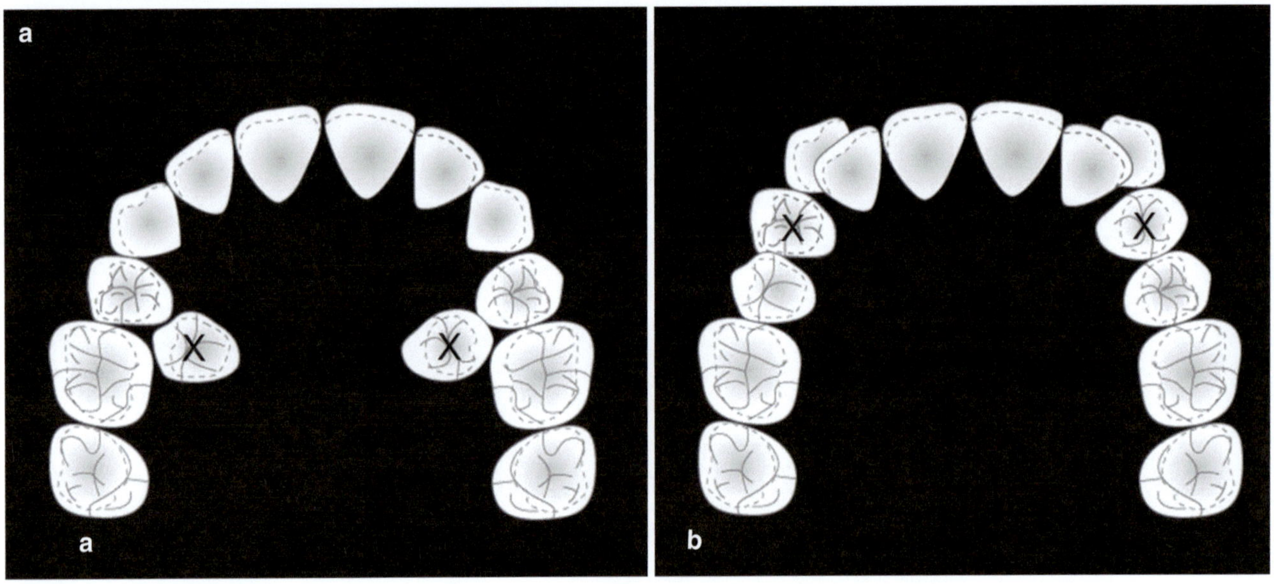

Fig. 9.3 Limitation of conventional approach. Scenario 3. (**a**) Two cases A and B which have different anchorage needs after extraction but look the same on the space analysis form. (**b**) If all premolars are 7 mm wide, both cases present with 14 mm of crowding which can be relieved by the extraction of one premolar on each side. Therefore, the first molars are not allowed to move forward a single millimeter. The form cannot help deciding the anchorage need. (**c**) Extra information for treatment planning. If the treatment objective is to keep upper incisors where they are, since the canine relationship is class I for case A and class II for case B, after the extraction of one premolar on each side, case B needs absolute anchorage to retract 13 and 23 along the arch (blue arrow). Therefore, case B is far more difficult than case A

b **Modified Royal London Space analysis form**

	Lower	Upper
Lower arch	+/-mm	+/-mm
Crowding/spacing		-14
Level curve of Spee		
Arch width change		
Incisor AP change		
Tip/torque change		
Tooth reduction/Enlargement		
Extractions		+14
Space opening for replacement		
Molar distalization		
Molar mesialization		
TOTAL (should = 0)	0	0

+ = Space available or gained
- = Space required or lost
Overjet - lower incisor AP change/2 - 2 = Overjet to be corrected
Overjet to be correct × -2 = upper incisor AP change

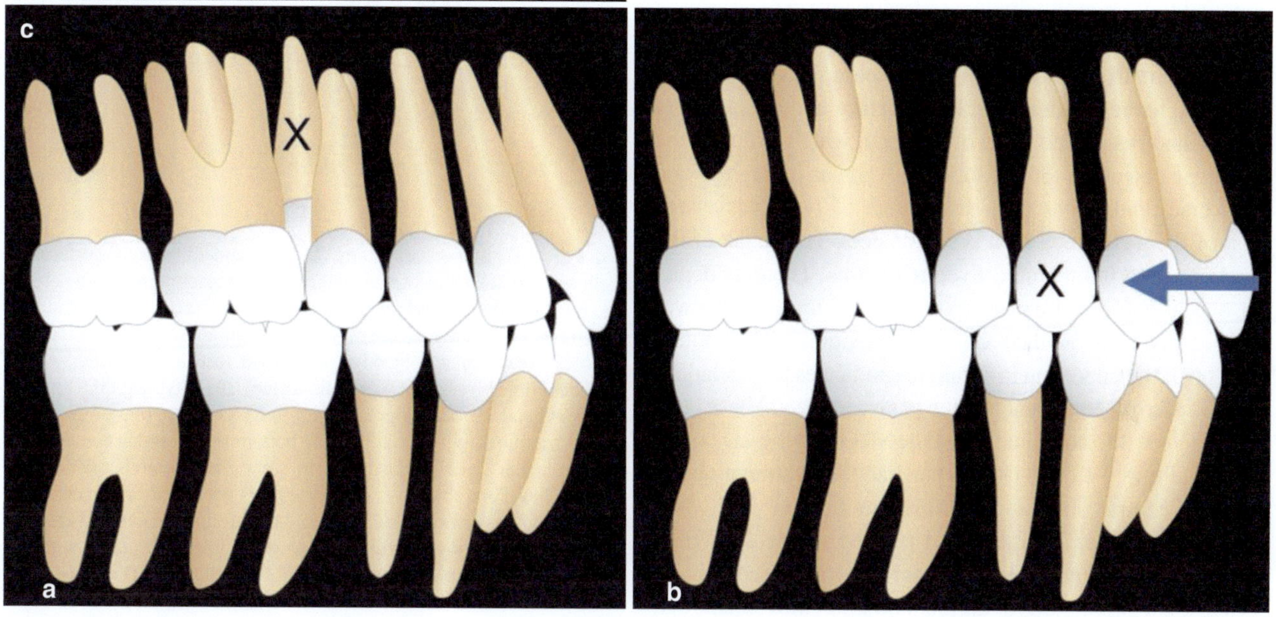

Fig. 9.3 (continued)

9.3 VTO and Occlusogram

Burstone introduced the use of visual treatment objectives (VTO) and 2D occlusogram for diagnosis and treatment planning in 1961 [10, 11]. The procedure can now be done by a computer software (t3DO) (True3d Occlusogram, IOSS, GmbH) which is developed by Giorgio Fiorelli [12], and the 3D occlusogram can be generated on virtual dental models (DDP-Ortho) (DDP-Ortho, Ortolab Sp. Z o.o.) [9] (Fig. 9.4).

VTO consists of the patient's tracing of pretreatment lateral cephalogram which is modified to demonstrate movements of incisors and first molars and/or surgical changes in sagittal and vertical dimensions, based on the facial treatment objectives [13]. Therefore, it is a face-driven approach of treatment planning which contrasts to the conventional lower incisor-driven approach [9, 14].

Furthermore, the procedure is a tool for risk management as the movement of the incisor roots confine to the envelope of the alveolar process [15]. Any violation of the root position to the supporting bone can be seen immediately which suggests to the clinician to rethink the treatment objectives and treatment plan to prevent gingival recession, root resorption, and tooth non-vitality due to treatment [15].

The information of the VTO is then transferred to the occlusogram. 2D occlusogram is a graphic representation of the dental arches from the occlusal surface and is essentially a simplified diagnostic setup of the teeth which indicates the treatment objectives of the tooth movement in sagittal and transverse dimensions [13]. It consists of two lines where each of them is joined by a series of dots. The shape of the two lines describe the objective arch forms. The dots depict the mesial and distal contact points of the upper and lower teeth respectively at their objective positions. The mutual position of the upper and lower arches indicates their relationship in space with reference to the jaws and cranial base [12].

Therefore, the combination of the VTO and the 2D occlusogram allows the clinician to visualize the treatment objectives of central incisors and first molars in 3D while movement of other teeth can be visualized only in 2D. When virtual models and 3D occlusograms are used, three-dimensional simulations of all planned tooth movements can be performed [9].

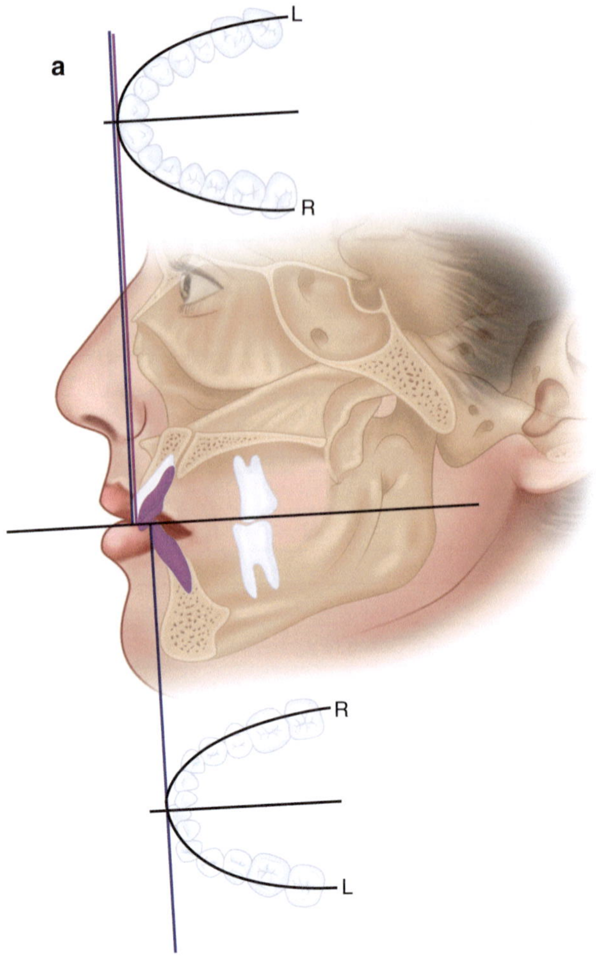

Fig. 9.4 VTO and occlusogram. (**a**) Pretreatment occlusal surfaces of teeth and the 2D occlusograms indicate the contact points of the objective position of teeth and the intended shape of the arches (top and bottom images). Tracing of lateral cephalogram and the shaded incisors indicate the treatment objective position of teeth and is called visual treatment objectives (VTO) (middle image). (**b**) A typical t3DO generated VTO and 2D occlusogram report (left). Occlusogram of the lower arch is traditionally viewed from the bottom so that it can be superimposed on the upper occlusogram to show the interarch relationship (right). Therefore, the lower occlusogram is presented in mirror image to the occlusal view of clinical photo. In the following cases (Figs. 9.5, 9.6, and 9.7), the lower occlusograms were flipped to match with the occlusal view of clinical photos to avoid confusion. (**c**) 2D occlusogram from t3DO as shown in (**b**) is transferred to virtual dental models (DDPOrtho) as a 3D occlusogram

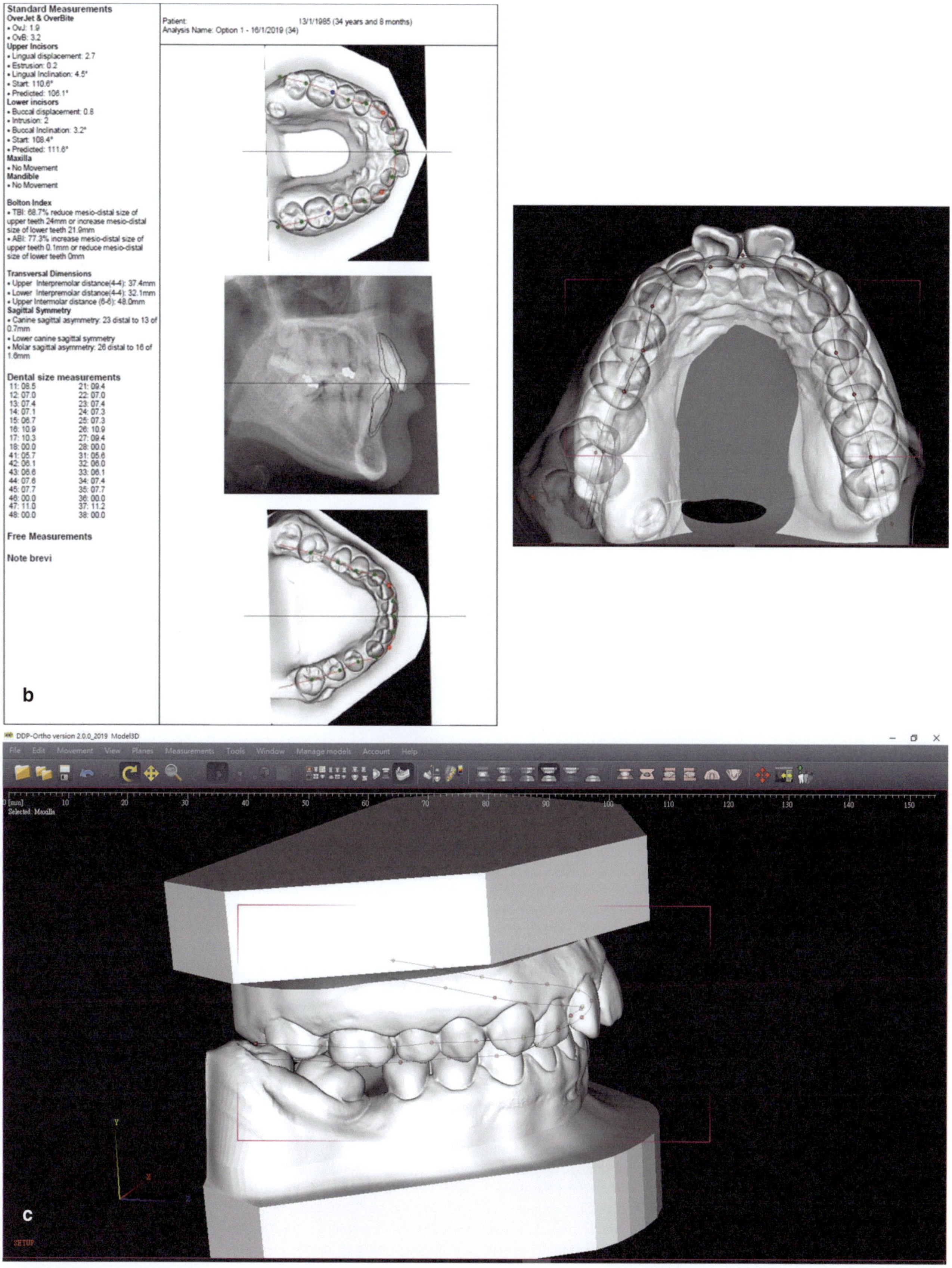

Fig. 9.4 (continued)

Furthermore, the latest version of virtual models (DDP-Ortho) allows full diagnostic setup of teeth based on the 3D occlusogram so that the relative position of individual teeth between pretreatment to objectives can be shown even more clearly. Figure 9.5 illustrates an example of using a combination of VTO with a 3D occlusogram for treatment planning.

9.4 Construction of VTO and Occlusogram by DDP-Ortho and t3DO

During VTO and occlusogram construction, the clinician has to go through a series of procedures to define the treatment objectives which lead to a treatment plan simulation [9, 12]. Therefore, they are excellent tools to learn and execute treat-

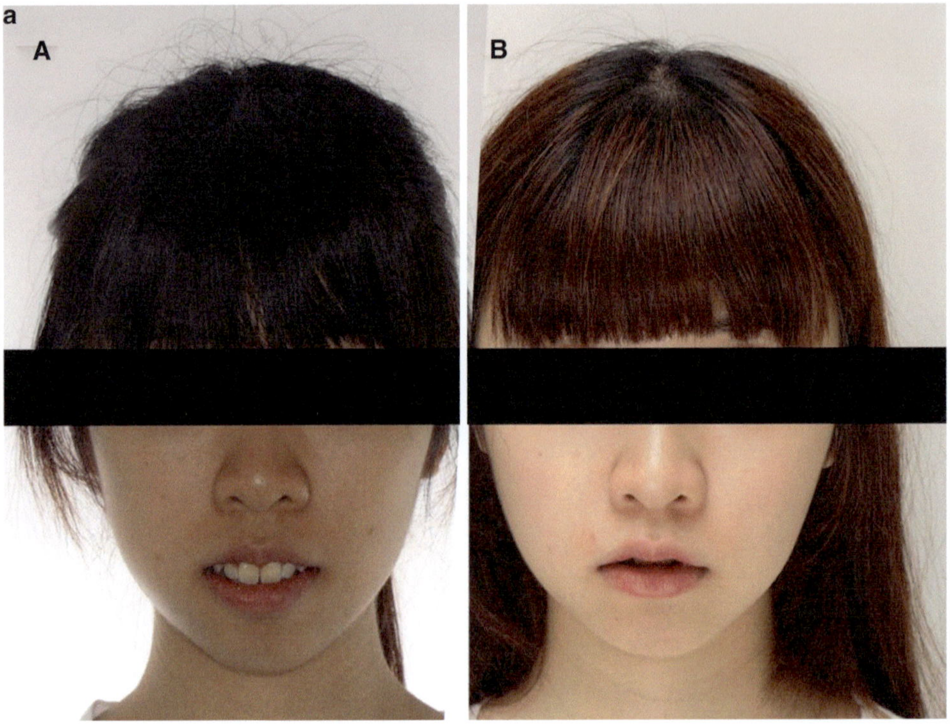

Fig. 9.5 Case NGM treated by Dr. Franklin She. Face-driven treatment planning by VTO of an orthodontic camouflage case with straight wire mechanics, extraction, and the use of TADs. (**a**) Frontal facial photos. A: Pretreatment. Rest incisal exposure and lip separation 10 mm B: After treatment: Rest incisal exposure and lip separation 3 mm. (**b**) Three-quarter smile photos. A: Pretreatment. Maxillary dentoalveolar excess in AP and total vertical. Gingival exposure at emotional smile at central incisor region 6 mm, premolar region 5 mm. B: After treatment: Intrusion and retraction of anterior teeth and intrusion of posterior teeth improved protrusion and gummy smile. (**c**) VTO: Upper central incisors were intruded 4 mm and retracted 7 mm. Upper first molars were intruded 4 mm. Counterclockwise rotation of mandible 3°. Lower central incisors were extruded 2 mm and retracted 5 mm. (**d**) VTO as a tool to test biological limit. A: Cortical bone on the palatal side is perforated by bodily retraction of upper central incisor by 7 mm. B: Since the shape of anterior dentoalveolar process of the maxilla resembles a funnel, a different incisor movement can be planned to avoid violating the biological limit. Retracting the upper central incisor by controlled tipping with the same amount of retraction (7 mm) as in A, and intrusion 4 mm as measured at the incisal edge, prevent perforation of cortical bone of the palatal side. (**e**) Pretreatment virtual dental models of DDP-Ortho. (**f**) Superimposition of virtual dental models to the lateral cephalogram. Simulation of change of occlusion in response to 3° counterclockwise rotation of mandible on virtual articulator of DDP-Ortho. (**g**) Occlusion in response to 3° counterclockwise rotation of mandible on virtual articulator of DDP-Ortho. (**h**) 2D occlusograms: Lines in red indicate objective arch form. Dots in pink, green, and red indicate contact points of incisors, canines, and second premolars and molars, respectively. Dots in blue indicate mesial contacts of first molars. A: Upper arch: Retraction of upper central incisors 7 mm and extraction of upper first premolars. Upper first molars move mesial 2 mm and canines move distal 5 mm, which indicates maximum anchorage. B: Lower arch: Retraction of lower central incisors 5 mm and extraction of lower left second and right first premolars. Upper first molars move mesial 2 mm and canines move distal 5 mm, which indicates maximum anchorage. (**i**) 3D occlusograms of the upper and lower arches which are viewed below the dental models in occlusion. (**j**) Virtual ideal setup based on 3D occlusogram of the right side of the upper arch. Teeth in transparent yellow color indicate pretreatment positions. Teeth in white color indicate the objective positions. The arrows in red indicate the movement of upper right first molar, second premolar, and canine. (**k**) Occlusal view of the virtual ideal setup. (**l**) Treatment progress 1: Orthodontic miniscrews (Orlus, Ortholution) were inserted at 16, 26 mesial buccal (1O16107) and distal palatal (1O18208) regions, between 11, 21 and 31, 41 (1O14107). Smartclip® brackets (3M Oral Care) in MBT® prescription were installed. Powerchains were used to move the teeth toward the miniscrews to achieve the objective positions. Stainless steel 0.036″ transpalatal and lingual arches were used for transverse control. (**m**) Treatment progress 2: Space closure by powerchain with reciprocal anchorage after intrusion. Extensive remodeling of the maxillary dentoalveolar process can be seen. (**n**) End of treatment. Gingivectomy was performed by Dr. Tak On Ryan, Tse

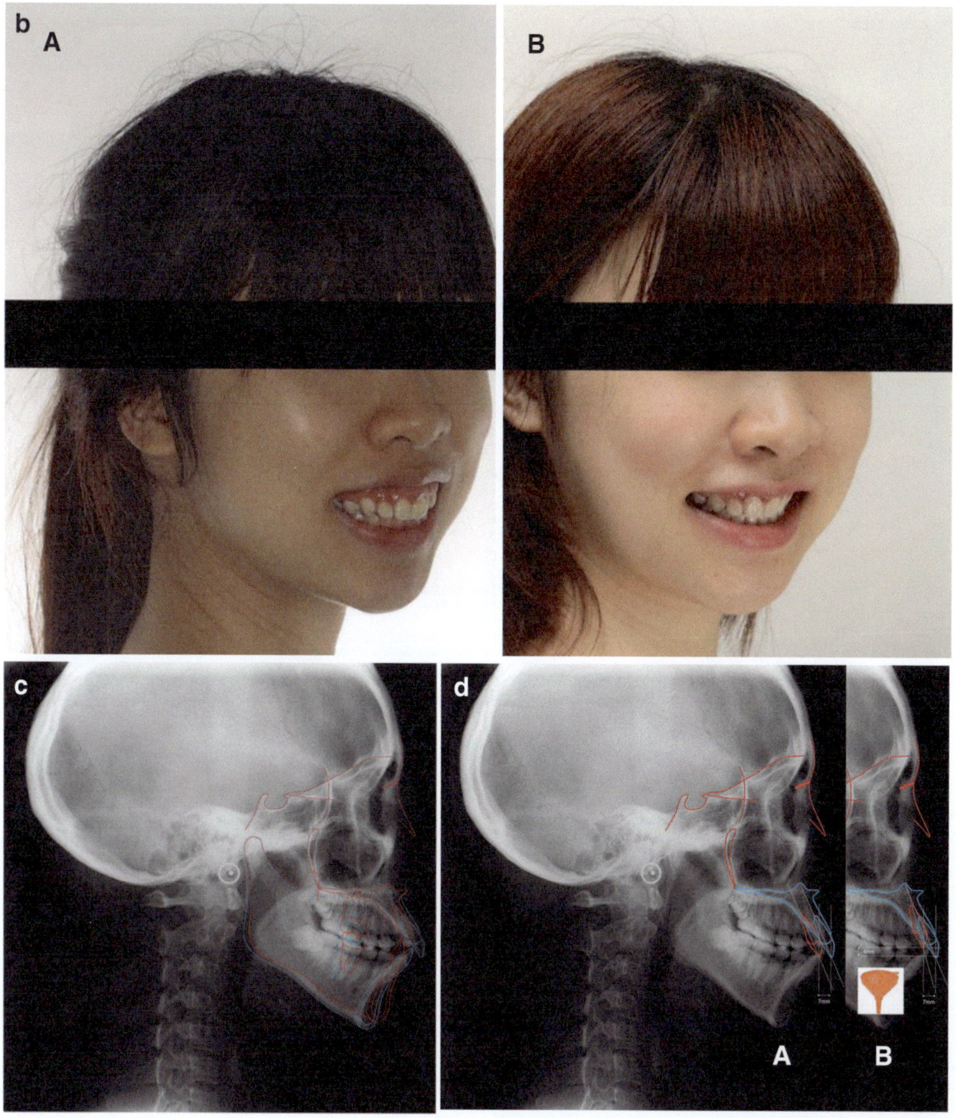

Fig. 9.5 (continued)

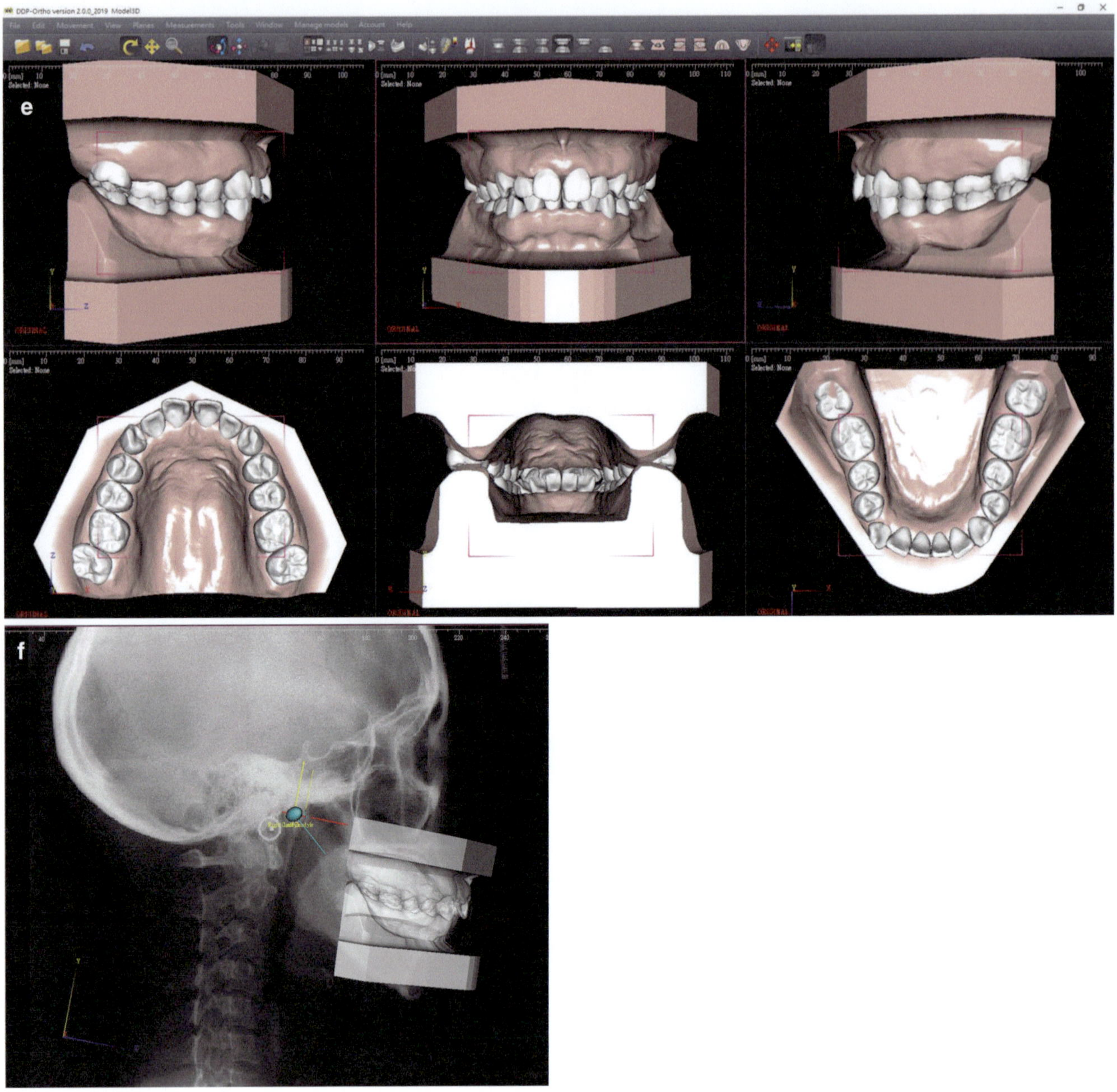

Fig. 9.5 (continued)

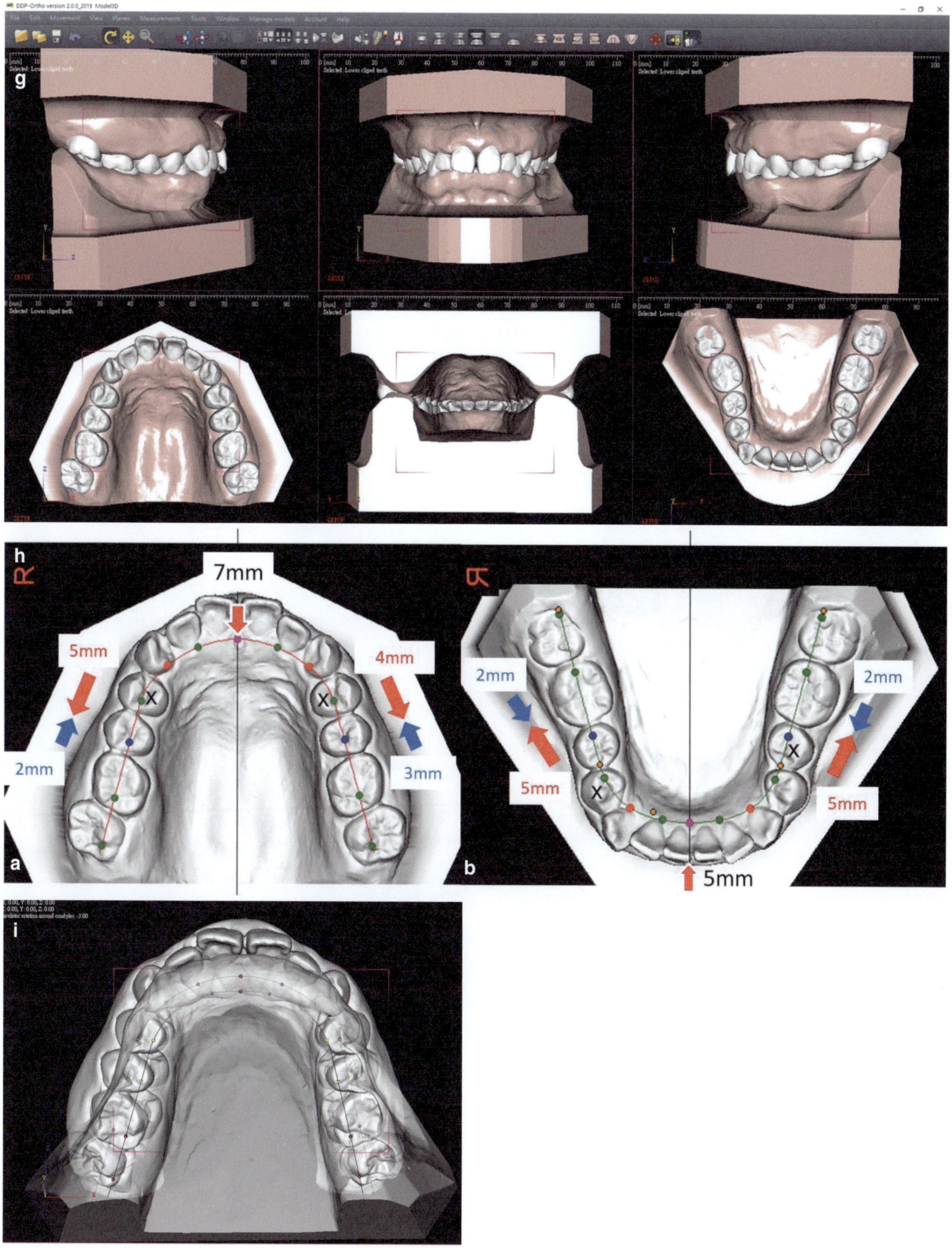

Fig. 9.5 (continued)

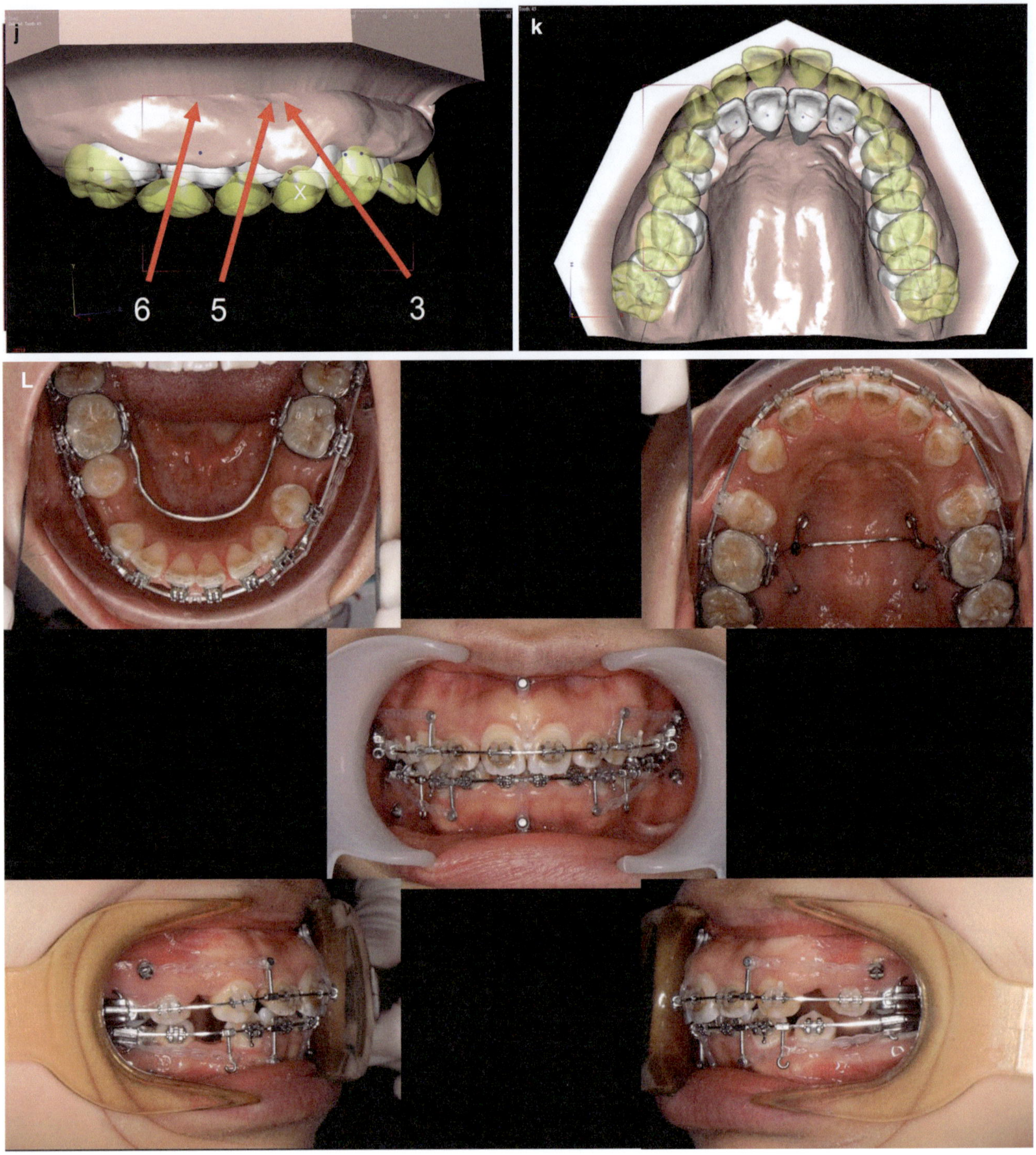

Fig. 9.5 (continued)

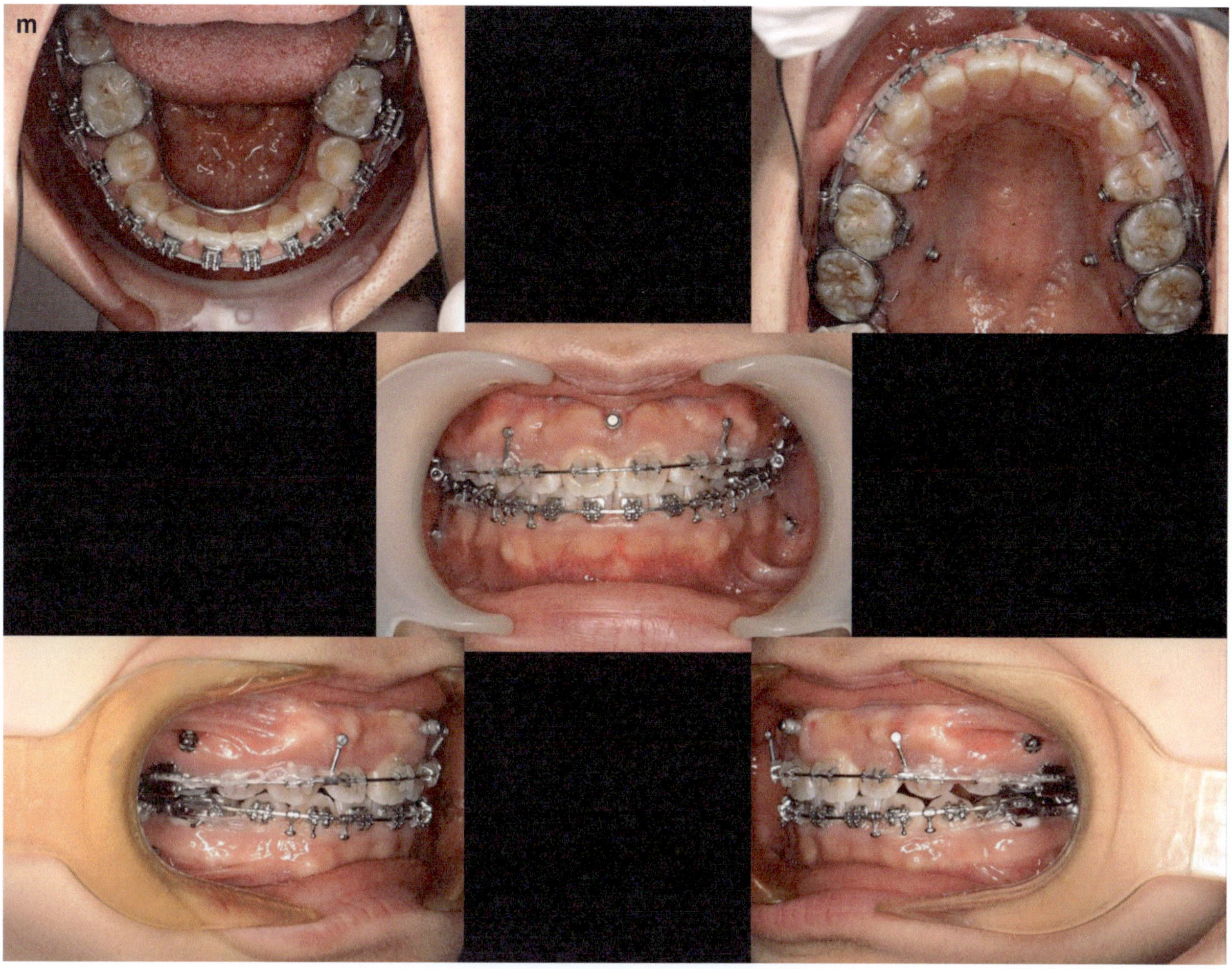

Fig. 9.5 (continued)

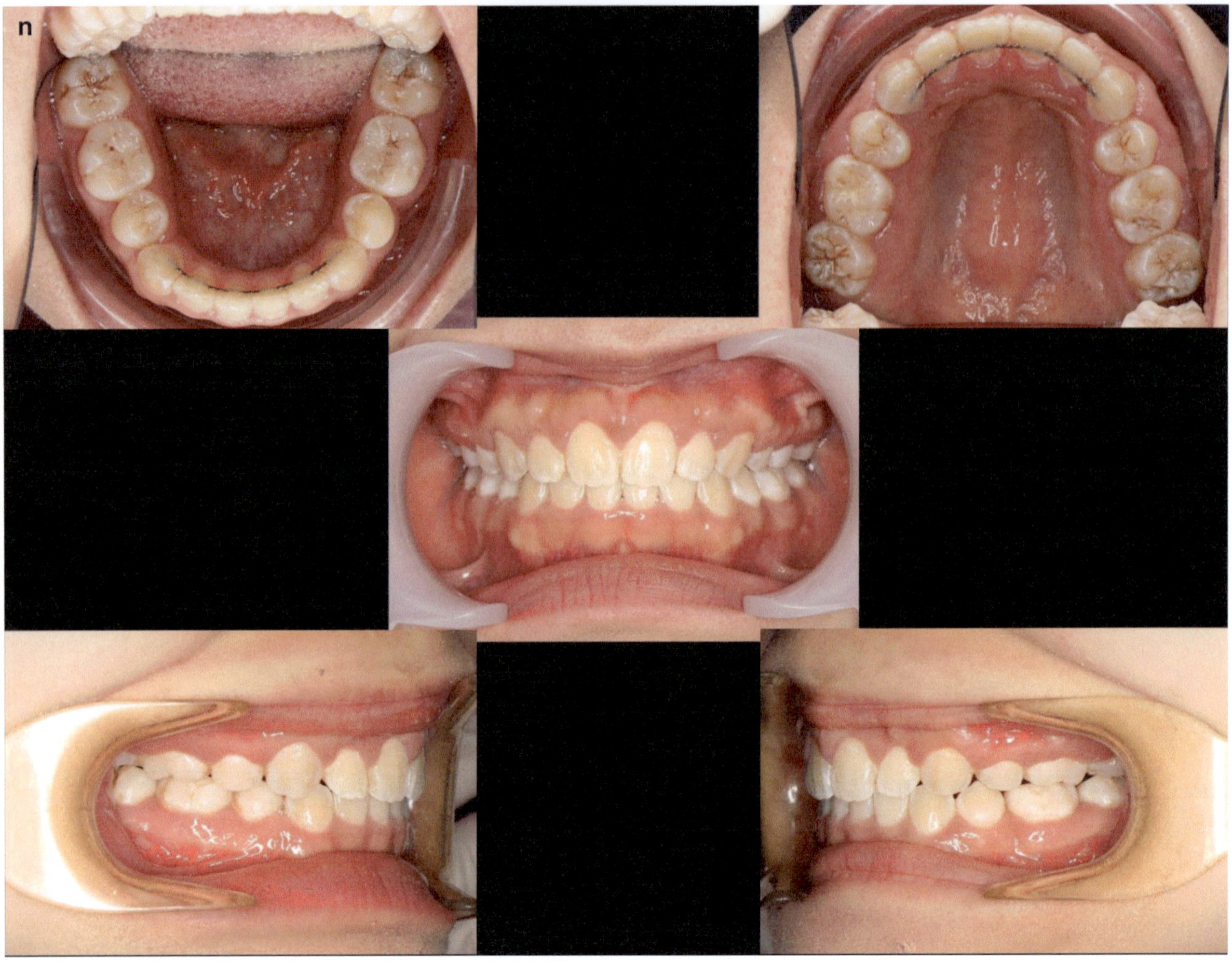

Fig. 9.5 (continued)

ment planning in a systematic way. On each treatment simulation, VTO and occlusogram will allow the clinician to (Fig. 9.6 illustrates an example of the steps below):

1. Simulate the pretreatment jaw relationship and occlusion
2. Visualize the change of jaw relationship due to orthognathic surgery or mandibular repositioning, e.g., after molar intrusion by TADs
3. Define symmetry axis, detect asymmetry of dental arches
4. Identify individual teeth or segments of teeth which are displaced from the objective arch form
5. Perform space analysis
6. Estimate tooth size/arch size discrepancies
7. Assess the changes needed in the length and the width of dental arches
8. Simulate the tooth movements in 3D
9. Define the active and reactive dental units
10. Define the force systems (force and moment) necessary for the planned tooth movements [16, 17]
11. Evaluate the anchorage requirements

It is an iterative process where each parameter, such as the final position of the incisors, arch shape, symmetry line, and extraction plan must be tested repeatedly so that the outcome is rational and practical to the existing condition of patient. The advantages of the computerized procedure are a reduction in execution time, improved accuracy, and, especially, the possibility of simulating different treatment options by changing just a single input parameter. In fact, once the first treatment plan is simulated, the clinician may explore other options by changing one of the parameters, and the software will recalculate the whole treatment simulation immediately. Figure 9.7 demonstrates the importance of defining the symmetry line during the treatment planning phase.

9.5 Application of VTO and 2D and 3D Occlusograms on Diagnosis and Treatment Planning

VTO and occlusogram are very useful for planning difficult cases such as:

1. Dental asymmetries
2. Surgical orthodontics
3. Orthodontic camouflage with TADs to create orthognathic surgery-like results [14, 18]
4. Interdisciplinary treatment, e.g., hypodontia [19, 20], temporomandibular disorder [21], and rehabilitation of pathologically migrated dentition [22–25]

These cases can be divided into two categories based on the age of the patients. The first group consists of young adults with dentofacial deformities. Extensive tooth movements are required to camouflage the existing basal discrepancy or to remove the dentoalveolar compensations in preparing for orthognathic surgery. The second group consists of older adults with degenerated or mutilated dentition due to tooth loss and periodontal breakdown. Extensive tooth movements are required to bring the drifted teeth back to the original position and open space for tooth replace-

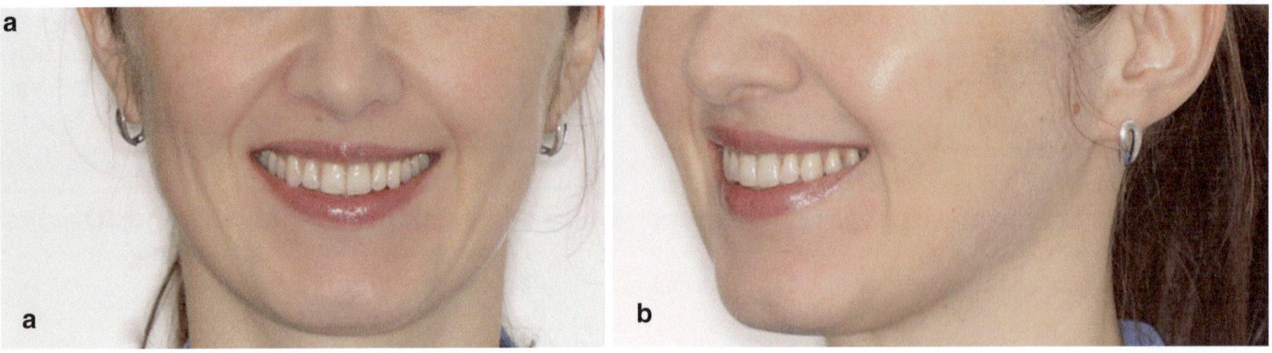

Fig. 9.6 Case AA treated by Dr. Giorgio Fiorelli: A temporomandibular disorder (TMD) patient presented with severe headaches and reciprocal clicks on the right temporomandibular joint (TMJ). (**a**) Posttreatment extra-oral photos. (**b**) Pretreatment occlusion: Asymmetrical occlusal relationship: Right side: Class II molar and canine relationship. Left side: Class I molar and canine relationship. Lower dental midline deviated to right side. Deep overbite with increased curve of Spee. Retroclined upper incisors. (**c**) Case AA: Deviation of chin to the right side can be seen on the front view of 3D volume rendering of dentofacial complex from CBCT data. (**d**) Simulation of mandibular reposition on DDP-Ortho software. Step 1: Superimposition of the virtual dental models to the frontal and lateral views of 3D volume rendering of dentofacial complex by the DDP-Ortho software. The position of the condyles were located on the images to calibrate the virtual articulator. (**e**) Simulation of mandibular reposition on DDP-Ortho software. Step 2: The virtual articulator simulated the occlusion when patient wore the stabilization splint which relieved the signs and symptoms of temporomandibular disorder (TMD). It is where the mandible was rotated around left condyle 1.8° on the articulator and the lower dental and facial midlines coincide to the upper midlines. (**f**) Simulation of mandibular reposition on DDP-Ortho software. Step 3: Simulated occlusion was saved in DDP-Ortho software and imported into t3DO software. (**g**) Construction of 2D occlusogram by t3DO. Step 1: Definition of symmetry axis. Symmetry axis (in blue color) of the dental arches is the objective midline which is defined by the clinician. It is often coincided with the facial midline along the median raphe of the palate unless there is a yaw rotation of the maxilla. A reference line (in red color) is formed by selecting two points on the upper arch which is considered symmetrical in one of the dental arches. The symmetry axis (in blue color) is constructed automatically which is perpendicular to and bisects the red reference line. Step 2: Alignment of the virtual dental models to the lateral cephalogram. The blue dots are registered along the symmetry axis by the clinician in the software which indicate incisal edges of upper and lower central incisors before treatment. (**h**) Construction of 2D occlusogram by t3DO. Step 2 (continued): The incisal edges (blue dots) of the upper and lower central incisors before treatment were transferred to the lateral cephalogram which is generated from the 3D image. Alignment of the virtual dental models to the lateral cephalogram is completed by registering the functional occlusal plane (in red color) on the lateral cephalogram. Step 3: Registration of the positions of upper and lower central incisors on the lateral cephalogram. Root apexes (green dots) of the upper and lower central incisors before treatment were registered to indicate the length and inclination of the central incisors and thus the images of central incisors are generated automatically (blue lines). (**i**) Construction of 2D occlusogram by t3DO. Step 4: Location of objective position of upper and lower central incisors (in red color) by the clinician with the consideration of biological limits. In this case, inclination of upper central incisor is changed by uncontrolled tipping (Torque). Lower central incisor was planned to move labial and apically without any change of inclination (Bodily movement). (**j**) Construction of 2D occlusogram by t3DO. Step 5: Definition of arch width and shape on the automatically generated 2D occlusogram. Since the contact points and the width of individual teeth were located and calculated by DDP-Ortho service provider, upper and lower occlusograms (red lines with dots in green, red and blue colors) are generated once the previous steps were completed. The objective arch width and shape can be modified by the clinician with the consideration of biological limits. The space analysis is done automatically and in real time when the width and shape of the objective arch form is modified (A). The software offers to indicate the alignments of individual teeth before treatment (blue lines) for clearer comparison with their objective position (B). (**k**) Construction of 2D occlusogram by t3DO. Step 6: Management of tooth size discrepancy, tooth extraction, or open space for tooth replacement. Individual tooth size can be seen in the chart, and the Bolton analysis is generated for reference. The software offers to show both upper and lower occlusograms on the same arch to illustrate inter-arch relationship. In this case, 1 mm tooth width was added to the upper lateral incisors (blue rectangle) to improve the molar relationship in sagittal dimension from half unit class II to full unit class I (compare relationship of blue dots on the occlusograms which indicate mesial contact points of first molars. Blue circle, before adjustment. Red circle, after adding 1 mm on each lateral incisors). If extraction is needed, the width of extracted teeth will be deduced from the arch length immediately by removing the tick in the checker box. (**l**) Diagnosis of tooth displacement by 2D occlusogram. Treatment objectives of the buccal tooth segments on sagittal and transverse dimensions were indicated. (1) Proclination of upper central incisors (orange). (2) Unilateral distalization of the right side of the upper arch (blue). (3) Unilateral expansion on the left side of the upper arch (red). (4) Unilateral expansion and mesialization on the right side of the lower arch (green). Lines of force which produce the objective tooth segment movements are indicated by arrows in colors representing the respective segments. (**m**) Construction of 3D occlusogram by t3DO. The position of the 2D occlusogram in the vertical plane of space is registered on the buccal and frontal view of the digital dental models in t3DO, and the data is transferred back to DDP-Ortho to generate the 3D occlusogram. (**n**) A: 3D occlusogram on the simulated occlusion of mandibular reposition on DDP-Ortho software. Pretreatment tooth position (yellow), lower teeth at the objective position (blue outline), lines of force to produce the individual objective position (red arrows). The need for tipping, intrusion, or extrusion of clinical crowns of buccal segments can be shown more clearly with the help of 3D occlusogram. (B) Virtual ideal setup which is based on the 3D occlusogram can be done either manually or semi-automatically. Objective tooth position (white). (**o**) Treatment progress 1: 3 months after mandibular repositioning by Triad® gel (Dentsply Sirona). Asymmetric expansion of upper right and lower left buccal segments by beta-titanium 0.036″ palatal and lingual arches. Orthodontic miniscrew (68.99.28A) (The Aarhus System, American Orthodontics) was used to fixed the position of 36, lingual arch was activated. Another miniscrew will be inserted to fix the position of 16 (68.99.30A), by that time palatal arch will be activated. (**p**) Treatment progress 2: Beta-titanium 0.017 × 0.025″ cantilever was used to tip 17, 16, and 15 distally. Beta-titanium 0.017 × 0.025″ box loop was used to move 23 labial. Vertical elastics were used to extrude buccal segments of the upper and lower arches reciprocally for occlusion setting. (**q**) Treatment progress 3: Beta-titanium 0.017 × 0.025″ cantilever was used to procline upper incisors. Beta-titanium 0.017 × 0.025″ box loop was used to extrude 35 34 and 33 for occlusion setting. (**r**) Treatment progress 4: Beta-titanium 0.017 × 0.025″ cantilever was welded on the TMA 0.036″ transpalatal arch to move 27 by extrusion and palatal tipping. Beta-titanium 0.017 × 0.025″ box loop was used to derotate and extrude 14. (**s**) Treatment progress 5: Beta-titanium 0.017 × 0.025″ box loops were used to intrude 21 to level the gingival margin with 11 and derotate 42. Beta-titanium 0.017 × 0.025″ cantilever was extended from the miniscrew at 16 region to 11 distal to counteract the side effect of the box loop to the 13 to 11 segment. (**t**) Posttreatment photos

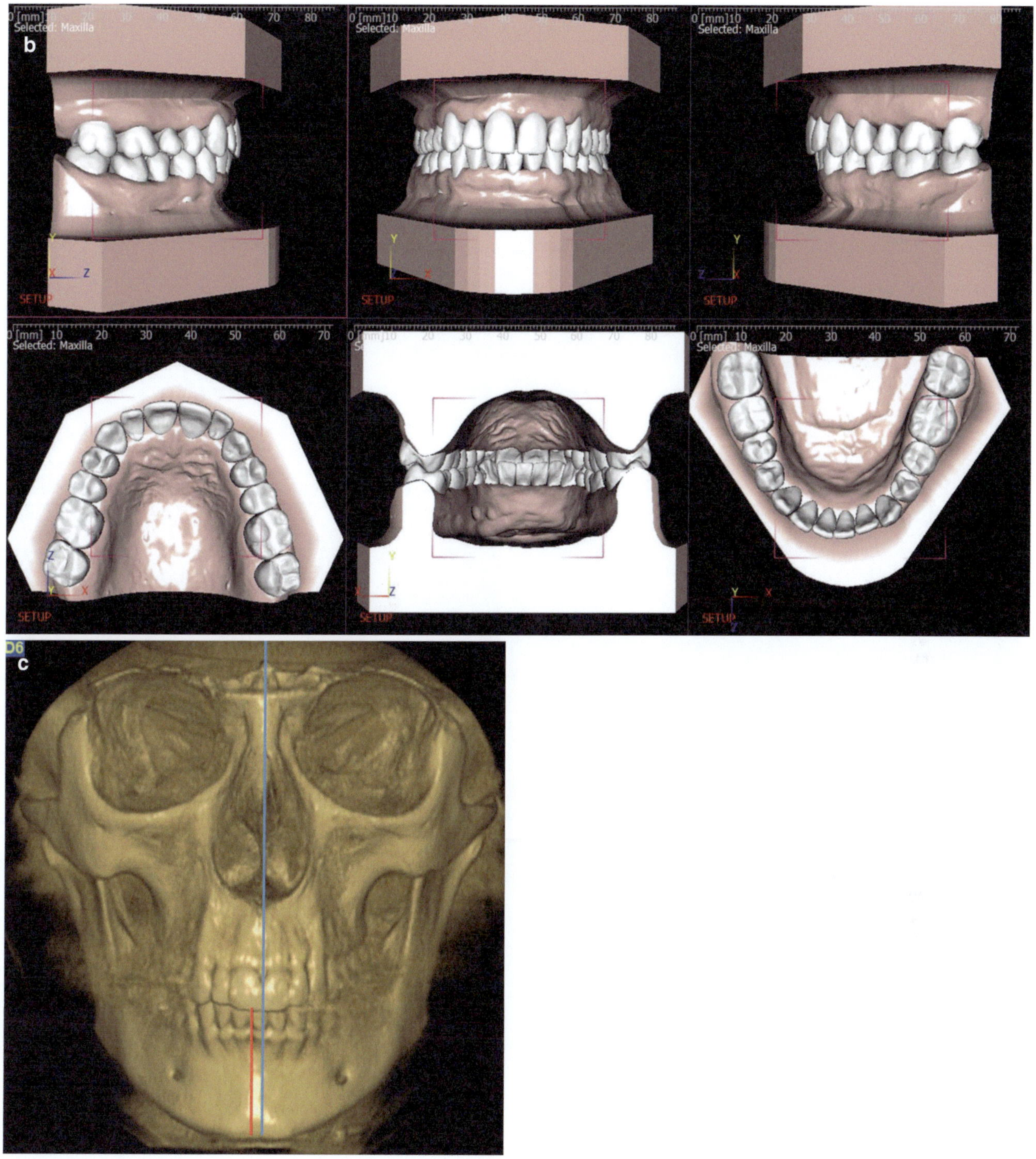

Fig. 9.6 (continued)

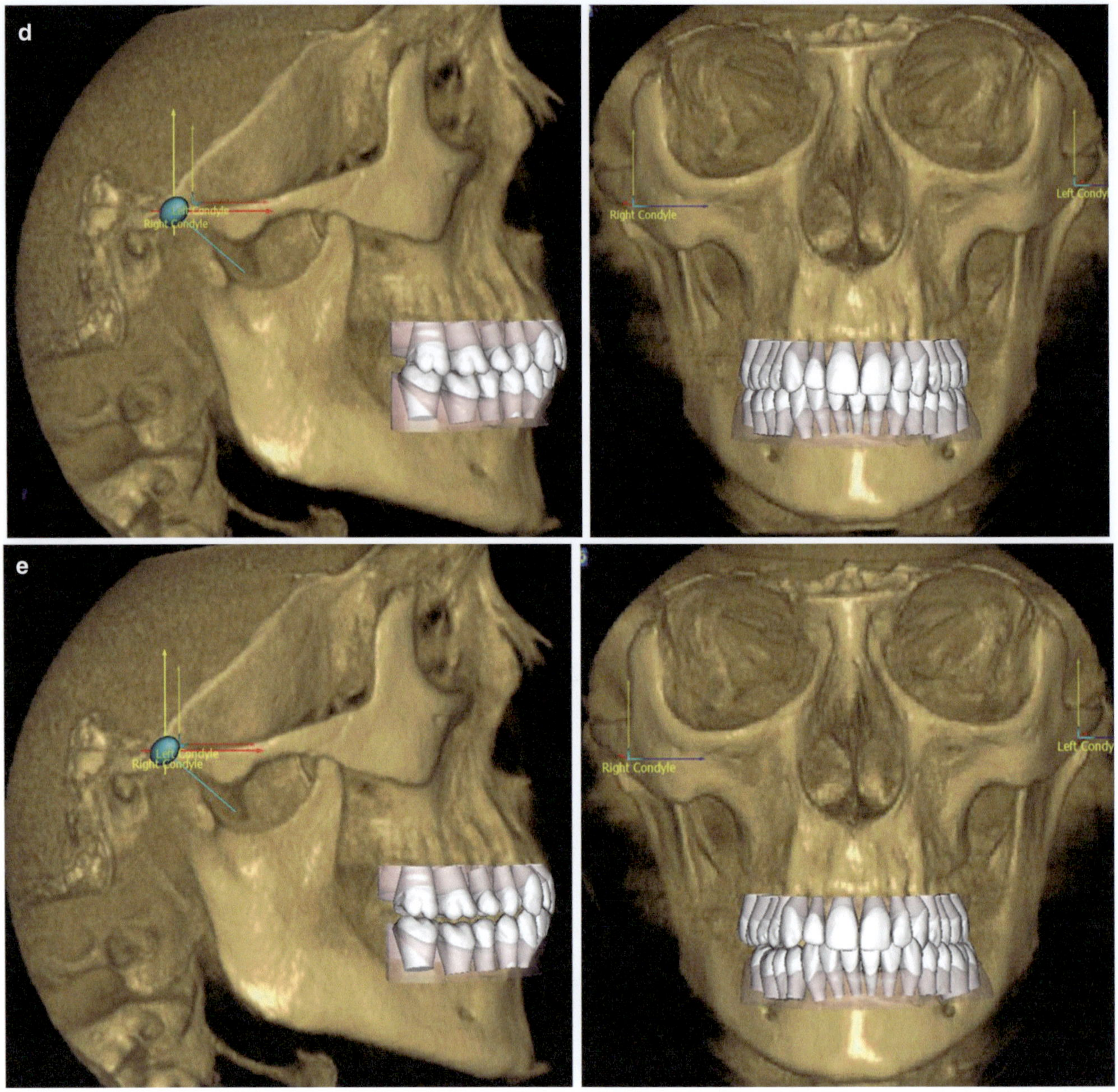

Fig. 9.6 (continued)

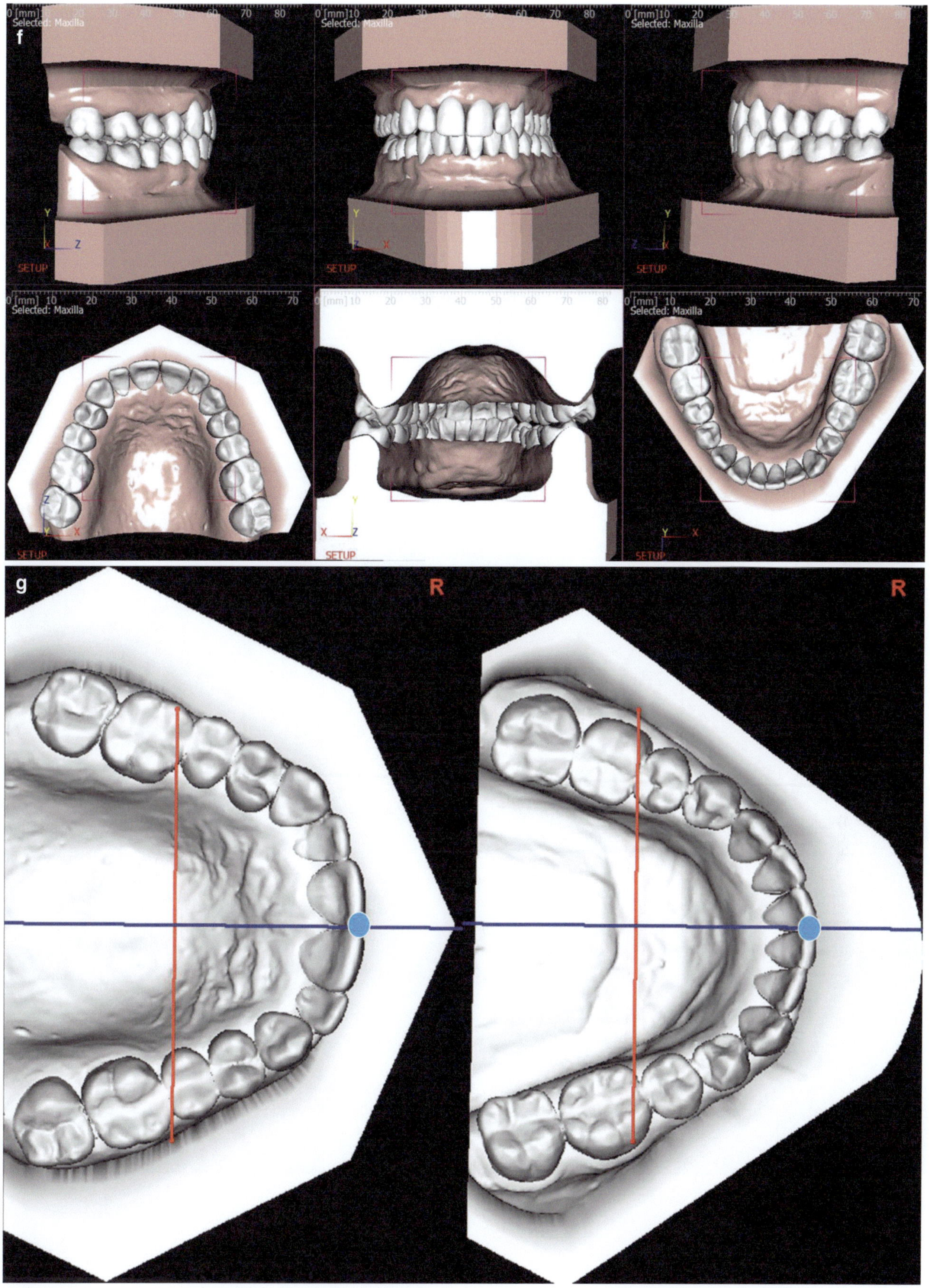

Fig. 9.6 (continued)

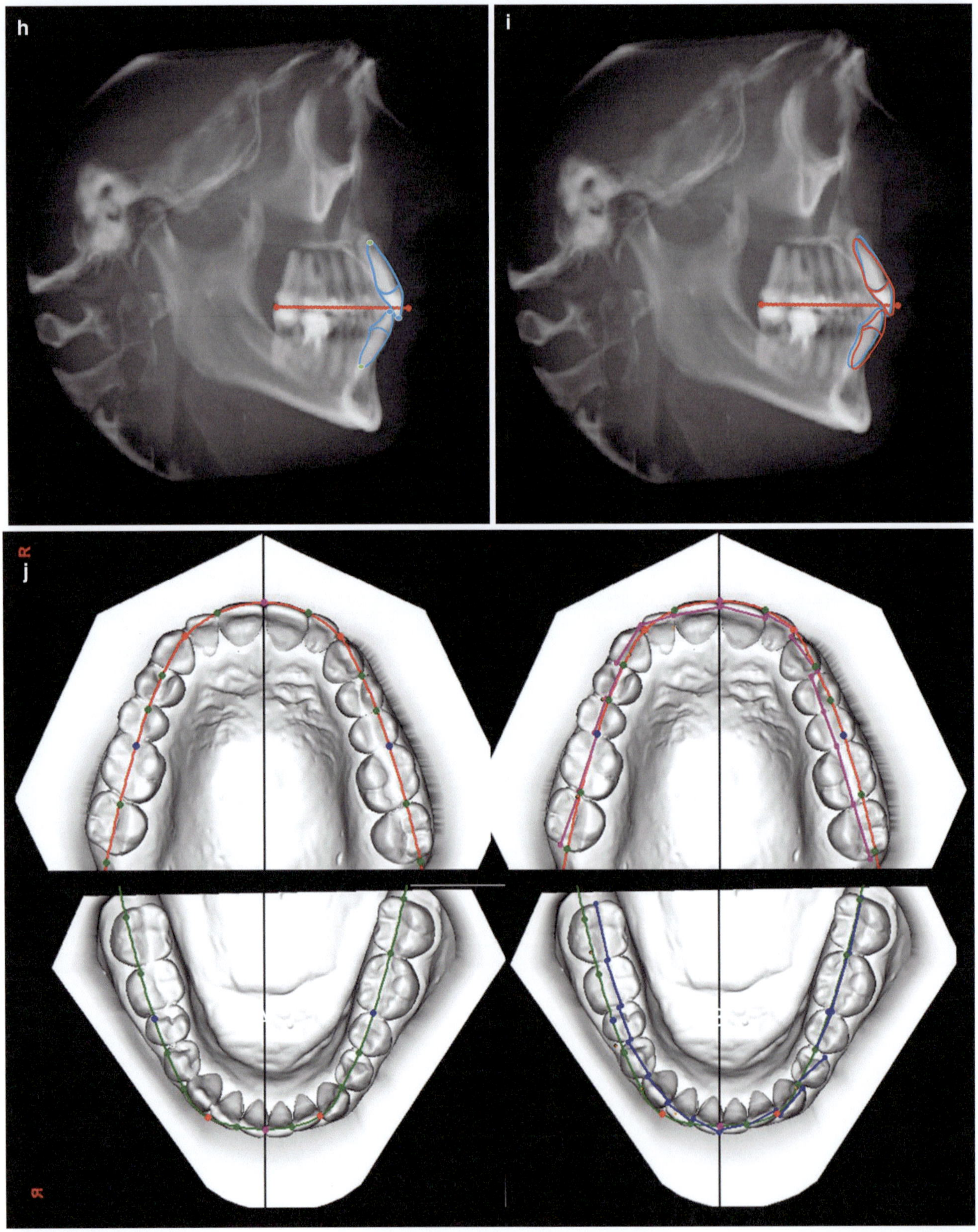

Fig. 9.6 (continued)

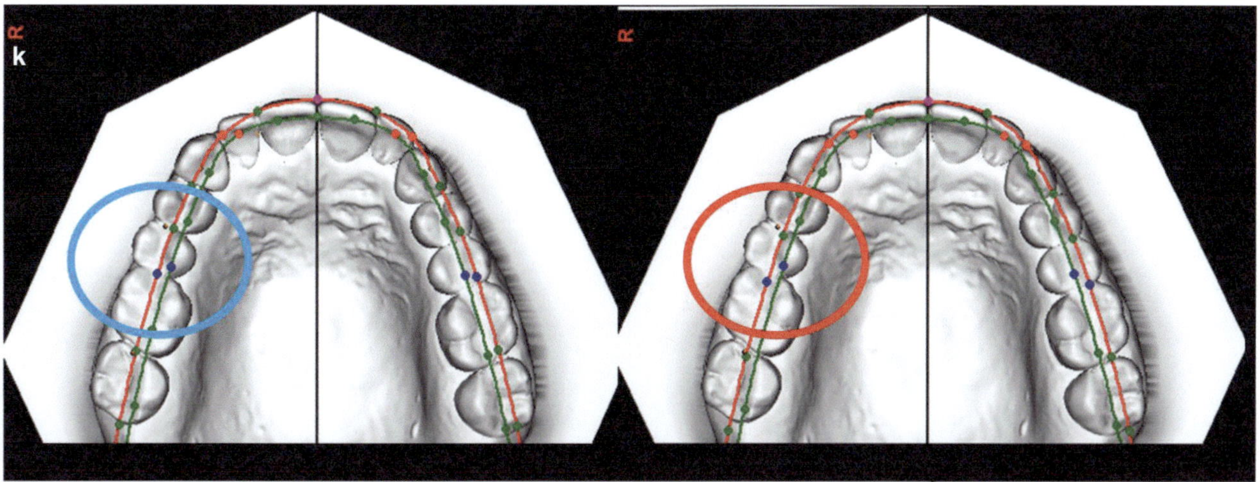

Measurements

	meas.	var.		meas.	var.		meas.	var.		meas.	var.
11	8,14	0	21	7,98	0	31	4,91	0	41	5,19	0
12	5,59	1	22	5,61	1	32	5,68	0	42	5,54	0
13	7,5	0	23	7,31	0	33	6,26	0	43	6,37	0
14	5,94	0	24	6,28	0	34	6,66	0	44	6,81	0
15	6,26	0	25	6,2	0	35	7,26	0	45	6,26	0
16	10,09	0	26	9,81	0	36	10,7	0	46	8,21	0
17	9,7	0	27	9,84	0	37	9,63	0	47	9,94	0
18	0	0	28	0	0	38	0	0	48	0	0

Bolton Index

- TBI: 92,1% increase mesio-distal size of upper teeth 0,7mm or reduce mesio-distal size of lower teeth 0,7mm
- ABI: 80,6% increase mesio-distal size of upper teeth 1,8mm or reduce mesio-distal size of lower teeth 1,4mm

Transversal Dimensions

- Upper Interpremolar distance(4-4): 35,7mm

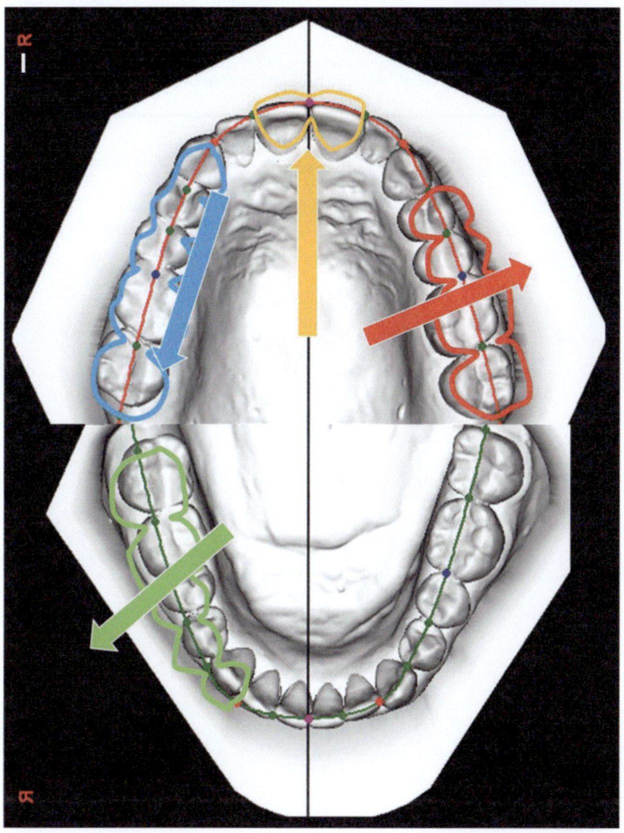

Fig. 9.6 (continued)

m

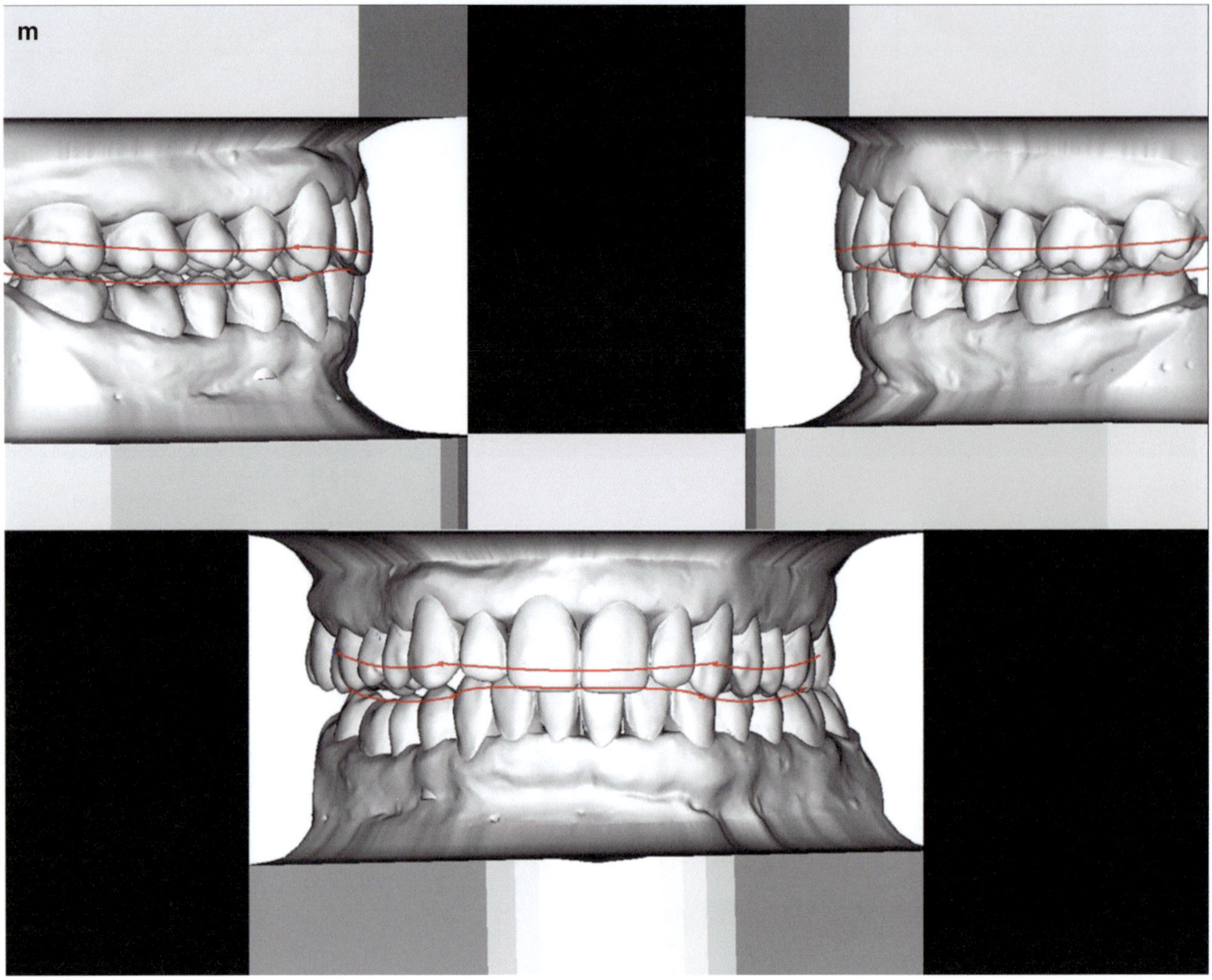

Fig. 9.6 (continued)

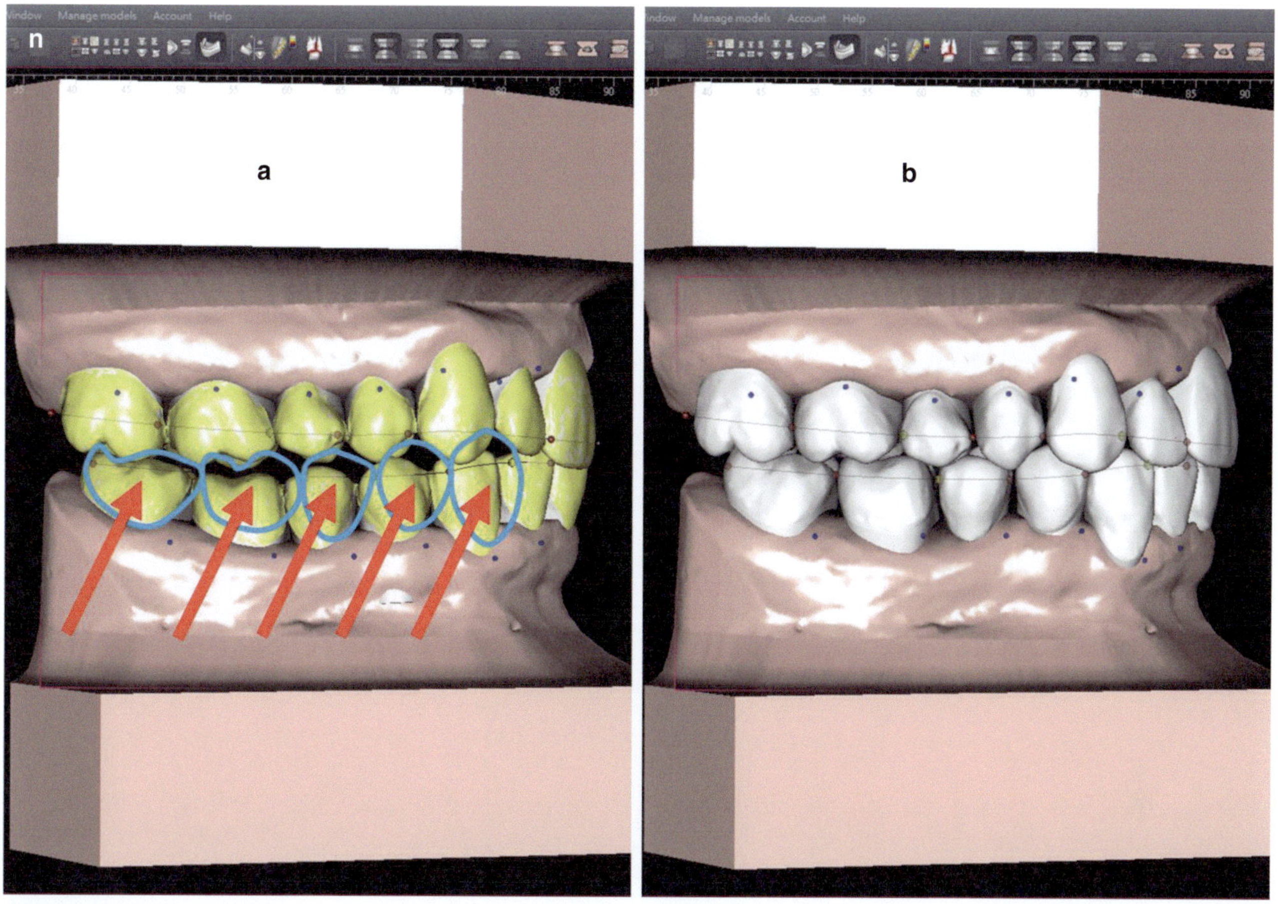

Fig. 9.6 (continued)

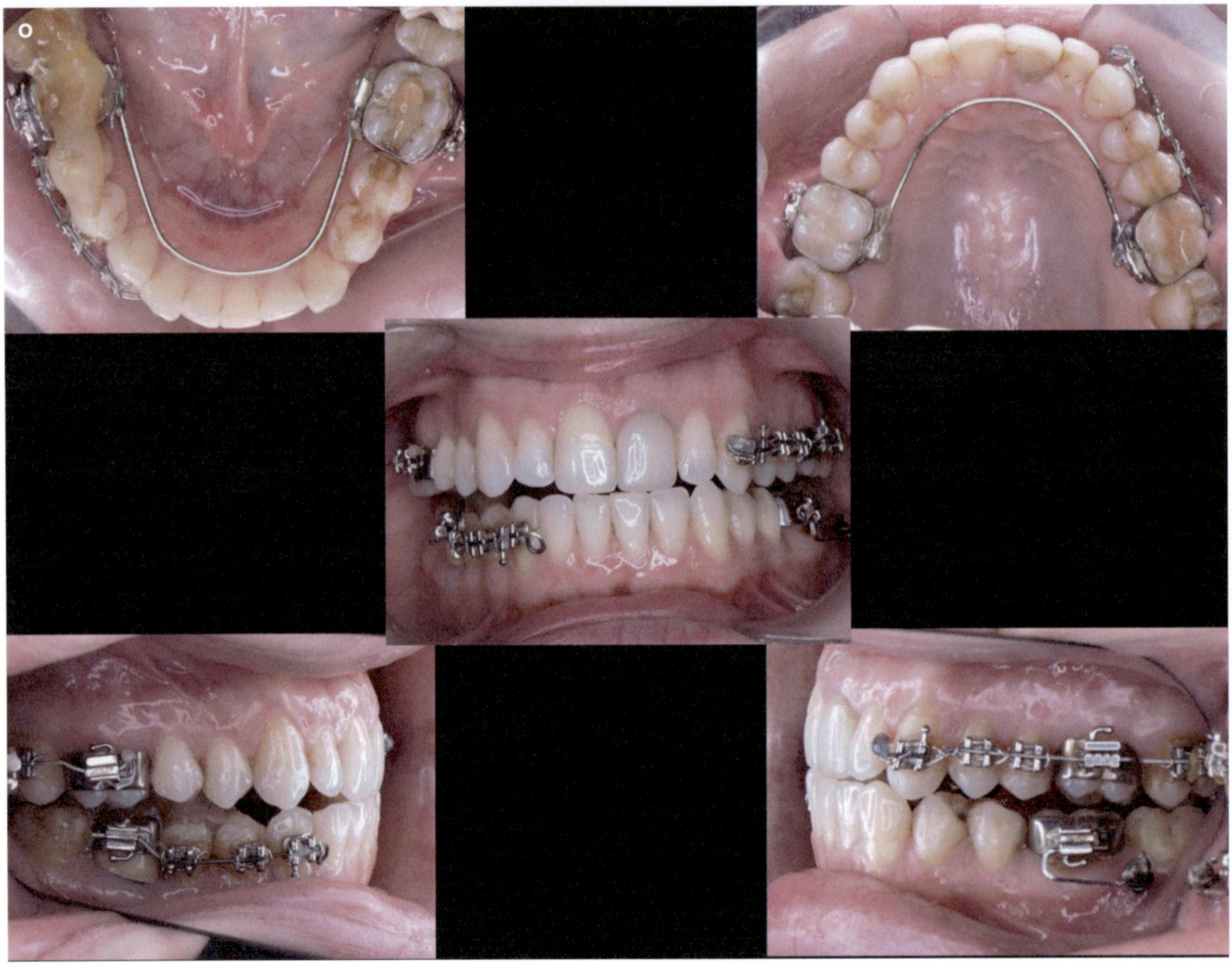

Fig. 9.6 (continued)

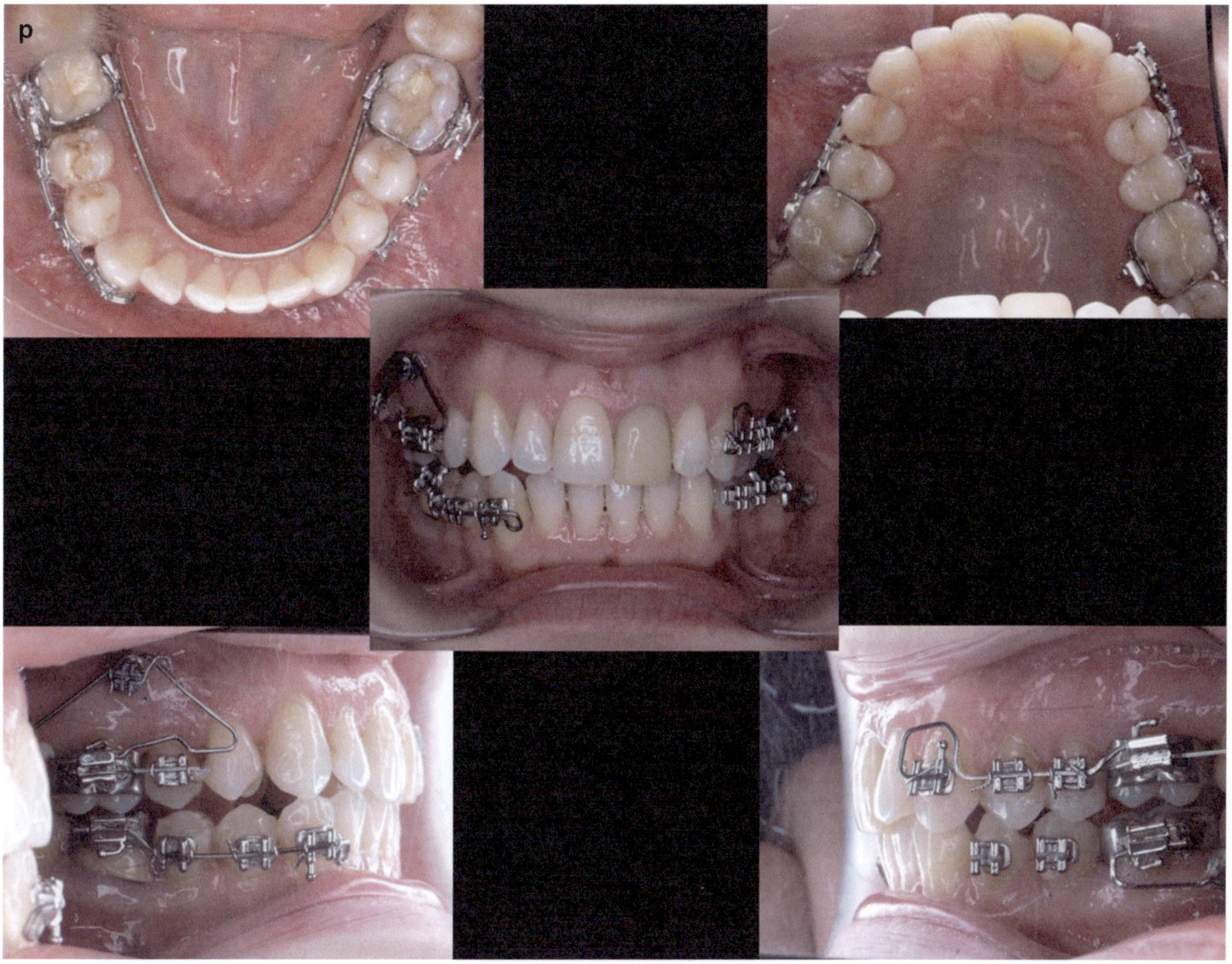

Fig. 9.6 (continued)

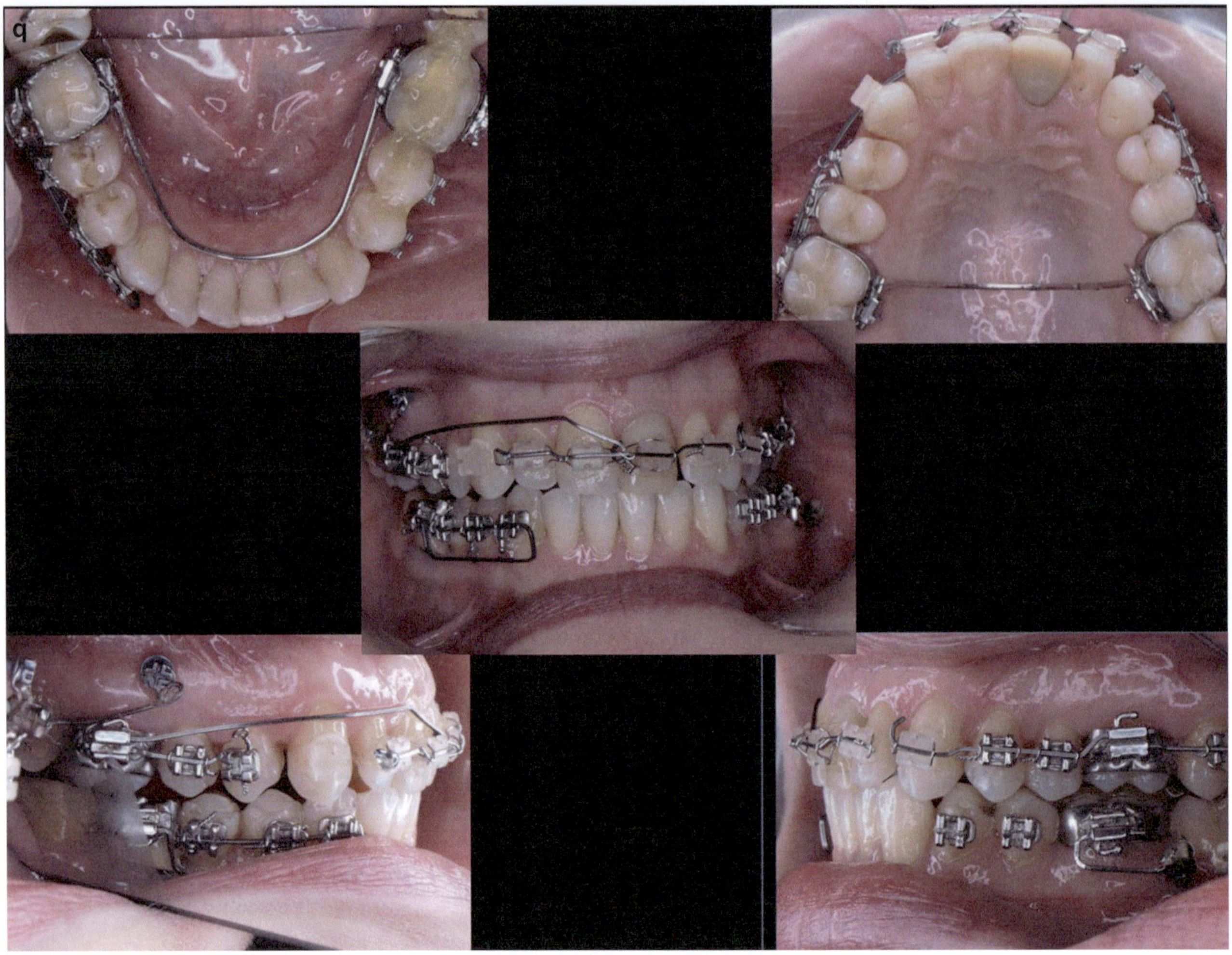

Fig. 9.6 (continued)

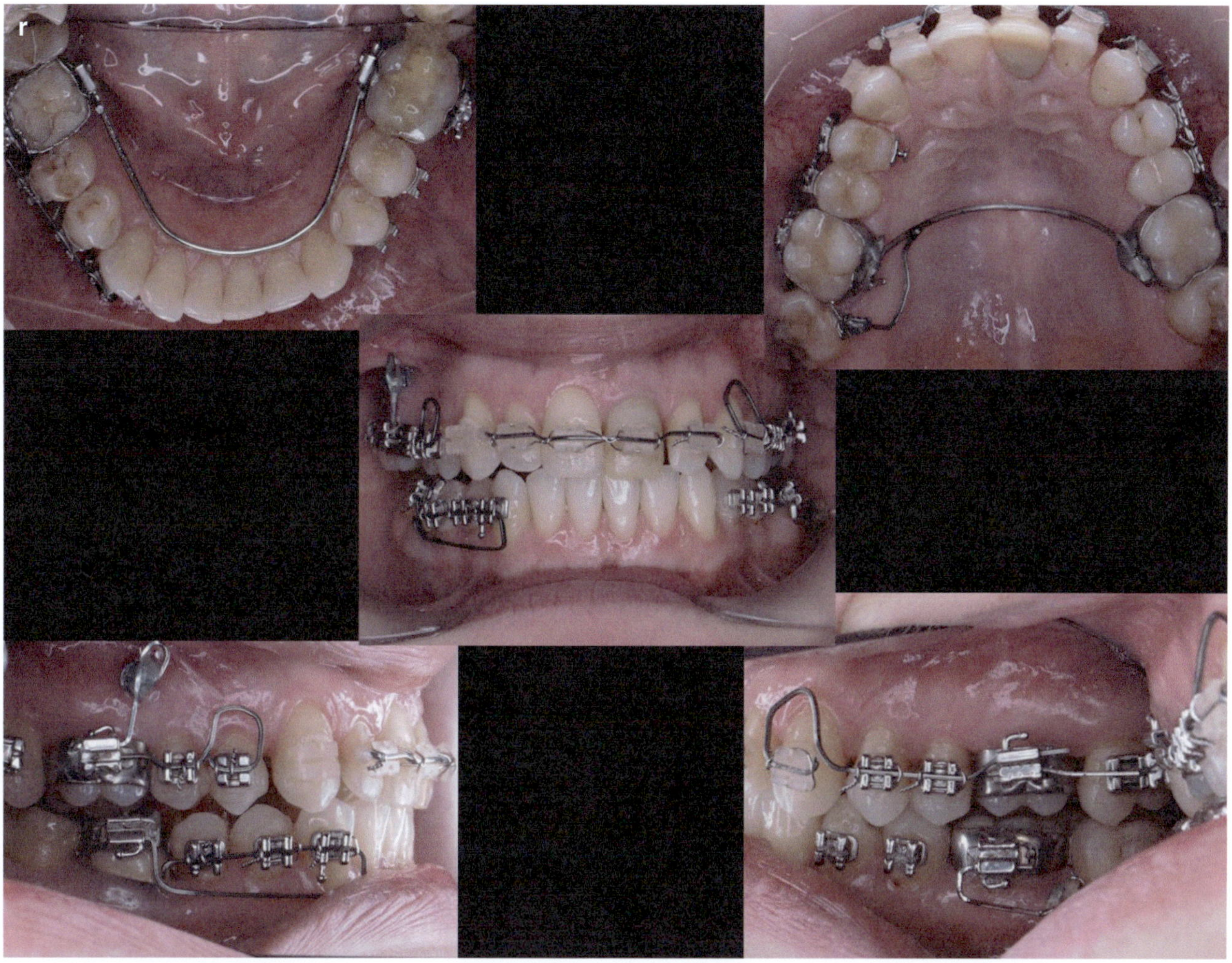

Fig. 9.6 (continued)

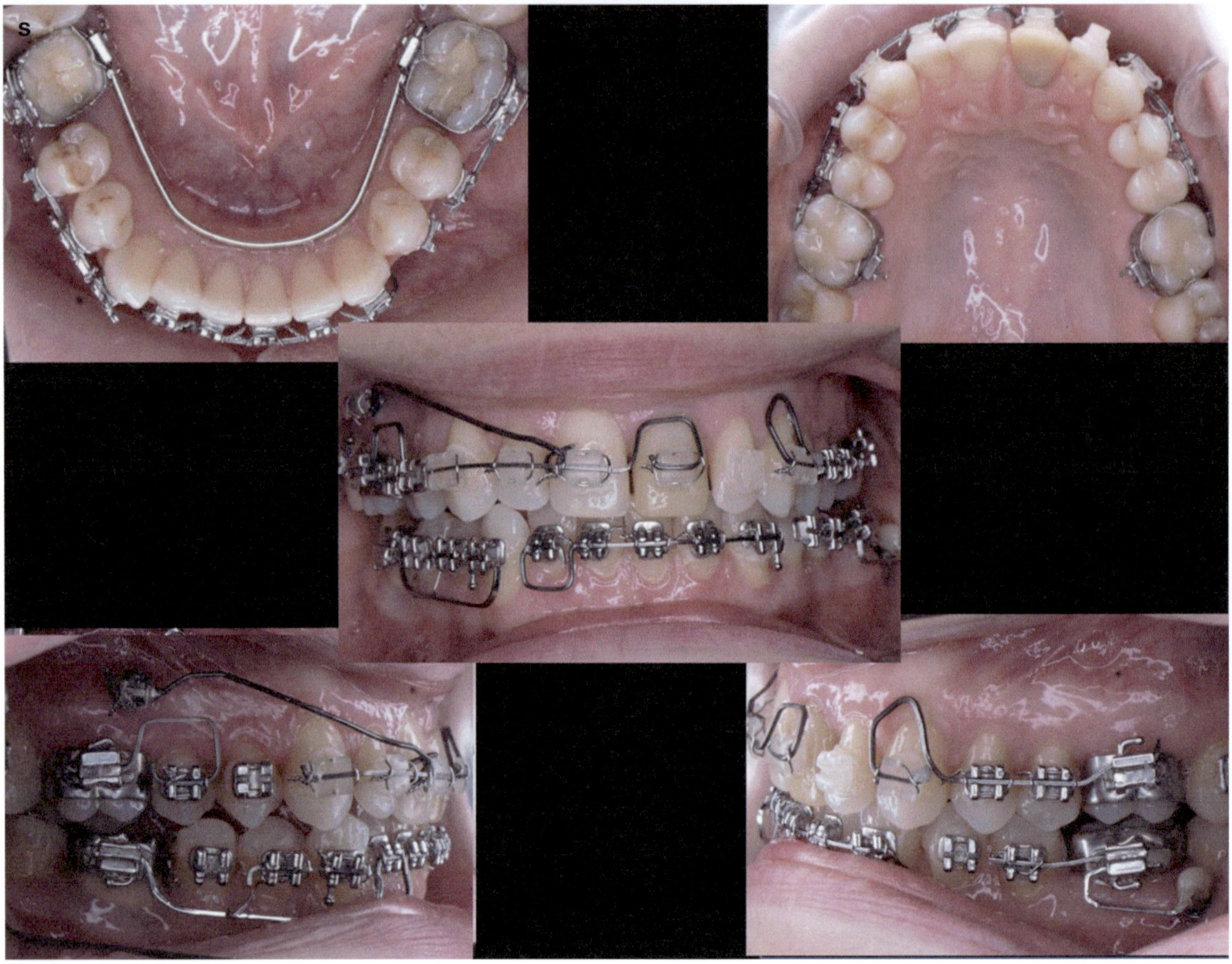

Fig. 9.6 (continued)

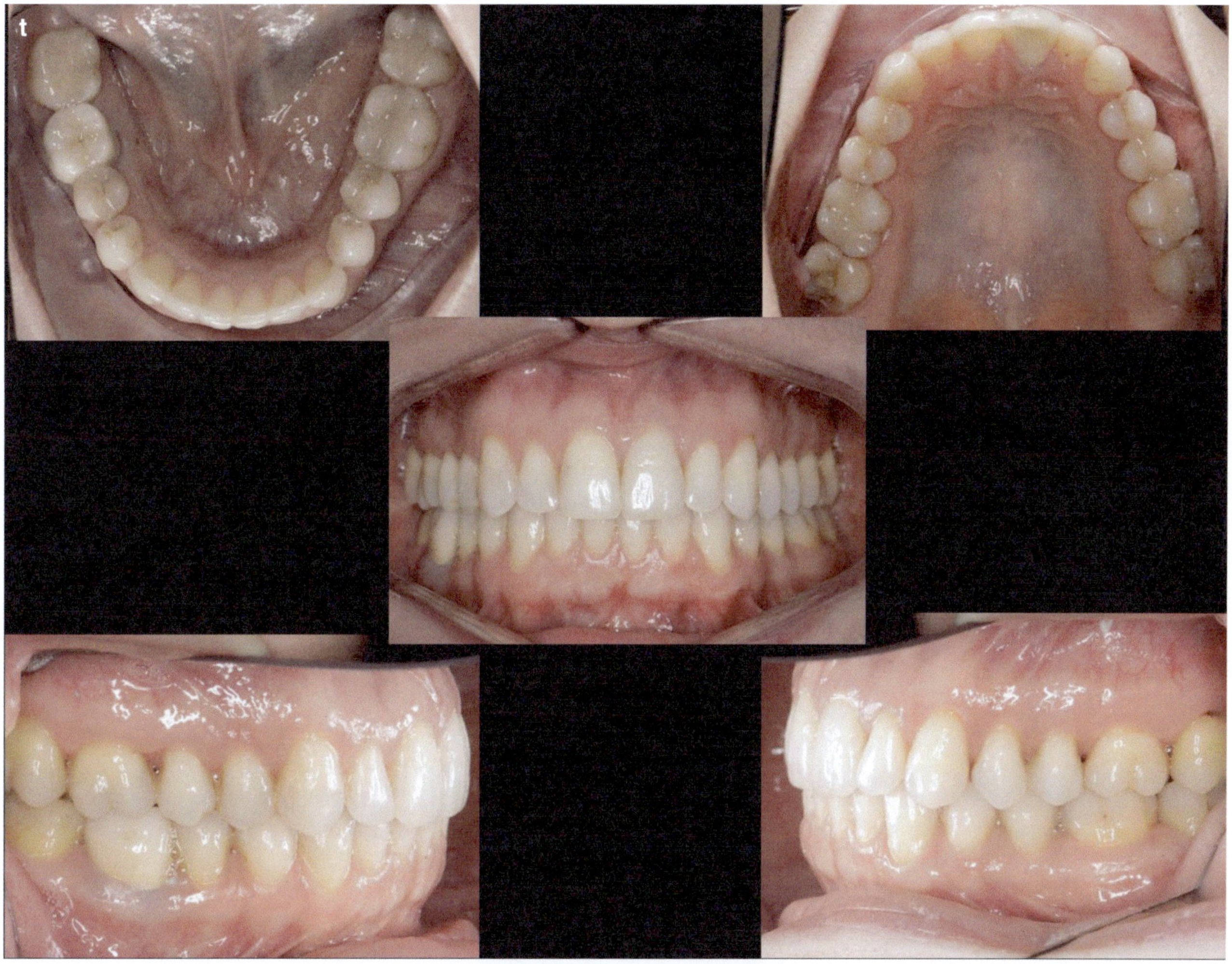

Fig. 9.6 (continued)

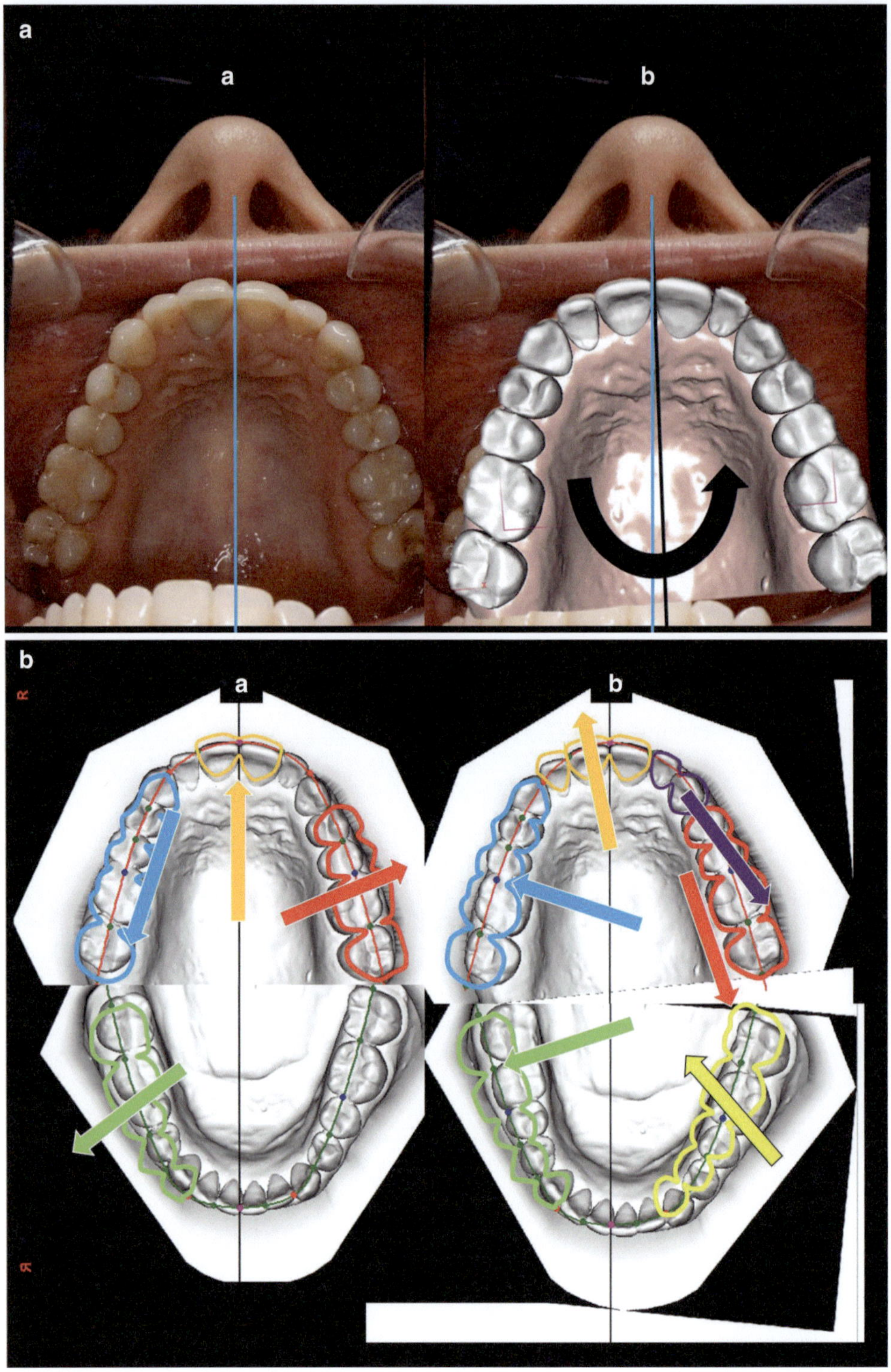

Fig. 9.7 Case AA: Significance of defining the symmetry axis. (**a**) Photos taken from submental region to show the relationship of the maxilla to the face. (A) The original case AA with facial midline coincides with the dental midline anteriorly and the symmetry is aligned along the median raphe of the palate. (B) The same case with a simulated counterclockwise yaw rotation of the maxilla with the facial midline coincides with the dental midline anteriorly, and the symmetry axis is in an angle with the median raphe. (**b**) 2D occlusograms. (A) Original symmetry axis. Movement of individual tooth segments as shown on Fig. 9.6k. (B) Alternate symmetry axis to camouflage yaw rotation of maxilla as shown on (**a**). Lines of force that produce the objective tooth segment movements are indicated by arrows in colors, representing the respective segments. Movement of individual segments are completely different compared to A and are likely to violate biological limits especially on quadrant 4. Based on the treatment simulation of two different options, the clinician can decide to accept the yaw rotation or consider orthognathic surgery

ment. Sometimes, the dental movement must go further to compensate for the existing basal discrepancy to improve stability and function. There is a much narrower margin of error of the force system which the orthodontic appliance can deliver in these two groups of patients. It is because they are lacking favorable growth, normal oral function, and bone support to overwhelm the side effects which can be produced by the nonspecific force system generated by the straight wire mechanics. Therefore, clearly defined treatment objectives on the VTO and the occlusogram are beneficial to the design of the appropriate treatment mechanics which deliver the correct force system to the active unit and prevent anchorage loss of the reactive unit. Straight wire appliance and clear aligners with special treatment sequences, application of TADs, or even customized segmented arch appliances are needed to reduce round tripping and other complications, improve treatment efficiency, and achieve good results (Fig. 9.8).

For growing patients, their dentofacial development and oral function make errors of the force systems delivered more forgiving. However, there are issues which have to be considered during treatment planning, for example, extraction vs non-extraction, space closure vs tooth replacement in fixed appliance therapy. Furthermore, the clinicians have to assess the treatment outcome of growth modification with favorable growth and good compliance and prepare the con-

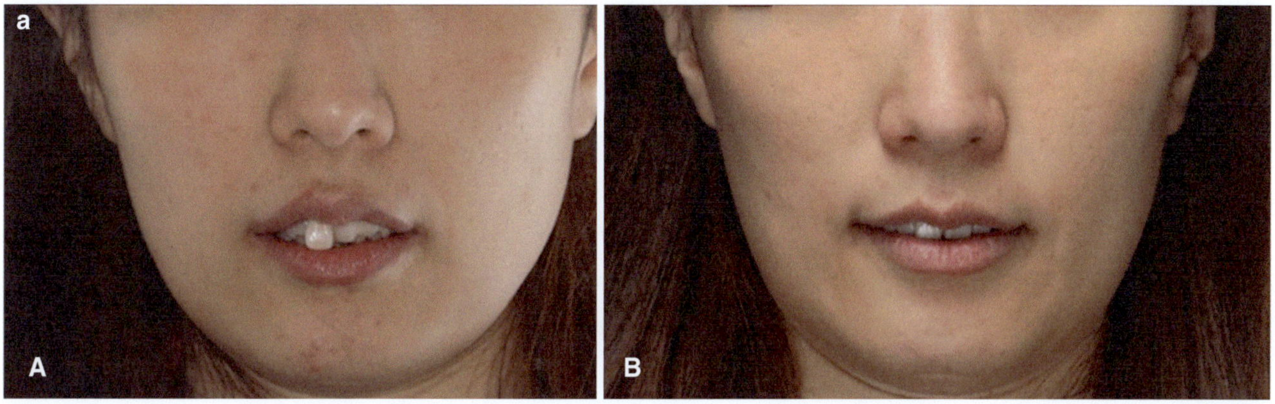

Fig. 9.8 Case LS treated by Dr. Franklin She: A case with pathologically migrated incisors due to periodontal disease. (**a**) Frontal facial photos. (A) Pretreatment. (B) Posttreatment. (**b**) Three-quarter smile photos. (A) Pretreatment. (B) Posttreatment. (**c**) Pretreatment virtual dental models on DDP-Ortho. (**d**) Sectioning of upper model at middle of 11 on sagittal plane to study the inter-incisal relationship. (**e**) 21 was planned to retract 7 mm and intrude 2 mm. After subtracting the width of 24 for extraction, occlusogram indicates moderate anchorage need on closing space at 16 and 24 regions. (**f**) Lower incisors are planned for proclination of 2 mm and intrusion of 2 mm with extraction of 32 to relieve crowding. Objective position of 36 (yellow). Distal buccal derotation of 36 is indicated with the center of rotation located at its mesial contact point (black dotted circle). (**g**) Use of a software Dental Movement Analyzer (IOSS, GmbH) to calculate the line of force to intrude 11 to the objective position. A three-piece intrusion and retraction arch was used to produce the planned line of force. (**h**) Ideal virtual setup based on 3D occlusogram shows clearly that after extraction of 32, sequential intrusion of 31, 33, 41, 42, and 43 are required as they present with different level of extrusion. Pretreatment position (yellow). Objective tooth position (white). Sequence of intrusion (A) 31, 41, and 42 (red arrows), (B) 33, 31, and 43 (blue arrows), (C) 43 (green arrow). (**i**) Pretreatment photos. Aggressive periodontitis was treated and monitored by Dr. Siu Keung Kenny, Tong. (**j**) Treatment progress 1: Upper arch: Beta-titanium 0.017 × 0.025″ T loops were used to close space at 16 and 24 region. Ligature wires were used to tip incisors distal during space closure. Lower arch: Beta-titanium 0.017 × 0.025″ three-pieces intrusion and retraction arch was used for proclination and intrusion of lower incisors. A passive stainless steel 0.036″ lingual arch and a stainless steel 0.019 × 0.025″ archwire were used to splint lower premolars and first molars together as an anchorage unit. (**k**) Treatment progress 2: Upper arch: Beta-titanium 0.017 × 0.025″ three-pieces intrusion and retraction arch was used to intrude and retract 11. Lower arch: Beta-titanium 0.018″ archwire was used to hold the position of 41 and 42. Beta-titanium 0.017 × 0.025″ box loop was used to intrude 31. A beta-titanium 0.017 × 0.025″ archwire was connected with two orthodontic miniscrews (68.99.28A) (The Aarhus System, American Orthodontics) at 33 and 43 regions. It served as anchorage to intrude 33 and 43. Another Aarhus screw was used to fix the position of 36 with stainless steel 0.019 × 0.025″ archwire and a beta-titanium 0.036″ lingual arch was used to derotate 46. (**l**) Treatment progress 3: Upper arch: Intrusion and retraction of 11 was in progress. Lower arch: 32 and 43 were leveled. 46 was derotated and was fixed by an Aarhus screw at 46 region. The beta-titanium 0.036″ lingual arch which was fixed by Aarhus screws at 36 and 46 regions and was used as an anchorage to further intrude 33 on the lingual side. The labial wire which was fixed by Aarhus screws at 33 and 43 regions were to be used as an anchorage to further intrude 33 on the labial side. (**m**) Treatment progress 4: Upper arch: Intrusion and retraction of 11 were completed. Lower arch: Lower incisors and canines intrusion were completed. A super-elastic nickel-titanium 0.017 × 0.025″ archwire was inserted for the alignment of lower teeth. (**n**) Treatment progress 5: Upper arch: Bracket of 11 was rebonded to the normal position. A stainless steel 0.019 × 0.025″ archwire was inserted. Closure of anterior spaces were done by bonding lingual buttons on 13–23 and powerchains. The line of force of space closure is closer to center of resistance which reduced friction. A stainless steel 0.019 × 0.025″ archwire was inserted on lower arch, and sliding mechanics was performed to close residual spaces. (**o**) Treatment progress 6: Upper arch, upper incisors and canines were cemented by a cobalt-chromium cast splint with extensions to direct the line of space closure force at the level of center of resistance of teeth with reduced bone support. Reciprocal anchorage was used for space closure as planned. (**p**) Posttreatment photos. Treatment was terminated before complete space closure due to periodontal flare-up. Periodontal condition was stabilized after debonding

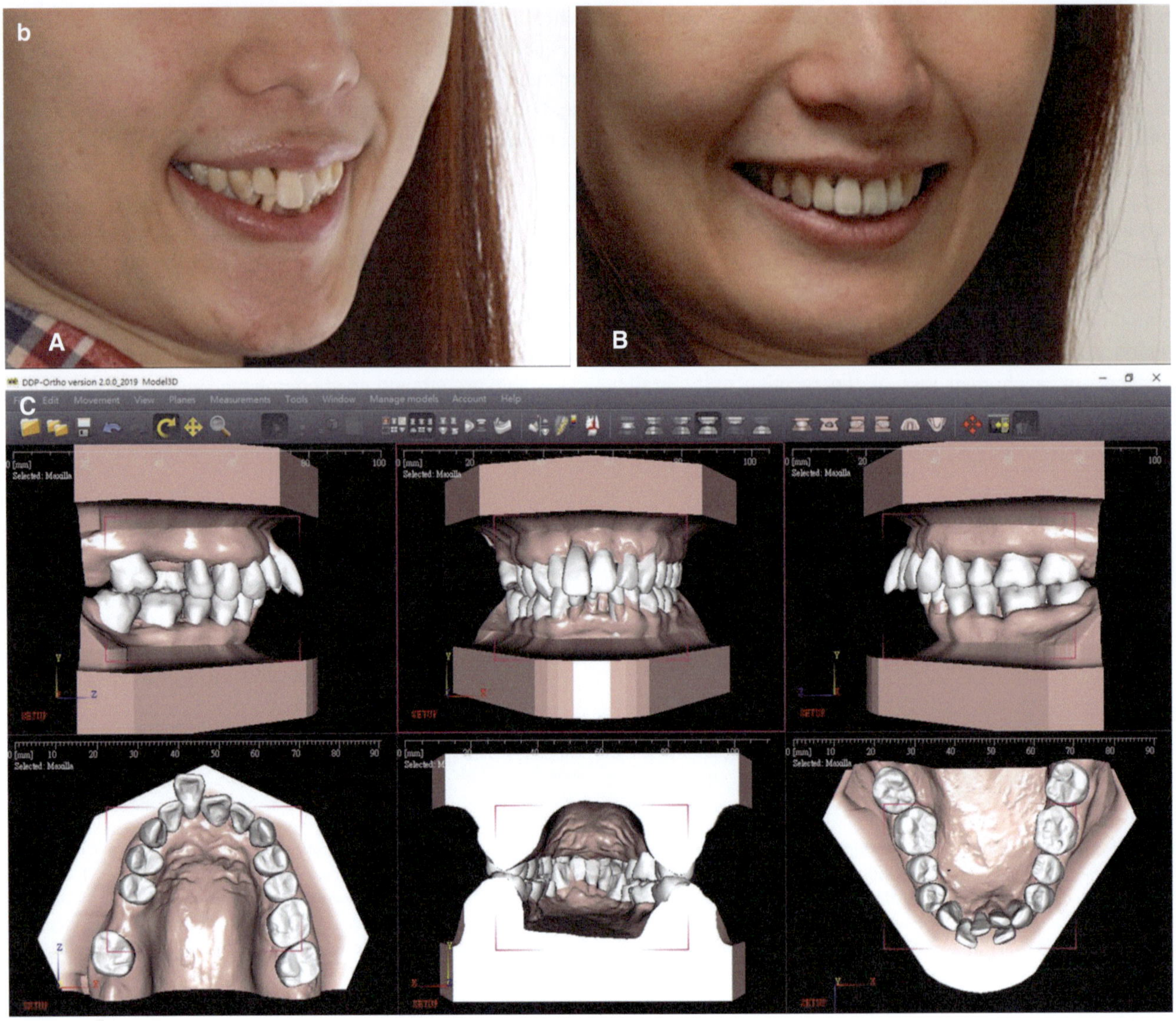

Fig. 9.8 (continued)

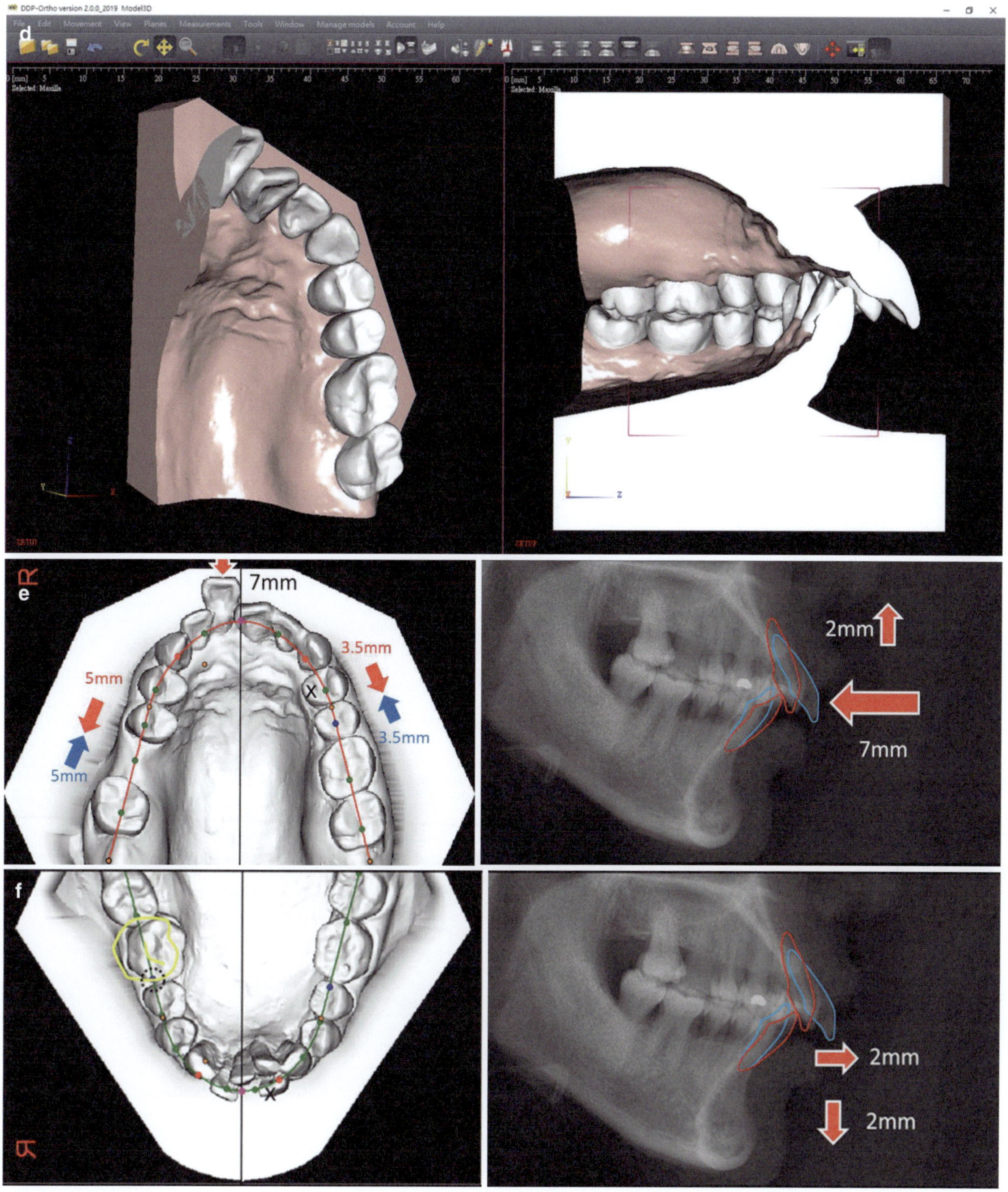

Fig. 9.8 (continued)

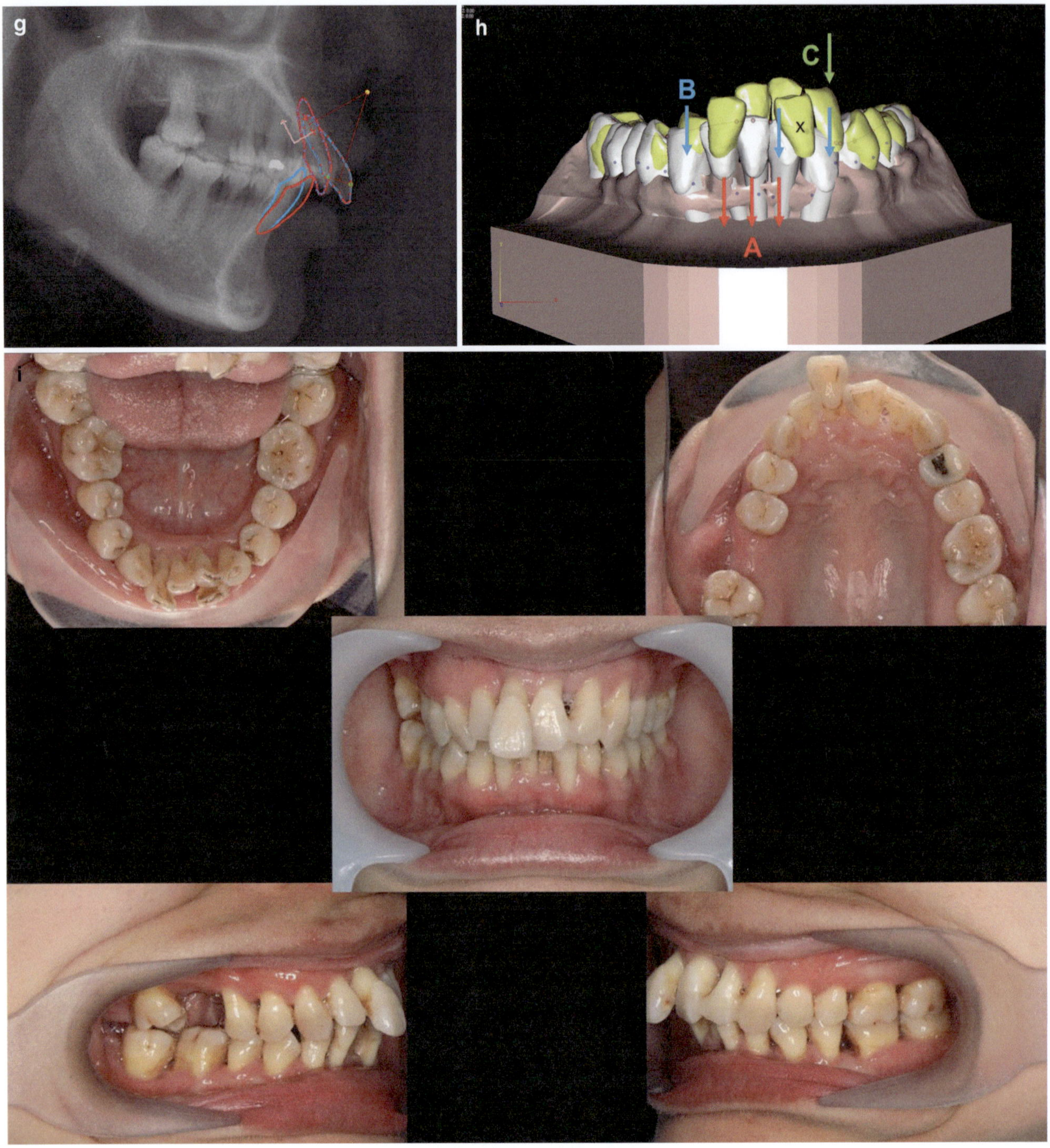

Fig. 9.8 (continued)

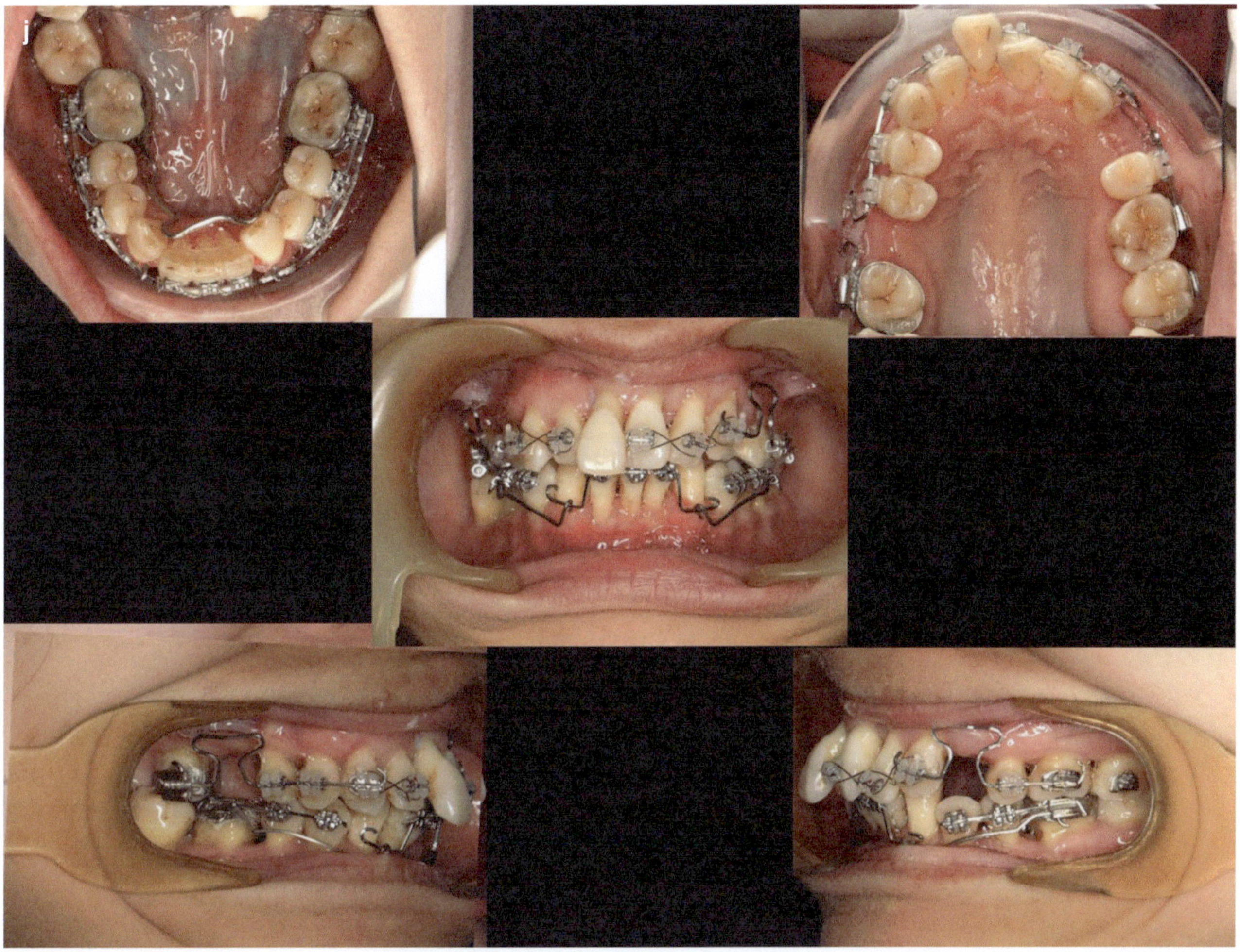

Fig. 9.8 (continued)

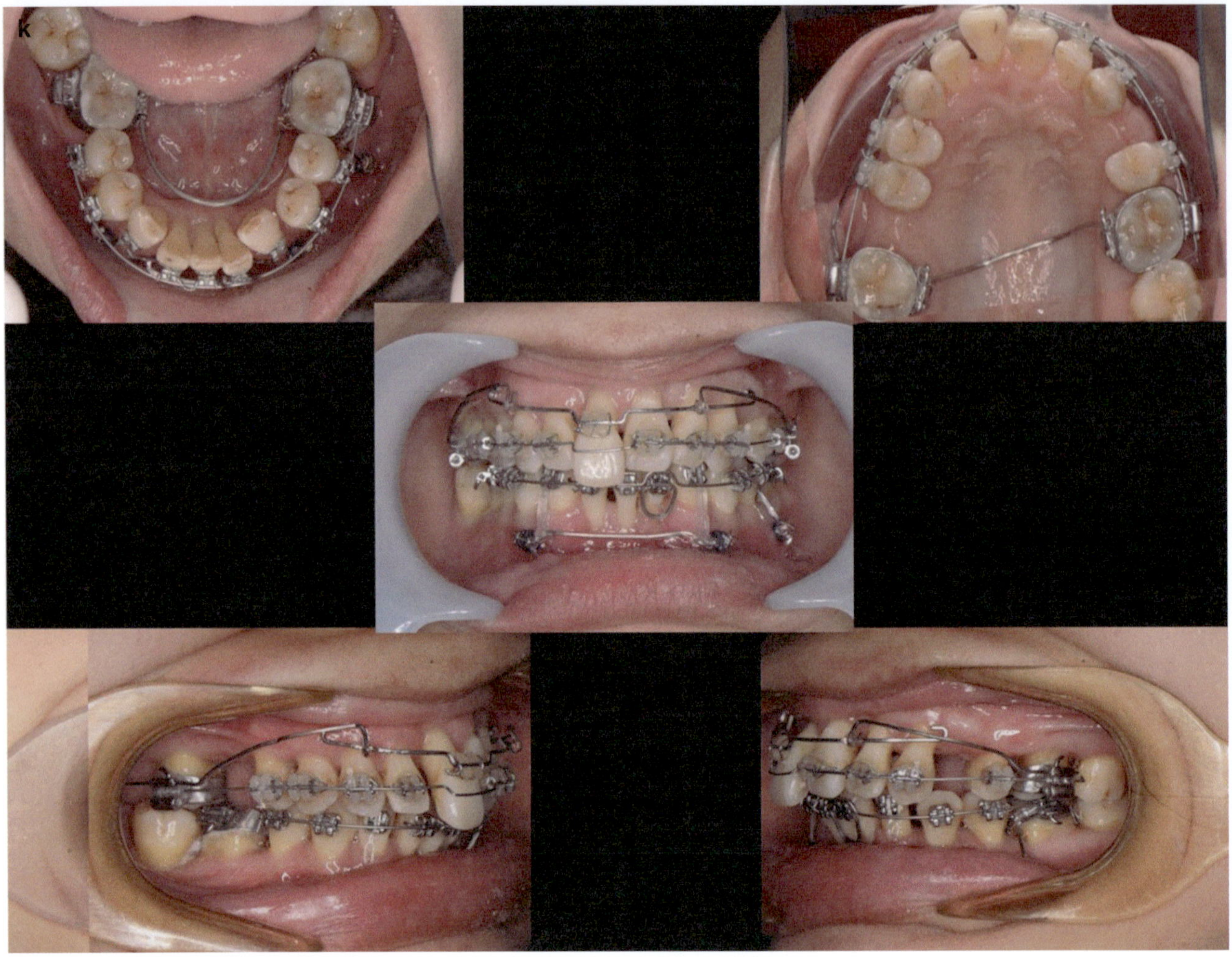

Fig. 9.8 (continued)

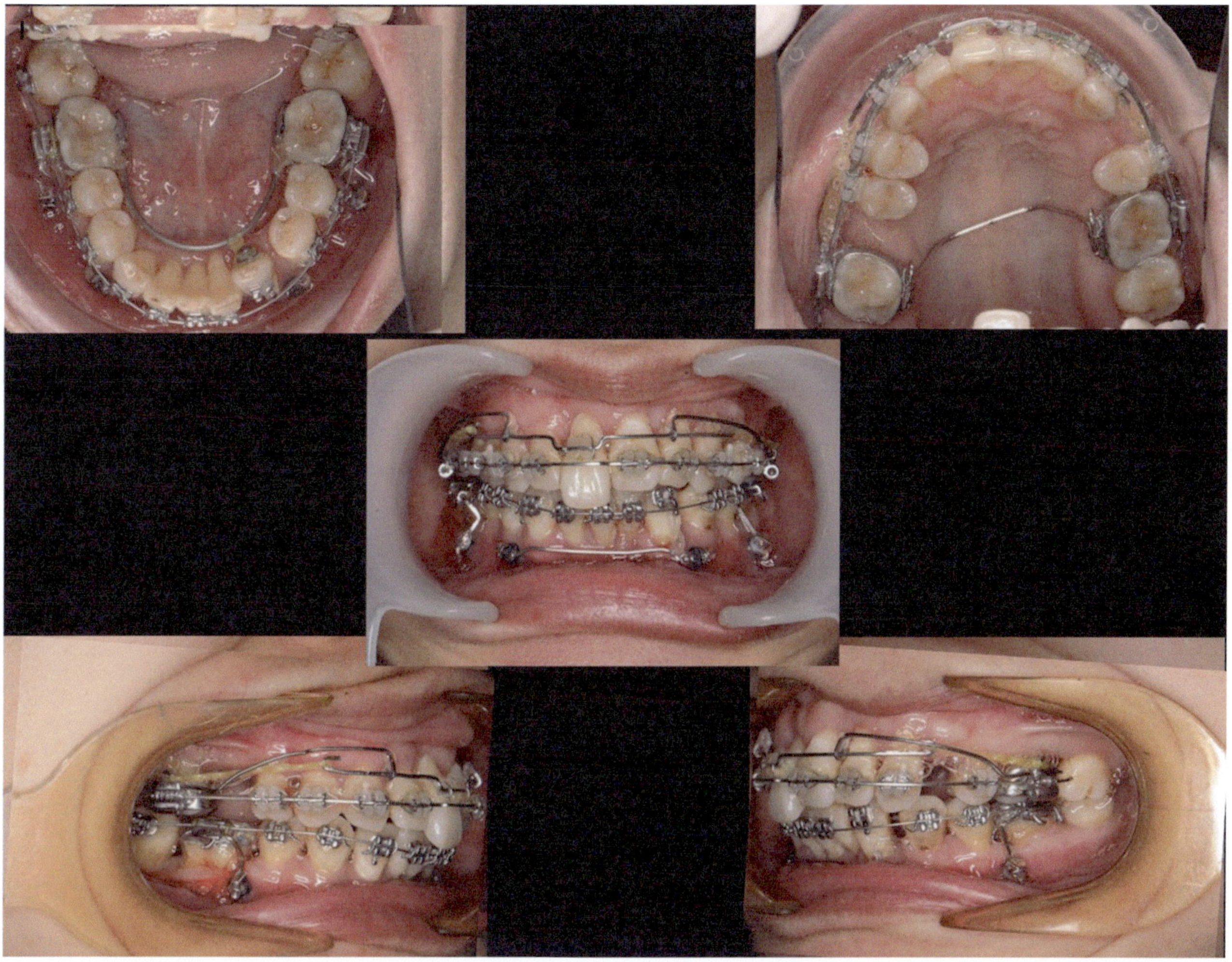

Fig. 9.8 (continued)

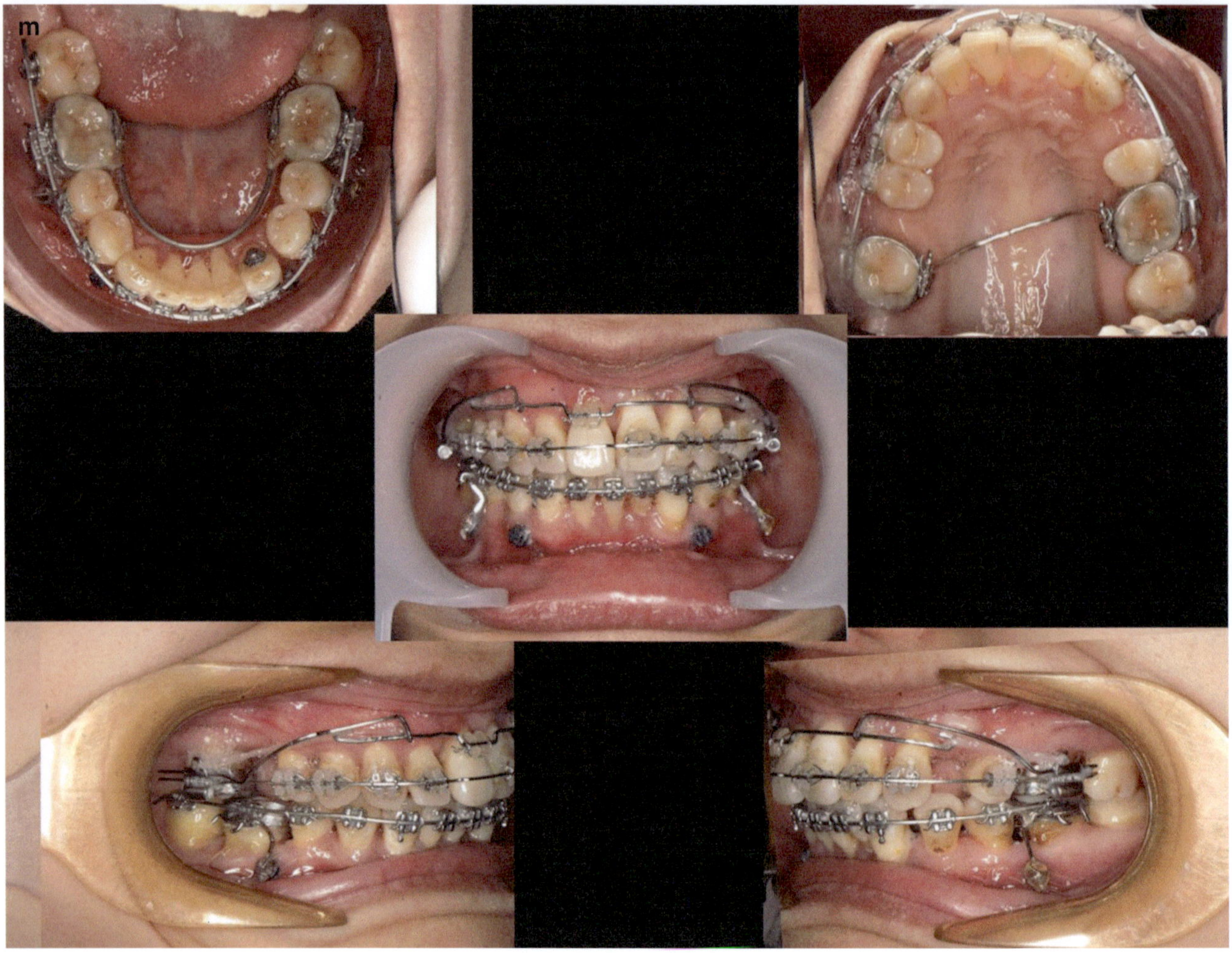

Fig. 9.8 (continued)

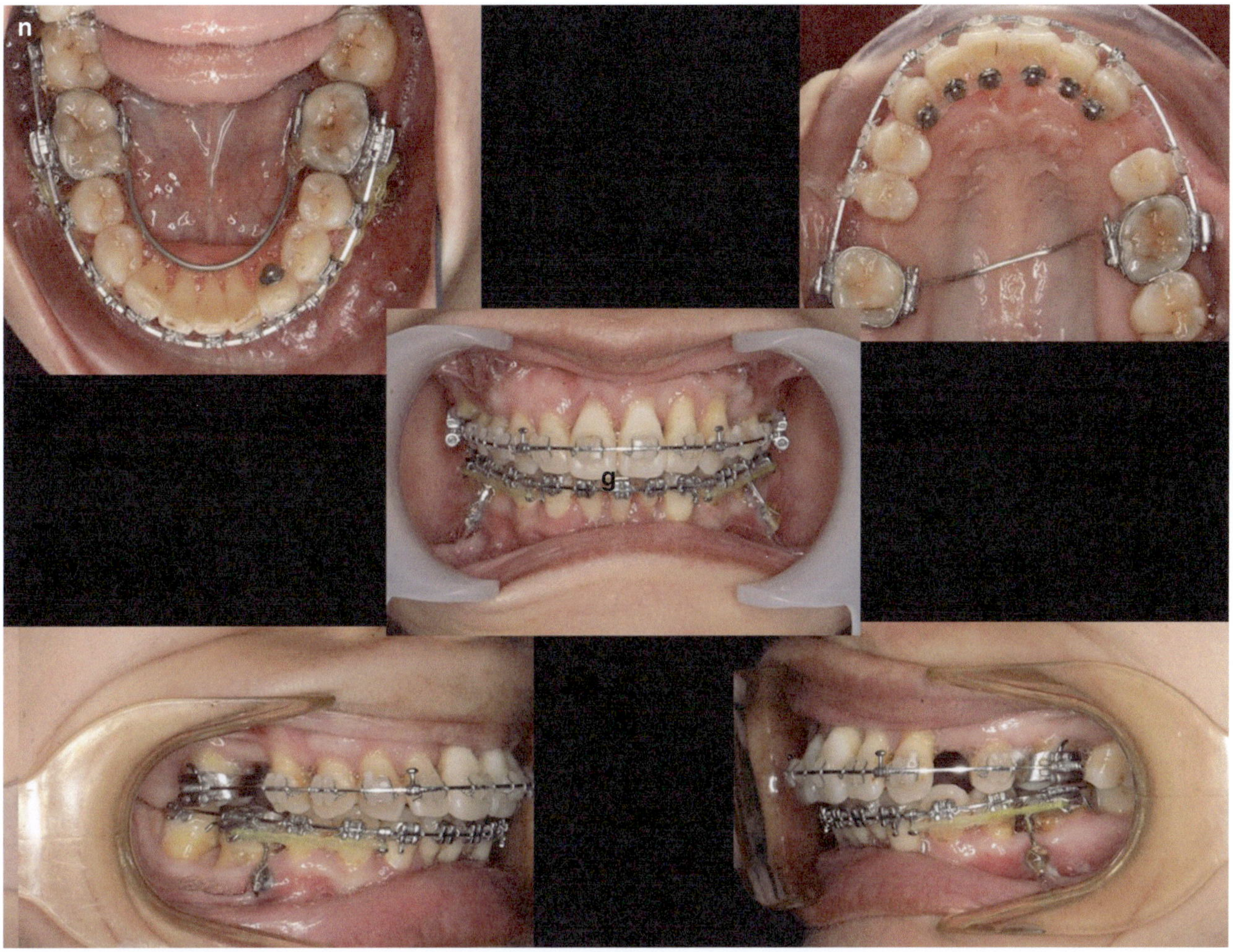

Fig. 9.8 (continued)

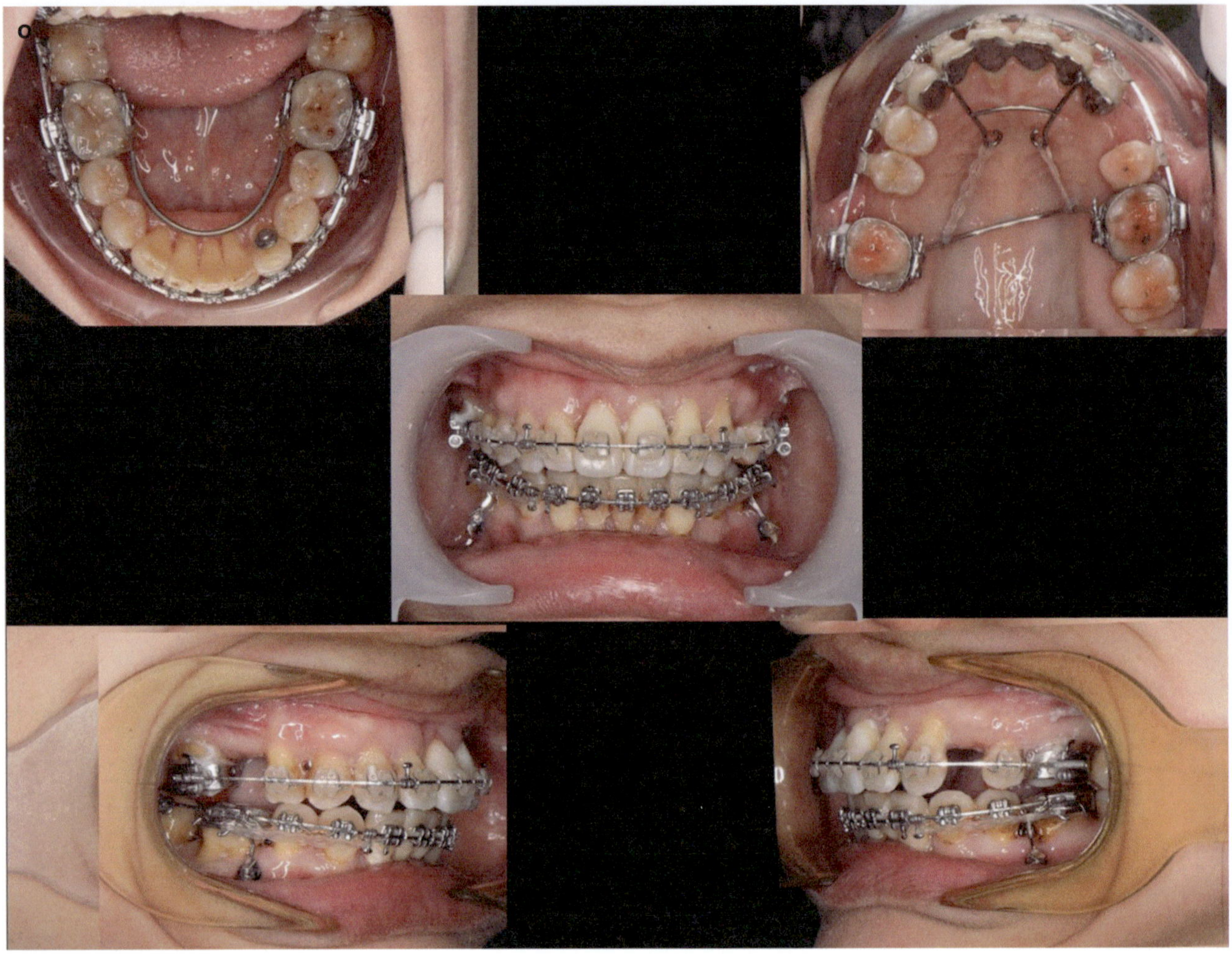

Fig. 9.8 (continued)

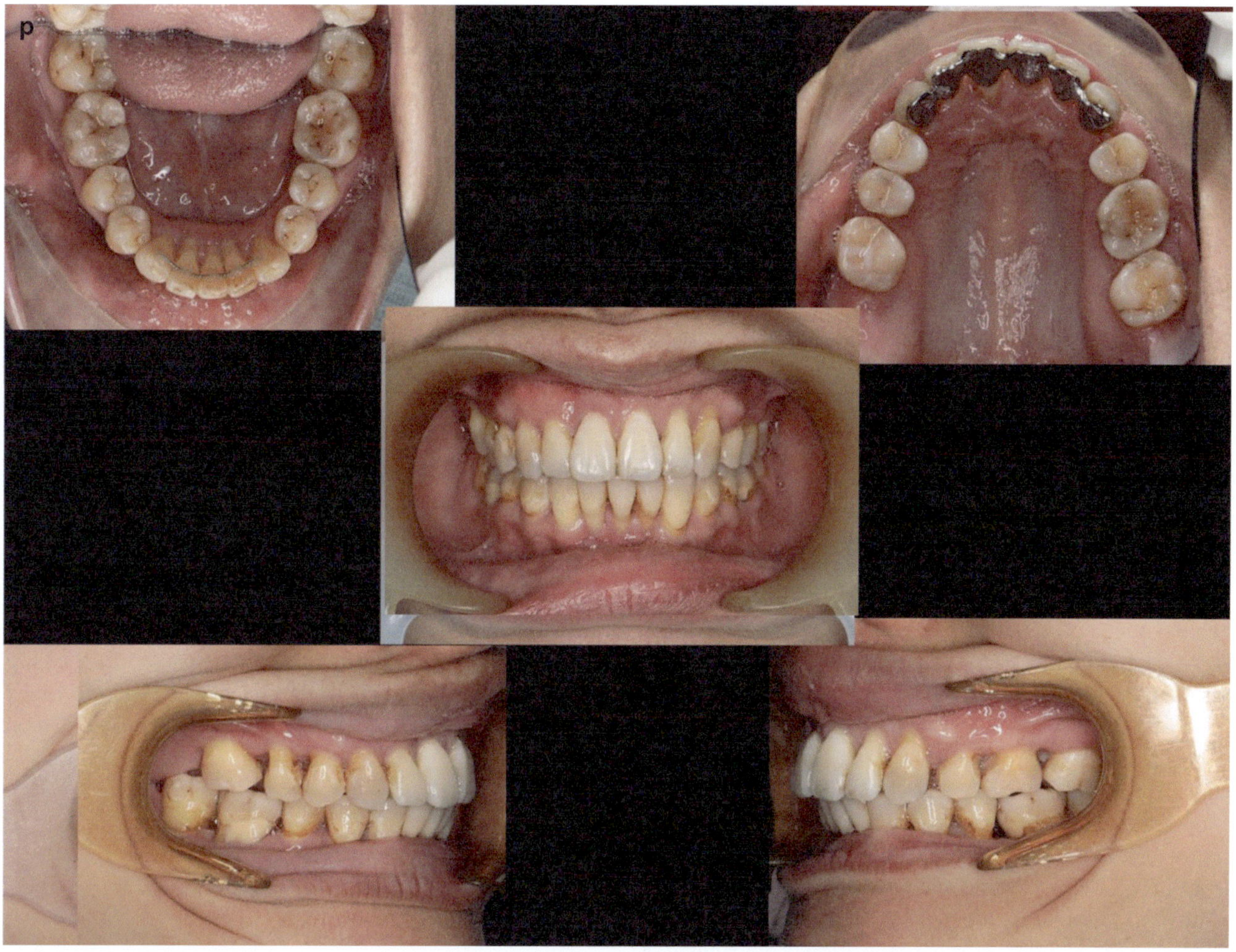

Fig. 9.8 (continued)

tingency plan in case of poor response and cooperation from the patients. This is where the use of the VTO and the occlusogram facilitate the treatment planning as these tools can simulate treatment results in different scenarios. In addition, the VTO and the occlusogram facilitate communication between the orthodontist, members of the treatment team, patients, and parents. This allows the different parties to "see" the outcome in advance, so they are able to comprehend the options more clearly.

9.6 Future Developments

9.6.1 Reducing Risk of Violation of Biological Limit

Conventional VTO can be used as a risk management tool to explore the biological limit of tooth movement which is the envelope of alveolar process [15]. However, it can only be applied on the central incisors in sagittal and vertical dimensions. Therefore, the next rational move is to superimpose a virtual dental model to CBCT images which is now a common feature of many dental implant and orthognathic surgery treatment planning software. At the time of writing this chapter, there is one commercially available planning software targeting clinicians as end users which can merge the image of clinical crowns from virtual models to the roots from CBCT images to facilitate virtual diagnostic setup [26]. However, the software is not able to show the supporting bone, and the accuracy of superimposition is not studied. At the same time, there is ongoing research working to overcome the limitations. For instance, researchers are now using professional engineering software to validate the accuracy of superimposition of 3D facial images, CBCT images, and virtual dental models [27]. In the future, software that supports accurate superimpositions of multiple structures will allow clinicians to compare all the teeth in the virtual setup to the existing supporting alveolar process and vital structures, e.g., incisive canal [28, 29] to explore their limitations to tooth movement in 3D. On the other hand, further research is required to address a very important question: What limits the orthodontic tooth movement? To be more specific, we need to know if we can manipulate bone growth in buccal and lingual directions by orthodontic tooth movement. Some clinical studies have shown an indirect proof of manipulated bone growth by preserving gingival attachment on labial lower incisor bodily movement with the use of segmented arch mechanics [30, 31], but this has to be investigated further using CBCT.

9.6.2 Improving Control of Tooth Movement and the Selection of Orthodontic Appliance

The next move after the success of superimposing CBCT to virtual dental models and the diagnostic setup based on the 3D occlusogram is the improved accuracy of estimating the position of centers of resistance of individual teeth. Our current understanding considers the center of resistance as a 3D volumetric center instead of a pinpoint because periodontal ligament and bone support are different in different directions [32, 33]. If the 3D volumetric center of resistance can be mapped, by comparing the change of position of individual teeth to the treatment objectives, the force system that leads to the shortest path of the planned tooth movement can be worked out more precisely [17]. This information can be input to the finite element analysis which is customized to individual patients in the future. This facilitates the design of the most suitable orthodontic appliance to achieve the treatment objectives which includes determination of position of TAD placement [34]. Therefore, it helps by determining which cases are best to be treated by straight wire fixed appliance, clear aligners, or customized segmented arch appliances.

9.6.3 Improving Patient Communication and Soft Tissue Change Prediction Due to Treatment

Software is now available which combines 2D and 3D facial imaging and simple digital ideal setup of front teeth to show the clinician and patient how the treatment would affect the smile [35, 36]. It helps with planning very simple orthodontic cases which involves minor anterior tooth movement which does not affect the lip and facial profiles [37]. Otherwise, this software is more of a sales tool which forms a part of so-called emotional dentistry and has a risk of giving unrealistic expectations to the patients. On the other hand, even if we can superimpose the 3D facial image, CBCT, and comprehensive digital setup of the teeth based on the occlusogram, it is still difficult to predict the soft tissue change in response to orthognathic surgery or extensive orthodontic tooth movement with TADs anchorage [38]. This is partly due to the fact that there have not been enough studies that included enough sample sizes on the soft tissue change in response to different treatments [39–41]. Also, soft tissue changes are subjected to huge individual variations [42, 43]. Therefore, further research is required to produce more viable data that would make the prediction of soft tissue changes more reliable. This will allow us to give a more accurate assessment of soft tissue change to different treatment options in the future.

9.7 Conclusions

Use of the VTO and the 2D and 3D occlusograms helps treatment planning in various ways. First, they provide an algorithm for the clinician to practice diagnosis and treatment planning in a rational and systematic way. Second, they allow visualization of treatment objectives. This reduces the risk of violating biological limits and facilitates the design of orthodontic appliances to deliver specific force systems which in turn improves treatment efficiency. Furthermore, it improves communication between members of the treatment team, parents, and patients.

References

1. Proffit WR, Sarver DM, Ackerman JL. Orthodontic diagnosis—the problem-oriented approach. In: Proffit WR, Fields HW, Sarver DM, editors. Contemporary orthodontics. 5th ed. Philadelphia, IL: Elsevier; 2013. p. 150–219.
2. Andrews LF. The six keys to normal occlusion. Am J Orthod. 1972;62(3):296–309.
3. Barber S. Shared decision-making in orthodontics: are we there yet? J Orthod. 2019;46(1_Suppl):21–5.
4. Kirschen RH, O'Higgins EA, Lee RT. The Royal London Space Planning: an integration of space analysis and treatment planning: part I: assessing the space required to meet treatment objectives. Am J Orthod Dentofac Orthop. 2000;118(4):448–55.
5. Kirschen RH, O'Higgins EA, Lee RT. The Royal London Space Planning: an integration of space analysis and treatment planning: part II: the effect of other treatment procedures on space. Am J Orthod Dentofac Orthop. 2000;118(4):456–61.
6. Al-Abdallah M, Sandler J, O'Brien K. Is the Royal London Space Analysis reliable and does it influence orthodontic treatment decisions? Eur J Orthod. 2008;30(5):503–7.
7. Grewal B, Lee RT, Zou L, Johal A. Royal London space analysis: plaster versus digital model assessment. Eur J Orthod. 2017;39(3):320–5.
8. McLaughlin RP, Bennett JC. The dental VTO: an analysis of orthodontic tooth movement. J Clin Orthod. 1999;33(7):394–403.
9. Melsen B, Fiorelli G. Treatment planning: the 3D VTO. In: Melsen B, editor. Adult orthodontics. Chichester: Wiley-Blackwell; 2012.
10. Marcotte MR. The use of the occlusogram in planning orthodontic treatment. Am J Orthod. 1976;69(6):655–67.
11. Burstone CJ, Marcotte MR. Problem solving in orthodontics: goal-oriented treatment strategies. Chicago: Quintessence Pub. Co.; 2000. vii, 267 pp
12. Fiorelli G, Melsen B. The "3-D occlusogram" software. Am J Orthod Dentofac Orthop. 1999;116(3):363–8.
13. Daskalogiannakis J. Glossary of orthodontic terms. Chicago, IL: Quintessence Books; 2000. ix, 296 p.p.
14. She TT, Chow RL. Aggravation of gummy smile by straight-wire mechanics and its management with or without orthognathic surgery up to 10-year follow-up. APOS Trends Orthod. 2018;8(2):96–109.
15. Handelman CS. The anterior alveolus: its importance in limiting orthodontic treatment and its influence on the occurrence of iatrogenic sequelae. Angle Orthod. 1996;66(2):95–109; discussion –10.
16. Burstone CJ, Choy K. The biomechanical foundation of clinical orthodontics. Chicago, IL: Quintessence Publishing; 2015.
17. Fiorelli G, Melsen B. Biomechanics in orthodontics. Wollerau: International Orthodontic School and Services; 2014.
18. She TT, Seto AWC, Chong MM. Interdisciplinary management of gummy smile. Hong Kong Med Diary. 2017;2(1):11–6.
19. Fiorentino G, Melsen B. Asymmetric mandibular space closure. J Clin Orthod. 1996;30(9):519–23.
20. Fiorentino G, Vecchione P. Multiple congenitally missing teeth: treatment outcome with autologous transplantation and orthodontic space closure. Am J Orthod Dentofac Orthop. 2007;132(5):693–703.
21. She TT, Wong ATY. Interdisciplinary management of an orthodontic patient with temporomandibular disorder. APOS Trends Orthod. 2017;7(5):230–41.
22. Bassarelli T, Melsen B. Expansion: how much can the periodontium tolerate? Clin Orthod Res. 2001;4(4):235–41.
23. Cacciafesta V, Melsen B. Mesial bodily movement of maxillary and mandibular molars with segmented mechanics. Clin Orthod Res. 2001;4(3):182–8.
24. Kalia S, Melsen B. Interdisciplinary approaches to adult orthodontic care. J Orthod. 2001;28(3):191–6.
25. Melsen B, Klemt B. Adjunctive orthodontics as part of interdisciplinary treatment: a case report. Int J Adult Orthodon Orthognath Surg. 1997;12(3):233–42.
26. Perri A, Gracco A, Siviero L, Parenti IS, Ippolito DR. Customized orthodontics: the Insignia System. Int J Orthod Milwaukee. 2014;25(4):17–20.
27. Xiao Z, Liu Z, Gu Y. Integration of digital maxillary dental casts with 3D facial images in orthodontic patients: a three-dimensional validation study. Angle Orthod. 2020;90(3):397–404.
28. Chung CJ, Choi YJ, Kim KH. Approximation and contact of the maxillary central incisor roots with the incisive canal after maximum retraction with temporary anchorage devices: report of 2 patients. Am J Orthod Dentofac Orthop. 2015;148(3):493–502.
29. Pan Y, Chen S. Contact of the incisive canal and upper central incisors causing root resorption after retraction with orthodontic mini-implants: a CBCT study. Angle Orthod. 2019;89(2):200–5.
30. Allais D, Melsen B. Does labial movement of lower incisors influence the level of the gingival margin? A case-control study of adult orthodontic patients. Eur J Orthod. 2003;25(4):343–52.
31. Melsen B, Allais D. Factors of importance for the development of dehiscences during labial movement of mandibular incisors: a retrospective study of adult orthodontic patients. Am J Orthod Dentofac Orthop. 2005;127(5):552–61; quiz 625.
32. Viecilli RF. 3D concepts in tooth movement. In: Burstone CJ, Choy K, editors. The biomechanical foundation of clinical orthodontics. Chicago, IL: Quintessence Publishing; 2015. p. 193–8.
33. Viecilli RF, Budiman A, Burstone CJ. Axes of resistance for tooth movement: does the center of resistance exist in 3-dimensional space? Am J Orthod Dentofac Orthop. 2013;143(2):163–72.
34. Roberts WE, Viecilli RF, Chang C, Katona TR, Paydar NH. Biology of biomechanics: finite element analysis of a statically determinate system to rotate the occlusal plane for correction of a skeletal

Class III open-bite malocclusion. Am J Orthod Dentofac Orthop. 2015;148(6):943–55.
35. Omar D, Duarte C. The application of parameters for comprehensive smile esthetics by digital smile design programs: a review of literature. Saudi Dent J. 2018;30(1):7–12.
36. Charavet C, Bernard JC, Gaillard C, Le Gall M. Benefits of digital smile design (DSD) in the conception of a complex orthodontic treatment plan: a case report-proof of concept. Int Orthod. 2019;17(3):573–9.
37. On Tse RT. Merging clear aligner therapy with digital smile design to maximize esthetics and minimize tooth reduction. Compend Contin Educ Dent. 2019;40(2):100–6.
38. Ullah R, Turner PJ, Khambay BS. Accuracy of three-dimensional soft tissue predictions in orthognathic surgery after Le Fort I advancement osteotomies. Br J Oral Maxillofac Surg. 2015;53(2): 153–7.
39. Akin N. Change in the soft tissue profile during and after orthodontic treatment. J Marmara Univ Dent Fac. 1993;1(4):347–53.
40. Peng MH, Meng QJ, Wang LC. [The soft tissue change of Angle's Class II division 1 malocclusion patients with vertical growth pattern after tooth extraction orthodontic treatment]. Hua Xi Kou Qiang Yi Xue Za Zhi. 2010;28(4):399–403, 7.
41. Wu YT, Sun J, Li YL, Chen LQ, Chen C. [Three dimensional study on change ratios of hard and soft tissue after orthognathic surgery]. Shanghai Kou Qiang Yi Xue. 2019;28(2):158–64.
42. Burns NR, Musich DR, Martin C, Razmus T, Gunel E, Ngan P. Class III camouflage treatment: what are the limits? Am J Orthod Dentofacial Orthop. 2010;137(1):9.e1–13; discussion 9–1.
43. Khamashta-Ledezma L, Naini FB. Systematic review of changes in maxillary incisor exposure and upper lip position with Le Fort I type osteotomies with or without cinch sutures and/or VY closures. Int J Oral Maxillofac Surg. 2014;43(1):46–61.

Three-Dimensional Treatment Simulation for Predictable Orthodontic Treatment Planning and Implementation

10

Jean-Marc Retrouvey, Yona R. Vandersluis, John Kaku, and Sivabalan Vasudavan

10.1 Introduction

The orthodontic profession has observed a significant paradigm shift in the delivery of orthodontic care, as evolving technological advances have been incorporated into our specialty practice. The implementation of digital diagnostic procedures has expanded the capabilities of the orthodontist to make more informed treatment decisions as it allows for the fusion of data obtained from different digital sources. The main files used for data analysis are the STL (Standard Tessellation Language) files, obtained from intraoral scanning of the dentition, and the DICOM (Digital Imaging and Communications in Medicine) files, from the cone beam computed tomography (CBCT) (Fig. 10.1). Combining these two files into diagnostic software allows for a three-dimensional analysis of the malocclusion that can be used to diagnose and plan treatment effectively [1–3]. Digital diagnosis is especially important as it provides the clinician with the opportunity to perform treatment simulations prior to and during treatment. Additionally, each patient file is instantaneously retrievable chairside for consultation during treatment, and treatment progress can be continuously monitored through the use of sequential intraoral scans. The software used for digital diagnostic procedures also allows for precise measurement of tooth movement, which facilitates accurate treatment planning and execution.

10.2 Digital Dental Casts and Diagnostic Measurements

Obtaining and analyzing orthodontic models is an essential part of orthodontic diagnosis and treatment planning. Digital models can be obtained from either intraoral scans using laser or structured light [4] or scans of plaster models obtained from alginate impressions (Fig. 10.2). Both have inherent advantages over conventional dental casts [5–7]. Conventional impressions from alginate or PVS material have several shortcomings including patient discomfort during the impression recording procedure, need for physical storage, material-related issues such as bubbles, time sensitivity, and distortion inaccuracies, and risk of breakage or loss of the models [3, 8]. Digital models obtained from intraoral scanning mitigate these disadvantages by providing improved patient comfort and experience during the intraoral scanning process and by allowing for subsequent digital storage of STL files. Digital casts are also obtained much more rapidly than conventional models and can be easily shared with the patient, other clinicians, and the dental laboratory for the fabrication of appliances [3, 9]. Additionally, studies have shown that digital models are as accurate as dental casts obtained from conventional impressions [10–12], which makes the use of digital models an easy diagnostic choice.

Similar to plaster models, two dimensional static measurements such as arch length, estimation of dental crowding, and estimation of rotations can be performed using digital casts. However, with digital models, these estimations can be transformed into much more precise computer-assisted measurements that can be stored in the patient database [11]. Several software programs are available which can be utilized to predictably measure the virtual files of dental casts in order to perform common orthodontic model analy-

J.-M. Retrouvey (✉)
Leo Rogers Endowed Chair and Professor, Department of Orthodontics, University Missouri Kansas City, Kansas City, MO, USA
e-mail: jean-marc.retrouvey@umkc.edu

Y. R. Vandersluis
Discipline of Orthodontics, Faculty of Dentistry, University of Toronto, Toronto, ON, Canada

J. Kaku
Private Practice, Tokyo, Japan

S. Vasudavan
Private Practice, Perth, WA, Australia
e-mail: drsiva@smilewithconfidence.com.au

J.-M. Retrouvey, M.-N. Abdallah (eds.), *3D Diagnosis and Treatment Planning in Orthodontics*,
https://doi.org/10.1007/978-3-030-57223-5_10

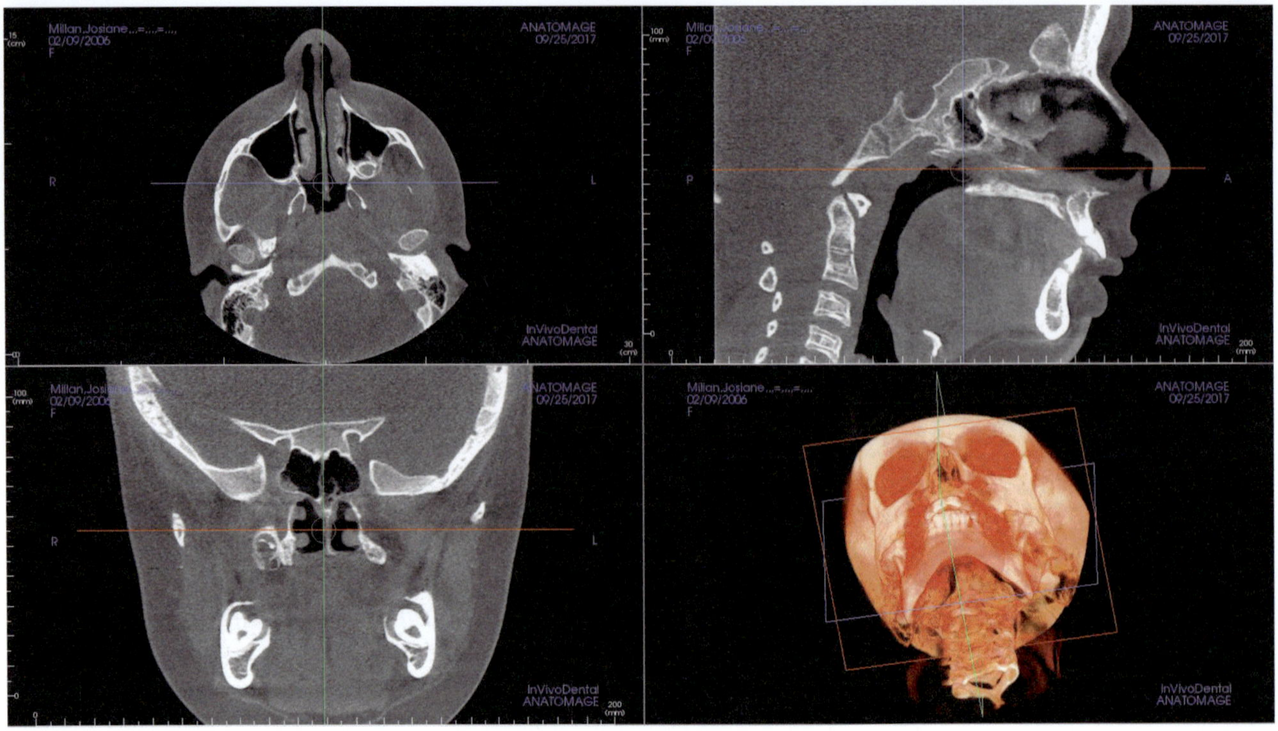

Fig. 10.1 Cone beam CT of a patient showing the three planes and the 3D reconstruction

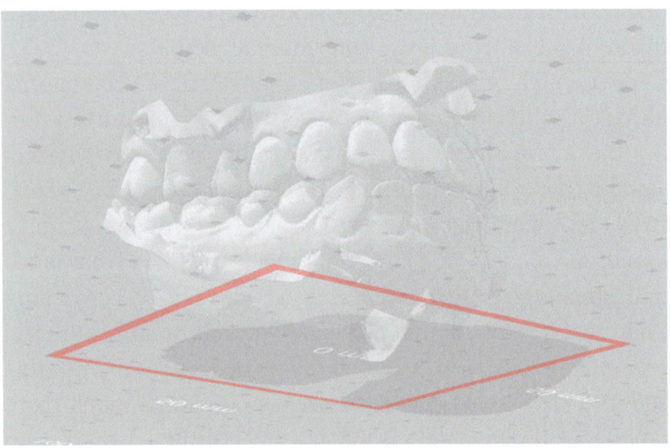

Fig. 10.2 STL file of a dentition obtained from a scan with a mask applied to show the surface. The mask covers the triangles

ses [13]. OrthoCAD™, affiliated with Invisalign, was one of the first developed software programs and can be utilized to perform several diagnostic measurements such as space analysis, Bolton analysis, overbite, and overjet [14] (Fig. 10.3). Other software that offer the most commonly used orthodontic measurements include 3Shape™, Orchestrate 3D™, and Maestro 3D™. As dental cast measurements are an essential part of orthodontic diagnosis and treatment planning, the ability to perform these measurements on digital casts allows for an accurate, efficient, and thorough digital diagnostic process.

10.3 Assessment of Dental Movement Through Superimposition

Digital models obtained from intraoral scanning can be utilized to assess tooth movement and treatment progress. By taking sequential scans as the patient's treatment progresses, superimposition of the different stages of treatment is possible (Fig. 10.4). This allows the practitioner to assess the amount and direction of tooth movement that has occurred between different timepoints and to determine if the intended tooth movement has occurred. Superimposition of scans is also important as it allows the clinician to assess the efficacy of their biomechanical plan.

10.4 STL Segmentation

An STL file is a cloud of points joined to form triangles, which describes the surface geometry of three-dimensional objects, such as the teeth, but does not have any color or texture [15]. As the STL file represents the natural curvature of the teeth by creating flat triangles, the accuracy of the STL file is largely influenced by the number and size of these triangles [16] (Fig. 10.5). STL files can be transformed by software into a specific file format [such as computer-aided design (CAD) files] that can be 3D printed by different methods [17, 18].

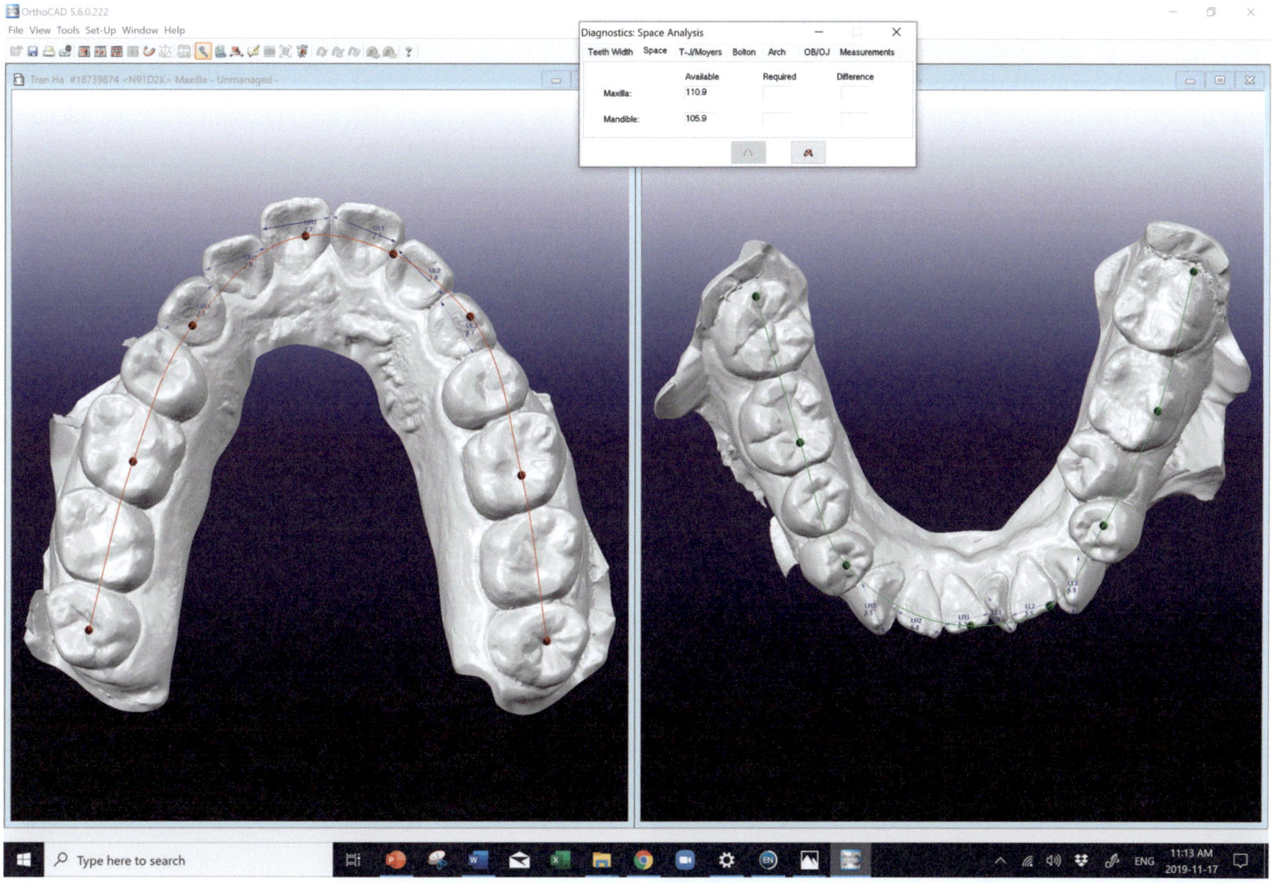

Fig. 10.3 OrthoCAD™ software, which allows for measurements of the dental casts

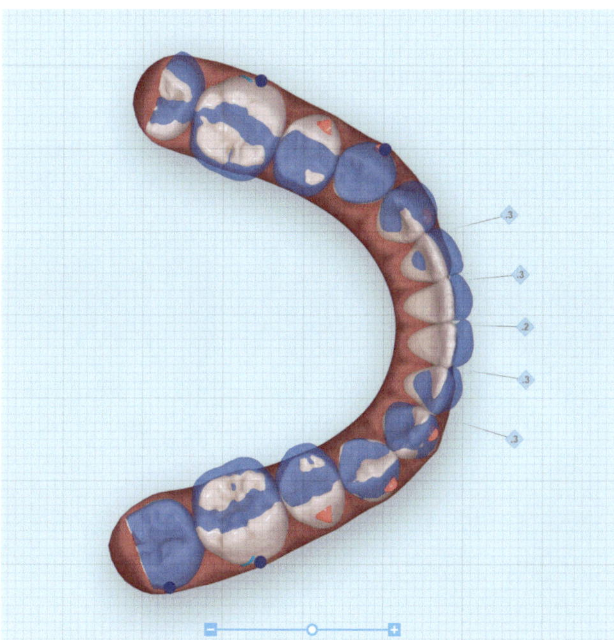

Fig. 10.4 Digital dental scans allow for superimposition of the dentition, allowing for the evaluation of treatment

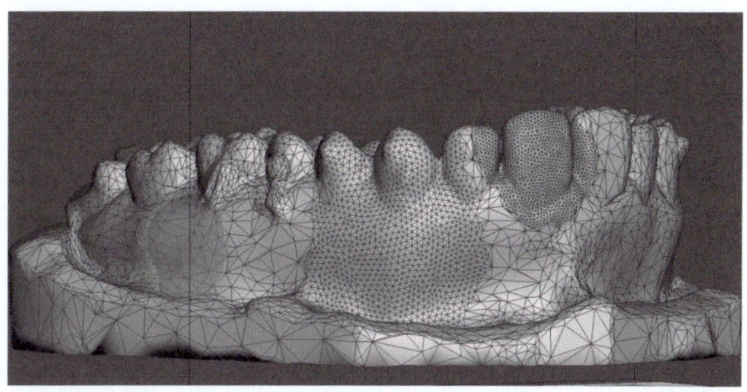

Fig. 10.5 The STL files may have different quantity and number of triangles. The more triangles that are present, the more precise the STL, but the larger the file

Virtual models obtained from STL files are extremely useful in orthodontics as they can be utilized for orthodontic treatment simulations via teeth segmentation (or surface cutting technique), which is a critical aspect of the preparation of the simulation files [19]. Segmentation involves partitioning the files either manually or automatically to create boundaries and to allow each tooth to become “free objects,” separated from the rest of the dental cast [20] (Fig. 10.6). Once segmented, the software enables the user to select one tooth and move it with six degrees of freedom using the computer mouse. The movements can be recorded and accurately measured in all three planes of space. Incremental tooth movement can be performed by positioning the virtual dental casts with the segmented teeth into maximum interdigitation and uploading them into proprietary software [21]. The software programs record tooth movements individually and in relation to the rest of the dentition. The clinician can assess any potential collision that may occur and can also maintain an ideal occlusal plane.

Several software programs, including Maestro 3D™ and DDP-Ortho™, allow the user to stitch radicular CBCT data to the intraoral scan to simulate a more realistic environment for tooth movement. Software such as DDP-Ortho™ allows the user to locate the instantaneous center of rotation (Fig. 10.7). Locating the center of rotation enables the clinician to better assess the needed tooth movement and to determine the force system that must be applied for the intended tooth movement [22].

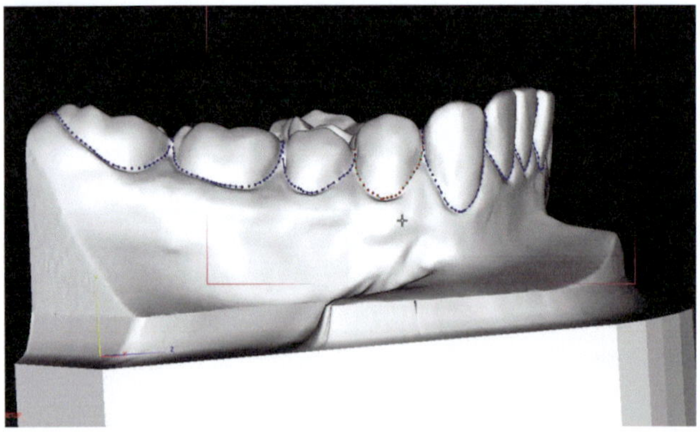

Fig. 10.6 Automatic segmentation of the dentition using the 3Shape™ software

10.5 Simulated Tooth Movement Using Digital Models

A main advantage of STL-driven digital study cast analysis is the ability to move each segmented tooth to a different position incrementally and precisely [21, 23]. As all orthodontic tooth movements are a combination of translation and rotation [24], software companies have built these movements into their interfaces to allow the teeth to be tipped, translated or rotated around instantaneous centers of rotations [25]. While each software program uses different methods to move teeth to their desired location, most programs allow for mesio-distal, labio-lingual, and vertical linear movements, as well as rotational movements, around the long axis of the tooth [26, 27]. Most software has built-in constraints, which will warn the practitioner if the programmed tooth movement is excessive or interferes with the dental occlusion [28, 29] (Fig. 10.8).

10.6 Dental Collisions

During simulated tooth movements, interproximal and occlusal collisions may occur, and computer assisted design (CAD) files used to simulate tooth movement need to be formatted to

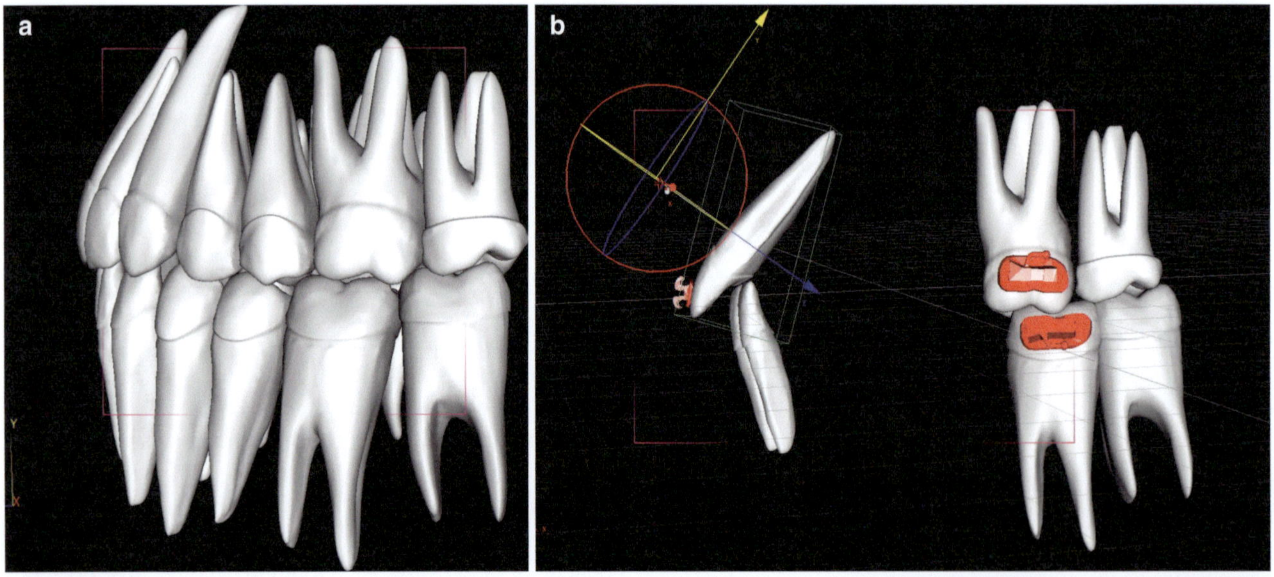

Fig. 10.7 (**a**) Visualization of the crowns and roots to calculate center of rotation. (**b**) Imaging of the center of rotation of orthodontic movements

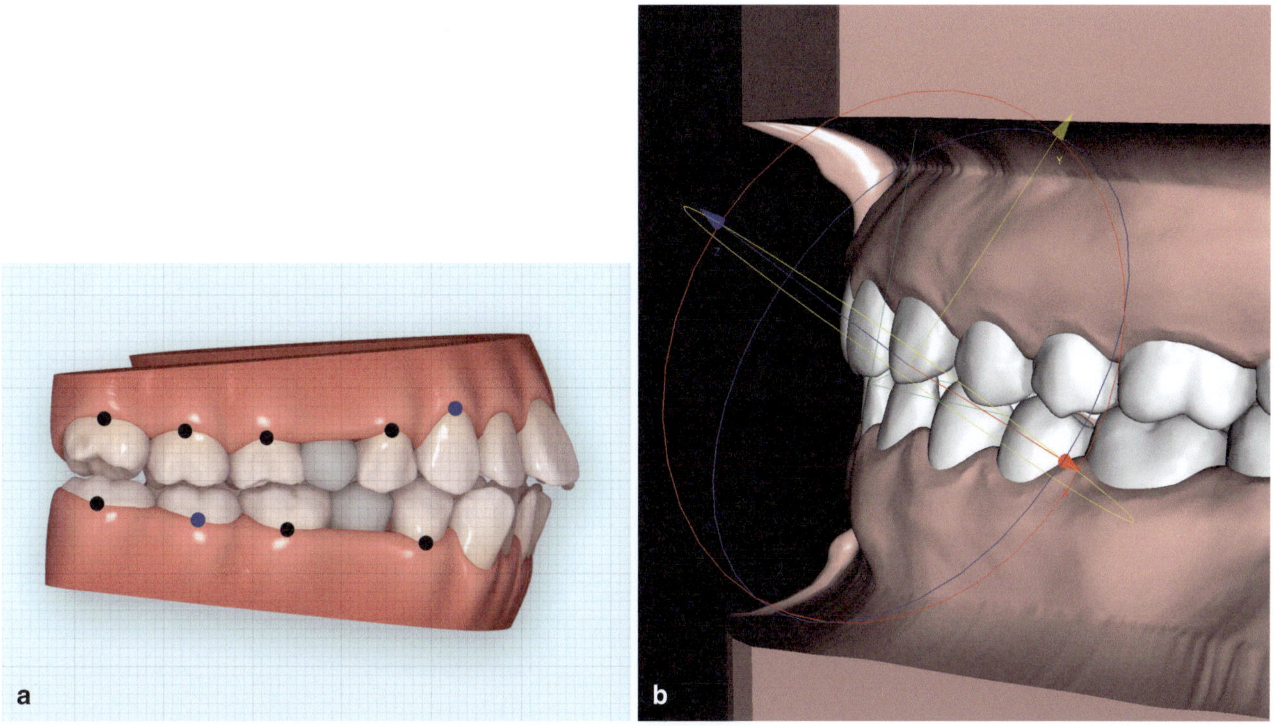

Fig. 10.8 (**a**) New software updates now indicate the boundaries of desired treatment. (**b**) The software allows for individual tooth movement and records the amount of movement in three planes of space

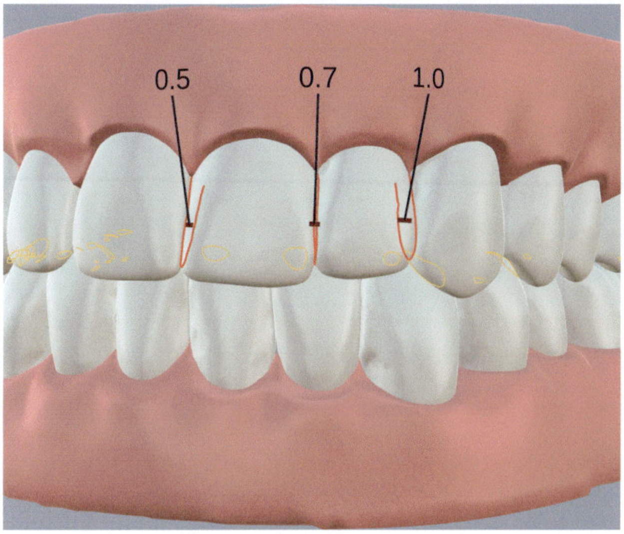

Fig. 10.9 Software program showing the collision between teeth during movement

be able to detect these collisions [30]. For example, during tooth alignment, if the teeth are arranged along a smaller arch form, collisions will occur between the teeth as they will end up occupying a smaller space. Complex algorithms are necessary to accurately document these collisions and to apply the necessary steps to eliminate them [31, 32].

Various software programs are capable of both detecting these collisions and quantifying the amount of overlap that is occurring (Fig. 10.9). With this information, the orthodontist can make informed decisions as to whether the teeth should be moved into different positions (usually labial or buccal displacements) or whether interproximal reduction (IPR) to reduce the mesio-distal dimensions of the teeth or if extractions should be performed in order to obtain the desired alignment [33].

10.7 Assessment of Occlusal Contacts

Several software programs can detect and provide information about occlusal contacts in maximum intercuspation, which helps with the detection of premature or heavy contacts (Fig. 10.10). Providing this information to the practitioner allows for the correction of premature or heavy contacts in order to create a balanced occlusion with even contacts [28].

10.8 Detection of Dynamic Mandibular Movements

SICAT-Dentsply™ is a unique software that combines data from the CBCT, the intraoral scan, and a mandibular tracking device. This combination of data allows for the visualization of dynamic excursive mandibular movements and condylar movements and allows the user to detect abnormal patterns of mandibular motion. When combined with the static regis-

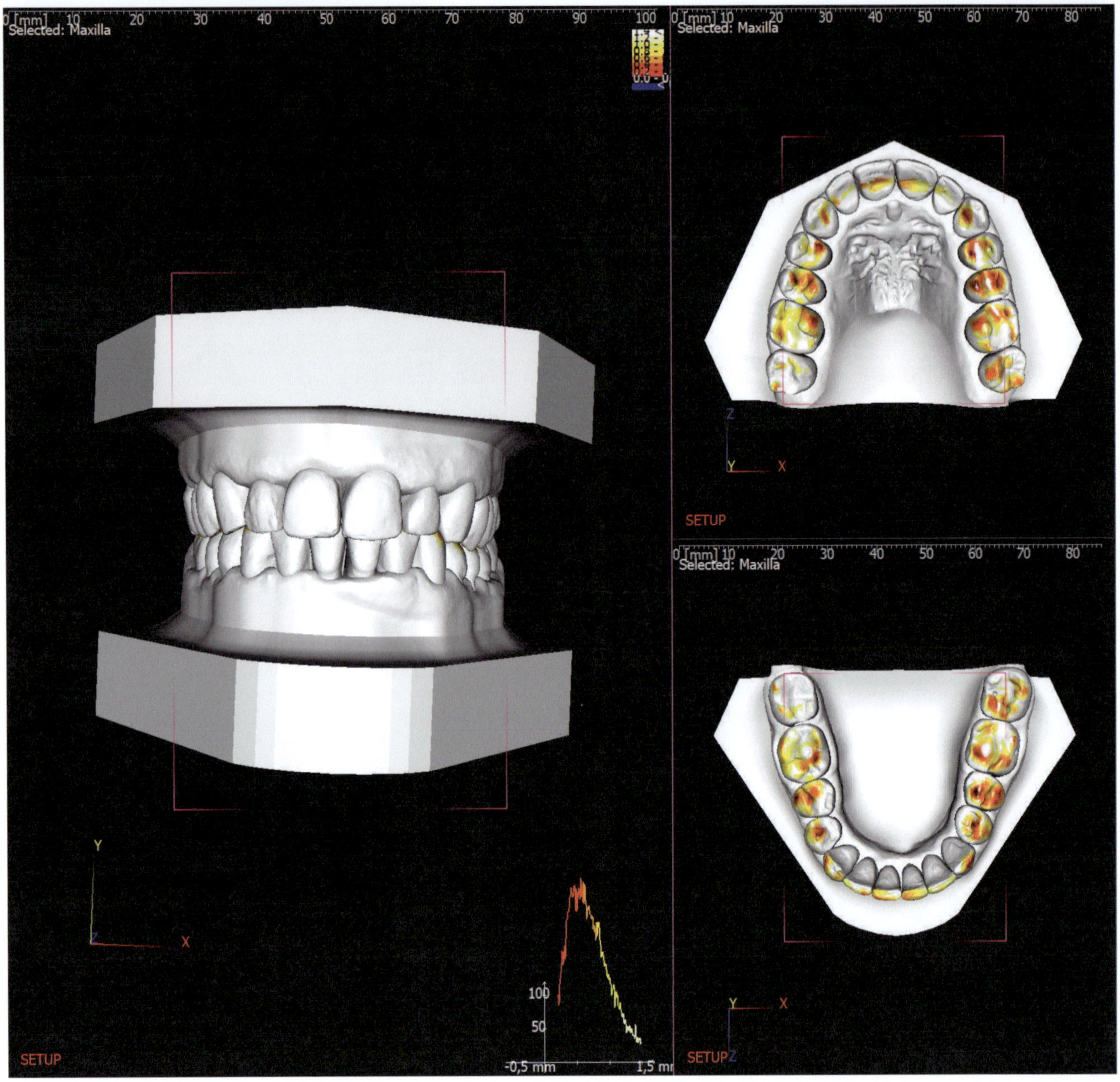

Fig. 10.10 Simulation software has the capabilities to record occlusal contacts in maximum interdigitation

tration of centric relation, the SICAT-Dentsply™ software provides information on normal and abnormal condylar motion and can be used to assist the practitioner in the treatment of cases with severe asymmetries and/or facial trauma.

10.9 Creating Space for Tooth Movements

In the early aligner systems, limitations within the software capabilities allowed only for the application of simple forces that pushed on the crown of teeth [34]. Therefore, the alignment of the dentition was mainly obtained by dentoalveolar expansion. Due to advancements in the software, current software programs offer more options to optimize dental alignment, such as IPR, distalization, or uprighting of posterior teeth [35] (Fig. 10.11). Using these techniques alone or in combination provides the practitioner with a variety of methods to create space without excessively relying on dentoalveolar expansion. This is important as studies have shown that excessive dentoalveolar expansion, especially in the premolar region, can promote bone loss [36].

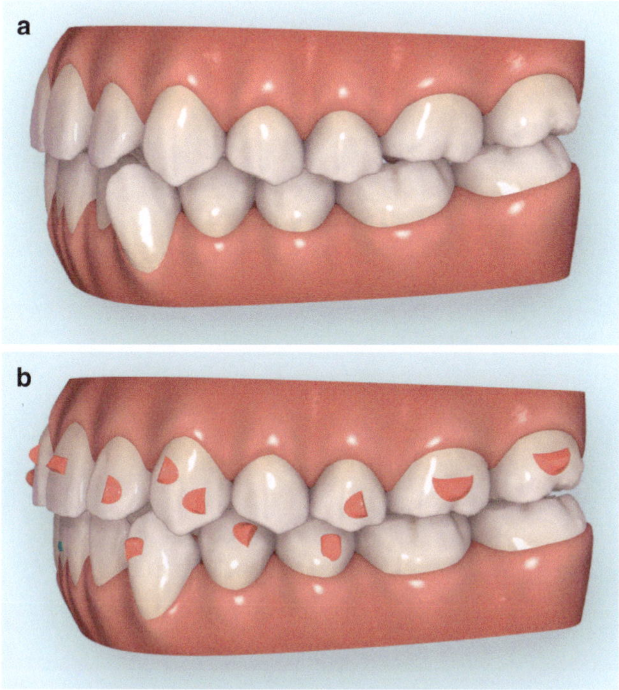

Fig. 10.11 (**a**) Simulation software allows for sequential and programmed dental movements. (**b**) After the first sequence of aligners, notice that the anterior teeth have remained in their original position

10.10 Staging

With conventional straight wire fixed orthodontic appliance systems, most orthodontists routinely place orthodontic brackets on all teeth and engage the wires in as many brackets as possible to achieve leveling and alignment of the dentition [37]. With this method, no specific individual tooth movement predictions can be built in, but rather the shape and energy that is stored in the wire dictate the final position of the teeth. This movement is described as a statistically indeterminate system, where the force systems cannot be accurately measured due to too many unknown variables, and the forces are for the most part uncontrolled [38, 39]. This leveling and aligning method is therefore more of a mechanistic stepwise approach, where the orthodontist moves from one wire to another, observes the result of the preceding action, and adjusts the mechanical approach accordingly.

One of the main advantages of treating with aligners is the ability to plan movements of a single tooth or a group of teeth without affecting the whole dentition (Fig. 10.12). This feature allows for the occlusion to be modified or maintained depending on the treatment requirements established by the orthodontist [40, 41]. With aligner therapy, teeth can also be aligned and moved sequentially in a process called aligner staging [42]. Currently, only a few software companies allow the aligner staging process to be modified. When modifiable, the orthodontist is able to move every single tooth or a group of teeth in three dimensions to correct the malocclusion with pre-planned mechanics. This staging method is then automatically applied by the software to obtain a sequence of aligners, which will correct the malocclusion with the desired mechanics [43].

For those programs that allow for individualized aligner staging modification, the software does not provide any guidance on staging modifications and the staging changes rely only on operator experience. Additionally, the software programs are currently unable to record the efficacy of the planned movements and therefore cannot be used to assist with future treatment planning. Both of these factors illustrate that operator experience and knowledge are essential for orthodontic treatment, even with the advanced digital technology that accompanies aligner therapy.

10.11 3D Orthodontic Brackets and Robot-Formed Wires (SureSmile® System)

SureSmile® is an integrated digital technology platform that allows for the diagnosis and design of a customized therapeutic treatment plan, through the fabrication of prescription archwires for the patient [44]. During orthodontic treatment with conventional fixed orthodontic appliances, brackets often need to be repositioned, or wires need to be bent by hand, to properly detail and finish the occlusion [44–46]. Additionally, bracket slots in conventional straight-wire appliances have been found to have poor tolerances, which can lead to imprecise tooth movement [44]. Both of these factors can unnecessarily prolong treatment time [44–46]. The customized prescription archwire eliminates this issue as the 3D planned treatment is utilized to create the customized prescription archwire [44] (Fig. 10.13). It has been reported that the robotic bends are very precise, with linear bends having a ±0.1 mm precision, and torsional and angular bends having a ±1° precision [47, 48]. This precision in appliance design helps to eliminate the reactive elements of orthodontic treatment and therefore may shorten treatment time [44]. However, this must be interpreted with caution as recent reports have questioned the accuracy of third order movement (labio-lingual torque) using the technology [49].

The 3D virtual imaging module in the software allows for a more precise and predictable treatment plan as the dentition can be visualized and measured in all three planes of space [44]. Furthermore, the software allows for decisions to be made through interactive simulations, which helps the clinician to both visualize and validate their proposed treatment plan [44]. As the software also has built-in workflow automation and standardized checklists, patient care can be planned sequentially, and errors can be minimized [44, 50].

Patients can be shown computer simulations of the proposed plan and can also be involved in the design of the sim-

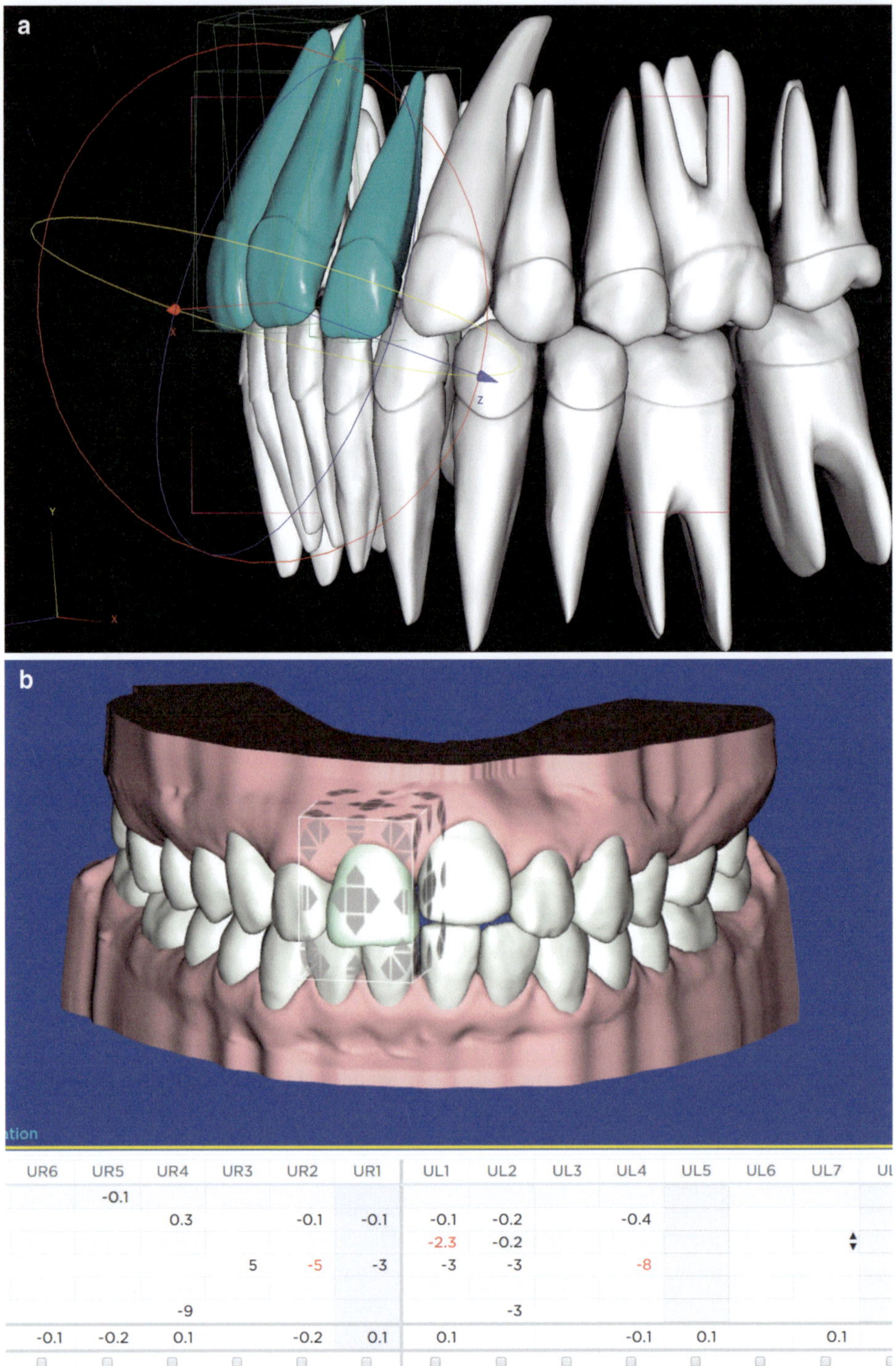

Fig. 10.12 (**a**) A group of teeth may be displaced as a unit to mimic orthodontic movement with a wire. (**b**) A single tooth can be moved at a time and its movements accurately recorded

ulated plan [44]. Showing the patient computer simulations has advantages as it has been found that patients who have seen computer simulations of their treatment have a better understanding of the treatment plan and may become more compliant [51, 52]. The software also allows the proposed treatment plan to be shared with other clinicians when required to facilitate interprofessional collaboration [44].

10.12 Clinical Cases

Four clinical cases will be presented below to illustrate the use of 3D diagnostics and treatment simulations in the development and implementation of a comprehensive and predictable treatment plan.

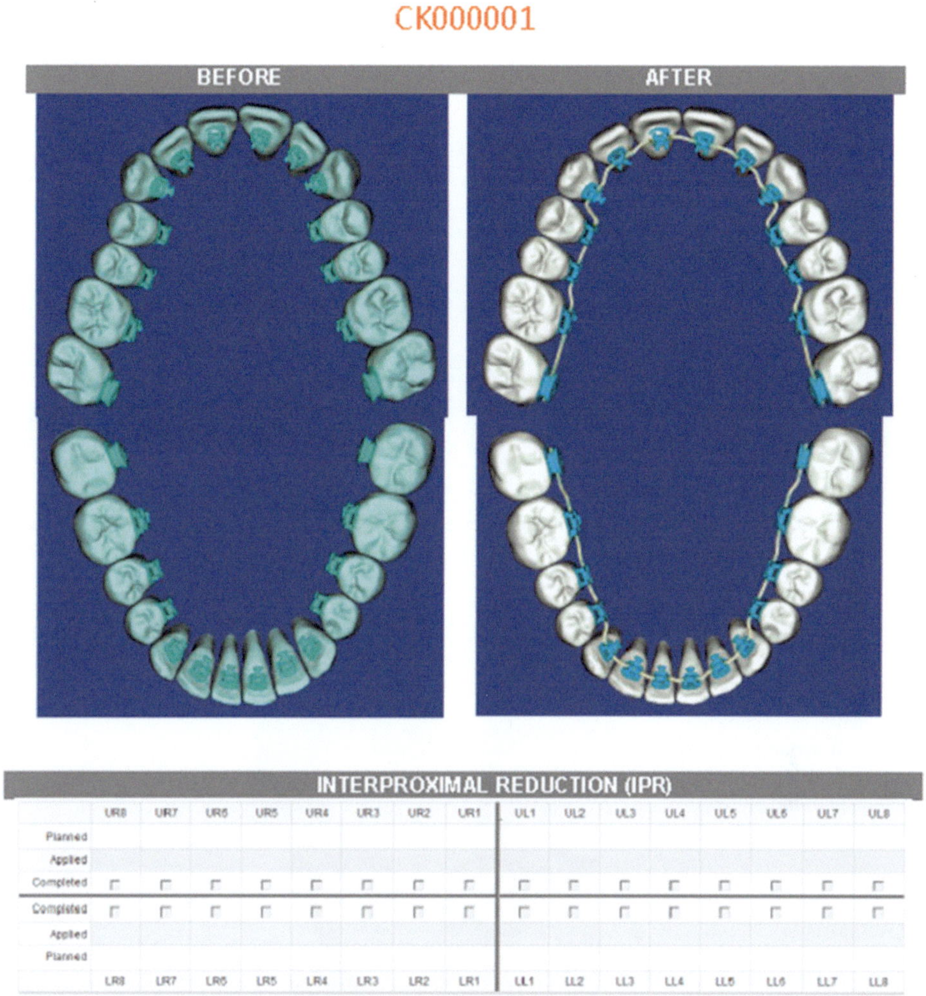

Fig. 10.13 Recording of movements built in the lingual SureSmile® software. These simulated movements are used to produce a preprogrammed wire to apply these movements to the dentition

Case 1: 3D Treatment Planning Using Simulations and Robotic Wires

A 15-year-old male patient presented with class II, division 1 malocclusion and a missing upper left lateral incisor with a significant maxillary midline deviation to the left (Fig. 10.14). Due to the missing left lateral incisor, the posterior dentition on the left side shifted more mesially than the right-side dentition, leading to more significant class II on the left side (Fig. 10.15a). The available space for the missing left lateral incisor was inadequate (Fig. 10.15b).

In cases with missing maxillary lateral incisors, two treatment options are possible: (1) closing the space with canine substitution or (2) opening the space for an implant-supported lateral incisor [53, 54]. Due to facial and occlusal considerations, in this case the decision was made to open the space for an implant in the lateral incisor position.

Using a treatment simulation picture provided by the SureSmile® simulation software, the malocclusion was corrected virtually and a pontic tooth was added in the left lateral incisor position. The position of the dentition relative to the face was verified by superimposing the treatment simulation image on the facial picture (Fig. 10.16).

For enhanced biomechanical advantage in both the correction of the class II malocclusion and the opening of the left maxillary lateral incisor space, the plan was to use a palatally positioned mini implant-supported appliance to distalize the molars into a class I position [55] (Fig. 10.17). For bracket placement, a simulation model was designed to correctly position the brackets to ensure the best possible root parallelism (Fig. 10.18). The correct occlusion was determined through the treatment simulation and all recorded measurements.

The final intraoral treatment photos show that the predicted and anticipated result was obtained, with adequate posterior occlusion, as well as anterior coupling, coincident midlines, and ideal overbite and overjet (Fig. 10.19). Adequate space was opened for the implant, and root parallelism was achieved (Fig. 10.20). This case illustrates that excellent outcomes can be achieved with 3D diagnostics and predictive software.

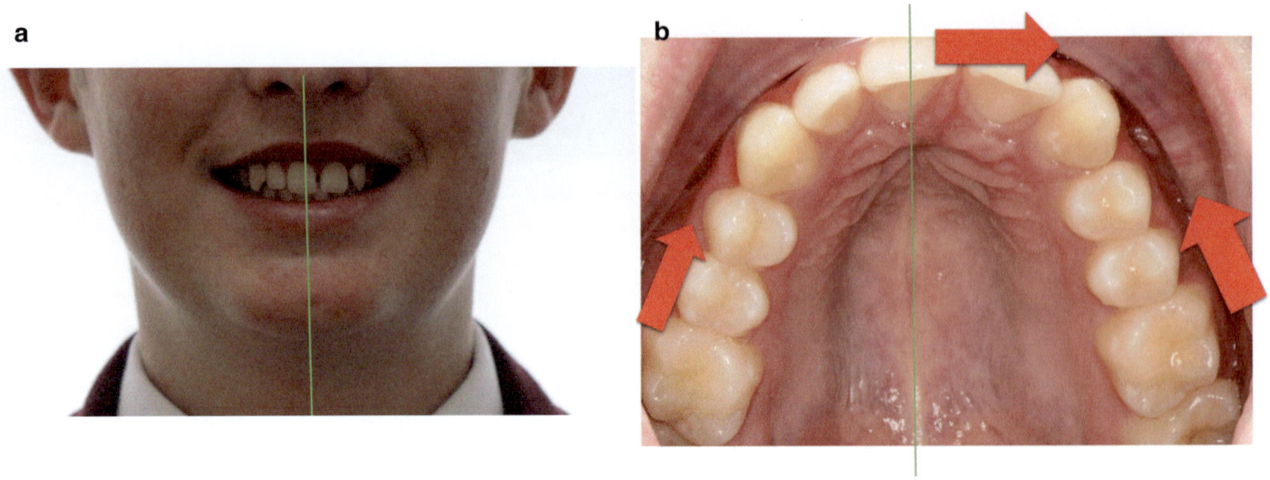

Fig. 10.14 (**a**) Smile line showing a significant deviation of the maxillary midline to the left. (**b**) Same deviation is observed when the palatal raphe is used as a reference line

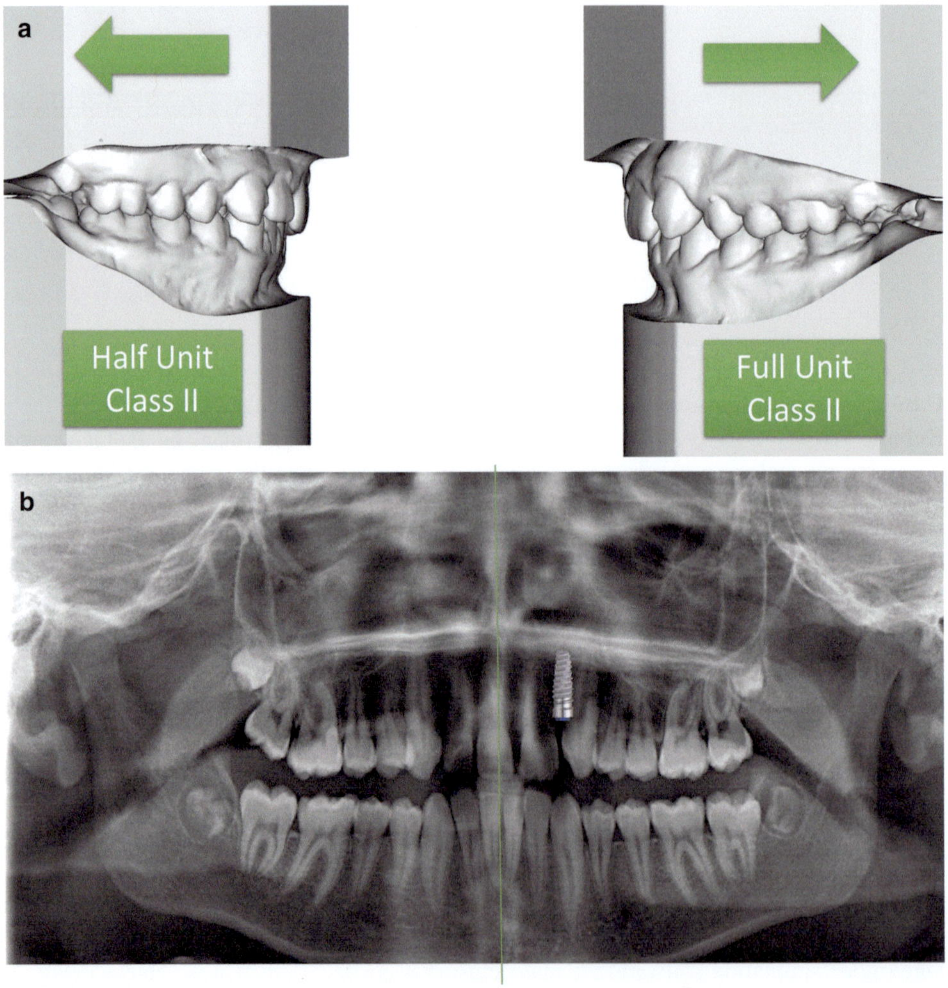

Fig. 10.15 (**a**) Lateral views of the dental casts showing the class II molar relationship. (**b**) The planned position and orientation of the future implant

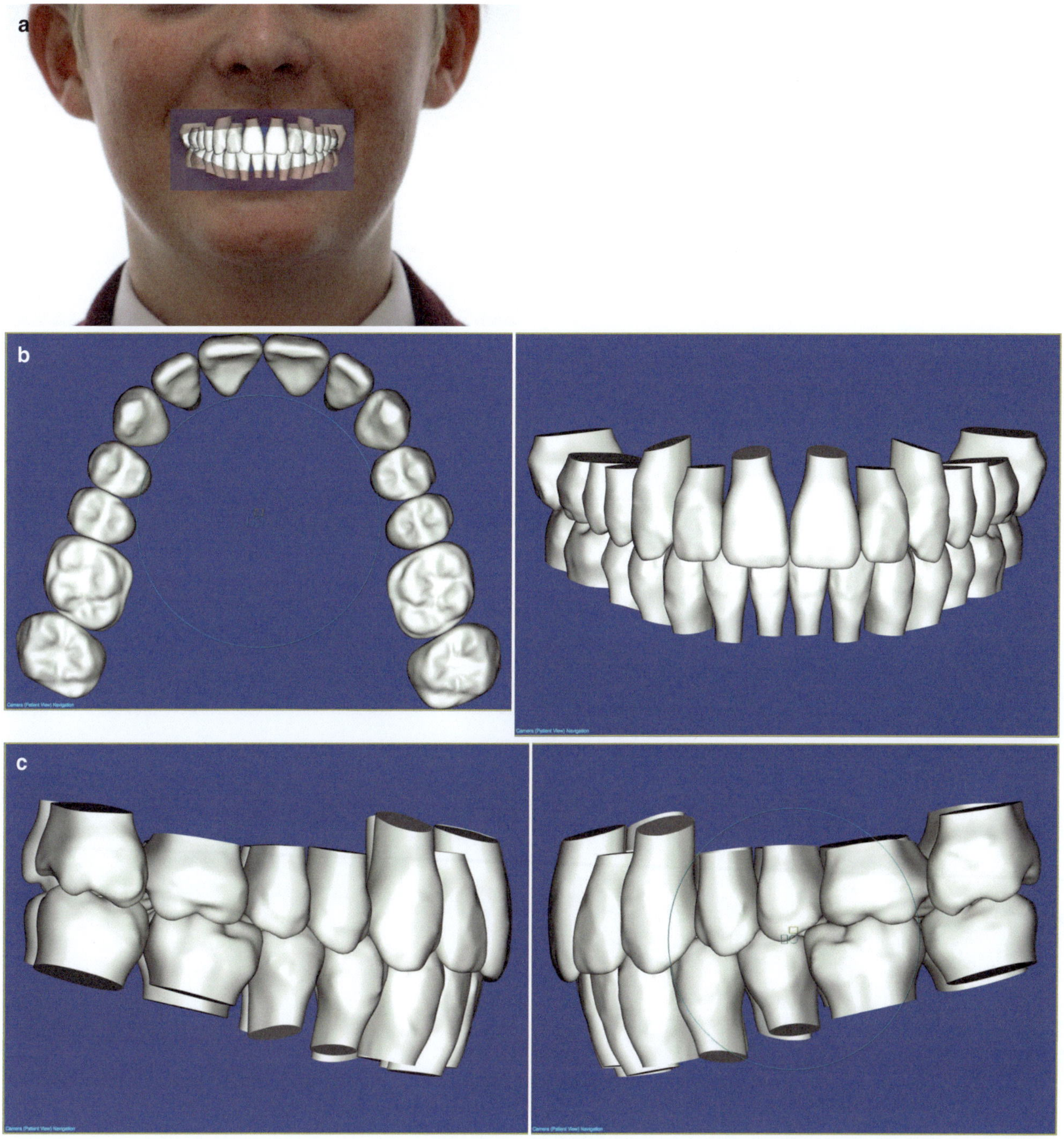

Fig. 10.16 (a) Insertion of the simulated result in the facial frontal picture. (b) Occlusal and frontal views of the simulated treatment with the pontic tooth incorporated. (c) Right and left lateral views of the simulated treatment

10.12.1 Canine Substitution: Assessment of Tooth Reduction and Shape Using Open Source Software

Although canine substitution was not chosen for case 1, 3D diagnostics and treatment simulations can be very helpful in the planning of canine substitution treatment. While the decision to open a missing lateral incisors space for an implant or close with canine substitution is based on the dental arch space available, the presented malocclusion, the patient's preference, and the facial profile [53, 56], canine substitution is often the preferable treatment option since it eliminates the need for an implant in this esthetically sensitive zone [57]. However, for canine substitution, the canine must have a shape and color that is amenable to modification into a lateral incisor [53].

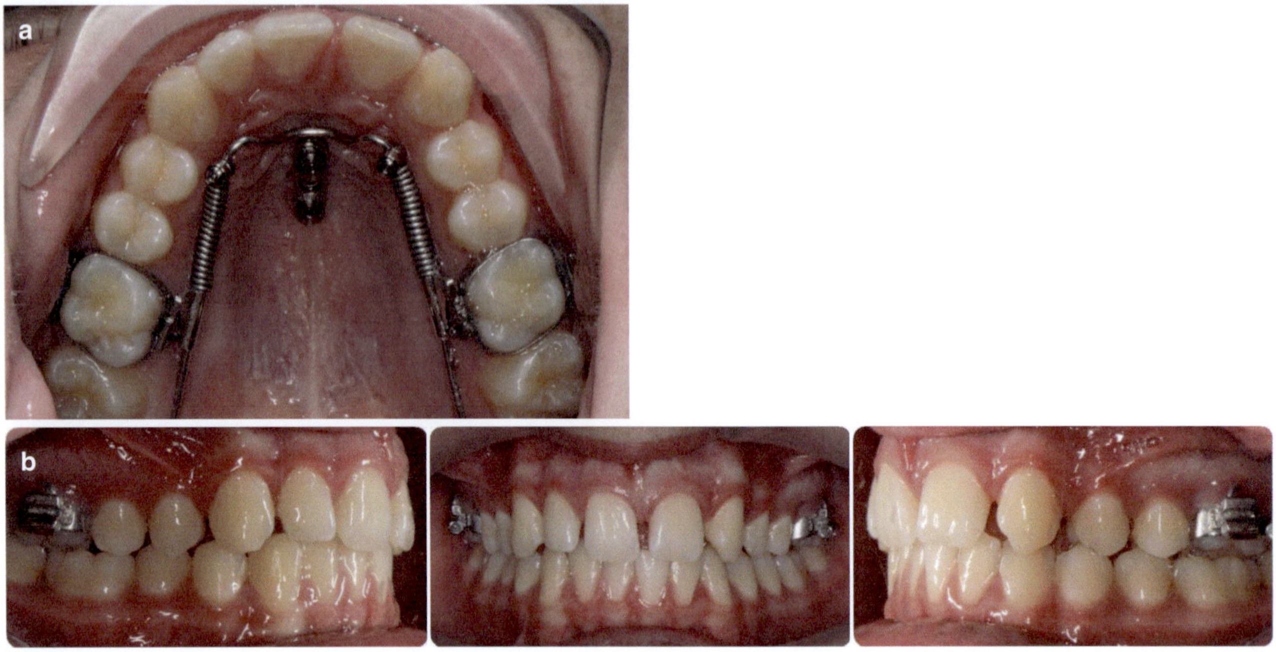

Fig. 10.17 (**a**) Occlusal view showing the implant supported distalizer appliance. (**b**) Frontal and lateral views with the distalizer

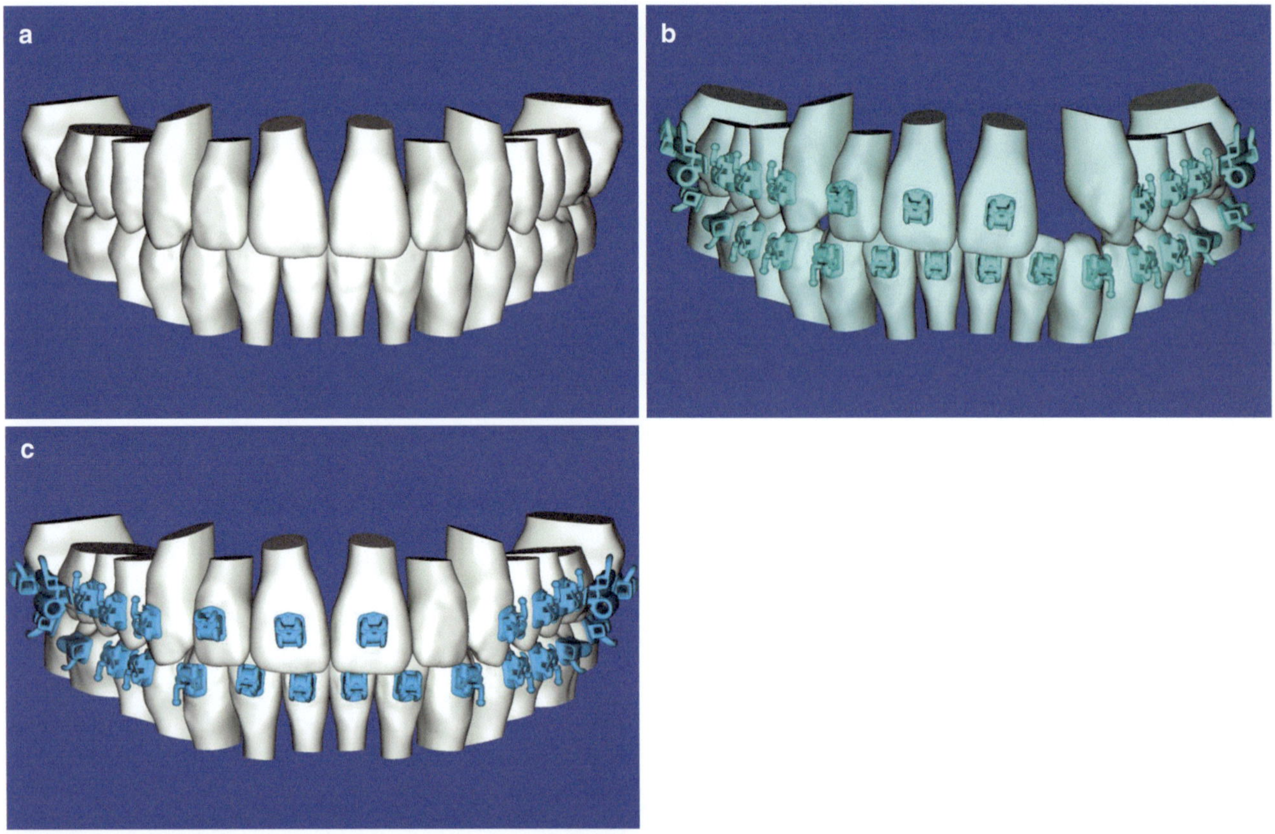

Fig. 10.18 Therapeutic simulation model. (**a**) Frontal view of the simulated treatment. (**b**) Virtual placement of brackets after molar distalization. (**c**) Simulation of treatment and correct positioning of brackets. (**d**) Frontal view of the therapeutic model. (**e**) Occlusal view of the therapeutic model. (**f**) Lateral view of the simulation model. (**g**) Occlusal view of the simulation model

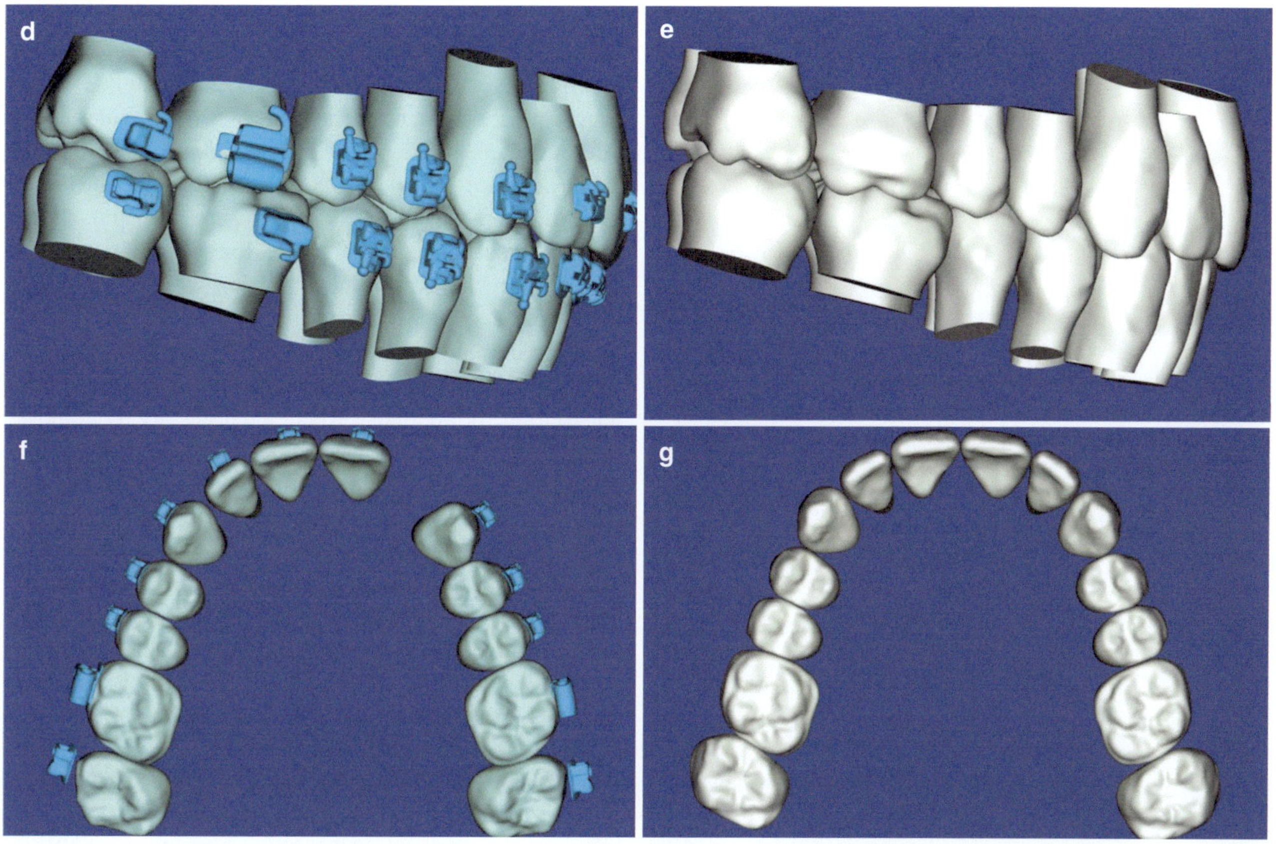

Fig. 10.18 (continued)

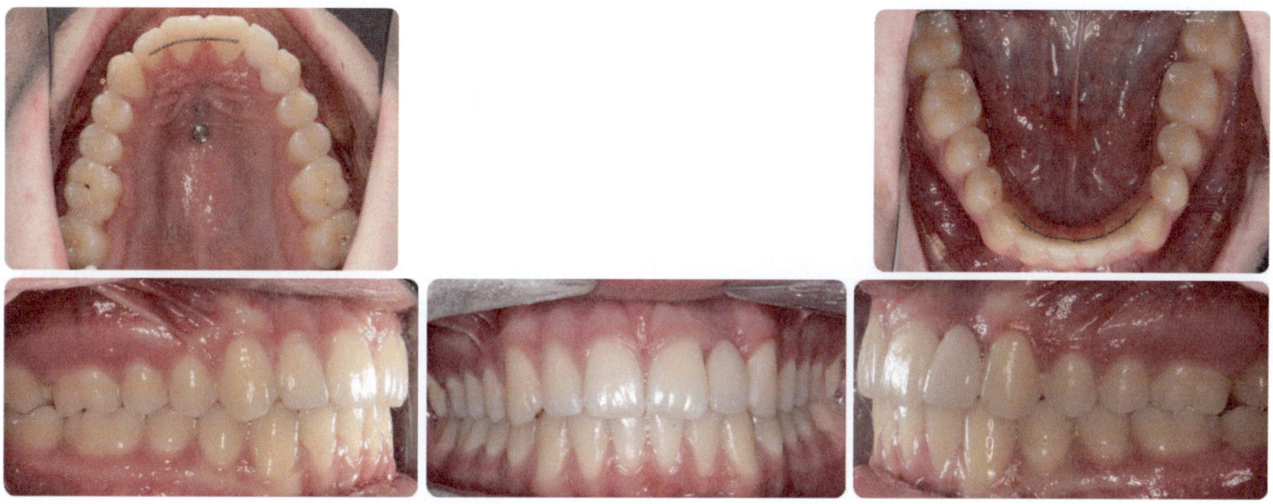

Fig. 10.19 Composite view of the treatment result

The therapeutic approach of reducing the size of the canine to match a lateral incisor is usually completed without 3D measurements or assessments, relying solely on the practitioner's experience [58]. An advantage of 3D software in canine substitution cases is that the software can be utilized to volumetrically reduce and reshape the canine, which allows the practitioner to assess the treatment needs and limitations (Fig. 10.21). An intraoral scan or a CBCT is needed to obtain 3D rendering files of the specific canine. The contralateral lateral incisor can then be used as a mirror template, or a virtual shape can be designed to create the desired future shape of the substituting canine. Once the shape and

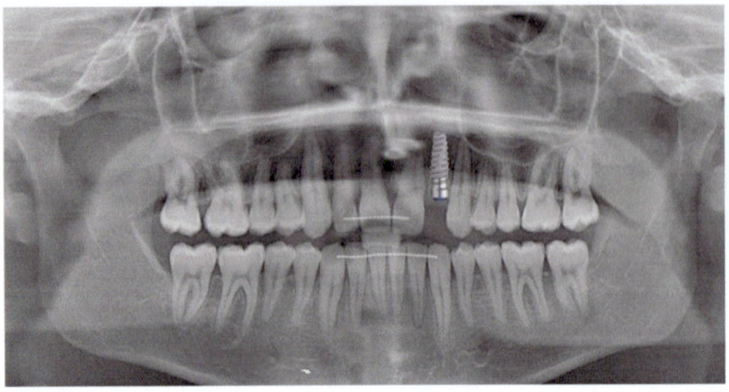

Fig. 10.20 Posttreatment panoramic radiograph

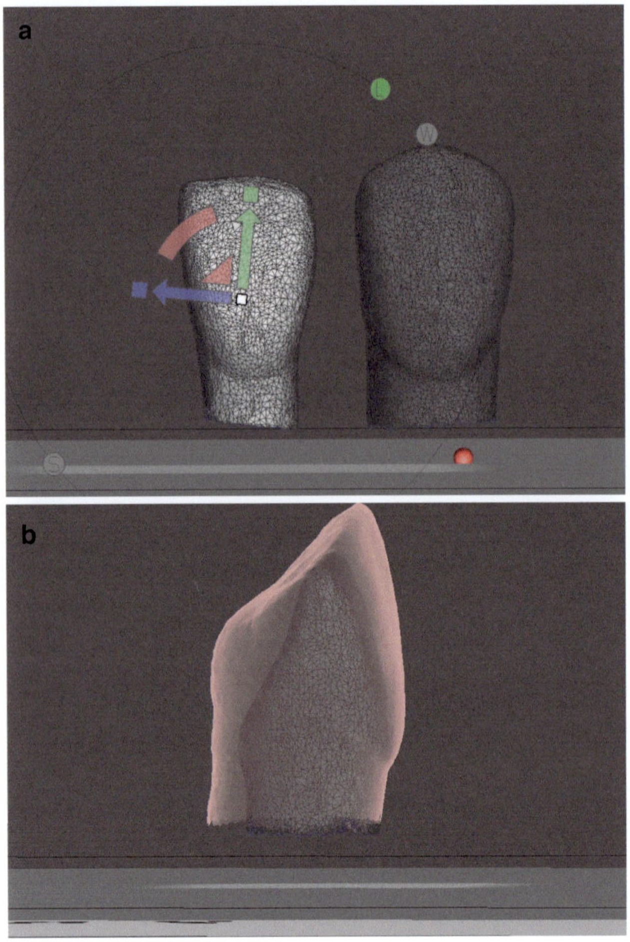

Fig. 10.21 (**a**) Frontal 3D rendering illustrating the differences in size and shape of an average lateral and canine. (**b**) Lateral 3D rendering illustrating the differences in size and shape of an average lateral and canine

Case 2: CBCT Digital Models Used for Planning Biomechanical Setup of Impacted Canines

The treatment of impacted canines is challenging [59], and conventional 2D diagnostic methods may not provide enough information about the position of the canine or its effects on the adjacent teeth [60, 61]. Impacted canines can lead to root resorption of adjacent lateral incisors, and this is not always properly visualized on 2D images [62]. Additionally, with 2D imaging, the exact canine position within the alveolar bone is not well-defined, and the superimposition of structures prevents an accurate diagnosis.

Impacted canines present complex biomechanical challenges to the orthodontist, where the necessary tooth movements must be carefully planned in order to both avoid root damage and to position the tooth optimally within the arch [63]. These canines require careful movement in all three planes of space and, if they are rotated, will require derotation which adds to the complexity of the procedure [29]. 3D imaging and the use of specialized software allow for proper visualization of the impacted tooth in all three dimensions of space, which provides an accurate diagnosis of the impacted tooth position (Fig. 10.22). The ability to visualize, assess, and measure the proposed tooth movement before the initiation of treatment is also a significant advantage as the prognosis and complexity of treatment can be assessed before the surgery is scheduled, which can decrease the morbidity of the orthodontic exposure and traction procedure [64].

To properly visualize impacted canines and to plan their movement, an open source software (3D slicer) can be used to segment the canines and several maxillary teeth from the CBCT DICOM file (Fig. 10.23).

This new data file can then be exported as an OBJ file into Meshmixer™, where a duplicate of the impacted canine anatomy is produced, and the duplicated tooth can be positioned in the correct position within the arch in the 3D rendering. DMA-DDP-Ortho™ software can then be used to calculate the most efficient force system to seamlessly move the impacted tooth into the desired position. Once the ideal size have been chosen, the crowns of the teeth are segmented, and the desired lateral incisor-shaped tooth is incorporated into the 3D rendering of the canine to assess the reduction that must be performed. This simple method helps the orthodontist to better visualize the most appropriate approach and to assess the feasibility of the canine substitution plan.

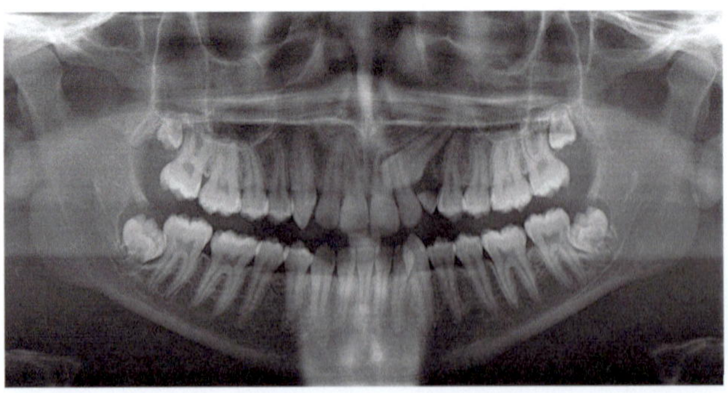

Fig. 10.22 (**a**) A panoramic view of an upper left impacted canine. (**b**) A frontal view of the cone beam CT rendering. (**c**) Palatal view. (**d**) Lateral view

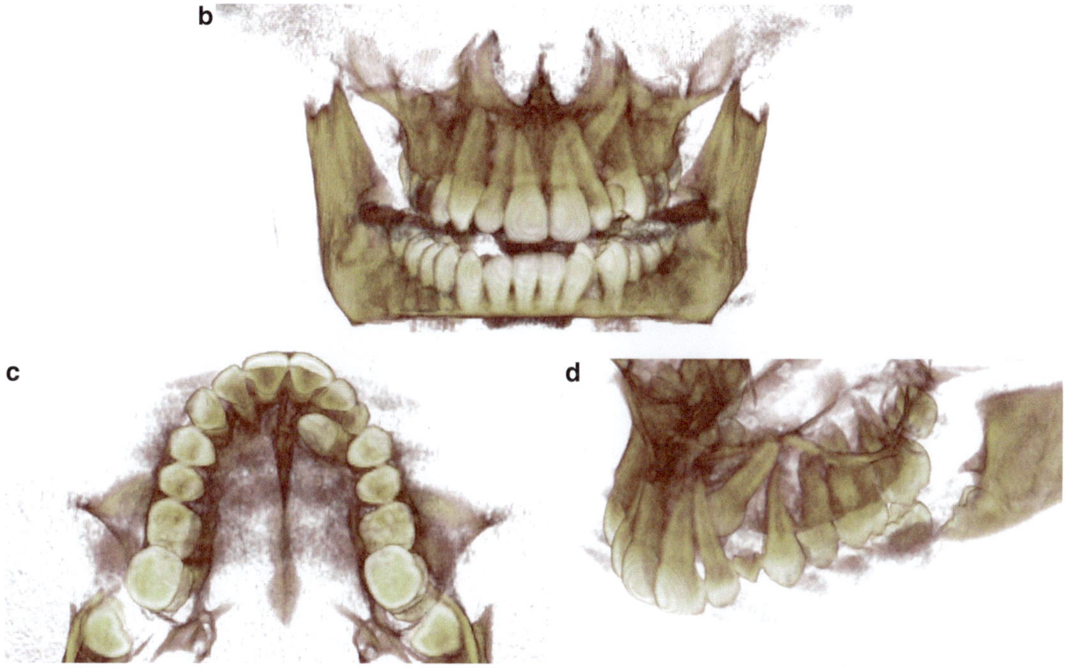

Fig. 10.22 (continued)

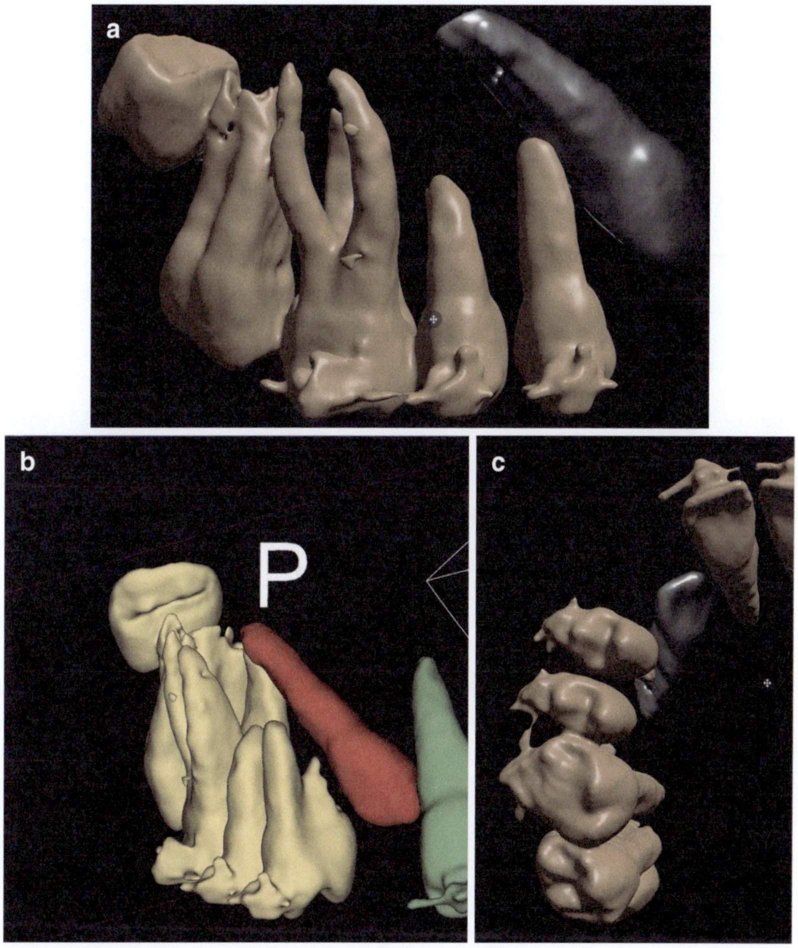

Fig. 10.23 Reformatting of the cone beam CT image of an impacted canine. (**a**) Lateral view. (**b**) Oblique view. (**c**) Occlusal view

force system is determined, this information can be used to design an appliance that will deliver this force to the canine crown with maximum effectiveness [65, 66]. Figure 10.24 shows the DICOM conversion to STL files when uploaded in Meshmixer™ and DMA-DDP-Ortho™, which allows for the center of rotation to be predicted and for the most appropriate force system to be determined.

A 15-year and 8-month-old male patient presented with a palatally impacted left permanent maxillary canine and a retained primary canine (Fig. 10.25a, b). A CBCT was per-

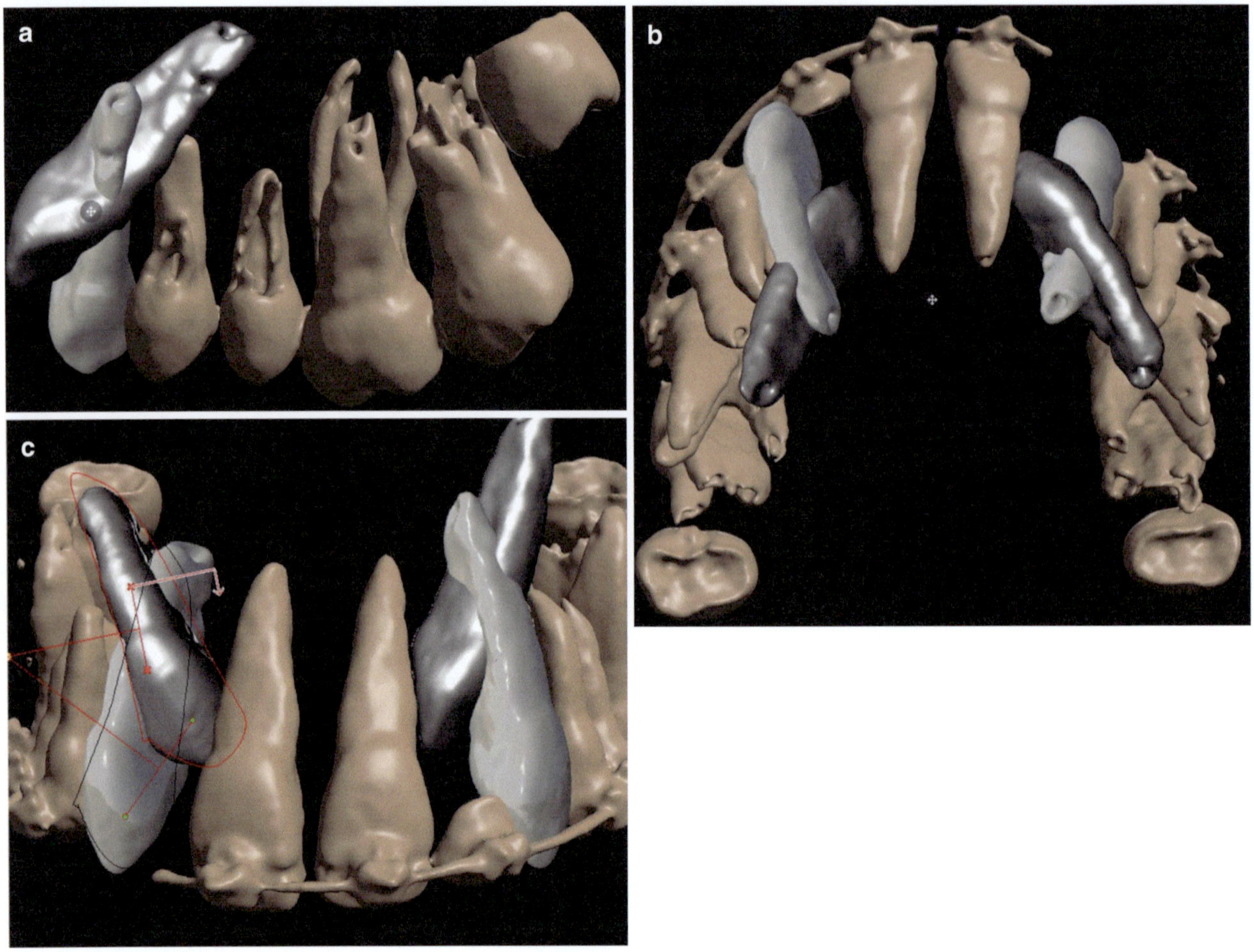

Fig. 10.24 The initial and desired position of the canine has been incorporated in a single 3D file. (**a**) Lateral view. (**b**) Occlusal view. (**c**) Correct force system applied (DMA-DDP-Ortho™ software)

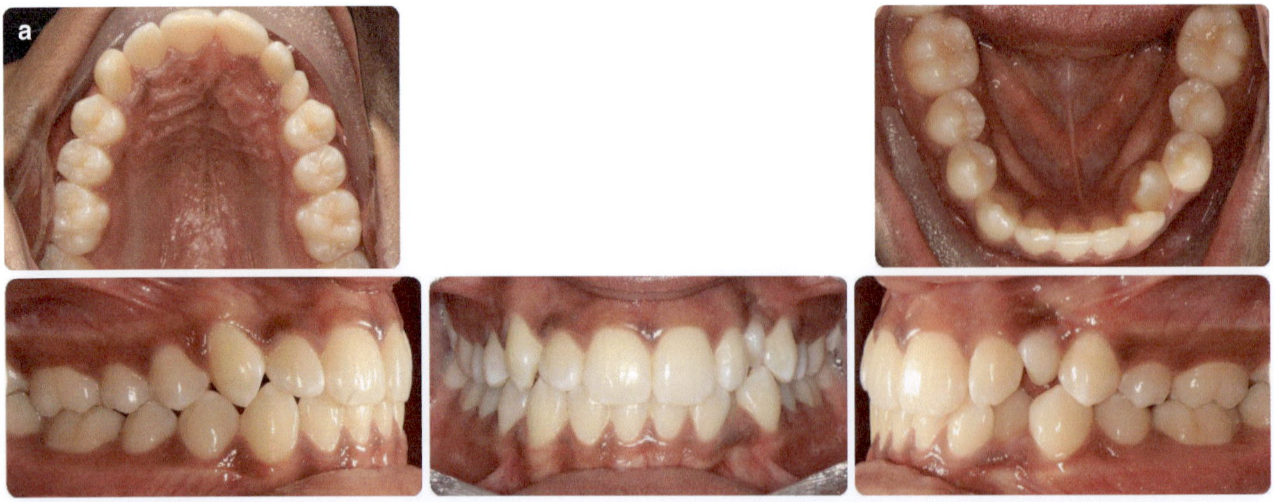

Fig. 10.25 (**a**) Pretreatment photographs. (**b**) Pretreatment digital models. (**c**) Biomechanical considerations and creation of the force system. (**d**) Cantilever design with the appropriate force system

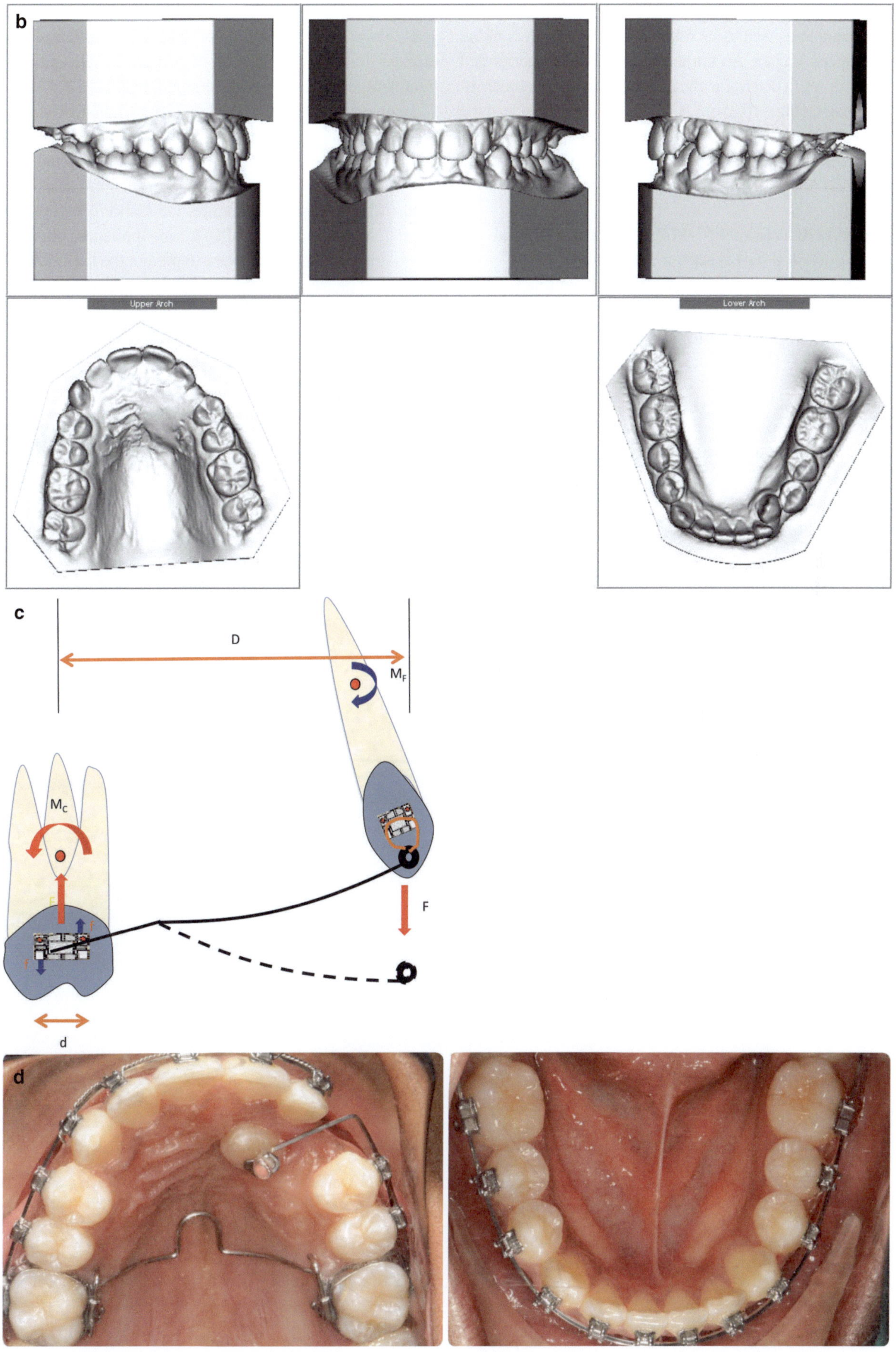

Fig. 10.25 (continued)

formed to determine the exact position and angulation of the impacted canine as well as its relationship to the crown of the adjacent lateral incisor. An intraoral scan was also performed and was utilized to determine the most appropriate biomechanical approach (Fig. 10.25c). A single-force cantilever-type mechanical system was then designed in order to apply the most appropriate force system for the impacted canine (Fig. 10.25d).

Case 3: Hybrid Treatment—Molar Distalization and Rotation Followed by Invisalign Therapy

The combination of two different treatment approaches during a patient's orthodontic treatment is often beneficial to the patient. For example, in certain cases, limited bracketing, growth modification, or the use of specific appliances can be utilized prior to the initiation of comprehensive orthodontic treatment to obtain the best treatment results [67].

In growing patients with class II malocclusion where distalization of the upper first molars is appropriate, it is beneficial to distalize these molars before the eruption of the second molars [68] (Fig. 10.26b). Several appliances may be used for this purpose, including the Carriere motion appliance™, headgear, and the Pendulum appliance, among others. Using simulation software to predict the treatment result of the first phase of treatment (distalization) may be of great benefit in the planning of the second phase of treatment.

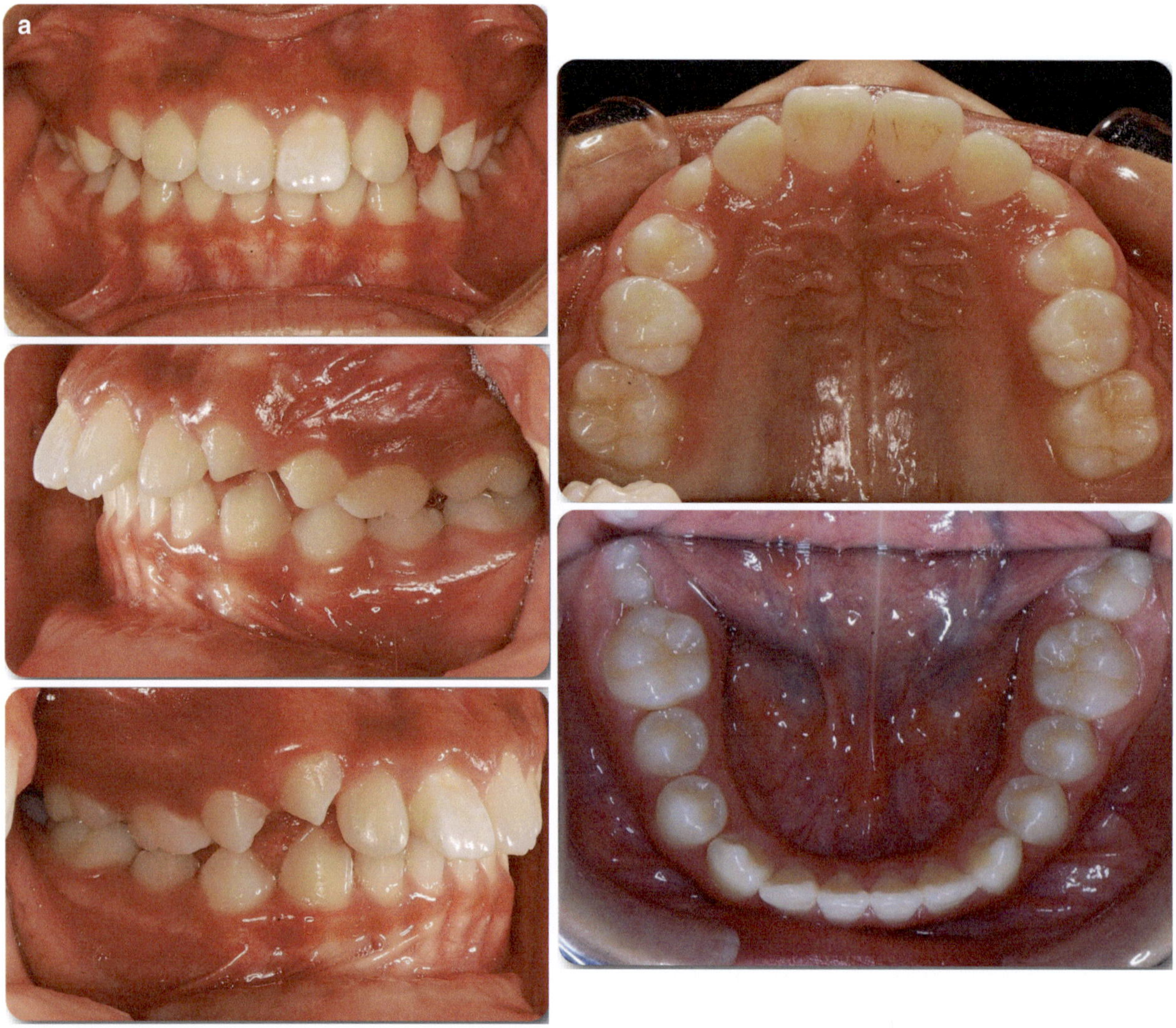

Fig. 10.26 (**a**) Pretreatment photographs. (**b**) Treatment needs and calculations of molar and incisor movement. Group 1, without second molar; Group 2, with second molar. It shows that the best time for molar distalization without loss of anchorage of anterior incisors is before second molar eruption [69]. (**c**) The predicted effect of the Carriere motion appliance™ (occlusal view). Occlusal view to visualize arch development with the Carriere motion appliance™. Please note that V-shaped arch form is changed to U-shaped arch form after distalization with the Carriere motion appliance™. The ball joint on the molar pads produces distal rotation during distalization. (**d**) The Carriere motion appliance™ from the lateral view. Please note that molar uprighting can happen from the ball joint on the molars while the canine moves distally with more bodily movement. (**e**) Result of the Carriere motion appliance™ treatment after 3 months. The canine position (blue line) can be compared with the incisor position (yellow line). The vertical position of canine moved into solid class I relationship and extruded within 3 months. (**f**) The first ClinCheck™ showing 39 aligners. (**g**) Calculations of the amount of distalization movement. (**h**) Final treatment outcomes

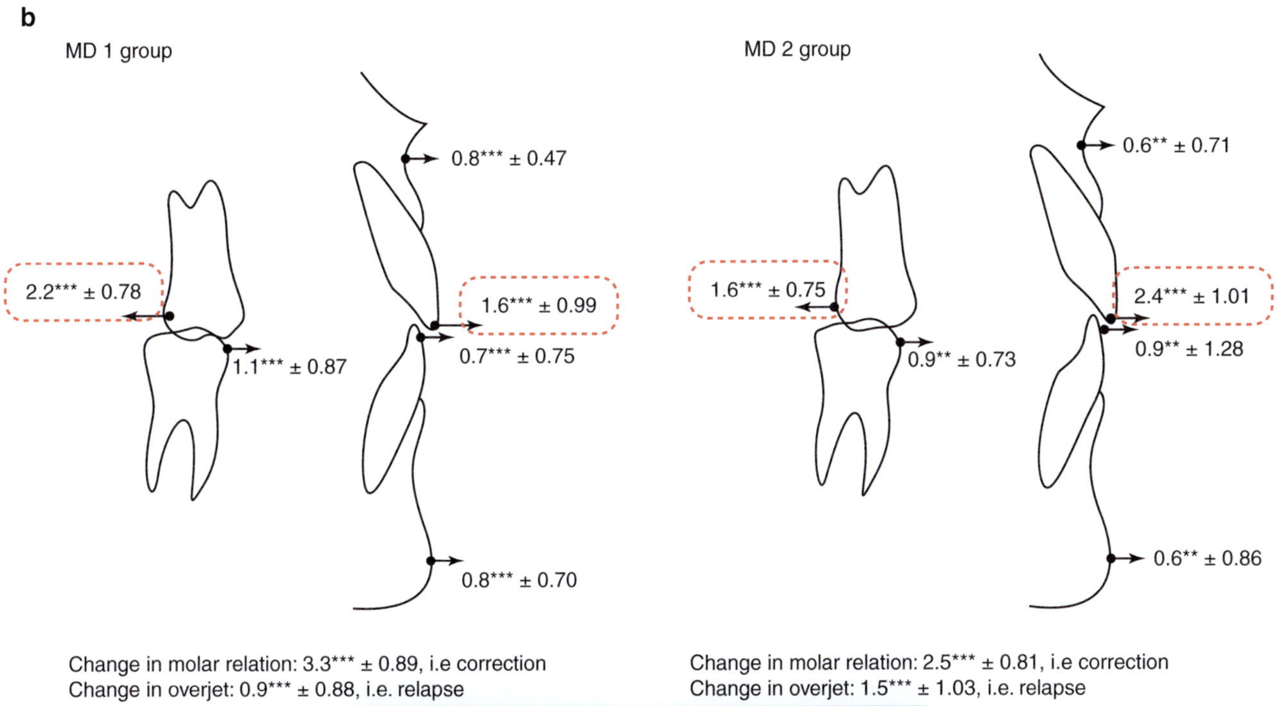

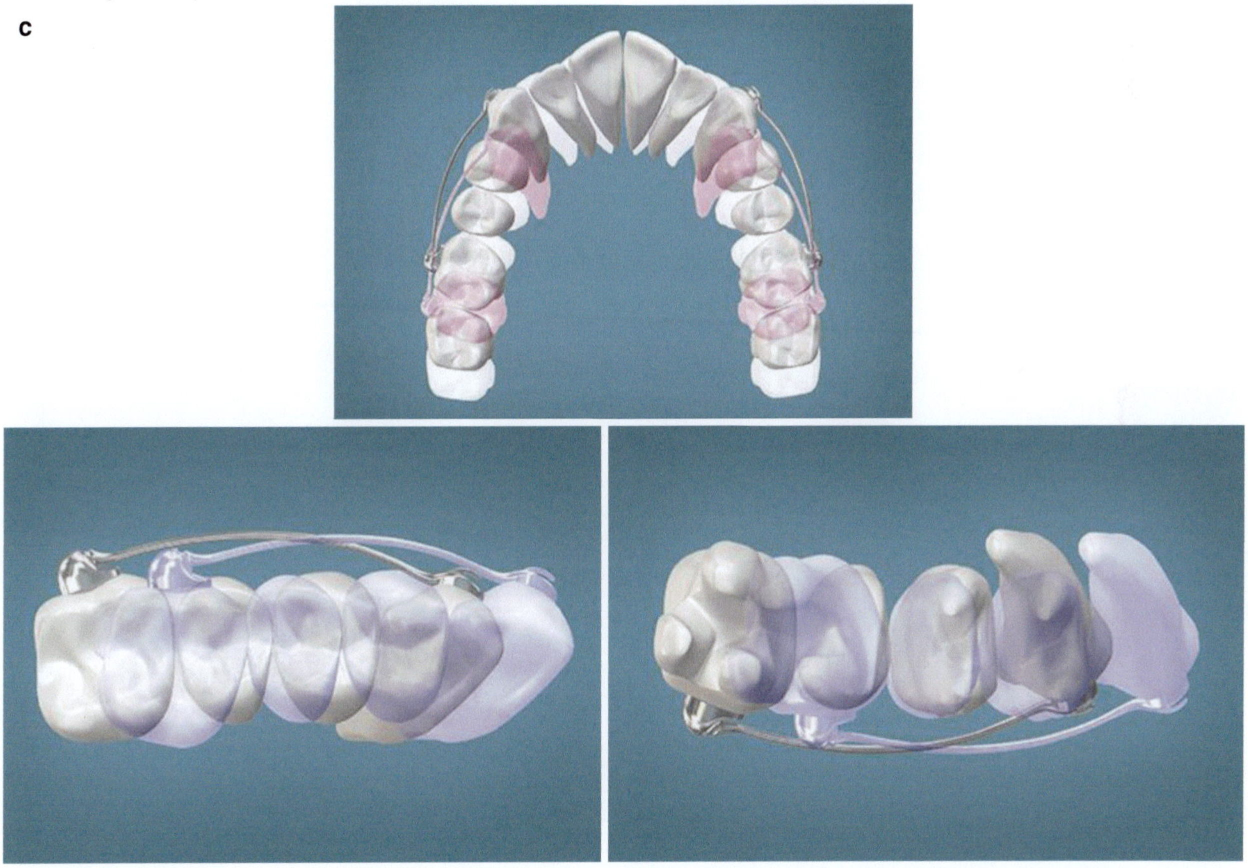

Fig. 10.26 (continued)

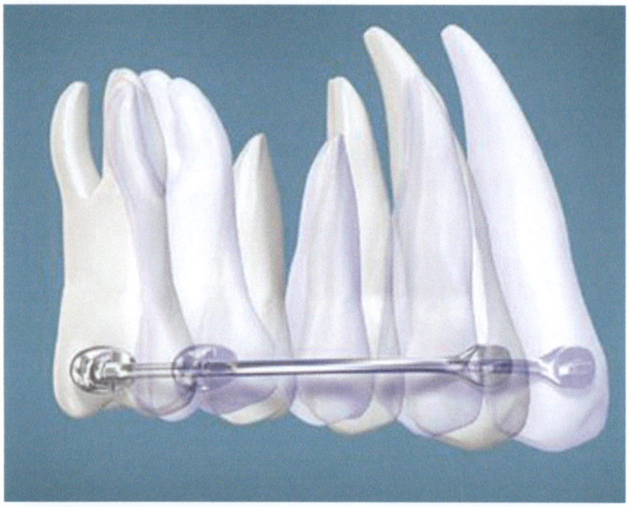

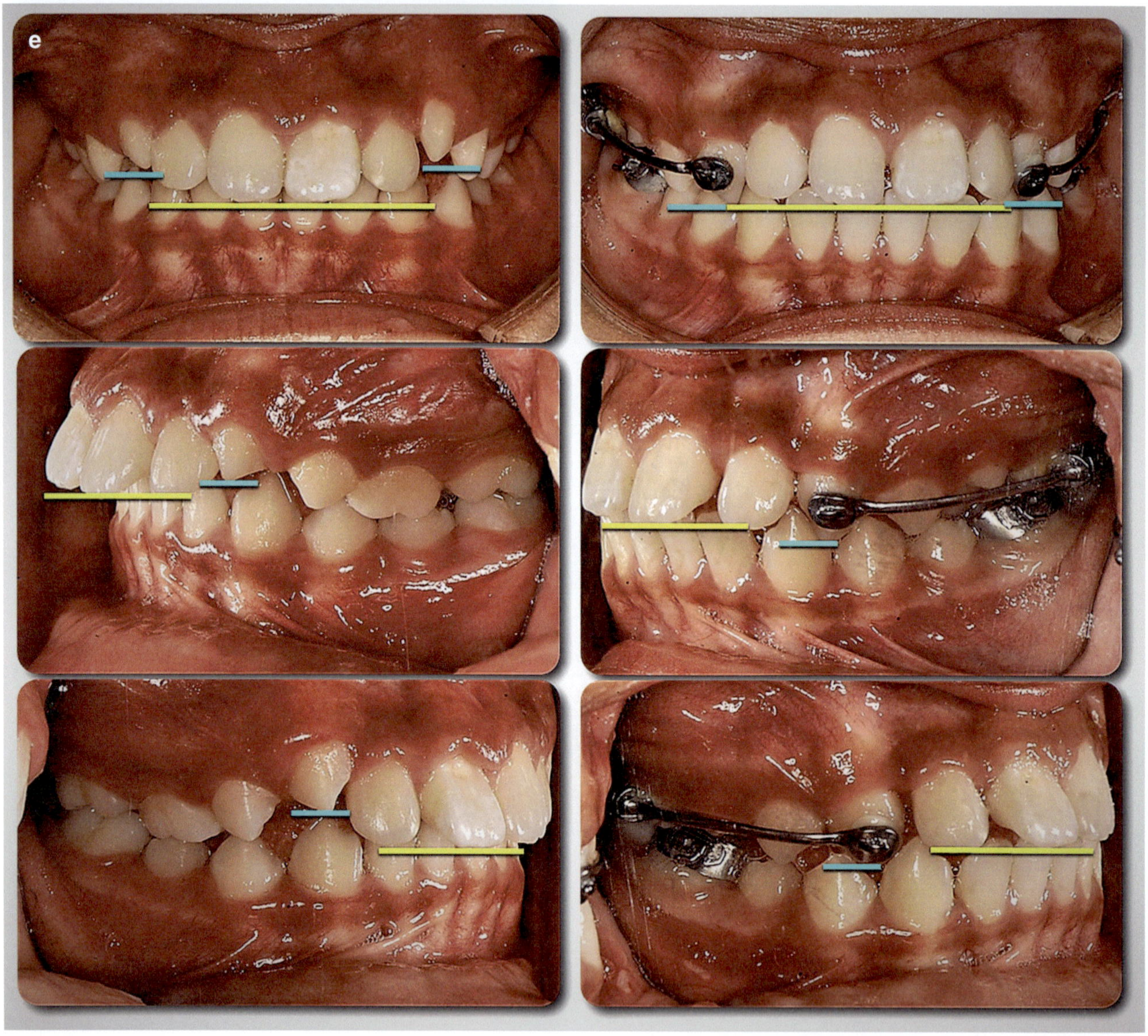

Fig. 10.26 (continued)

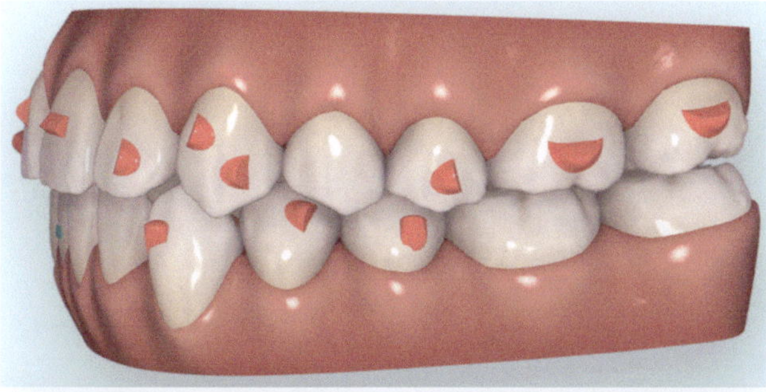

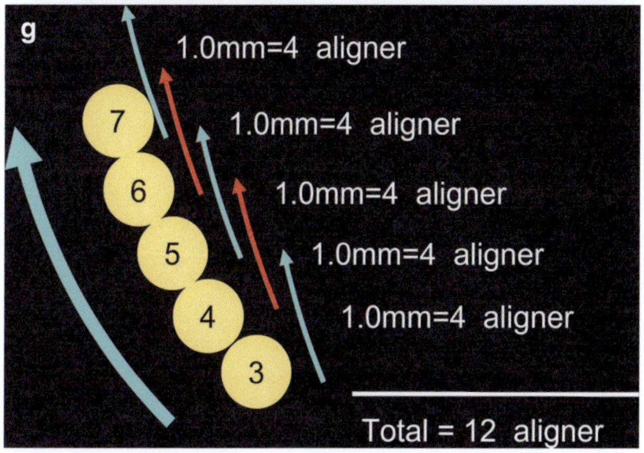

Fig. 10.26 (continued)

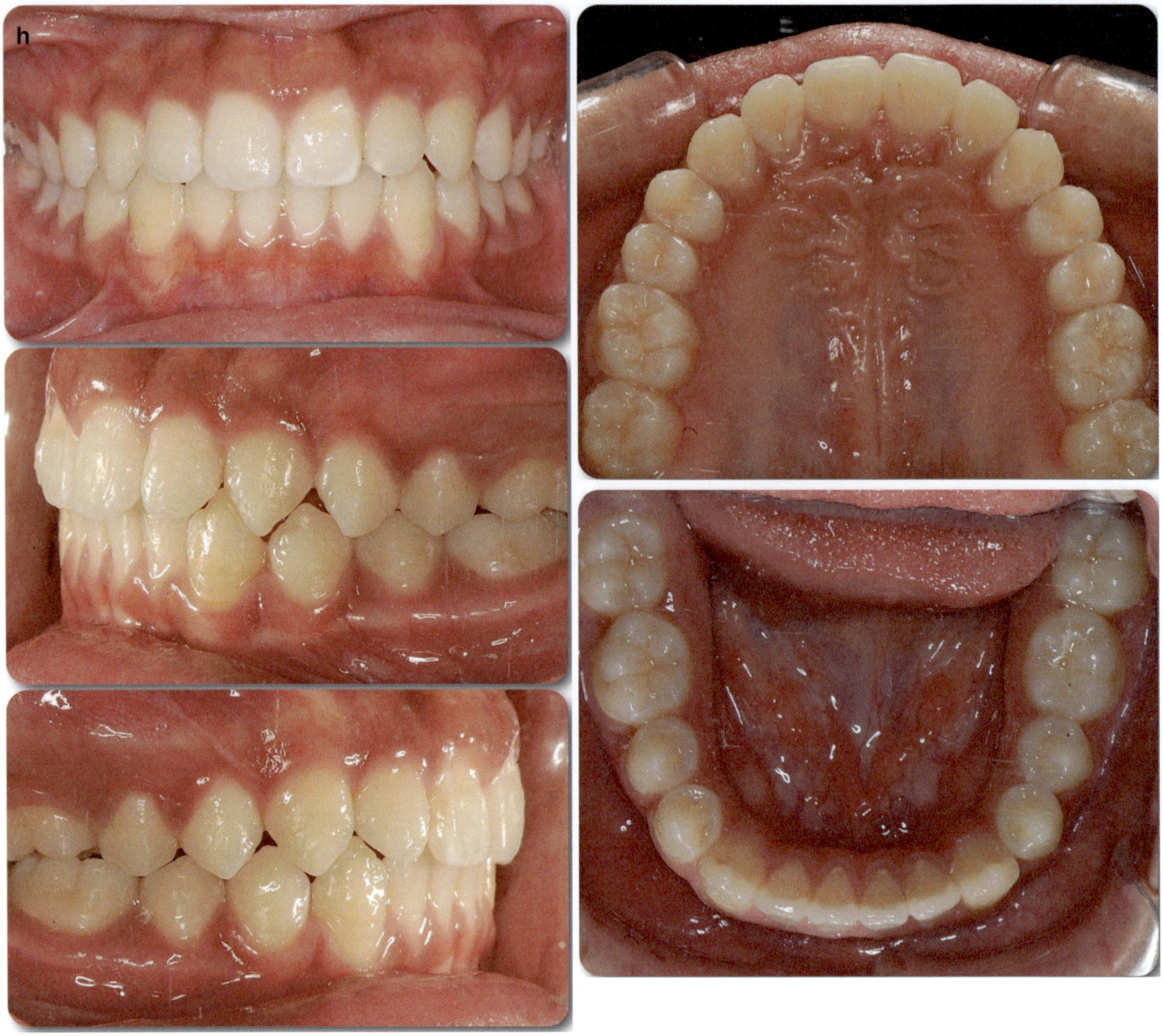

Fig. 10.26 (continued)

Case 3 was a 13-year-old male patient who presented with a class II, division 1 malocclusion and proclined upper incisors (Fig. 10.26a). The Carriere motion appliance™ was considered in order to first address the sagittal discrepancy. A prediction of the potential posterior tooth movements with the Carriere motion appliance™ was performed using imaging software [70] (Fig. 10.26b, c). As the prediction showed that the amount of distalization would be adequate, this therapeutic approach was retained.

Once the distalization was achieved (Fig. 10.26e), another intraoral scan of the patient was taken, and the virtual dental casts were uploaded to the ClinCheck™ software from Align™ technology. The software was used to evaluate the potential alignment of the dentition and the dental occlusion that would be obtained from the use of orthodontic aligners, which was chosen as the modality of treatment in this case (Fig. 10.26f, g). This prediction allowed the treating orthodontist to decide the most appropriate course of treatment in a proactive way.

Figure 10.26h shows the final intraoral photos, where a class I molar occlusion was achieved with adequate overbite and overjet and coincident midlines. The total treatment time was 21 months. This case illustrates the advantages of using the predictive capabilities of 3D software in the simulation of two-phase treatment options and in designing the most appropriate treatment approach.

Case 4: 3D Simulation of Extraction Versus Non-extraction Case

The decision to treat patients with or without premolar extractions is complex and not always clear-cut, as both the approaches present with advantages and disadvantages [71]. Having the capacity to assess and evaluate both the treatment options and their outcomes before starting the treatment is an asset in the determination of the most appropriate treatment plan [72].

A 13-year-old female patient with a class II, division 1 malocclusion presented for orthodontic assessment. The patient was a vertical grower, had moderate crowding in both arches (with buccally positioned upper left, upper right, and lower right canines), and a 3 mm mandibular midline deviation to the right (Fig. 10.27a, b).

An occlusogram was performed following the facial analysis, which indicated that repositioning the upper incisors 1.5 mm lingually and incorporating 1 mm of intrusion would result in the most esthetic treatment outcome (Fig. 10.27e). Intraoral scanning was performed, and STL files of the dentition in occlusion were uploaded to the DMA-DDP-Ortho™ software in order to perform the two treatment simulations (Fig. 10.27c).

In the first simulation, 4 second premolars were extracted, and the spaces were closed, respecting the initial occlusogram (Fig. 10.27c). In the extraction simulation, a significant amount of protraction in the lower arch was required, which made this option more complex than anticipated (Fig. 10.27d).

The second simulation used a non-extraction approach (Fig. 10.27c) and quantified the movements that were necessary to reposition the lower midline and to align the dentition. The planned occlusogram could not be used for the maxillary incisor position in this treatment option, as no lingual movement of the upper incisors was planned with this

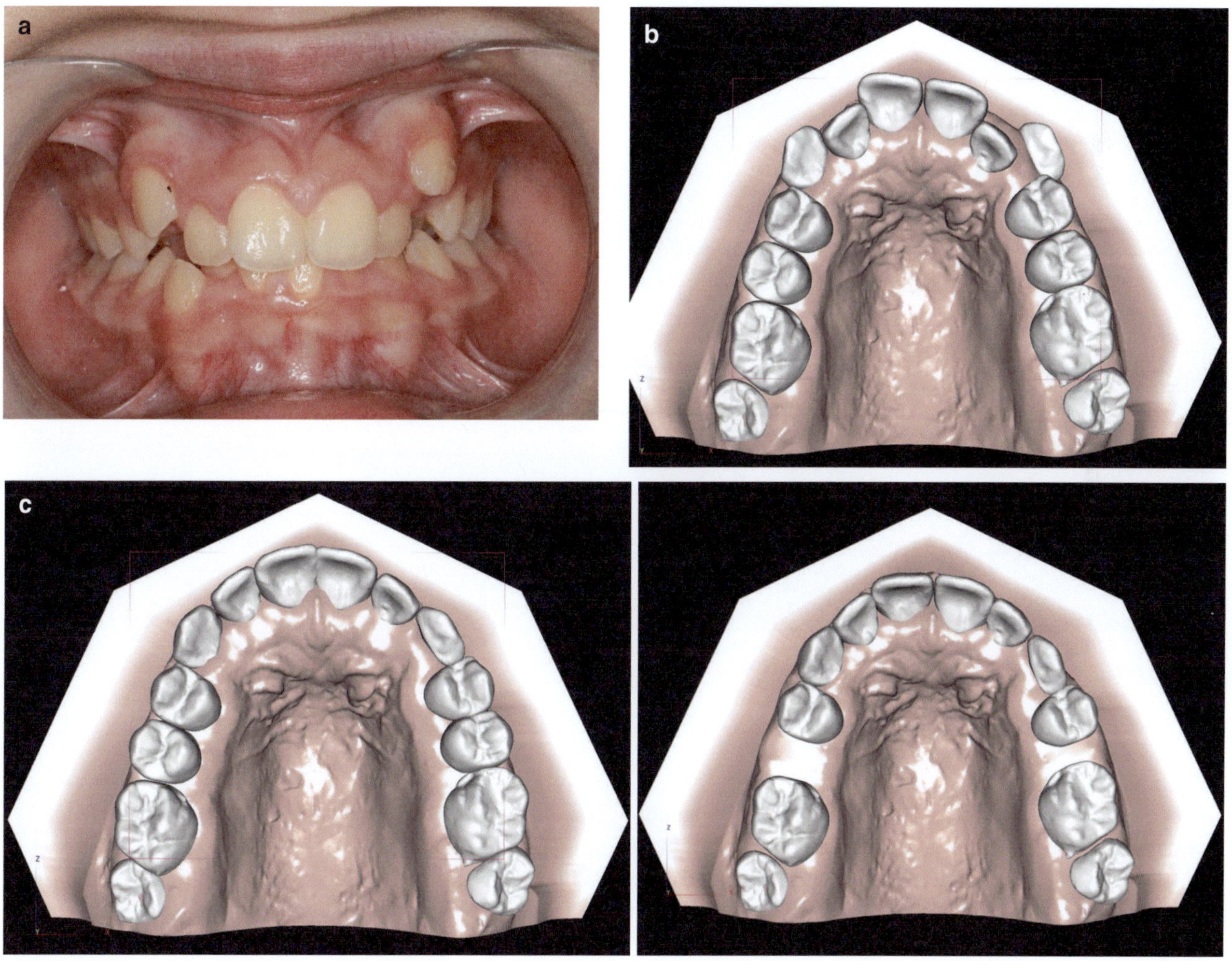

Fig. 10.27 (**a**) Frontal view of malocclusion showing the lower midline deviation and blocked out upper canines. (**b**) Occlusal view of the virtual models. (**c**) Simulation of extraction and non-extraction protocols. (**d**) Models showing the amount of protraction necessary to solve the malocclusion. (**e**) Cephalometric radiograph showing the desired position of the incisors

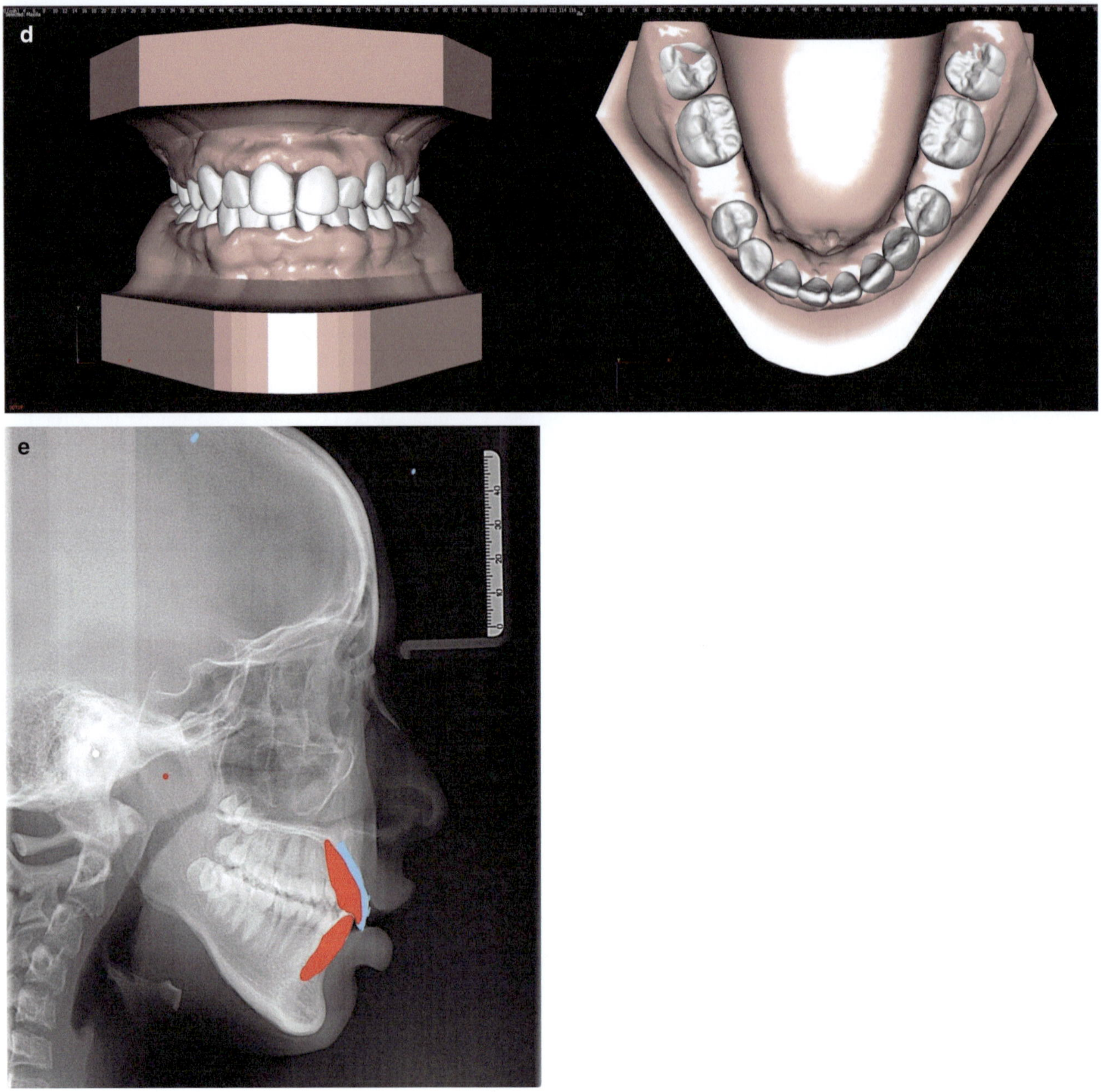

Fig. 10.27 (continued)

approach. In the non-extraction approach, the midline correction was better visualized, and a significant amount of correction was achieved by uprighting the lower left canine and premolars. This uprighting motion was quantifiable in the simulation and was deemed to be achievable by the treating orthodontist.

Figure 10.28 demonstrates the results of the non-extraction treatment at 1 year post-debond. The non-extraction approach allowed for lower midline correction and provided a satisfactory result without extractions.

10.13 Future Directions

While 3D diagnostics and treatment planning are promising, further development and advancement in artificial intelligence will still be required to create an ideal system. With the possible potential provided through the use of "big data" and neural networks, future diagnostic processes and treatment planning simulations in orthodontics may provide orthodontists with enhanced capabilities to both diagnose and predict treatment outcomes correctly and accurately.

Fig. 10.28 (**a**) Final intraoral pictures taken 12 months posttreatment showing a slight relapse of the class II on the left side. (**b**) Occlusal views. (**c**) Cephalometric radiograph 12 months posttreatment

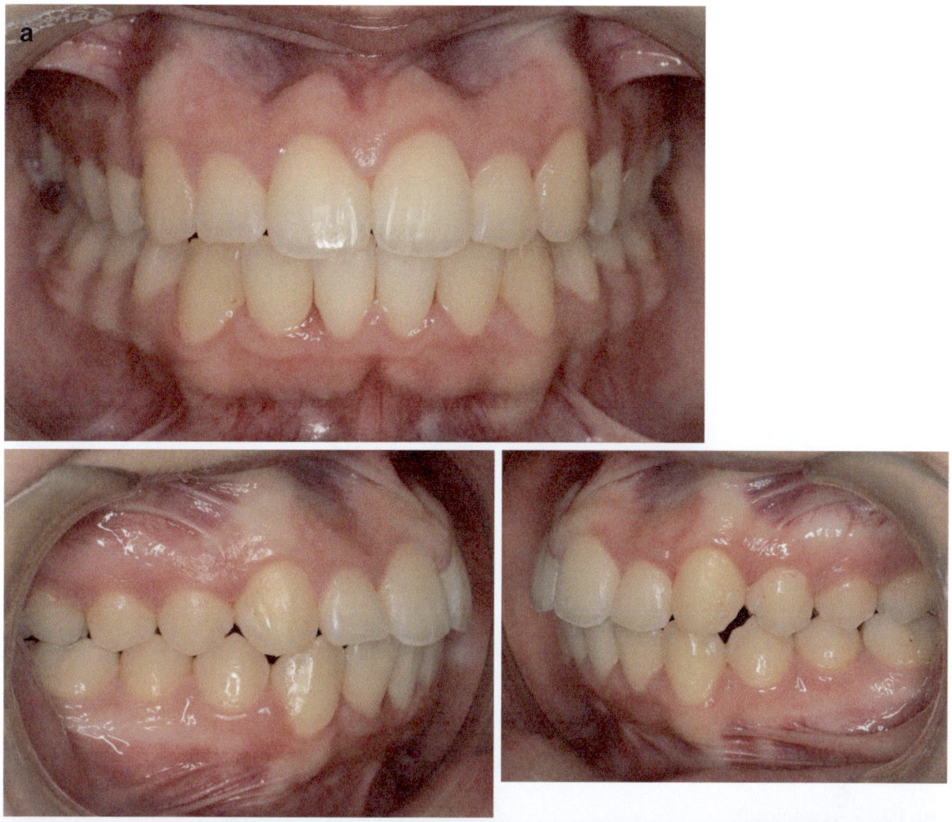

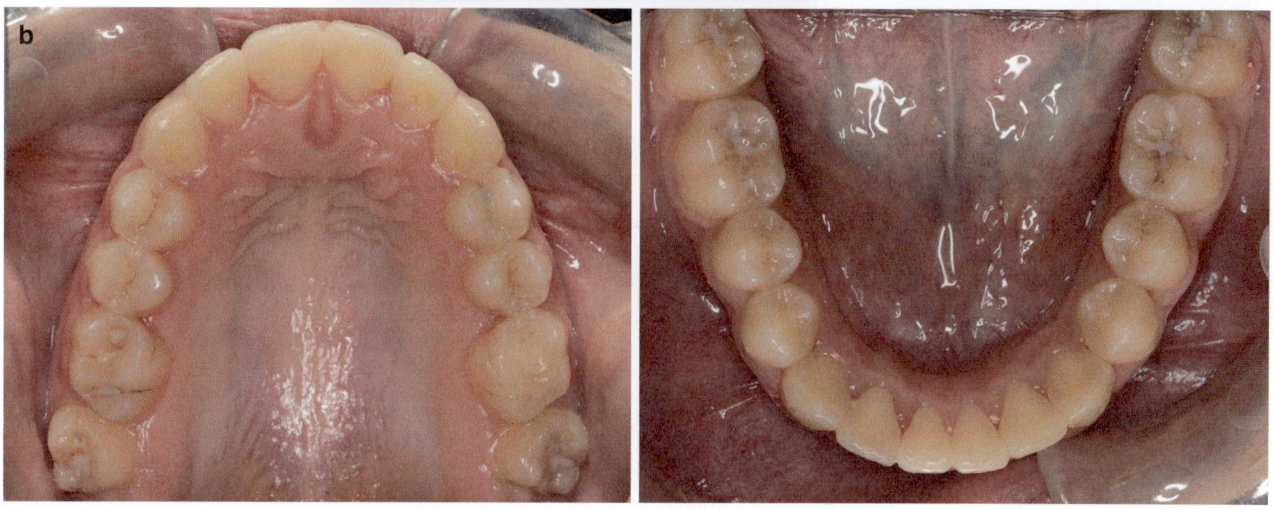

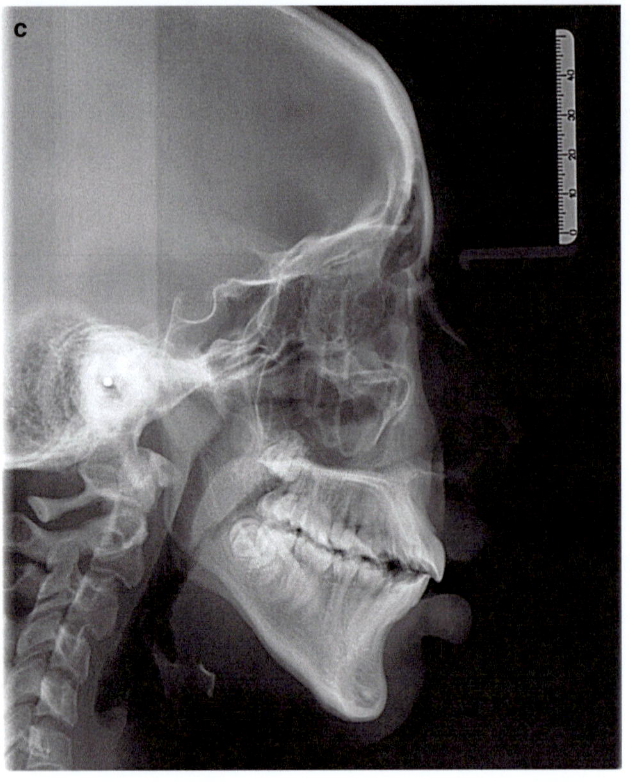

Fig. 10.28 (continued)

References

1. Plooij JM, Maal TJ, Haers P, Borstlap WA, Kuijpers-Jagtman AM, Bergé SJ. Digital three-dimensional image fusion processes for planning and evaluating orthodontics and orthognathic surgery. A systematic review. Int J Oral Maxillofac Surg. 2011;40(4):341–52.
2. Joda T, Gallucci GO. The virtual patient in dental medicine. Clin Oral Implants Res. 2015;26(6):725–6.
3. Kravitz ND, Groth C, Jones PE, Graham JW, Redmond WR. Intraoral digital scanners. J Clin Orthod. 2014;48(6): 337–47.
4. Figliuzzi M, Mangano F, Mangano C. A novel root analogue dental implant using CT scan and CAD/CAM: selective laser melting technology. Int J Oral Maxillofac Surg. 2012;41(7):858–62. https://doi.org/10.1016/j.ijom.2012.01.014.
5. Imburgia M, Logozzo S, Hauschild U, Veronesi G, Mangano C, Mangano FG. Accuracy of four intraoral scanners in oral implantology: a comparative in vitro study. BMC Oral Health. 2017;17(1):92.
6. Fleming P, Marinho V, Johal A. Orthodontic measurements on digital study models compared with plaster models: a systematic review. Orthod Craniofac Res. 2011;14(1):1–16.
7. Kau CH, Littlefield J, Rainy N, Nguyen JT, Creed B. Evaluation of CBCT digital models and traditional models using the Little's Index. Angle Orthod. 2010;80(3):435–9.
8. Jones P. The iTero optical scanner for use with Invisalign: a descriptive review. Dent Implantol Updat. 2008;19:1–4.
9. Martin CB, Chalmers EV, McIntyre GT, Cochrane H, Mossey PA. Orthodontic scanners: what's available? J Orthod. 2015;42(2): 136–43. https://doi.org/10.1179/1465313315Y.0000000001.
10. Luu NS, Nikolcheva LG, Retrouvey J-M, Flores-Mir C, El-Bialy T, Carey JP, et al. Linear measurements using virtual study models: a systematic review. Angle Orthod. 2012;82(6):1098–106.
11. Wiranto MG, Engelbrecht WP, Nolthenius HET, van der Meer WJ, Ren Y. Validity, reliability, and reproducibility of linear measurements on digital models obtained from intraoral and cone-beam computed tomography scans of alginate impressions. Am J Orthod Dentofac Orthop. 2013;143(1):140–7.
12. Yilmaz H, Ozlu FC, Karadeniz C, Karadeniz EI. Efficiency and accuracy of three-dimensional models versus dental casts: a clinical study. Turk J Orthod. 2019;32(4):214–8. https://doi.org/10.5152/TurkJOrthod.2019.19034.
13. Zhang F, Suh K-J, Lee K-M. Validity of intraoral scans compared with plaster models: an in-vivo comparison of dental measurements and 3D surface analysis. PLoS One. 2016;11(6):e0157713.
14. Joffe L. Current products and practices OrthoCAD™: digital models for a digital era. J Orthod. 2004;31(4):344–7.
15. Ciobota N-D. Standard tessellation language in rapid prototyping technology. National Institute of Research and Development for Mechatronics and Measurement Technique, Bucuresti, The Scientific Bulletin of Valahia University–Materials and Mechanics. 2012(7).
16. Valentan B, Brajlih T, Drstvensek I, Balic J. Basic solutions on shape complexity evaluation of STL data. J Achiev Mater Manuf Eng. 2008;26(1):73–80.
17. Hazeveld A, Huddleston Slater JJ, Ren Y. Accuracy and reproducibility of dental replica models reconstructed by different rapid prototyping techniques. Am J Orthod Dentofac Orthop. 2014;145(1):108–15. https://doi.org/10.1016/j.ajodo.2013.05.011.
18. Ventola CL. Medical applications for 3D printing: current and projected uses. Pharm Therap. 2014;39(10):704.
19. Sinthanayothin C, Tharanont W, editors. Orthodontics treatment simulation by teeth segmentation and setup. In: 2008 5th international conference on electrical engineering/electronics, computer, telecommunications and information technology, IEEE; 2008.
20. Lee S-H, Kim H-C, Hur S-M, Yang D-Y. STL file generation from measured point data by segmentation and Delaunay triangulation. Comput Aided Des. 2002;34(10):691–704.
21. Yaqi M, Zhongke L, editors. Computer aided orthodontics treatment by virtual segmentation and adjustment. In: 2010 international conference on image analysis and signal processing, IEEE; 2010.
22. Yau H-T, Yang T-J, Chen Y-C. Tooth model reconstruction based upon data fusion for orthodontic treatment simulation. Comput Biol Med. 2014;48:8–16.
23. Keilig L, Piesche K, Jäger A, Bourauel C. Applications of surface–surface matching algorithms for determination of orthodontic tooth movements. Comput Methods Biomech Biomed Engin. 2003;6(5–6):353–9.
24. Smith RJ, Burstone CJ. Mechanics of tooth movement. Am J Orthod. 1984;85(4):294–307.
25. Burstone CJ, Pryputniewicz RJ. Holographic determination of centers of rotation produced by orthodontic forces. Am J Orthod. 1980;77(4):396–409.
26. Hennessy J, Al-Awadhi EA. Clear aligners generations and orthodontic tooth movement. J Orthod. 2016;43(1):68–76.
27. Kravitz ND, Kusnoto B, BeGole E, Obrez A, Agran B. How well does Invisalign work? A prospective clinical study evaluating the efficacy of tooth movement with Invisalign. Am J Orthod Dentofac Orthop. 2009;135(1):27–35.
28. Chang YB, Xia JJ, Gateno J, Xiong Z, Zhou X, Wong ST. An automatic and robust algorithm of reestablishment of digital dental occlusion. IEEE Trans Med Imaging. 2010;29(9):1652–63. https://doi.org/10.1109/TMI.2010.2049526.
29. Cheng C, Cheng X, Dai N, Liu Y, Fan Q, Hou Y, et al. Personalized orthodontic accurate tooth arrangement system with complete teeth model. J Med Syst. 2015;39(9):84.
30. Rodrigues MAF, Silva WB, Neto MEB, Gillies DF, Ribeiro IM. An interactive simulation system for training and treatment planning in orthodontics. Comput Graph. 2007;31(5):688–97.

31. Im J, Cha J-Y, Lee K-J, Yu H-S, Hwang C-J. Comparison of virtual and manual tooth setups with digital and plaster models in extraction cases. Am J Orthod Dentofac Orthop. 2014;145(4):434–42.
32. Qiu N, Fan R, You L, Jin X. An efficient and collision-free hole-filling algorithm for orthodontics. Vis Comput. 2013;29(6–8):577–86.
33. Missier MS, George AM, Vardhan A. Estimating the amount of crowding in different occlusal patterns. Estimating the amount of crowding in different occlusal patterns. Int J Res Pharm Sci. 2018;9(4):1611–5.
34. Phan X, Ling PH. Clinical limitations of Invisalign. J Can Dent Assoc. 2007;73(3):263–6.
35. Simon M, Keilig L, Schwarze J, Jung BA, Bourauel C. Treatment outcome and efficacy of an aligner technique–regarding incisor torque, premolar derotation and molar distalization. BMC Oral Health. 2014;14(1):68.
36. Morais JF, Melsen B, de Freitas KM, Castello Branco N, Garib DG, Cattaneo PM. Evaluation of maxillary buccal alveolar bone before and after orthodontic alignment without extractions: a cone beam computed tomographic study. Angle Orthod. 2018;88(6):748–56.
37. Creekmore TD, Kunik RL. Straight wire: the next generation. Am J Orthod Dentofac Orthop. 1993;104(1):8–20.
38. Fiorelli G, Melsen B, Modica C. The design of custom orthodontic mechanics. Clin Orthod Res. 2000;3(4):210–9.
39. Burstone CJ, Koenig HA. Force systems from an ideal arch. Am J Orthod. 1974;65(3):270–89.
40. Chisari JR, McGorray SP, Nair M, Wheeler TT. Variables affecting orthodontic tooth movement with clear aligners. Am J Orthod Dentofac Orthop. 2014;145(4):S82–91.
41. Rossini G, Parrini S, Castroflorio T, Deregibus A, Debernardi CL. Efficacy of clear aligners in controlling orthodontic tooth movement: a systematic review. Angle Orthod. 2015;85(5):881–9.
42. Bowman SJ, editor. Improving the predictability of clear aligners. Seminars in orthodontics. Saunders: Elsevier; 2017.
43. Morton J, Derakhshan M, Kaza S, Li C, editors. Design of the Invisalign system performance. Seminars in orthodontics. Elsevier; 2017.
44. Sachdeva RC, Aranha SL, Egan ME, Gross HT, Sachdeva NS, Frans Currier G, et al. Treatment time: SureSmile vs conventional. Orthod Art Pract Dentofac Enhanc. 2012;13:72.
45. Raphael E, Sandrik JL, Klapper L. Rotation of rectangular wire in rectangular molar tubes: part I. Am J Orthod. 1981;80(2):136–44.
46. Matasa CG. Bracket angulation as a function of its length in the canine distal movement. Am J Orthod Dentofac Orthop. 1996;110(2):178–84.
47. Sachdeva R. Integrating digital and robotic technologies. Diagnosis, treatment planning, and therapeutics. In: Orthodontic current principles and techniques; 2012, 5.
48. Mah J, Sachdeva R. Computer-assisted orthodontic treatment: the SureSmile process. Am J Orthod Dentofac Orthop. 2001;120(1):85–7.
49. Nguyen T, Jackson T, editors. 3D technologies for precision in orthodontics. Seminars in orthodontics. Elsevier; 2018.
50. Hales BM, Pronovost PJ. The checklist—a tool for error management and performance improvement. J Crit Care. 2006;21(3): 231–5.
51. Almog D, Marin CS, Proskin HM, Cohen MJ, Kyrkanides S, Malmstrom H. The effect of esthetic consultation methods on acceptance of diastema-closure treatment plan: a pilot study. J Am Dent Assoc. 2004;135(7):875–81.
52. Morisky DE, Malotte CK, Choi P, Davidson P, Rigler S, Sugland B, et al. A patient education program to improve adherence rates with antituberculosis drug regimens. Health Educ Q. 1990;17(3): 253–66.
53. Kokich VO Jr, Kinzer GA. Managing congenitally missing lateral incisors. Part I: canine substitution. J Esthet Restor Dent. 2005;17(1):5–10.
54. Kokich VO, Kinzer GA, Janakievski J. Congenitally missing maxillary lateral incisors: restorative replacement. Am J Orthod Dentofac Orthop. 2011;139(4):443.
55. Nanda R, Uribe FA, Yadav S. Temporary anchorage devices in orthodontics e-book. Elsevier Health Sciences; 2019.
56. Brough E, Donaldson AN, Naini FB. Canine substitution for missing maxillary lateral incisors: the influence of canine morphology, size, and shade on perceptions of smile attractiveness. Am J Orthod Dentofac Orthop. 2010;138(6):705.e1–9.
57. Schneider U, Moser L, Fornasetti M, Piattella M, Siciliani G. Esthetic evaluation of implants vs canine substitution in patients with congenitally missing maxillary lateral incisors: are there any new insights? Am J Orthod Dentofac Orthop. 2016;150(3):416–24.
58. Oliver R, Mannion J, Robinson J. Morphology of the maxillary lateral incisor in cases of unilateral impaction of the maxillary canine. Br J Orthod. 1989;16(1):9–16.
59. Mavreas D, Athanasiou AE. Factors affecting the duration of orthodontic treatment: a systematic review. Eur J Orthod. 2008;30(4):386–95.
60. Dalessandri D, Migliorati M, Visconti L, Contardo L, Kau CH, Martin C. KPG index versus OPG measurements: a comparison between 3D and 2D methods in predicting treatment duration and difficulty level for patients with impacted maxillary canines. Biomed Res Int. 2014;2014:537620.
61. Eslami E, Barkhordar H, Abramovitch K, Kim J, Masoud MI. Cone-beam computed tomography vs conventional radiography in visualization of maxillary impacted-canine localization: a systematic review of comparative studies. Am J Orthod Dentofac Orthop. 2017;151(2):248–58.
62. Alqerban A, Jacobs R, Lambrechts P, Loozen G, Willems G. Root resorption of the maxillary lateral incisor caused by impacted canine: a literature review. Clin Oral Investig. 2009;13(3):247–55.
63. Haney E, Gansky SA, Lee JS, Johnson E, Maki K, Miller AJ, et al. Comparative analysis of traditional radiographs and cone-beam computed tomography volumetric images in the diagnosis and treatment planning of maxillary impacted canines. Am J Orthod Dentofac Orthop. 2010;137(5):590–7.
64. Kapila S, Conley R, Harrell W Jr. The current status of cone beam computed tomography imaging in orthodontics. Dentomaxillofac Radiol. 2011;40(1):24–34.
65. Suri S, Utreja A, Rattan V. Orthodontic treatment of bilaterally impacted maxillary canines in an adult. Am J Orthod Dentofac Orthop. 2002;122(4):429–37.
66. Chandhoke TK, Agarwal S, Feldman J, Shah RA, Upadhyay M, Nanda R. An efficient biomechanical approach for the management of an impacted maxillary central incisor. Am J Orthod Dentofac Orthop. 2014;146(2):249–54.
67. Graber LW, Vanarsdall RL, Vig KW, Huang GJ. Orthodontics-E-book: current principles and techniques. Elsevier Health Sciences; 2016.
68. Kinzinger GS, Fritz UB, Sander F-G, Diedrich PR. Efficiency of a pendulum appliance for molar distalization related to second and third molar eruption stage. Am J Orthod Dentofac Orthop. 2004;125(1):8–23.
69. Karlsson I, Bondemark L. Intraoral maxillary molar distalization. Angle Orthod. 2006;76(6):923–9.
70. Hamilton C, Saltaji H, Preston C, Flores-Mir C, Tabbaa S. Adolescent patients' experience with the Carriere distalizer appliance. Eur J Paediatr Dent. 2013;14(3):219–24.
71. Luppanapornlarp S, Johnston LE Jr. The effects of premolar-extraction: a long-term comparison of outcomes in "clear-cut" extraction and nonextraction class II patients. Angle Orthod. 1993;63(4):257–72.
72. Xie X, Wang L, Wang A. Artificial neural network modeling for deciding if extractions are necessary prior to orthodontic treatment. Angle Orthod. 2010;80(2):262–6.

11 Digital Planning in Orthognathic Surgery

Marco Caminiti

11.1 Introduction

Planning OGS remains an important challenge for surgeons and orthodontists alike. The methods for proper diagnosis are well documented and have not changed with the development of technologies other than the facilitation of communication and ease of data capture. Conversely, the technical orthodontic and surgical aspects have not changed much over the past 20 years, and advances in materials and surgical outcomes are still related to experience and surgical planning. The current method of planning cases using 3D technologies has transformed the practice and the outcomes in surgical orthodontic treatment. Notwithstanding these improvements, errors do occur and are due to errors in judgment. Understanding the advantages of digital over analog surgical planning will demonstrate the benefit and accuracy of digital data acquisition and planning. It is the production of accurate interfaces that have allowed for improved outcomes [1–3].

The biggest change and improvement in the orthognathic process have occurred because of digital technologies in planning and splint (surgical guide) fabrication [3]. A variety of digital platforms can be used to improve the ability to accurately diagnose problems and to determine what movements are required—i.e., computer-aided design. These same digital platforms are then used to produce accurate interfaces that allow for improved outcomes using prefabricated surgical guides and splints—i.e., computer-aided manufacturing. Key steps in the digital workup for OGS will include digital panoramic and cephalometric analysis, digital occlusal scanning, recommended CT capture with the use of fiducial markers for complex cases, understanding the importance of obtaining a proper centric relation, uploading of data, and simplifying the online meeting or planning session. New developments that digital planning allows that was not previously available includes the determination of hinge axis to aid in vertical prediction, the ability to exactly pinpoint central incisor position (vertical, horizontal, and angular), surgical orthodontic preparation using clear aligner technology (while understanding the limitations and advantages), proper aids in estimating yaw deformities/deviations, the ease of mandible first double-jaw surgery and its advantages, and encouraging a degree of comfort in practitioners in the control of digitally set occlusions. The final decision requires a solid framework and disciplined execution which combines all the data and interprets the findings that are supported by a sound clinical examination. The eventual goal is to be able to attend the operating room with surgical guides in hand and a completed and well-documented patients' custom surgical plan. The focus of this chapter is describing to an orthodontic audience the methods and sequence to accurately position the maxillomandibular complex as followed in our surgical orthodontic center at the University of Toronto. The final decision requires a solid framework and disciplined execution which combines all the data and interprets the findings of the clinical examination.

It must be noted that creating surgical guides using analog methods (alginate impressions, stone models, articulators, semi-adjustable articulators (galletti), stone cutting, and luting of segmental stone models, acrylic, or PVS splint fabrication) is still commonplace and still has a role in simple single-jaw cases. The very early comparisons between analog and the rudimentary digital planning did not show that the digital technologies were adequate [4]. However, with time, the errors with the analog method when compared to the accuracy of digital planning eventually revealed a level of precision that is not comparable especially when dealing with double-jaw surgery [1, 3, 5, 6].

M. Caminiti (✉)
Oral and Maxillofacial Surgery, Faculty of Dentistry, University of Toronto, Toronto, ON, Canada

Oral and Maxillofaical Surgery, Humber River Hospital, Toronto, ON, Canada

Jaw Deformity Clinic, Holland Bloorview Kids Rehabilitation Hospital, Toronto, ON, Canada
e-mail: marco.caminiti@utoronto.ca

J.-M. Retrouvey, M.-N. Abdallah (eds.), *3D Diagnosis and Treatment Planning in Orthodontics*,
https://doi.org/10.1007/978-3-030-57223-5_11

The teeth guide the occlusion, but the occlusion is guided by the desired esthetics. The surgical orthodontic treatment plan is based on the position of the maxillary central incisor (angular, vertical, horizontal). This position is determined using the clinical, panoramic, cephalometric, and computed tomography. Esthetics starts with recognizing best esthetic relative to specific racial and gender norms, determining the vertical and horizontal position of the dentition as well as evaluation of the cant, occlusal plane, and incisor angulations and obviously patient expectations.

The intraoral examination in a surgical candidate is somewhat different from that in a nonsurgical orthodontic candidate in that in the former, the malocclusion is secondary to discrepancies in the maxillary and mandibular position. In other words, in a surgical candidate, the occlusion in situ is not representative of the orthodontic needs or “readiness.” Therefore, much of the needed information is obtained from a set of dental models (standard or digital), as these allow the clinician to hand-articulate them into a better sagittal relationship and assess a multitude of important orthodontic data. It is for this reason that in a surgical candidate, evaluation of dental models should be regarded *as part of the physical examination* and not an ancillary step.

Prior to making the esthetic diagnosis, it is important to recognize that facial esthetics is a subjective quality that is subject to change with time, gender, race, and cultural setting. The clinician must be cognizant of these variations and attempt to elicit as much information as possible during the initial patient interview. Key items in the esthetic evaluation are discussed below.

(a) Incisal display
An esthetically pleasing incisal display at rest is a key component to facial esthetics. There is some variability in age and gender, with a higher display range seen in younger patients and in females.
(b) Central incisor position and angulation
The horizontal position and angulation have a profound impact on the overall facial esthetics. The A-P position and angulation play a crucial role in upper lip support, which in turn play a central role in nasolabial esthetics. We clinicians must be able to reasonably *anticipate* the incisal position after presurgical orthodontics, surgery, and postsurgical orthodontics.
(c) Profile and nasolabial esthetics
A straight profile is generally preferred, and both qualitative (clinician’s subjective assessment) and objective quantitative (e.g., convexity angle [7]) can be used during the assessment. Elements that make up the profile silhouette include the nasal projection, upper lip projection and angulation, chin position, and morphology.

In this chapter, no single measurement is suggested. A dogmatic approach to esthetic determination is fraught with error, and determination of changes requires patient and clinician discussion as the definition of best esthetics is controversial [8]. For example, while a nasolabial angle of 90–105° is considered esthetically pleasing, the components that make up the nasolabial angle is arguably more important, i.e., nasal tip projection and lip position.

11.2 When Is the Ideal Age for OGS and How Can We Determine This with Our Digital Processes?

The combination of wrist films, superimposition of lateral cephalometry or spheno-occipital synchondrosis seen in CBCT guides to determine growth cessation. The surgical orthodontic team should get a good idea of the suitability for timing. In general, the ideal age for surgery appears in the realm of [9–12]:

- Severe class III mandibular excess: You can initiate phase 1 orthodontics with expansion and alignment. Delay surgery until demonstration of completion of mandibular growth. This could be as late as 22–24 years old.
- In severe asymmetry and unilateral hypertrophy, the surgery may need to be delayed until bone scans demonstrate cessation of growth activity of the hypertrophic condyle.
- In cases with vertical maxillary excess (class I + class II): The surgery can be considered before growth is complete when psychosocial factors dictate; however, these patients may require mandibular surgery in the future.
- In cases with maxillary transverse deficiency: Orthodontic expansion may be effective up to age 14 years (girls) and 16 years (boys). Thereafter, expansion of the maxilla may require either a surgical expansion (SARPE) or segmental osteotomy.
- Some mandibular deficiencies may be treated early as these patients will have the same class II relationships throughout growth. The mandibular advancement in this group is stable. However, younger patients do show greater changes than adult treated cases especially in larger movements.

Notwithstanding, the psychosocial needs and requirements of the patient may supersede these growth determinants, and close monitoring of mental maturity and preparedness is required. The influence of social media on our patients is a further element to be aware of when counseling is performed [13]. A fine balance between too early surgery resulting in a poorly prepared patient subjecting them to relapse and possible stunting subsequent growth needs to be tempered by performing surgery too late when orthodontic management, patient compliance, the effects of social stigma, and burnout lead to an unsatisfied patient.

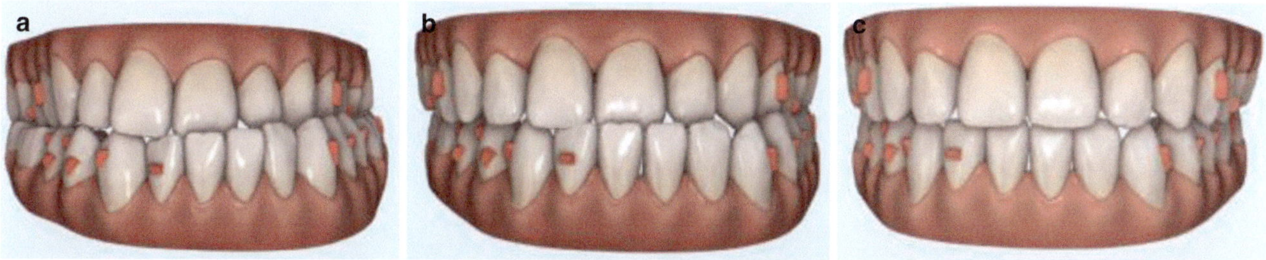

Fig. 11.1 There is uncertainty in planning for the transverse discrepancy seen in (**a**). Measurements showed an 8 mm too narrow maxilla. Whether a SARPE or segmental expansion or dental expansion was required was solved by a clear aligner "ideal diagnostic wax up". These realistic predictions showed that in (**b**) (pre-surgery with decompensations) the dentition did not require SARPE or Segmental Lefort. The image in (**c**) shows the post-surgical prediction with good transverse alignment. These predictions can be invaluable in surgical orthodontic planning

"*Readiness*" for surgery depends on three items:

1. Maturity/growth (including patient mental maturity)
2. Orthodontic preparedness for postoperative finishing
3. Requirements for successful surgical preparation and execution

11.3 When Are Patients Orthodontically Ready for Surgery?

This was once completely dependent on the orthodontic setup. Decompensation of the occlusion was the main objective. Teeth ideally should be placed over basal bone and in a stable position. Orthodontists must also minimize any excessive intrusive or extrusive movements or indeed even expansive movements outside of the alveolar envelope. It is important not to perform class II or class III elastic mechanics in correction.

With the push toward surgical first OGS [14], different mechanical systems (clear aligners, lingual orthodontics, Damon, Andrews, etc.) [15] and the movement to mandible first sequencing [16] what was once established protocol is no longer *de rigueur*. Orthodontic treatment to level and align the occlusion, the closure of all spaces, study model checks of the setup, and seeing if a perfect class I can be obtained is no longer a requirement. Current approaches to preparedness are whether the orthodontic team can *finish* postsurgical cases. The ideal A-P position with a class I canine, the securing of proper overbite, and no crossbites are the minimal needs for the orthodontist. Given these results, final alignment [12] or leveling may be facilitated after surgery, but the orthodontist needs to play a role in this decision.

Study models: Either stone (analog) or digital models physically produced are used to demonstrate the direction the presurgical orthodontic movements are taking. If patients are having the orthomechanics with clear aligners, then diagnostic working models can be virtually demonstrated to the surgical orthodontic team using the software interface used by the CAT provider (e.g., Invisalign and ClinCheck) (Fig. 11.1). However, the accuracy of ClinCheck with certain movements—especially in the transverse dimension—tends to be underestimated [17].

With time, the surgical execution of OGS and the associated osteotomies does usually not present with great challenges. It remains the planning, preparation, patient care, and vigilant follow-up that now have shifted our focus. Technologies have facilitated the preparation of the surgical plan unlike any other advancements in surgical orthodontics. Advances in materials (miniplates) and techniques (clear aligners) have made a significant difference in the way we practice, but by far the greatest improvement has been in the ease of planning and computer-aided simulated surgery (CASS) [3, 18].

11.3.1 Space Analysis, Arch Length, Incisor Position Angulations

It is important to quantify the amount of crowding or spacing within the dental arches because treatment will vary according to the severity of crowding or spacing. Space analysis is simply the difference between the space available and the space required. It can be performed directly on dental casts (by calipers) or on digital scans (by computer algorithm). In general, class II malocclusions tend to have multiple factors affecting space analysis because they have increased crowding in the mandible compared to the maxilla, and the maxillary incisors can have excess angulation (Division 1) or retroclination (Division 2). Most of the time, the incisor angulation is compensated with proclination, and most class II have an accentuated curve of Spee.

It is important to recognize that the incisor angulation affects the total space required. It is these measurements that

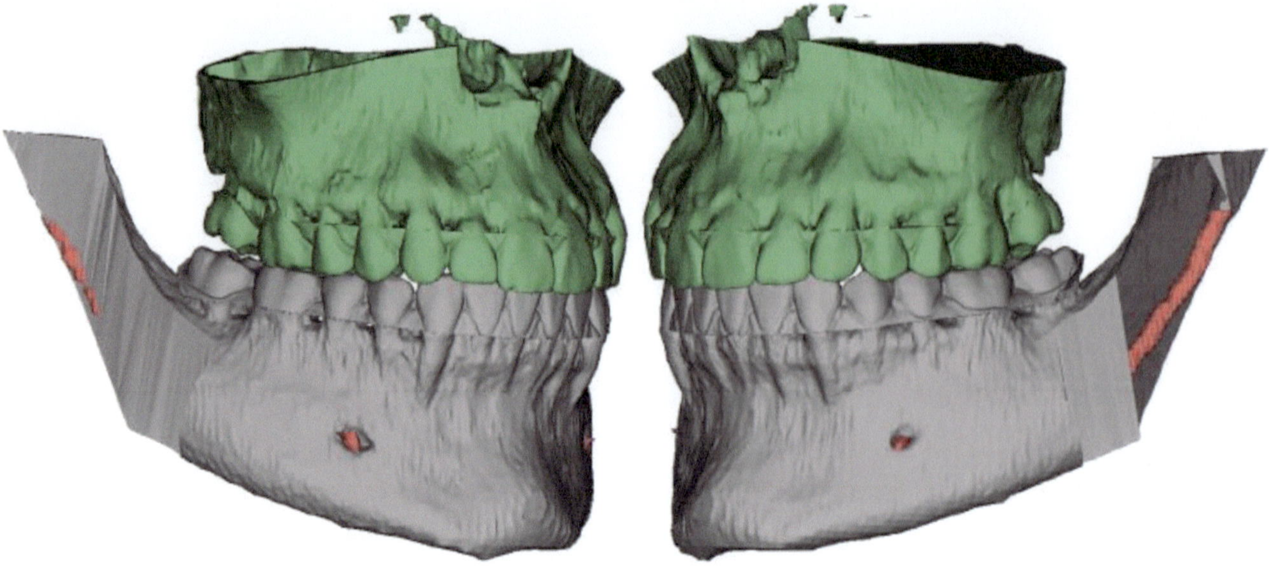

Fig. 11.2 These images demonstrate that even with the best intentions, tooth size discrepancies may not always be addressed orthodontically. Here the canines cannot be placed into a class I without segmentation of the maxilla—however, the already wide lateral incisors cannot afford to be cosmetically widened so the compromise is to leave the occlusion in this class II position

help the orthodontist decide on whether teeth are required to be extracted, proximally reduced, or merely tipped to gain or create space in the arch.

The classic method to determine these measurements was with stone models; however, contemporary and more accurate measurements are obtained with Digital Planning software and Clear Aligner Technology and the applied computer-aided simulations (i.e., ClinCheck) as shown in Fig. 11.1.

11.3.2 Bolton Analysis and Its Importance: Assess Tooth Size Discrepancies

The Bolton Analysis relates the mesiodistal width of the maxillary teeth compared with the mandibular teeth. The ratio of widths of the anterior six teeth (incisors and canines) is about **77.2%** (mandibular teeth/maxillary teeth) and the ratio of the widths of all teeth from first molar on the right side to the first molar on the left side is about **91.3%** (mandibular teeth/maxillary teeth) [19].

Approximately 5% of the population have some degree of tooth size discrepancy (TSD). A TSD of greater than 1.5 mm is considered clinically significant. And most of the clinically significant TSDs are in the anterior region and due to small maxillary laterals. If not accounted for, in the desire to establish an ideal overbite and overjet, it may result in a class II end-on buccal segment relationship [20]. The method in which to correct most TSD is by building up the maxillary lateral incisor, performing interproximal reduction of the anterior mandibular teeth, or even extracting a lower incisor (but this results in a challenge in canine coordination and leaves excess overjet at times).

The problem with the Bolton Analysis is that it should be used as a guide because it does not consider the labio-lingual thickness of incisors, the axial inclination of the incisors, nor the marginal ridge thickness (see Fig. 11.2). However, it must be recognized that almost 60% of surgical class II patients present with anterior Bolton excess [21].

11.4 Decompensation of the Occlusion

To perform stable and predictable orthodontics, the goals remain that to **aligning the arches, level the curve of Spee, and decompensate the dentition.** The general trend is to create a presurgical discrepancy that is at least as great as the underlying skeletal discrepancy. This will permit the use of the occlusion as a guide to position jaws during surgery. It maximizes surgical correction of the malocclusion.

Space may be required for ideal alignment in order to correct arch length deficiency (crowding), an accentuated curve of Spee, incisor proclination/protrusion, dental arch asymmetries/midline deviations, and as mentioned previously, tooth size discrepancy. The treatment options depend on the amount of space required, and in general [20], if the space required is ≤4 mm, then extractions are rarely indicated. These can be managed by expansion and/or IPR. Extractions may be considered in cases of severe incisor protrusion or vertical discrepancy [21, 22].

11.5 Leveling the Curve of Spee

The decision to level the curve of Spee before or after surgery should be based on planning for the desired vertical change. Presurgical leveling allows for mandibular advancement with minimal clockwise rotation of the mandible, which helps promote horizontal movement and chin prominence. Postsurgical leveling allows for mandibular advancement with increased clockwise rotation of the mandible, which helps promote vertical movement. The decision to the curve of Spee presurgically has an important impact on the lower face height and chin projection! [22]. In Low angle cases, the curve of Spee is not leveled in general. Steps are placed in all rectangular arch wires including the stabilizing arch wire. During surgery, the splint utilized tends to be thicker in premolar area. The overall movements of the mandible induce a clockwise rotation of mandible which will increase the mandibular angle and increase in lower face height. Post-surgically, the extrusion of premolars with reverse curve of Spee arch wires, intermaxillary vertical elastics, is performed, and the teeth will erupt faster without an opposing dentition.

In high-angle cases, the curve of Spee is leveled presurgically. This is done by intrusion of incisors with intrusive base arch, TADs. Sometimes, an anterior open bite may occur. During surgery, a thin splint and counterclockwise rotation of mandible is allowed, and this will decrease in lower face height and increase chin projection. Postsurgically, the extrusion of premolars is minimized, to prevent the development of an AOB and maintain chin projection and improves stability.

11.6 Quick Method to Measure Transverse Discrepancy

Discrepancies in sagittal position of the maxilla and the mandible alter the relative transverse relationship. When this relationship is corrected (via hand-articulation into a class I occlusion, which roughly "simulates" the anteroposterior surgical movements), the transverse relationship could change. Reversal of a transverse discrepancy on hand-articulation is then referred as a *relative* transverse discrepancy, and maintenance of a preexisting transverse discrepancy is referred as an *absolute* transverse discrepancy. In addition to the posterior transverse relationship, that in the anterior (i.e., canine region) must be analyzed. This is because strategies to address anterior and posterior maxillary constrictions differ, and the timing may be significantly impacted depending on the choice of treatment (e.g., surgically assisted rapid palatal expansion for anterior maxillary constriction) [23–25].

A simple assessment used by the author includes an algorithm that evaluates four elements: the absolute transverse measurement; the curve of Wilson; tooth-arch requirements (crowding); and the inclination of the buccal segments. By using the table in Fig. 11.3, the surgical-orthodontic team can be aided in the decision whether a case can be treated by segmentation of the maxilla during OGS or that a SARPE is needed prior to orthodontic level and alignment (Fig. 11.3 SARPE Score).

Obviously, it is the clinician's decision and comfort level that influence the final treatment plan. Other reasons that may influence the decision to perform a SARPE over a segmental Lefort include:

- Uncertainty of long-term stability (if expansion was done previously)
- Unstable presurgical orthodontic movements (closing an open bite for example)
- Large advancement of the maxilla is required (cases requiring large Lefort advancements (>5 mm) with the need to segment to expand are prone to relapse)

11.6.1 What Is Normal? Where Do the Central Incisors Belong?

An esthetically pleasing incisal display at rest is a key component to facial esthetics [26]. There is some variability in age and gender, with a higher range seen in younger patients and in females. In general, a favorable incisal display at rest for the young patient is accepted as 2–4 mm for males and slightly more for females [27]. It is important to recognize that incisal display at rest does not always correspond to incisal display on smile, as the latter is a dynamic measurement affected by how high or low an individual's smile line is. Therefore, the term "gummy smile" is not always equated to a vertical maxillary excess. There are no standardized and validated "numbers" to provide, but the evidence is clear that the most unesthetic position is where there is no tooth shown at rest [28–30].

Central incisor angulation has also been evaluated [31] with the ideal range being 103–108° in men and slightly flatter in women. A maxillary incisor that is upright or in slight lingual inclination is preferable, regardless of the AP position of the maxillary incisors. Labial inclination of the upper incisors could easily ruin a pleasing smiling appearance, and maxillary incisor protrusion is preferable to retruded incisors.

Score	**1**	**2**	**3**
Transverse measurement*	0-4mm	4-8mm	>8mm
Lingual Inclination of the Buccal Segment	Lingually inclined	Straight/Vertical	Buccally inclined
Tooth Arch discrepancy	Need to Extract teeth	Moderate: IPR	Mild: Non-Extraction
Curve of Wilson	Flat	Shallow/Mild	Deep
Total			

*measure the central fossa of the upper maxillary 1st molar compared to the distal buccal cusp of the lower mandibular 1st molar (or measure the relationship in the predicted (final) class I molar occlusion)

The SARPE Score table is a guide to help determine the management of transverse discrepancies.
The score is added for each row and the total score is applied to the decision range as follows:
<5 = manage orthodontically.
5-8= manage with a segmental Lefort
>8 = manage with a SARPE

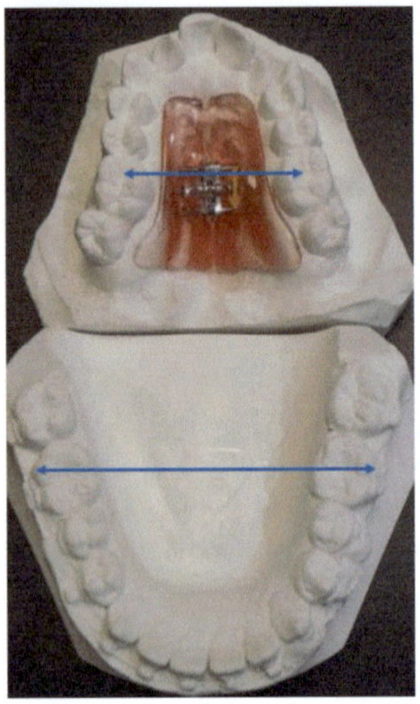

Fig. 11.3 This case indicates that the transverse measurement is 11 mm (3 points), the buccal segment is in a straight axial position(2 points); there is moderate crowding (2 points) and a mild curve of Wilson (2 points). Total 10 points—this helps support the clinical decision to first correct the maxillary transverse discrepancy with a Surgically Assisted Rapid Palatal Expander (A TAD retained appliance is shown) [25]

11.7 Profile and Nasolabial Esthetics

The profile and nasolabial esthetics are determined not only by horizontal incisor position but as well the angulation of the tooth and its role in the upper lip support. In general, a straight profile is preferred regardless of gender. Both qualitative (clinician's subjective assessment) and objective quantitative can be used in NLA assessment. The elements that make up the profile silhouette include the nasal projection, upper lip projection and angulation, chin position, and morphology. The clinician should correlate each region with the corresponding facial unit. This includes the A-P position of the central incisor relative to forehead (Andrews), the upper lip with the maxillary dentoalveolar unit (Steiner), and the chin position with the mandibular skeletal unit and Skeletal base (Holdaway) [32, 33].

If an acute nasolabial angle is deemed primarily due to a ptotic nasal tip (Fig. 11.4), strategies involving improving the nasal tip (e.g., maxillary advancement or rhinoplasty) should be considered, whereas if it is deemed secondary to a procumbent upper lip, consideration should be given to retract or upright the maxillary anterior teeth should be considered. This is especially important to determine in the initial consultation phase, as the decision to extract and retract

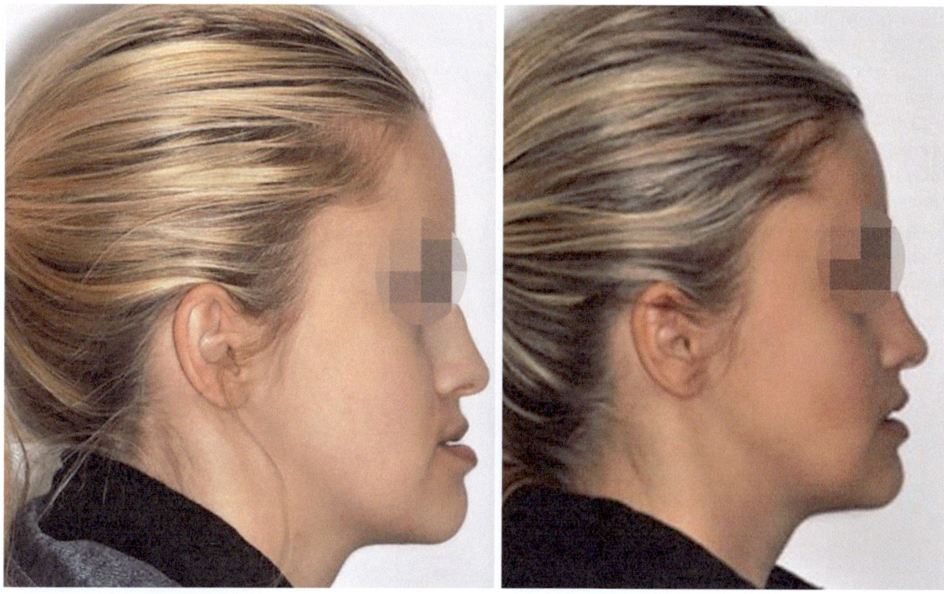

Fig. 11.4 In this case the NLA is considered acute. But the ptotic nasal tip can be manipulated by maxillary advancement which causes the nasal tip to rise while advancing the position of the upper lip into a more esthetically pleasing position

in the maxilla should be made as soon as possible to avoid unnecessary delays in treatment.

A challenge for patients, surgeons, and orthodontists is how and where to normalize structures while ensuring optimal esthetics. Blinded to soft tissue outcomes, establishing a "normal" occlusion—class I molar and proper overbite and overjet can easily be achieved. However, the difficulty is in determining where that maxillomandibular complex is positioned vertically, horizontally, angularly, and rotationally (the so-called pitch/yaw/roll or *x*–*y*–*z* axis positioning) [2, 3, 34].

11.8 Occlusal Esthetic Quartet: Incisor Angulation, Occlusal Plane Angle, Effectiveness of Pogonion and Fullness at Subnasale

The occlusal plane determination will influence many points (Figs. 11.5 and 11.6). For example, if the occlusal plane is increased during the digital planning session, then expect:

1. Upright proclined incisors
2. Increasing the fullness at Sn
3. Reducing the prominence of pogonion
4. Promoting an esthetic U-shaped smile[1]

Although these elements can be used in beneficial esthetic changes, it must be noted that they can quickly and easily ruin a well-executed plan. Simply increasing the occlusal plane to soften pogonion and ignoring that a patient has upright incisors, will induce a very unesthetic retroclined incisor look. Furthermore, over steepening the plane will cause unesthetic alterations to subnasale and cause the patient to have the appearance in the subnasal/labial area akin to the "Whoville" look [35].

Finally, consideration must be given for the age of the patient. Sarver has evaluated extensively the position of the teeth and gingiva and mandibular teeth. Over decades of evaluation, it is obvious that with aging there is less tooth display of the maxillary incisors and more tooth display of the mandibular incisors. To this effect, it should be noted that providing patients with more tooth display is more youthful [28].

11.9 Digital Aids to Planning

11.9.1 System Requirements for Complete Digital Recording, Transfer, Design, and Manufacturing

These include commonplace software and some specialized hardware that constantly evolve. Obvious requirements include some form of processing computer, whether desktop or laptop. With current cloud-based data storage (Dropbox, Sync, OneDrive, iCloud), the data can be kept secure and readily available.

Adobe Acrobat DC Pro: This enables the transformation of the images, PowerPoint slides, Word documents into and out of PDF with a broad range of functionality and security.

[1]The case in Fig. 11.5 shows how small changes in the occlusal plane and vertical increase show more tooth display, resulting in subtle esthetic improvements. A final (nonesthetic) change that occurs with occlusal plane alteration includes changing the occlusal function pattern.

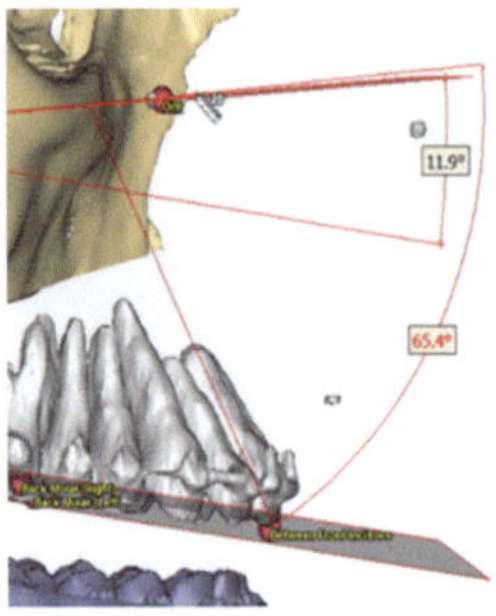

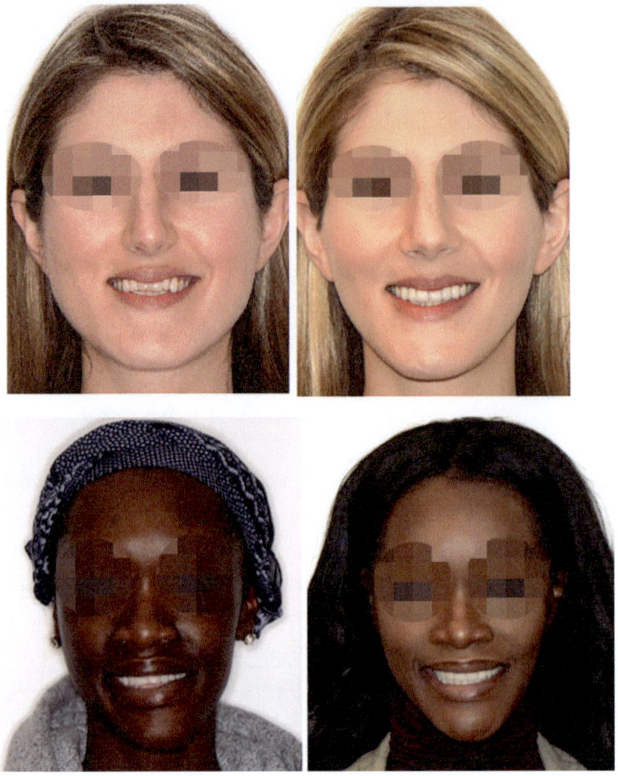

Fig. 11.5 A Skeletal Class III with anterior open bite corrected with maxillary advancement and downgraft with steepening of the occlusal plane. Both these cases show the smile is converted from and inverted U-shape to a more esthetic U-shape with the added vertical augmentation

Windows 7 or 10: This is dependent on the software preferences of the practitioner—in general, PC formats work well with the large file formats of the terabytes needed with radiographs and other imaging without compatibility issues.

PowerPoint: A simple and efficient program with significant flexibility to store high-quality images, videos, notations, and chart information. All images PDF, JPG, STL, and videos can be stored in this one. Cases are stored in a .pptx format, labeled, and indexed for ease of retrieval and research.

Fiducial Markers/Laser Leveler: Accurate registration of natural head position may be required. Most office panoramic/cephalometric machines or CBCTs will have vertical and horizontal lights that are projected on a patient's face to indicate the facial midline and Frankfort horizontal. Radiopaque fiducial markers can be added, and the image will have these points that facilitates the orientation of the head by the DPC engineers when they segment and clean the images (Fig. 11.7).

A Cephalometric Tracing Software with 2D or 3D Virtual treatment objective capability. These programs can also act as image storing, and higher-level in-house manufacturing of splints can be generated with some computing knowledge. Free online programs with limited capability are available, and for small fees, they can increase in sophistication.

SLR Digital Camera: Preferably a full-frame SLR camera with a 100-mm macro lens with no distortion; or recent mirrorless SLRs with super-sensitive image processors: Nikon Z, Sony Alpha. Handheld phone cameras may be enough to record video or quick photos, but standard esthetic facial images need to be created with proper lenses without distortion and reproducible lens ratios.

Dental Scanners/Intraoral Scanners [36]: Few scanners can reproduce accurately a dentition with orthodontic brackets in place. A recommended unit is the Trios scanner which is an open format STL video capture not needing powder coating. It is simple to use with a short learning curve [37–39].

STL Reader: This is not always required if the IOS images are fed directly to the digital planners. However, if storage of these in your database is of interest, then they need to be viewed. Software is available to download; however, there are many numerous free online versions.

Sync/Dropbox/OneDrive/iCLoud: Numerous safe, reliable, and dependable cloud-based storage methods are available. However, the encryption of your data may be required, and regional legislative requirements need to be followed and differ across countries.

Adaptable CAD/CAM Digital Manufacturer or the Digital Planning Company (DPC): The DPC engineers need to be

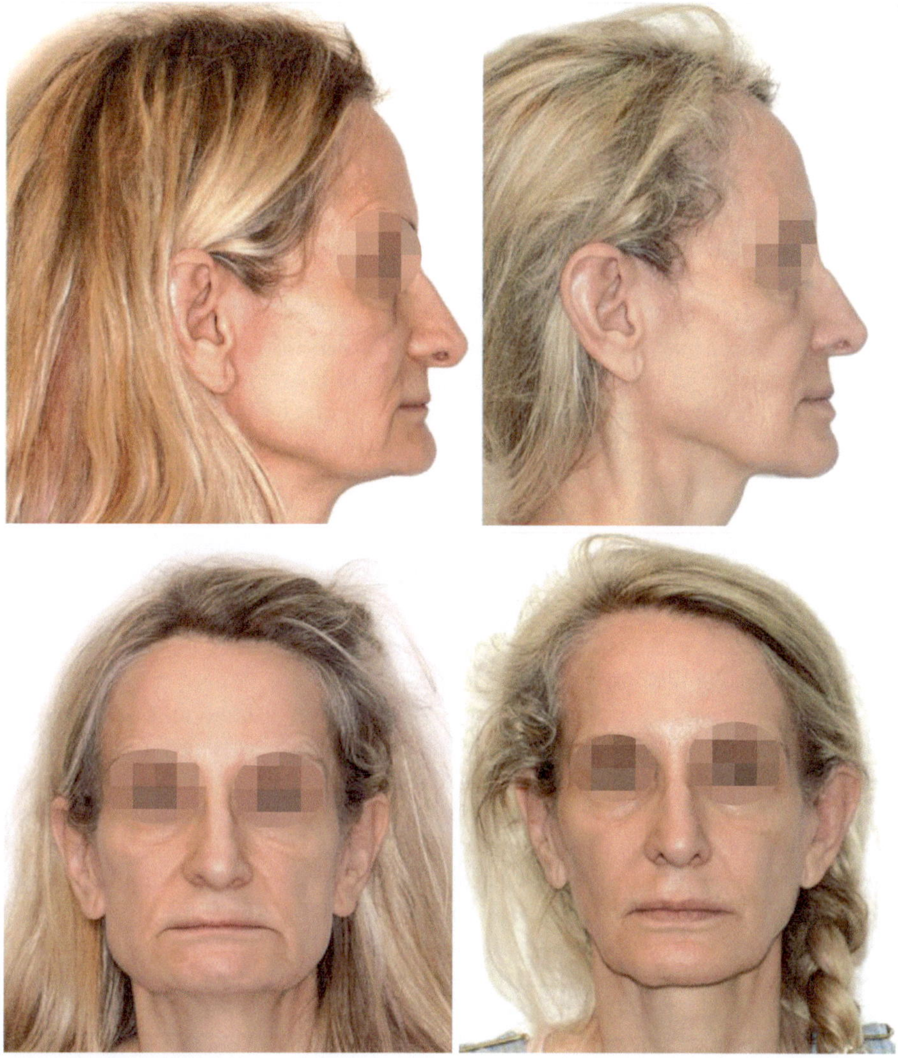

Fig. 11.6 The considerable esthetic and youthful improvements by vertical augmentation of facial structures

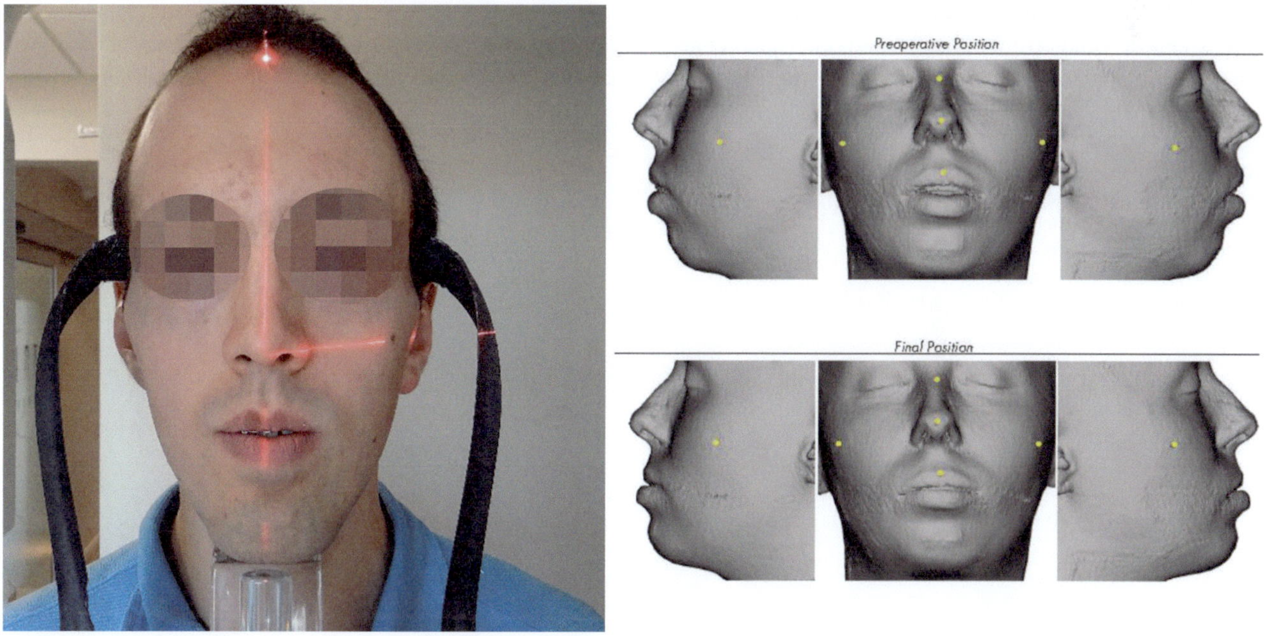

Fig. 11.7 Utilization of the CBCT or PAN/CEPH alignment lights to help determine natural head position and the midline. These are important in asymmetric case and large cants or yaws. Radiopaque markers are placed on the skin and these are transferred to the CT image which help the planning engineers zero and match the images and coordinate these positions

flexible to your needs and adapt to your "custom" flow and requirements. Currently available CASS include Dolphin 3D, 3D Systems, Materialise/PROPLAN, KLS Martin, Protomed, and Nemotec, but many more and many surgical-orthodontic teams now develop their own "home grown" processing and in-house printing.

Treatment Coordinator: Although this is not a "Digital Aid," it is a system requirement. A knowledgeable computer literate assistant is required to compile, collate, organize, prepare, upload and download, and basically keep track of all the different small bits of information that is distributed to the many members of the team. One person needs to hold this responsibility and collect all the data.

Reminders: The CAD/CAM process is nothing but a tool—a "fancy articulator." It should be an aid to support your diagnosis and plan, it provides excellent occlusal positioning, it accurately predicts the outcomes, and it significantly simplifies "model surgery" especially segmental surgery.

Centric relation is critical when bimaxillary surgery is performed with maxilla-first surgery. A misconception is that for mandible-first surgery, CR is not important (or can be eliminated). That is not entirely true because if we are generating our digital plan to position the maxillomandibular complex, your final splint still positions the maxilla according to the CR of the digital mandible. If your condylar positions (digital and operative) are not coincident, there will be changes in postoperative maxillary position (occlusion will still be good). This is only truly avoided by prefabricated plates and positioners, but then this will limit your vertical control for the maxillomandibular complex, and it is not favored by the author.

Intraoral scanners may provide better accuracy [40] in representing the occlusion when compared to scanned wax bites. Different registration methods and imaging can produce a centric relation that changes. Another challenge is that the imaging to reproduce the CR position can vary. Recently we evaluated that the CR record taken during the CT was more accurate in positioning the condyle in the fossa when compared to the CR record taken with an intraoral scan [41]. Although the method of digital planning with CAD/CAM format is accurate, intraoperative condylar positioning still presents as a challenge [6].

The reason centric relation is important is because regardless of position, it is reproducible and stable, so each practitioner may develop his or her own sense of centric relation. If it is reproduced at the time of surgery, then the planning will match [6]. The argument is not what the definition of centric relation is but rather its reproducibility at the time of surgery in order to make your splint ability accurate. In cases where there are significant cants or asymmetries, fiducial markers will be placed in the centric relation record as seen here.

Natural Head Position, like centric relation, has many definitions and practitioners use numerous data points. These range from the Natural Head Position obtained in a physical examination or clinical photographs, to cephalometric reference of Frankfort horizontal, and to the axis-orbital plane derived from articulated dental models. Some aids that are used to assess NHP may include laser light indicators (obtained from panoramic or cephalometric machines, gyroscopic positioners placed in the mouth and linked to electronic referencing devices or the placement of fiducial markers [42]. On average, the positioning of the head can produce differences by up to 8°, and this problem alone can be responsible for a 15% difference in maxillary projection between planned and actual outcomes [3, 18, 43–45].

Hinge Axis Determination: Not often required, this simple registration aids in the ability of the engineer and practitioners to determine where the hinge axis of the patient may be. This is helpful in cases where there is a large CR to CO shift, where there may be a habitual bite (dual bite) and when planning large vertical changes where an inaccurate hinge axis may produce unwanted horizontal changes (Fig. 11.8).

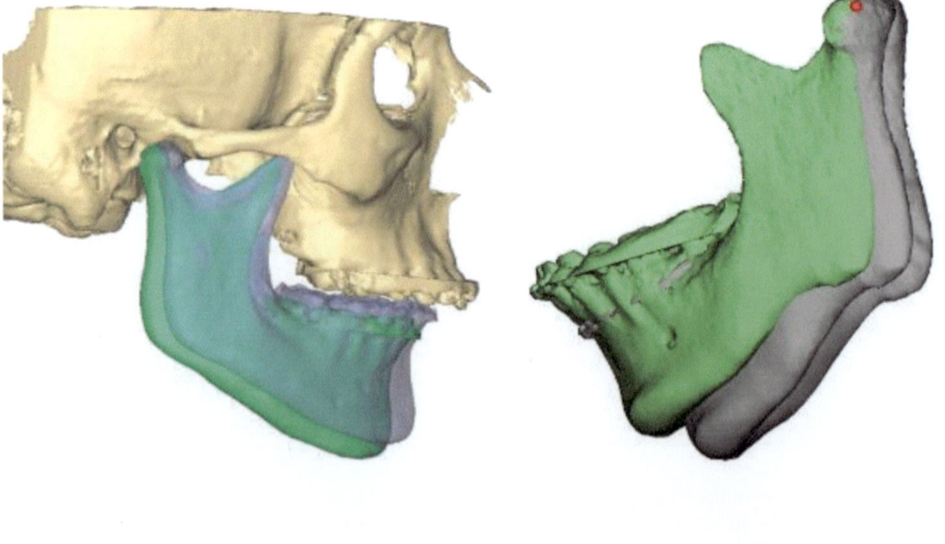

Fig. 11.8 The image shows the difference in the condylar position using two centric relation recording records. The condyles drift down and back before rotating. This small but subtle change is seen as a 4 mm discrepancy. On large vertical changes this difference will be magnified even more. Therefore, a good centric relation and hinge axis is required in large vertical impactions or downgrafts

11.9.1.1 Surgery First OGS

This topic is of great interest. It was introduced to eliminate the presurgical orthodontic phase and accelerate the management of dentofacial deformities by restaging the orthodontic decompensation until after surgery. Emerging data from the literature shows an overall decrease in treatment time, with stability comparable to that of the traditional "orthodontics-first" approach [14, 16, 46]. Despite these benefits, routine use of the surgery-first approach is often not feasible, as there are many difficulties in the planning phase that are not apparent in the traditional approach. Some malocclusions (anterior open bite extraction class II vertical divergent cases) may be more of a challenge with surgery first, whereas other cases (non-extraction class III corrections) are more easily approached.

Because the surgery-first approach involves no presurgical orthodontics, the skeletal movements must be planned with the final orthodontic outcome in mind. This can be extremely challenging if there are significant arch length/width discrepancies, asymmetries, and vertical discrepancies. There are technical disadvantages as well due to the absence of braces at the time of surgery; however, these are easily overcome using Clear Aligner technologies and the development of and use of clear aligner orthognathic splints [15]. Postoperatively, the clinician typically must deal with shifting occlusion with TADs or other anchors until such a time that the patient may be able to start orthodontic bonding.

Due to these challenges, case selection must be done with full understanding of the anticipated benefits, predictability, and the clinicians' comfort level.

11.10 Timeline Challenges with Digital Planning

Table 11.1 demonstrates a recommendation of the time required by both surgical and orthodontic teams to set up and prepare a case given the numerous steps necessary. In traditional model surgery, the lab time dictates the creation of the surgical splint. In digital planning, it is the transport of the material that is the rate-determining step. Obvious in-house methods of splint or surgical guide fabrication can shorten some steps.

Table 11.1 Orthognathic surgery workup timeline with digital planning technologies

Step	Plan	Timing
1	Surgical orthodontic diagnosis and preliminary surgical treatment plan and visual treatment objective	Initial consults
2	Orthodontic presurgical preparation	0–6 (for surgery first) to 12–18 months (for traditional set up)
3	Determination of suitability/readiness for surgery and establish a draft of the surgical treatment plan	4–6 months pre op
4	**Establish operating room time**	
5	Confirm appointments for hospital presurg/medical tests/exams/dental exam/hygiene/orthodontic visits/surgical work up	2 months pre op
	Presurgical preparation steps	
6	Orthodontic prep: remove attachments or add surgical wire	4 weeks pre op
7	Digital data gather, final counseling	4 weeks pre op
8	Distribute/upload digital material	3 weeks pre op
9	DPC video conference	2 weeks pre op
10	Confirmation of CASS plan	2 weeks pre op
11	Apply surgical hooks	1 weeks pre op
12	Collect splints/try in prn	1 weeks pre op
	Surgery	T0

11.11 Final Digital Planning Meeting: A Suggested Sequenced Approach

All these steps above are then combined and brought together during the virtual digital planning session. The decision of what gross movements in all axes must be determined **BEFORE** the digital planning session (DPS). The DPS is only a guide or confirmation of what you decided in the clinical examination and the 2D and 3D analyses. The influence of the movements must be tempered with surgical knowledge and the limitations of OGS. Movements to minimize relapse should be understood. Condylar positioning and its replication intraoperatively need to be coincident. Finally, application of rigid fixation techniques and occlusal stabilizations need to be mastered in order to avoid postsurgical complications. The sequence and appropriate images are shown in Fig. 11.9 and detailed below:

11.11.1 Determine the Need for Segmentalization and Where to Osteotomize

Most anterior open bites will require segmentation. Obvious transverse discrepancies will also require segmentation. However, many cases (subtle Bolton issues, crossbites in final occlusions) may be difficult to predict prior to the planning session. The team should share this with the DPC prior to the online meeting in order to allow them to prepare for this. Sometimes, the DPC determines that segmentation may be best, and a good working relationship needs to be established in order to relinquish this decision. Most often, segmentation is preferred between lateral and canines and rarely in the midline. Root divergence for possible segmentation is NOT recommended as this will distort planned occlusal rela-

Fig. 11.9 Digital planning steps

	TASKS: SET UP THE HEAD POSITION	
1	DETERMINE THE NEED FOR SEGMENTALIZATION AND WHERE TO OSTEOTOMIZE	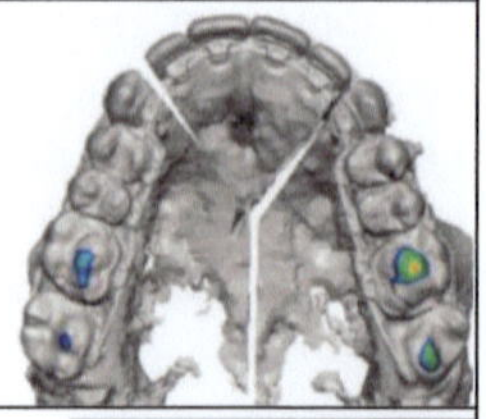
2	CHECK AND VERIFY THE NATURAL HEAD POSITION	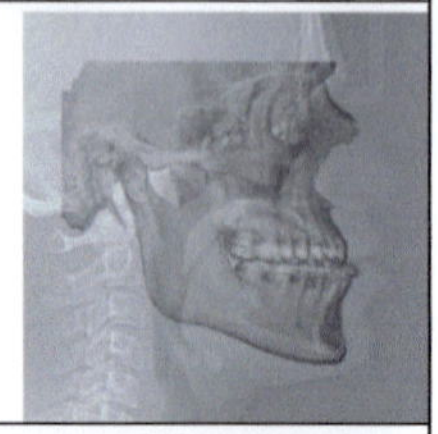
3	CHECK AND VERIFY THE CANT.	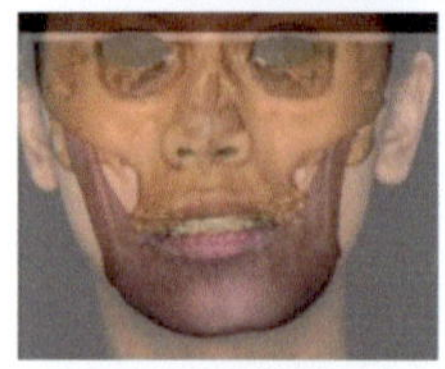
4	CHECK THAT THE MIDLINES ARE PROPERLY INDICATED/MARKED	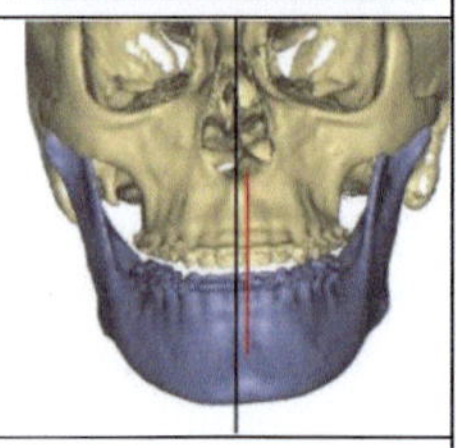
	TASK: EXECUTE MOVEMENTS	
5	ROTATE THE MAXILLA TO CORRECT THE CANT	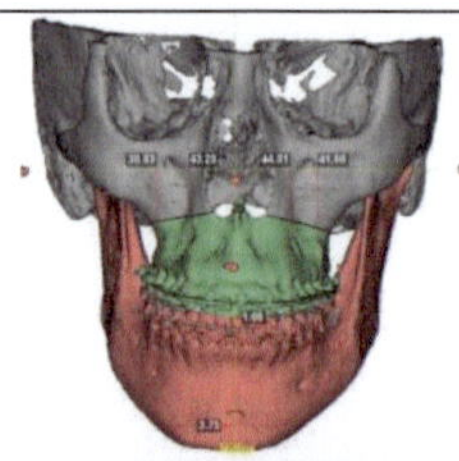
6	DETERMINE HINGE AXIS IF YOU HAVE LARGE VERTICAL CHANGES	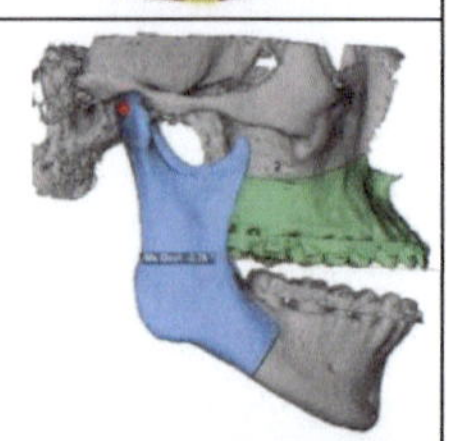
7	CENTRAL INCISOR POSITION BASED ON BEST ESTHETICS	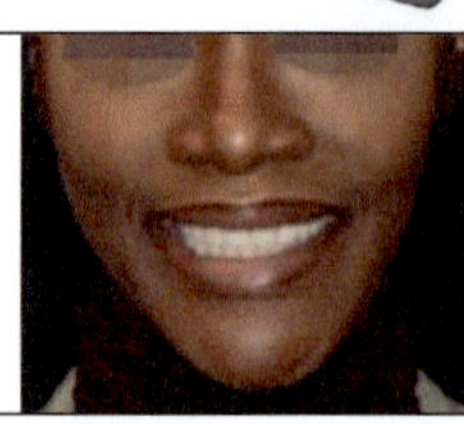

Fig. 11.9 (continued)

8	OCCLUSAL PLANE ALTERATION AND THE QUARTET EFFECT	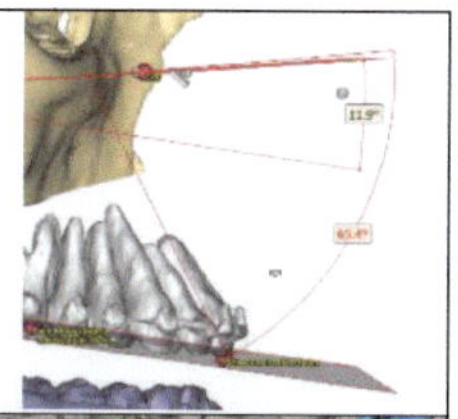
9	SET UP THE BEST OCCLUSION	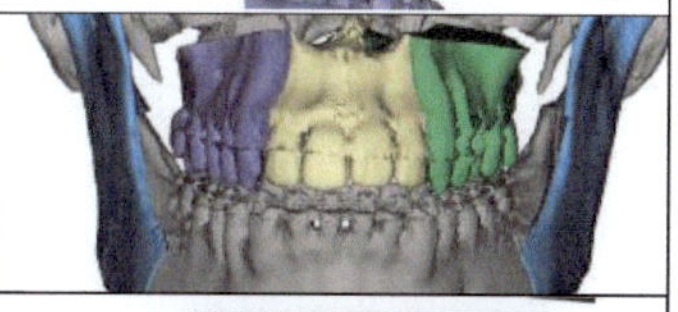
10	YAW CORRECTION; WORMS AND BIRDS EYE VIEW	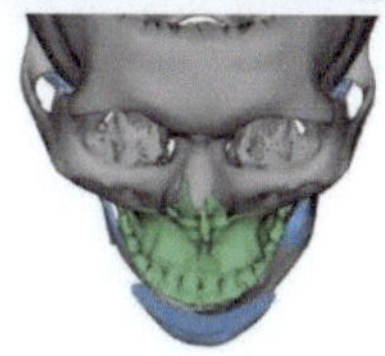
11	LOOK AT INTERFERENCES	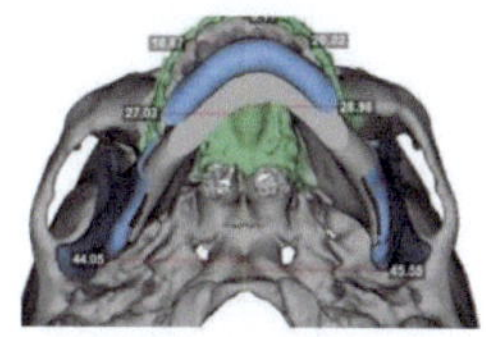
12	PLAN YOUR GENIOPLASTY	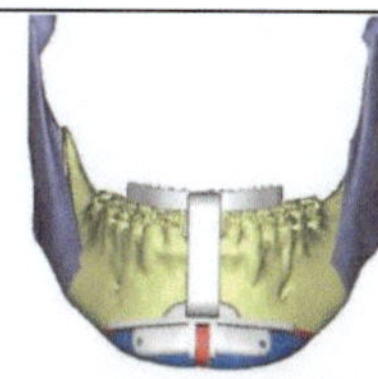
13	MANDIBLE OR MAXILLA FIRST?	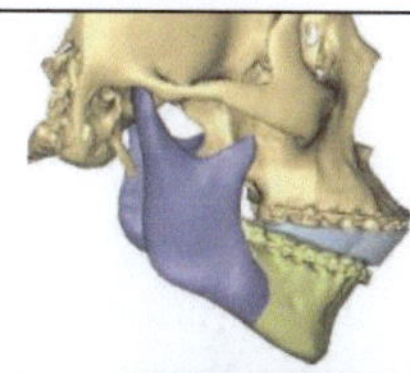
14	SPLINTS: GENERATE TYPE, THICKNESS, GUIDES, RETAINERS	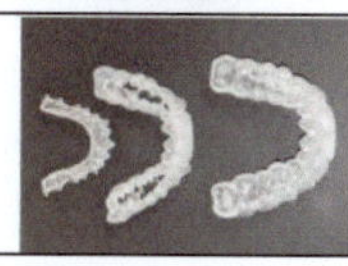

tionship (and we surgically “split” the alveolus rather than osteotomize through it).

11.11.2 Check Natural Head Position

There are many methods to obtain an accurate NHP as previously discussed. Confounding the issue is what position should you base the NHP and treatment on has no consensus. Frankfort horizontal may still be the most reliable method, but we use the image created from our lateral cephalogram. Whether you use an elaborate *XYZ* axis determination using gyroscopes, fiducial markers, occlusal radiopaque template, or simple laser levelers on most CBCT/ceph machines, you must be able to indicate to the DPC if the lateral head position is accurate. The author uses a transparent lateral ceph that is taken at the presurgical workup and quickly overlays this over the DPC CBCT/CT image and communicates whether to reposition in the *x*, *y*, or rotated axis. Eventually, it is the DPC that fuses the scans and radiographs [47, 48].

11.11.3 Check and Verify the CANT

This assessment must be correlated to the clinical examination. Virtual planners use the orbital rim to the canines or molars to make this assessment, and any bony abnormality/deformity will create inaccuracies. However, your clinical examination MUST supersede this. Facial CANTS are determined from the pupils to the occlusal plane and NOT the orbital rims. A quick overlay of the clinical photo over the DPC CBCT/CT will aid in communicating with the engineer to rotate the CBCT image to match your clinical CANT.

11.11.4 Check That the Midlines Are Properly Indicated

This, perhaps next to incisor show, is the most important element in planning any OGS case. The clinical determination of the midline is the veto over any midline determined from a radiograph. DO NOT let the DPC/engineers alter your midline position if you have a solid understanding of where it lies. In general, if the lips are anatomically correct (i.e., no previous surgeries, clefts, fillers), then use the midline of the philtrum as your reference. The figure shows the patients true clinical midline in red. The DPC engineers indicated that the facial midline was in black (following nasal spine). If the surgeon concedes and plans according to the DPC, then the midline would have been unesthetically shifted to the patients' right. These small subtleties are critical.

Steps 1–4 help with the orientation of the maxillomandibular complex and the occlusal relationships. The next steps deal with the planned movements which are based on the clinical plan and supported by imaging.

11.11.5 Rotate the Maxilla to Correct the CANT

The rotation point can be determined during the DPC session and can use various center of rotations. In general, it is easiest to place the center of rotation at the contact point of the central incisors. Large canted movements require the use of fiducial markers on the skin to obtain more accurate results.

11.11.6 Determine Hinge Axis

This is important only in cases where they may be large vertical changes. Any error in positioning the condyle during the VSP will create horizontal discrepancies (errors) because of the arc of rotation of the mandible may not always be accurate because true hinge axis is a soft tissue phenomenon and not simply based on a reformatted 3D image. The author uses two CR wax bites at tooth contact and 10 mm apart, and the intraoral scans of the two are sent to the DPC to calculate the HA.

11.11.7 Central Incisor Position

This is the central decision in ultrafine planning. It is a combination of the clinical, cephalometric, CBCT/CT position, but it must be matched to the understanding of the surgically induced soft tissue changes that each surgeon must develop an instinct for. Although many reports have been reviewed above, where the central incisor needs to be placed remains the "art" of OGS.

11.11.8 Occlusal Plane Alteration

Evaluation of the occlusal plane must be matched with incisor angulation, pogonion position, and subnasale prominence and cannot be left in isolation. It bears repeating that as the occlusal plane steepens, there is a quartet effect: the patient will tend to have the central incisors in a more upright position, the projection of Pogonion is softened, the area around SubNasale becomes fuller (which may require osteoplasty of the nasal sill), and finally the patients' occlusion will tend more toward a cuspid rise occlusion.

11.11.9 Best Occlusion

The fitting of the mandible into the best occlusion is the next step. The DPC can establish this with pre-set indices created by the surgical orthodontic team generated with articulators (wax bites, blue mousse bites, acrylic wafer, or any other material that will help the DPC provide for the best-fitting bite). Currently, most DPC will set the occlusion given the models provided, and they can share wherever the interferences may lie. The author now relies completely on the STL scanned dentition to be matched with the CBCT/CT and letting the DPC engineer "fit" the best occlusion. This is then reviewed during the online meeting. Particular attention must then be addressed if occlusal adjustments are required especially if greater than 1–1.5 mm. The DPC engineer must let you know if this is the case and you need to approve of this.

11.11.10 Yaw Correction

Looking at the maxillomandibular complex from an inferior or superior perspective (worms view and birds view) can address esthetic issues of yaw asymmetries as well as the shape of the inferior border of the mandible, the uneven fullness at the nostrils and most importantly the interferences that may occur as a result of the mandibular osteotomies.

11.11.11 Interferences

The DPC can immediately report on interferences at the pterygoid plates, the ramus, the BSSO sites, the maxillary movement osteotomy, genioplasty, and all boney contact points. Also, the occlusal map interferences is provided to trim the enamel for the splints to fit (and for the occlusion to fit!) This is a very helpful tool to make accurate adjustments.

11.11.12 Genioplasty

The final step of the session will be to demonstrate the possible bony changes with a genioplasty. DPCs all have different approaches,[2] but they only follow on the direction of the surgeon. The location of the osteotomies and the changes in boney positioned are discussed between the engineer and the surgeon. Clinical, cephalometric, and CBCT data will help with these movements. Most of the time, the DPC will demonstrate and indicate possible genioplasty movements as a form of record. At times, surgical cutting and positioning guides can be utilized. The author finds these useful when reducing pogonion transversely.

11.11.13 Mandible or Maxilla First?

Depending on the movements, the intermediate splint can be too bulky or cumbersome. For example, in mandible first surgery and large anterior open bite cases the splint is too thick. Conversely in maxilla first surgery for class II cases with maxillary advancements, the A-P splint length is a challenge to wire or position intraoperatively. The DPCs can quickly demonstrate the size of the splints to guide the surgeon to which direction they would like to go. This surgeon preference is to use mandible first for all cases however due to the numerous benefits.

11.11.14 Splints

Final step is to design the splints whether thick or thin, clear or opaque, flange or no flange, palatal shelf or strut. There are many variations, and the preferences are surgeon specific. A preference is to always use clear splints and no flange (unless there is a segmental that needs to be wired in place. The absence of a flange allows the operator to see that the cusp tips are fully engaged in the splint—remember—it is all about the occlusion.

[2]Currently there are many digital planning companies that provide the service for CAD/CAM fabrication of surgical guides or splints. They all work closely with surgical teams to develop good and consistent results but they are only as good as the information that is provided to them.

11.12 Conclusions

OGS brings together a complex set of domains which results in one of the more transformative outcomes in medicine. It is the outcome of a challenging and invasive surgical intervention. But before and after the surgery, there are so many people and so many steps involved in producing the best outcome possible. By understanding and scrutinizing the data and clinical examinations available, the planning team can provide for near perfect results with attention to detail. This chapter demonstrated that 3D planning is useful, and with some practice, the many layers, nuances, and steps involved become simple and rewarding. For the novice entrant into this realm, the establishment of a relation with a mentor is very helpful.

References

1. Sharifi A, Jones R, Ayoub A, et al. How accurate is model planning for orthognathic surgery? Int J Oral Maxillofac Surg. 2008;37(12):1089–93. https://doi.org/10.1016/j.ijom.2008.06.011.
2. Swennen GRJ, Mollemans W, Schutyser F. Three-dimensional treatment planning of orthognathic surgery in the era of virtual imaging. J Oral Maxillofac Surg. 2009;67:2080–92. https://doi.org/10.1016/j.joms.2009.06.007.
3. Sheng-Pin Hsu S, Gateno J, Bryan Bell R, et al. Accuracy of a computer-aided surgical simulation protocol for orthognathic surgery: a prospective multicenter study. YJOMS. 2013;71:128–42. https://doi.org/10.1016/j.joms.2012.03.027.
4. Eckhardt CE, Cunningham SJ. How predictable is orthognathic surgery? Eur J Orthod. 2004;26(3):303–9. https://doi.org/10.1093/ejo/26.3.303.
5. Quast A, Santander P, Witt D, et al. Traditional face-bow transfer versus three-dimensional virtual reconstruction in orthognathic surgery. Int J Oral Maxillofac Surg. 2019;48:347–54. https://doi.org/10.1016/j.ijom.2018.09.001.
6. De Riu G, Virdis PI, Meloni SM, Lumbau A, Vaira LA. Accuracy of computer-assisted orthognathic surgery. J Craniomaxillofac Surg. 2018;46(2):293–8. https://doi.org/10.1016/j.jcms.2017.11.023.
7. Legan HL, Burstone CJ. Soft tissue cephalometric analysis for orthognathic surgery. J Oral Surg (Chic). 1980;38(10):744–51.
8. Naini FB, Moss JP, Gill DS. The enigma of facial beauty: esthetics, proportions, deformity, and controversy. Am J Orthod Dentofac Orthop. 2006;130(3):277–82. https://doi.org/10.1016/j.ajodo.2005.09.027.
9. Alhazmi A, Vargas E, Palomo JM, Hans M, Latimer B, Simpson S. Timing and rate of spheno-occipital synchondrosis closure and its relationship to puberty. PLoS One. 2017;12(8):1–16. https://doi.org/10.1371/journal.pone.0183305.
10. Proffit WR, Phillips C, Turvey TA. Long-term stability of adolescent versus adult surgery for treatment of mandibular deficiency. Int J Oral Maxillofac Surg. 2010;39(4):327–32. https://doi.org/10.1016/j.ijom.2010.01.012.
11. Hassel B, Farman AG. Skeletal maturation evaluation using cervical vertebrae. Am J Orthod Dentofac Orthop. 1995;107(1):58–66. https://doi.org/10.1016/S0889-5406(95)70157-5.
12. Graber L. In: Graber LW, Vanarsdall R, Vig KWL, Huang GJ, editors. Orthodontic aspects of orthognathic surgery. Elsevier, St. Louis Missouri. 2017;6:708–11.
13. Montemurro P, Porcnik A, Per H, Otte M. The influence of social media and easily accessible online information on the aesthetic

plastic surgery practice: literature review and our own experience. Aesthetic Plast Surg. 2015;39(2):270–7. https://doi.org/10.1007/s00266-015-0454-3.
14. Peiró-Guijarro MA, Guijarro-Martínez R, Hernández-Alfaro F. Surgery first in orthognathic surgery: a systematic review of the literature. Am J Orthod Dentofac Orthop. 2016;149(4):448–62. https://doi.org/10.1016/j.ajodo.2015.09.022.
15. Caminiti M, Lou T. Clear aligner orthognathic splints. J Oral Maxillofac Surg. 2019;77(5):1071.e1–8. https://doi.org/10.1016/j.joms.2018.12.012.
16. Perez D, Ellis E. Sequencing bimaxillary surgery: mandible first. J Oral Maxillofac Surg. 2011;69(8):2217–24. https://doi.org/10.1016/j.joms.2010.10.053.
17. Houle J-P, Piedade L, Todescan R, Pinheiro FHSL. The predictability of transverse changes with Invisalign. Angle Orthod. 2017;87(1):19–24. https://doi.org/10.2319/122115-875.1.
18. Xia JJ, Gateno J, Teichgraeber JF. Three-dimensional computer-aided surgical simulation for maxillofacial surgery. Atlas Oral Maxillofac Surg Clin North Am. 2005;13(1 Spec. ISS):25–39. https://doi.org/10.1016/j.cxom.2004.10.004.
19. Bolton WA. The clinical application of a tooth-size analysis. Am J Orthod. 1962;48:504–29. https://doi.org/10.1016/0002-9416(62)90129-X.
20. Proffitt W, Fields HW, Larson BE, Sarver DM. Contemporary orthodontics. 6th ed. St. Louis: Mosby, Inc.; 2018.
21. Hanna A, Iii EE. Tooth-size discrepancies in patients requiring mandibular advancement surgery. J Oral Maxillofac Surg. 2016;74(12):2481–6. https://doi.org/10.1016/j.joms.2016.08.003.
22. Larson BE. Orthodontic preparation for orthognathic surgery. Oral Maxillofac Surg Clin N Am. 2014;26:441–58. https://doi.org/10.1016/j.coms.2014.08.002.
23. Betts NJ. Surgically assisted maxillary expansion. Atlas Oral Maxillofac Surg Clin North Am. 2016;24(1):67–77. https://doi.org/10.1016/j.cxom.2015.10.003.
24. Suri L, Taneja P. Surgically assisted rapid palatal expansion: a literature review. Am J Orthod Dentofac Orthop. 2008;133(2):290–302. https://doi.org/10.1016/j.ajodo.2007.01.021.
25. Caminiti MF, Marko JM, Metaxas A. TAD retained acrylic palatal expander for SARPE. J Oral Maxillofac Surg. 2017;75(10):e349–50. https://doi.org/10.1016/j.joms.2017.07.041.
26. Schlosser JB, Preston CB, Lampasso J. The effects of computer-aided anteroposterior maxillary incisor movement on ratings of facial attractiveness. Am J Orthod Dentofac Orthop. 2005;127(1):17–24. https://doi.org/10.1016/j.ajodo.2003.11.025.
27. Caramello F, Bittencourt MAV, Machado AW. Influence of maxillary incisor level of exposure on the perception of dentofacial aesthetics among orthodontists and laypersons. J World Fed Orthod. 2015;4(3):108–13. https://doi.org/10.1016/j.ejwf.2015.06.002.
28. Sarver DM. Interactions of hard tissues, soft tissues, and growth over time, and their impact on orthodontic diagnosis and treatment planning. Am J Orthod Dentofac Orthop. 2015;148(3):380–6. https://doi.org/10.1016/j.ajodo.2015.04.030.
29. Panossian AJ, Block MS. Evaluation of the smile: facial and dental considerations. YJOMS. 2010;68:547–54. https://doi.org/10.1016/j.joms.2009.09.021.
30. Sarver D, Jacobson RS. The aesthetic dentofacial analysis. Clin Plast Surg. 2007;34(3):369–94. https://doi.org/10.1016/j.cps.2007.05.008.
31. Naini FB, Manouchehri S, Al-Bitar ZB, Gill DS, Garagiola U, Wertheim D. The maxillary incisor labial face tangent: clinical evaluation of maxillary incisor inclination in profile smiling view and idealized aesthetics. Maxillofac Plast Reconstr Surg. 2019;41(1):31. https://doi.org/10.1186/s40902-019-0214-4.
32. Andrews WA. AP relationship of the maxillary central incisors to the forehead in adult white females. Angle Orthod. 2008;78(4):662–8. https://doi.org/10.2319/071307-329.1.
33. Ellis HS, Hamidzadeh F, Stefanos SM, Rouhanian M, Huber JH, Arena ME, Ye L. The effects of computer-aided anteroposterior maxillary incisor movement on ratings of facial attractiveness. J Dent Oral Heal. 2017;3(5):2–6.
34. McCormick SU, Drew SJ. Virtual model surgery for efficient planning and surgical performance. J Oral Maxillofac Surg. 2011;69(3):638–44. https://doi.org/10.1016/j.joms.2010.10.047.
35. Seuss D. How the Grinch stole Christmas. (BookSources, ed). New York: Random House; 1957.
36. Kravitz N, Groth C, Jones P, Graham J, Redmond R. Intraoral digital scanners. J Clin Orthod. 2014;48(6):337. www.jco-online.com. Accessed 4 Apr 2019.
37. González de Villaumbrosia P, Martínez-Rus F, García-Orejas A, Salido MP, Pradíes G. In vitro comparison of the accuracy (trueness and precision) of six extraoral dental scanners with different scanning technologies. J Prosthet Dent. 2016;116(4):543–550.e1. https://doi.org/10.1016/j.prosdent.2016.01.025.
38. Kim JH, Park YC, Yu HS, Kim MK, Kang SH, Choi YJ. Accuracy of 3-dimensional virtual surgical simulation combined with digital teeth alignment: a pilot study. J Oral Maxillofac Surg. 2017;75(11):2441.e1–e13. https://doi.org/10.1016/j.joms.2017.07.161.
39. Rangel FA, Maal TJJ, Bronkhorst EM, et al. Accuracy and reliability of a novel method for fusion of digital dental casts and cone beam computed tomography scans. PLoS One. 2013;8(3):e59130. https://doi.org/10.1371/journal.pone.0059130.
40. Nilsson J, Richards RG, Thor A, Kamer L. Virtual bite registration using intraoral digital scanning, CT and CBCT: in vitro evaluation of a new method and its implication for orthognathic surgery. J Craniomaxillofac Surg. 2016;44(9):1194–200. https://doi.org/10.1016/j.jcms.2016.06.013.
41. Lee R, El-Rabbany M, Kienle F, Caminiti M. Accuracy of centric relation record derived from intraoral scan versus computed tomography in condylar positioning for computer assisted surgical simulation. J Oral Maxillofac Surg. 2019;77(9):e5–6. https://doi.org/10.1016/j.joms.2019.06.021.
42. Bobek S, Farrell B, Choi C, Farrell B, Weimer K, Tucker M. Virtual surgical planning for orthognathic surgery using digital data transfer and an intraoral fiducial marker: The charlotte method. J Oral Maxillofac Surg. 2015;73(6):1143–58.
43. Xia JJ, Gateno J, Teichgraeber JF. New clinical protocol to evaluate craniomaxillofacial deformity and plan surgical correction. J Oral Maxillofac Surg. 2009;67:2093–106. https://doi.org/10.1016/j.joms.2009.04.057.
44. Bell RB. Computer planning and intraoperative navigation in orthognathic surgery. J Oral Maxillofac Surg. 2011;69(3):592–605. https://doi.org/10.1016/j.joms.2009.06.030.
45. Plooij JM, Maal TJJ, Haers P, Borstlap WA, Kuijpers-Jagtman AM, Bergé SJ. Digital three-dimensional image fusion processes for planning and evaluating orthodontics and orthognathic surgery. A systematic review published by Elsevier Ltd on behalf of International Association of Oral and Maxillofacial Surgeons. J Oral Maxillofac Surg. 2010;40:341–52. https://doi.org/10.1016/j.ijom.2010.10.013.
46. Uribe FA, Farrell B. Surgery-first approach in the orthognathic patient. Oral Maxillofac Surg Clin North Am. 2020;32(1):89–103. https://doi.org/10.1016/j.coms.2019.08.009.
47. De Waard O, Baan F, Verhamme L, Breuning H, Kuijpers-Jagtman AM, Maal T. A novel method for fusion of intra-oral scans and cone-beam computed tomography scans for orthognathic surgery planning. J Craniomaxillofacial Surg. 2016;44(2):160–6. https://doi.org/10.1016/j.jcms.2015.11.017.
48. Uechi J, Tsuji Y, Konno M, et al. Generation of virtual models for planning orthognathic surgery using a modified multimodal image fusion technique. Int J Oral Maxillofac Surg. 2015;44(4):462–9. https://doi.org/10.1016/j.ijom.2014.11.007.

3D Planning for Complex Cases in Orthognathic Surgery

12

Marco Caminiti and Tiantong Lou

12.1 Introduction

Rapid advancements in three-dimensional (3D) imaging technology has revolutionized the fields of orthodontics and orthognathic surgery [1, 2]. The advent of 3D imaging allows for more accurate diagnosis and more predictable treatment planning [3]. Building on the concepts previously discussed, this chapter showcases four complex cases that effectively utilize the concept of 3D treatment planning and surgery. The first case shows combined clear aligner therapy with orthognathic surgery; the second case demonstrates a complex orthodontic case involving osteochondroma requiring total joint replacement; the third case illustrates the benefits of using a surgery-first approach; the final case shows the posttreatment management of idiopathic condylar resorption.

12.2 Role of Clear Aligners in Orthognathic Surgery

Due to an ever-increasing demand among perspective orthodontic patients for more esthetic and comfortable treatment options, clear aligner therapy (CAT) has rapidly increased in popularity and quickly became a mainstay in contemporary orthodontics [4–7]. The challenge of adopting this technology for patients requiring orthognathic surgery has only been discussed to a limited extent [8]. In a recently published article, we proposed the use of a 3D printed clear aligner orthognathic splint (CAOS) for intraoperative control of the occlusion during surgery [9]. The following case demonstrates the use of this appliance as well as several other techniques that are helpful in the adoption of CAT to OGS.

12.3 Case Report

A 25-year-old healthy male patient presented with a class III malocclusion of skeletal and dentoalveolar etiology for orthodontic treatment. Extraorally, the patient had a prognathic facial type with a concave profile. Intraoral examination revealed a slightly constricted maxillary arch with mild crowding and a moderately crowded mandibular arch with excess negative overjet (Fig. 12.1). A non-extraction treatment plan using CAT was selected in conjunction with orthognathic surgery to advance the maxilla, rotate the occlusal plane, and set back the mandible.

The presurgical set of aligners consisted of only ten stages in total. Crowding in the lower anterior region was alleviated by proclination of the lower incisors. The presurgical phase was completed in approximately 3 months. Following decompensation, the method of temporary MMF used was with the aid of the CAOS splint and four temporary anchorage devices (TADs) (Fig. 12.2). The planned movements were a setback of the mandible of 4.5 mm and slight asymmetry correction followed by a 4 mm advancement and 3 mm impaction of the maxilla. The patient had all CAT attachments removed 1 month prior to surgery, and four passive aligners were delivered. These were to be worn for 1 month presurgery and 1 month postsurgery. During the first 2 weeks following surgery, the patient was kept on corrective elastics to maintain the occlusion, using the same TADs as points of attachment (Fig. 12.3). Following an uneventful postoperative course, the patient returned to clinic on week 2 and was scanned for the refinement set of aligners. The virtual treatment plan was performed in coordination with the surgeon and the orthodontist, resulting in 20 additional aligners delivered to the patient by approximately the fourth

M. Caminiti (✉)
Oral and Maxillofacial Surgery, Faculty of Dentistry, University of Toronto, Toronto, ON, Canada

Oral and Maxillofaical Surgery, Humber River Hospital, Toronto, ON, Canada

Jaw Deformity Clinic, Holland Bloorview Kids Rehabilitation Hospital, Toronto, ON, Canada
e-mail: marco.caminiti@utoronto.ca

T. Lou
Private Practice, Toronto, ON, Canada

J.-M. Retrouvey, M.-N. Abdallah (eds.), *3D Diagnosis and Treatment Planning in Orthodontics*,
https://doi.org/10.1007/978-3-030-57223-5_12

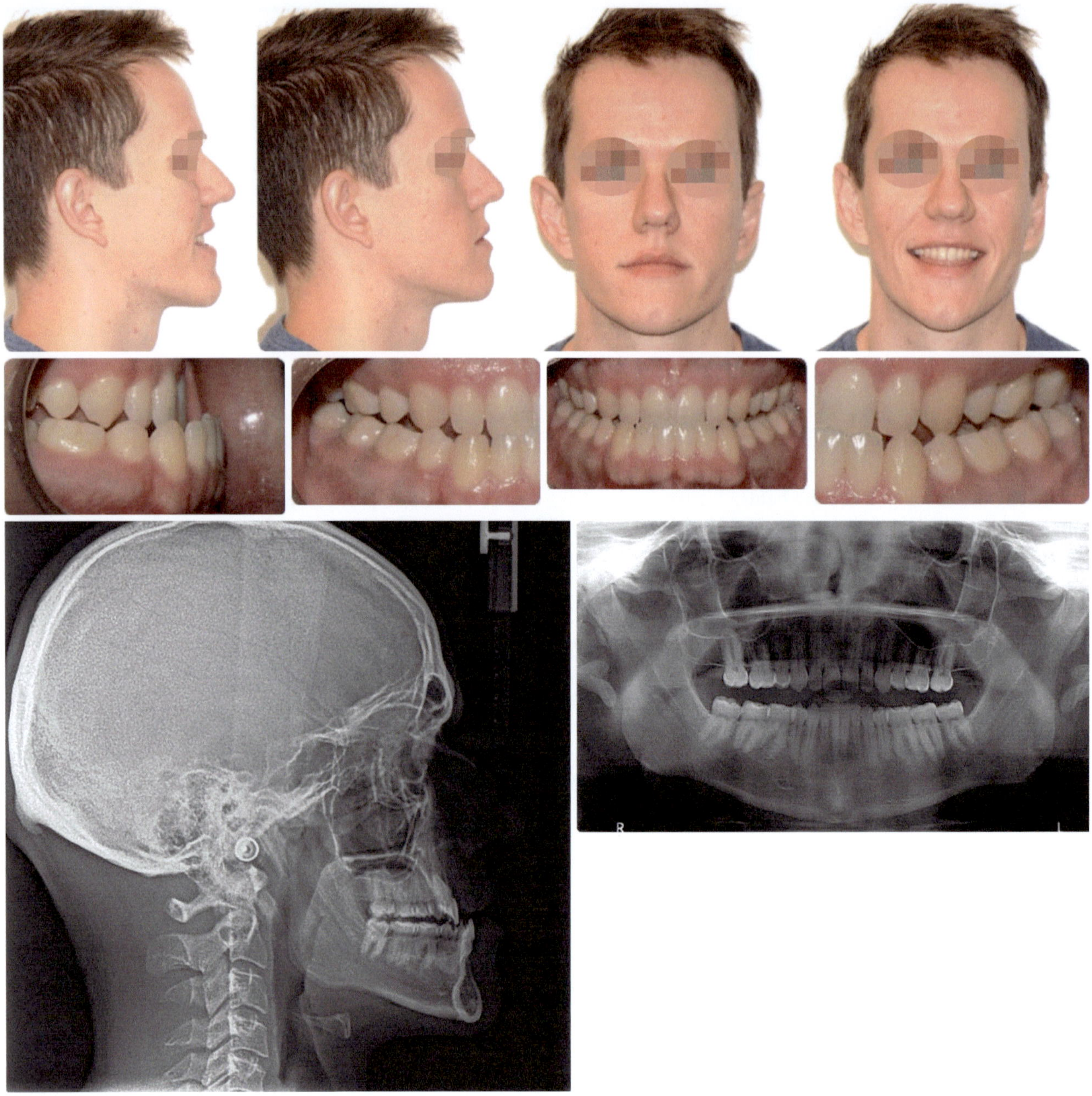

Fig. 12.1 Pretreatment records for case 1: extraoral photographs, intraoral photographs, and radiographs

week. The final occlusion was achieved after 11 months, with complete correction of the anterior-posterior and transverse deficiencies and satisfaction of the patient. The total treatment time was 16 months (Fig. 12.4).

12.4 Total Joint Replacement in Complex Ortho Treatment

Total joint replacement is a surgical approach to the treatment of a heterogenous group of pathologies involving the temporomandibular joint, collectively known as temporomandibular disorders (TMD) [10]. These disorders are the most frequent source of chronic orofacial pain and can have significant psychosocial impact for the affected individual [11]. There exist many conservative approaches to the treatment of TMD, including both articular and muscular, such as physiotherapy, various pharmacological agents, and occlusal splints [12, 13]. However, in cases of TMD that do not respond to traditional approaches or in cases involving structural anomalies, a surgical intervention may be necessary [14].

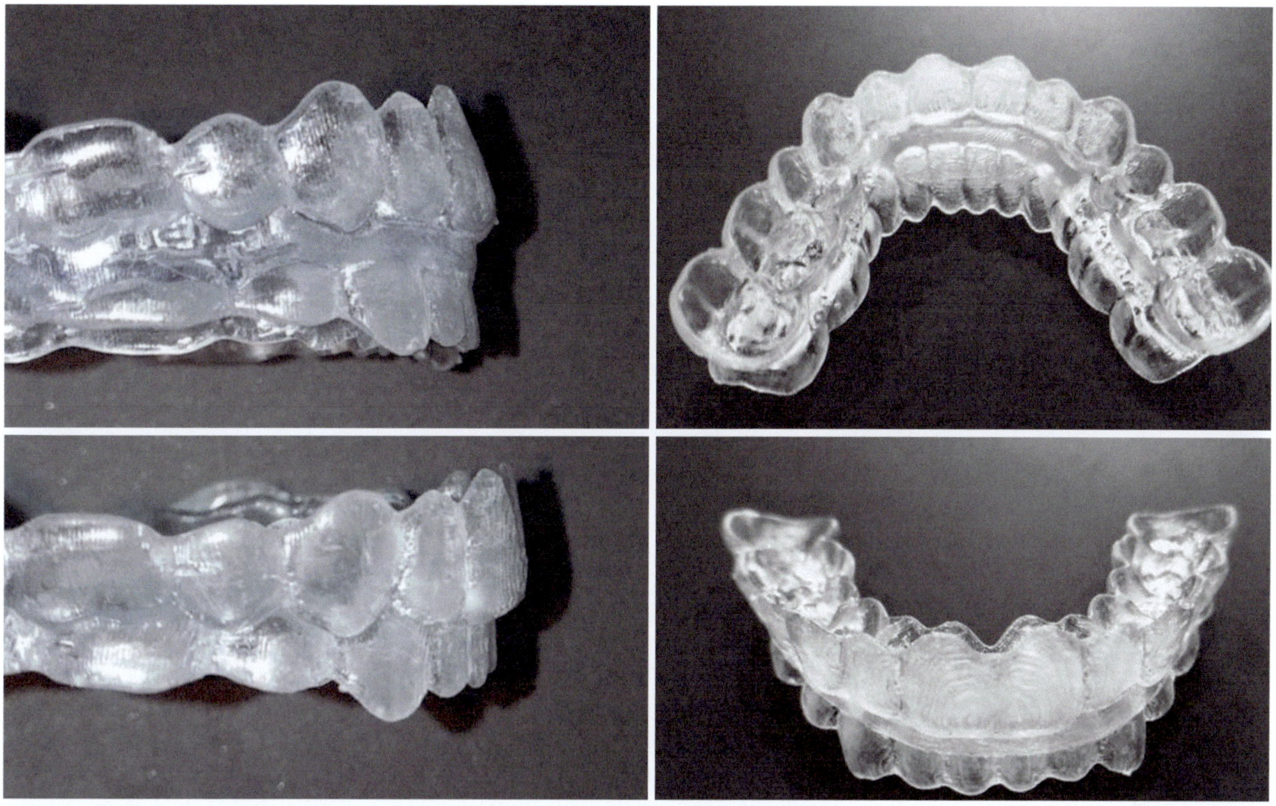

Fig. 12.2 The 3D printed clear aligner orthognathic splints (CAOS) used for achieving temporary maxillomandibular fixation intraoperatively

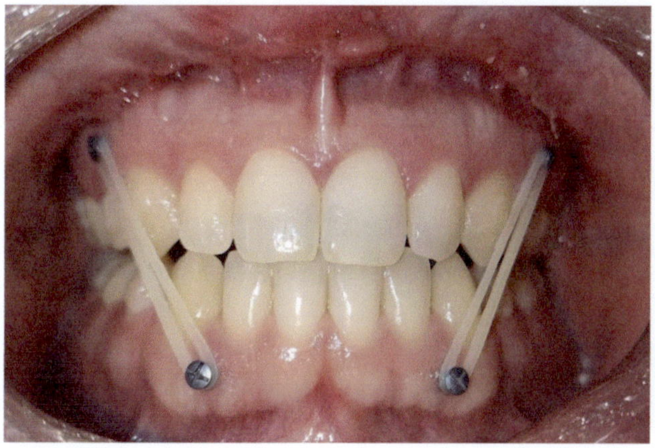

Fig. 12.3 Two-week postoperative result. Intraoral elastics were used to maintain and stabilize the occlusion using the same TADs that were placed during surgery

12.5 Case Report

This 47-year-old healthy female patient initially presented to the orthodontist for the treatment of her "facial asymmetry." Significant extra-oral findings included a maxillary cant with the right side being more superior, as well as a mandibular asymmetry with deviation toward the left hand side (Fig. 12.5). Intraorally, the patient had a class II malocclusion with both dentoalveolar and skeletal contributions. Upon further investigation and imaging, the etiology of the mandibular asymmetry was recognized to be due to an osteochondroma of the right condyle. This case was then subsequently referred to our center for further treatment.

The digital treatment planning for this case was aided by CASS and 3D printing, which can help with minimizing the errors of traditional analog methods. The treatment of the mandibular asymmetry involved an initial resection of the right mandibular condyle to remove the osteochondroma. Following 1 year of observation and no new growth, the planning for the reconstruction took place. This consisted of a total joint replacement using a custom joint, a LeFort osteotomy advancement and downgraft to correct the cant, and a BSSO to advance, rotate, and correct the cant of the mandible and establish an ideal occlusion. With the aid of 3D printing, the essential planning materials were developed: the surgical splints (intermediate and final) as well as surgical cutting guides can be accurately pre-fabricated. The TMJ components are custom titanium milled condylar prosthesis and a milled high-density polyethylene fossa (Fig. 12.6).

The surgery proceeded as planned and was uneventful. The access for the right TMJ was performed with an extra-oral approach requiring a preauricular incision superiorly to access the fossa and a retromandibular incision to access the ramus (Fig. 12.7). The maximum opening at the 3-week

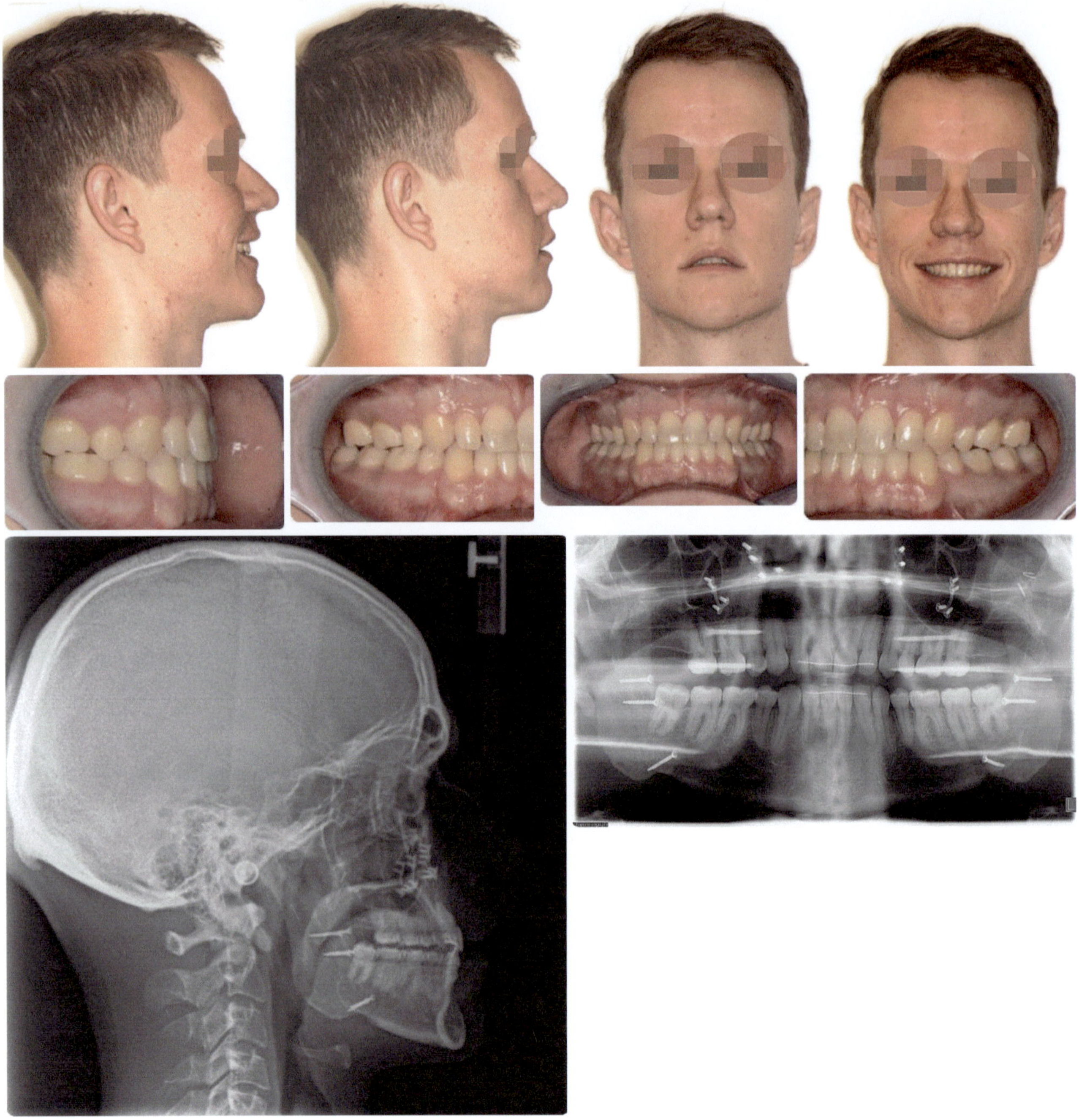

Fig. 12.4 Posttreatment records for case 1: extraoral photographs, intraoral photographs, and radiographs

postoperative follow-up was 46 mm and improved to more than 50 mm after 1 year. The incision site healed with minimal scarring and is well hidden under the patient's hairline (Fig. 12.8).

12.6 Surgery-First

The surgery-first approach (SFA) is a two-stage procedure where OGS is performed at the initial stage treatment, followed by a postsurgical phase orthodontic therapy [15]. Due to issues with occlusal instability and relapse, this method fell out of favor to the traditional three-stage conventional surgical orthodontic approach we have today [16]. With the rapid technological advances in 3D imaging techniques, there has been growing interest in the SFA [17]. Indeed, recent studies have shown that 3D imaging and simulation can allow for the clinician to treatment plan and diagnosis with better precision and accuracy [3]. Some of the benefits of the SFA include early improvements in facial esthetics, increased rate of orthodontic tooth movement due to the regional acceleratory phenom-

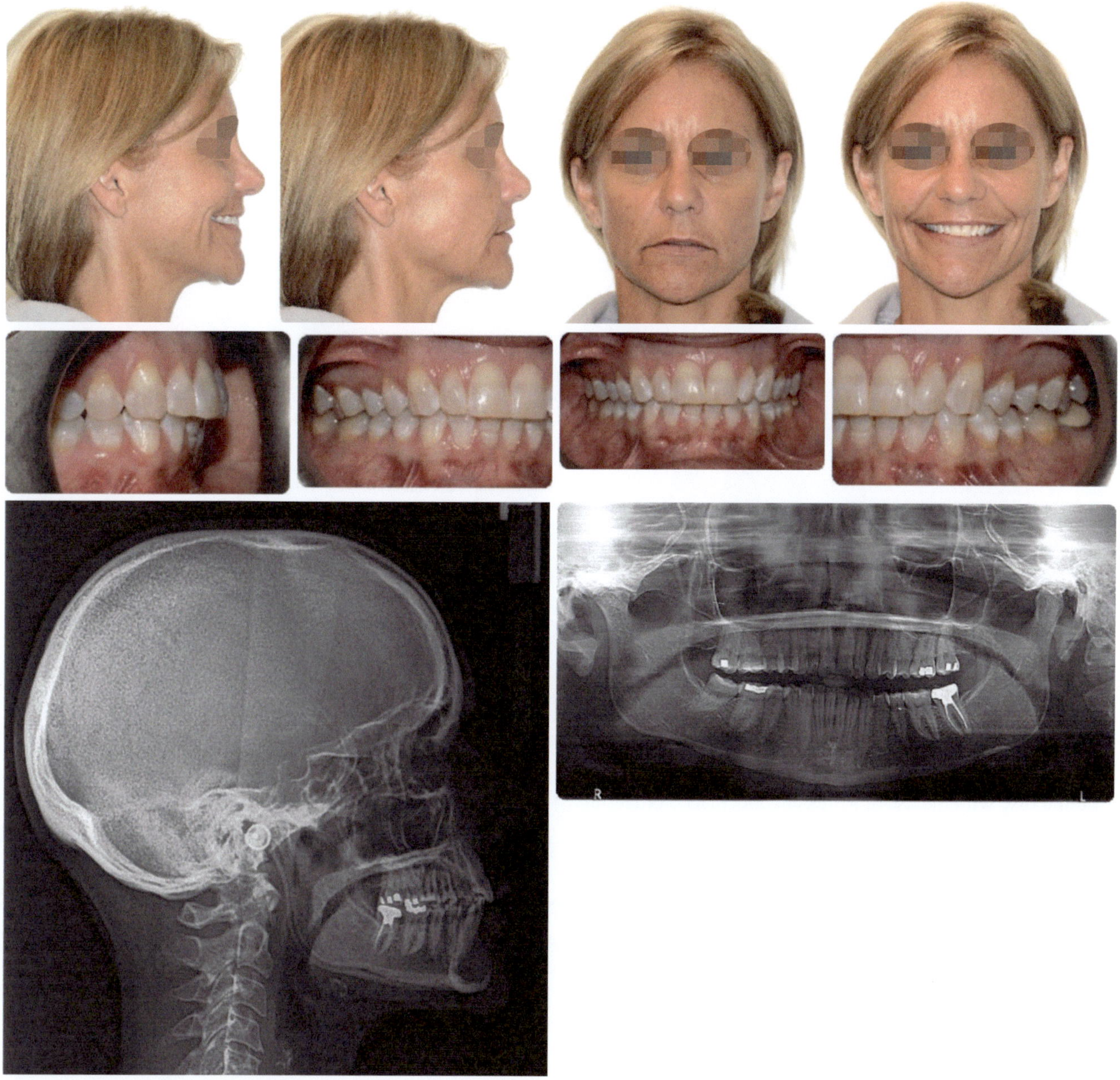

Fig. 12.5 Pretreatment records for case 2: extraoral photographs, intraoral photographs, and radiographs

enon, as well as improved stability and patient compliance [16, 18–20].

12.7 Case Report

A 24-year-old female patient who was previously treated with a functional appliance as a child presented to the orthodontist for retreatment with a chief concern of "limited mouth opening and a large overbite" (Fig. 12.9). Extraorally, she had a skeletal class II pattern associated with vertical maxillary excess, a retrognathic mandible, and retrognathic chin. Intraorally, she had a class II div 1 malocclusion with 8 mm of overjet. Functionally, her maximal opening was 29 mm, limited by pain, and her lateral excursions were limited bilaterally (2 mm only). She was ultimately diagnosed with bilateral anterior disc displacement without reduction.

Her treatment was a combined surgical orthodontic approach using clear aligner therapy and surgery first and management of her dislocated discs in order to improve her opening. The presurgical setup using virtual treatment planning software helped to involve the diagnostic predictions and aided in the decision to decompensate via extraction of the lower first bicuspids to maximize the surgical movements. Surgery involved two consecutive steps. The first was the TMJ surgery. This involved bilateral plication of the

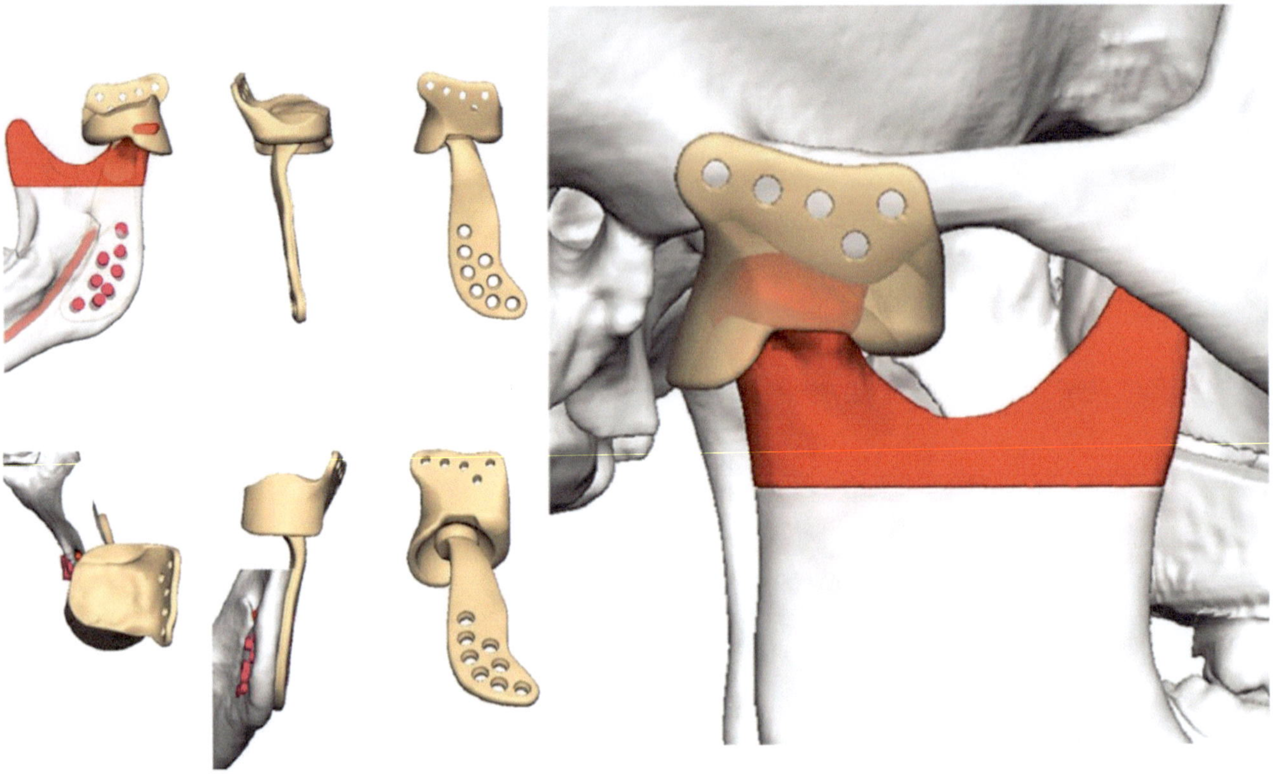

Fig. 12.6 Condylar prosthesis was digitally designed and custom milled from titanium, and the articular fossa was made from high-density polyethylene

articular disc with the use of Mitek anchors placed bilaterally in the condylar neck (Fig. 12.10). The orthognathic movements involved a 5 mm LeFort impaction, 4 mm of BSSO advancement, and a 3 mm sliding genioplasty (Fig. 12.11). Clear Aligner Orthognathic Splints were 3D printed to help facilitate the accurate transfer of the digitally planned movements during surgery.

The surgery proceeded uneventfully without complication, and intermaxillary fixation was achieved with 8 MMF screws. At the 2-week postoperative appointment, the patient's maximal opening was 24 mm (Fig. 12.12). The remaining lower spacing was closed during the postsurgical phase of orthodontic treatment with clear aligners. Following completion of treatment, the patient's maximal opening improved to 39 mm at the 1-year follow-up.

12.8 Idiopathic Condylar Resorption Following Orthognathic Surgery

Idiopathic condylar resorption (ICR) is a pathological condition that has been well documented throughout the literature yet poorly understood [21, 22]. It is described by condylar bone loss along with progressive alteration in condylar shape with no obvious underlying cause [21, 23]. The consequence of these changes include reduction of the posterior face height, anterior open bites, as well as TMJ dysfunction and pain [24]. This condition is often seen in young women between ages of 15 and 35 years and most common among teenage girls during the prepubertal growth spurt [21]. These patients are often dolichofacial with a skeletal class II relationship, vertical growth tendency, as well as history of TMJ-related disorders [22]. The treatment of ICR ranges from conservative management with occlusal splints to orthognathic surgery and/or prosthetic joint replacement [25–27].

12.9 Case Report

This case was selected to demonstrate the management of ICR following orthognathic surgery. A 22-year-old female patient presented with a hyperdivergent skeletal pattern, involving vertical maxillary excess as well as a retrognathic and clockwise-rotated mandible (Fig. 12.13). Medically she was a known Ehlers–Danlos syndrome patient but with no major systemic conditions. Intraorally, she had an anterior open bite along with two congenitally missing upper bicuspids and lower arch crowding. Her initial surgical-orthodontic treatment involved extraction of two lower biscuspids followed by orthodontic leveling and alignment and surgery which included a LeFort 1 osteotomy 4 mm impaction, a BSSO advancement of 1 mm, and a genioplasty of advance-

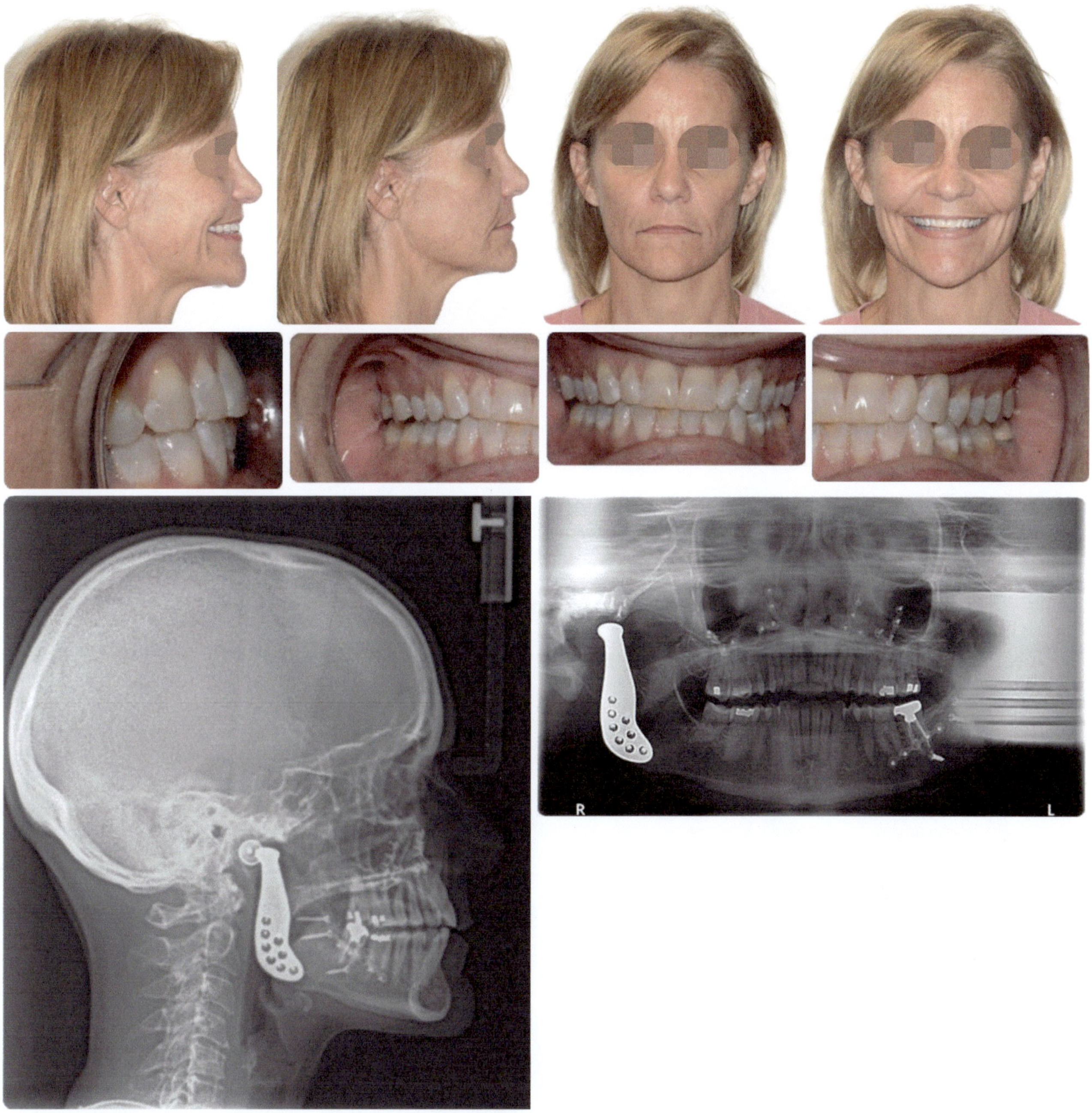

Fig. 12.7 Posttreatment records for case 1: extraoral photographs, intraoral photographs, and radiographs

ment of 6 mm. The patient was placed on the surgeon's anecdotal condylar resorption protocol.[1] Regardless, the surgery and immediate postop course was uneventful with good stability, and no complaints at the 1-year post-surgical follow-up. However, before the second-year postop examination, the patient began having painful joints and limited opening and evidence of relapse of the anterior open bite due to idiopathic condylar resorption (Fig. 12.14).

There are several ways to approach the treatment of this case, including re-osteotomizing the maxilla, the mandible, or a combination of both jaws. However, these approaches run the risk of further deterioration of the anterior open bite if the condylar resorption continues to advance. As a result, the final treatment plan selected for this case was resection

[1]*ICR Prophylaxis Protocol:*

1. *Vitamin D and $CaCO_3$ (chewable forms usually 600 mg tablets * BID OTC)*
2. *Meloxicam (Mobicox) 15 mg po OD (or Celebrex 200 mg po bid)*
3. *Omega 3 fatty acids (or fish oils 1000 mg)*
4. *Doxycycline 100 mg po OD*

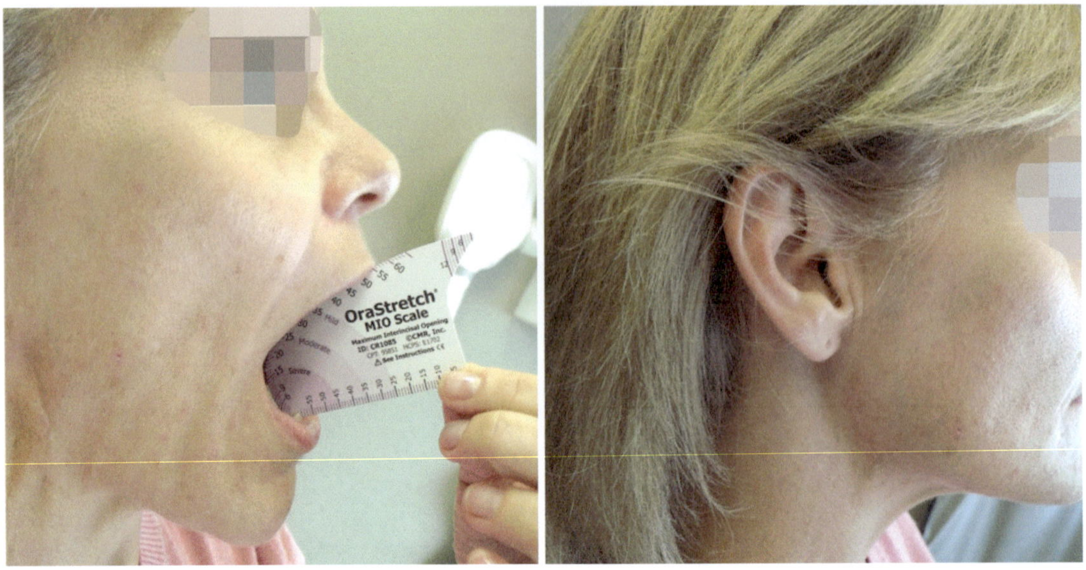

Fig. 12.8 One-year following demonstrating maximum opening of <50 mm (left) and minimal scarring at the incision site (right)

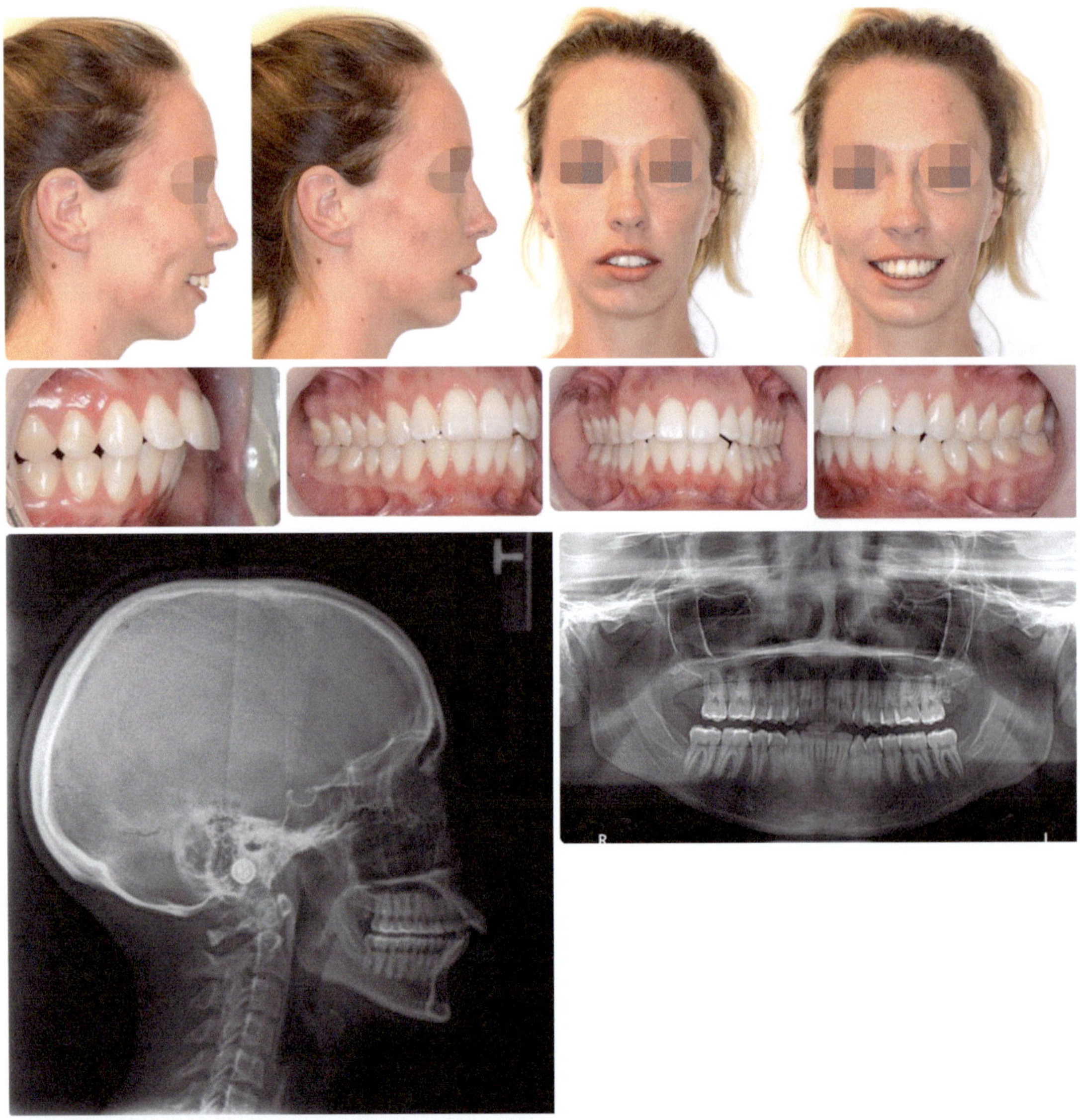

Fig. 12.9 Pretreatment records for case 3: extraoral photographs, intraoral photographs, and radiographs

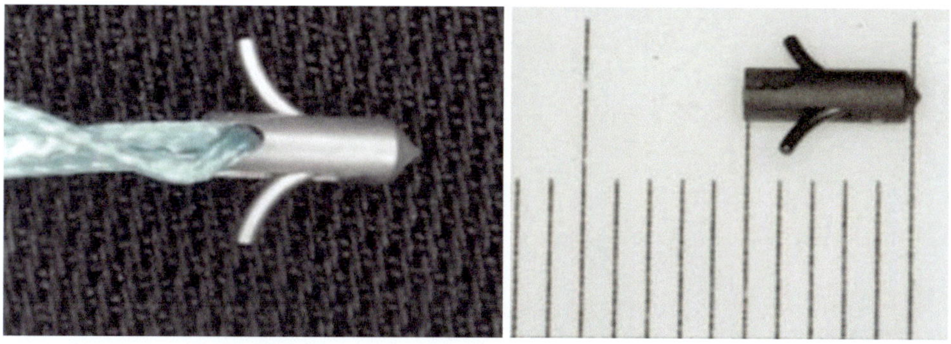

Fig. 12.10 Mitek anchor with prolene suture and ruler showing its 5-mm length

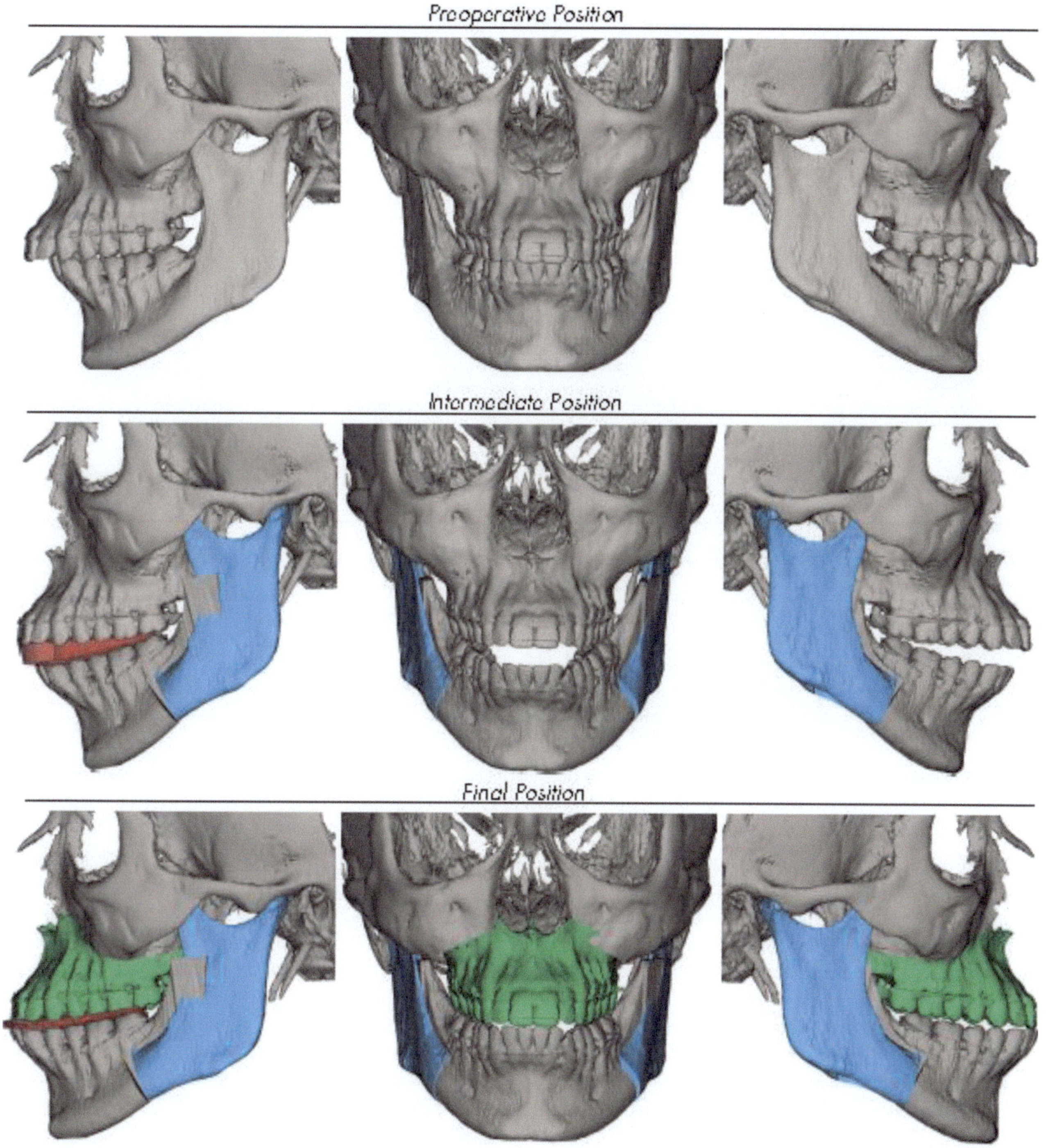

Fig. 12.11 Virtual surgical planning and setup for case 3

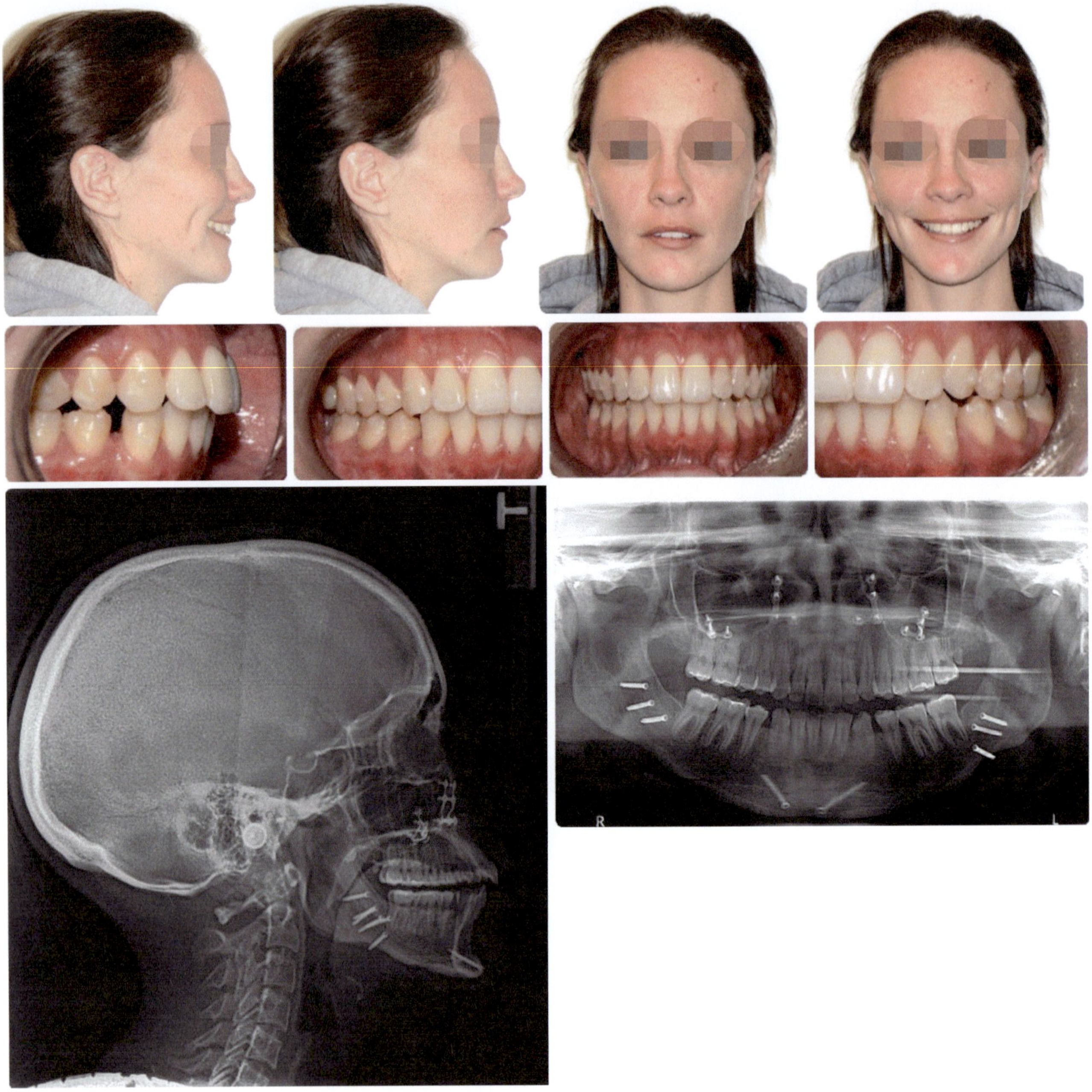

Fig. 12.12 Posttreatment records for case 3: extraoral photographs, intraoral photographs, and radiographs

and total joint replacement of both mandibular condyles. This case was visualized using CASS to facilitate virtual treatment planning. This process allows the surgeon to accurately locate critical anatomic structures such as the inferior alveolar nerve and design the appropriate appliances to avoid their injury (Fig. 12.15). The subsequent custom surgical guide, joint, and fossa implants were accurately fabricated via 3D printing.

The surgery proceeded successfully and uneventfully, with the occlusion being unchanged from the planned state at the 1-year follow-up (Fig. 12.16). This case demonstrates the importance of preoperative identification of at-risk patients of condylar resorption. Techniques that could reduce the risk of ICR includes limiting the mandibular advancement, minimizing counterclockwise condylar repositioning, passively seating the condyle, as well as early postoperative TMJ physical therapy and occlusal equilibration. Notwithstanding all these measures, for this specific case, however, the medical connective tissue disorder may have played a role in the development of the ICR.

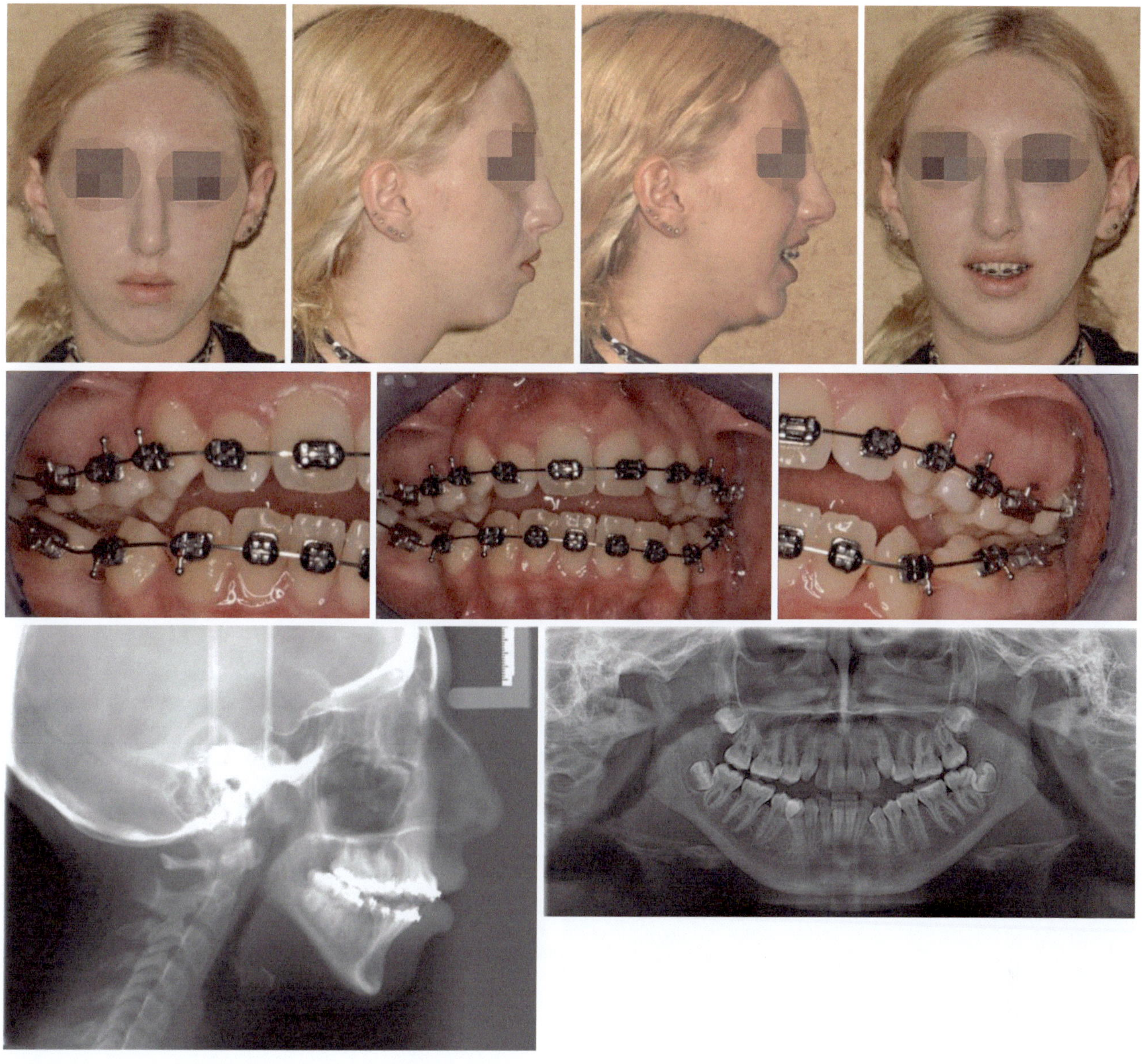

Fig. 12.13 Pretreatment records for case 4: extraoral photographs, intraoral photographs, and radiographs

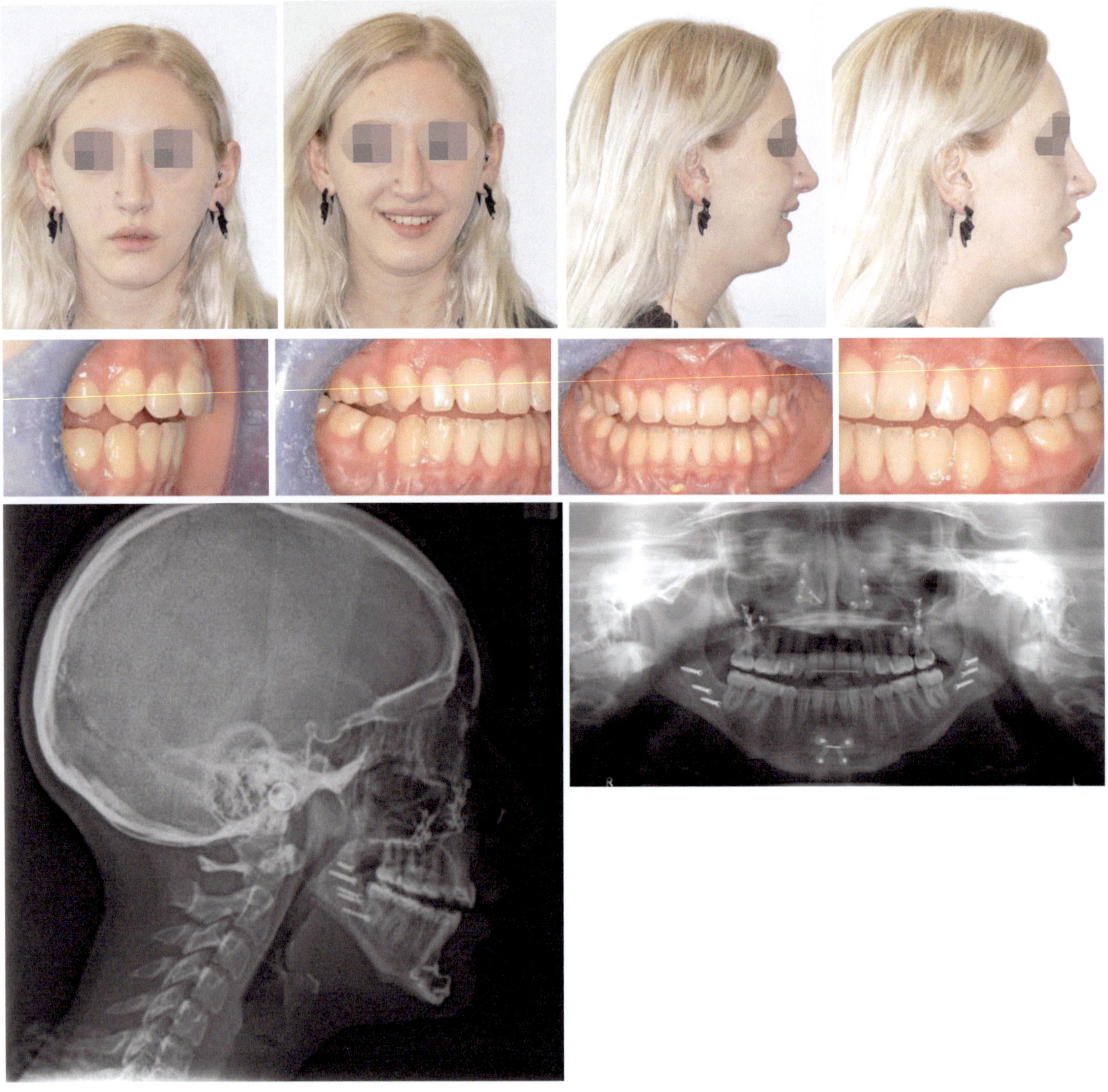

Fig. 12.14 Posttreatment records for case 4: extraoral photographs, intraoral photographs, and radiographs

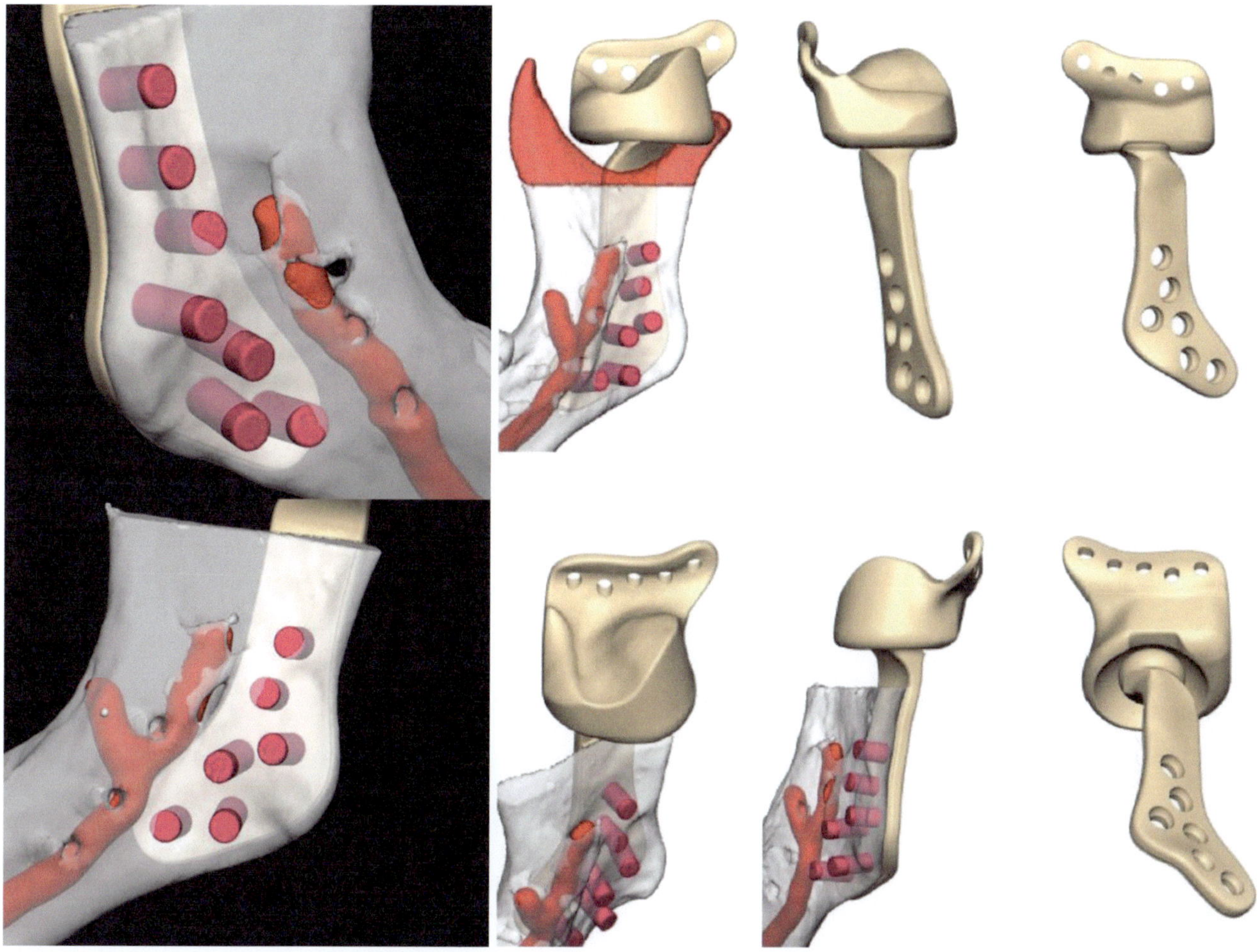

Fig. 12.15 Utilization of 3D planning to digitally design a prosthesis with care and attention to critical anatomical structures, such as the inferior alveolar nerve

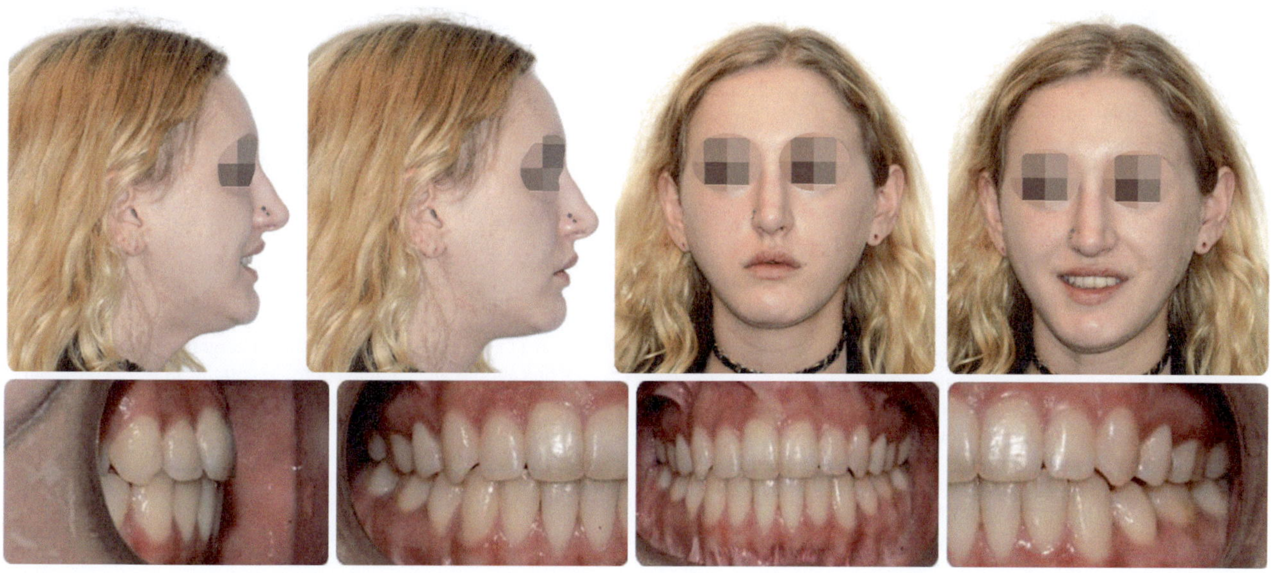

Fig. 12.16 Post-retreatment records for case 4: extraoral photographs, intraoral photographs, and radiographs

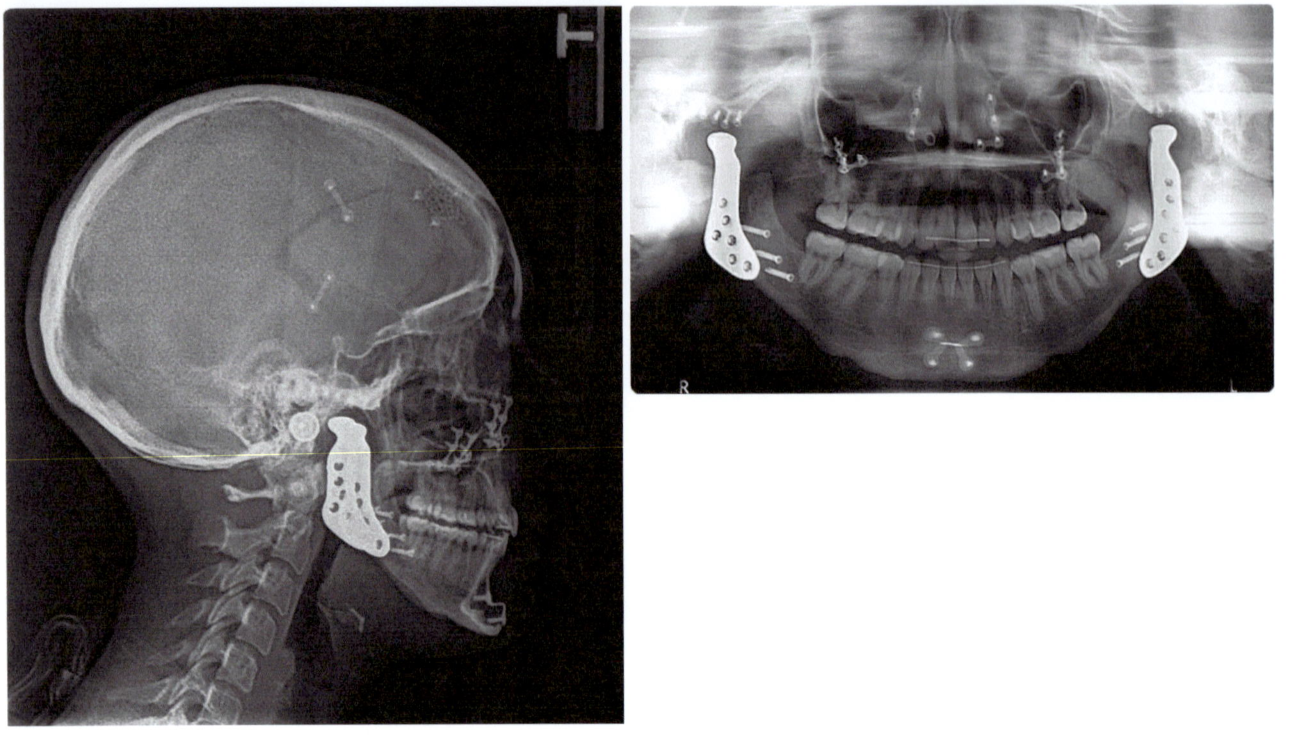

Fig. 12.16 (continued)

References

1. Harrell WE Jr. 3D diagnosis and treatment planning in orthodontics. Semin Orthod. 2009;15(1):35–41. https://doi.org/10.1053/j.sodo.2008.09.004.
2. Badiali G, Costabile E, Lovero E, Pironi M, Rucci P, Marchetti C, et al. Virtual orthodontic surgical planning to improve the accuracy of the surgery-first approach: a prospective evaluation. J Oral Maxillofac Surg. 2019;77(10):2104–15. https://doi.org/10.1016/j.joms.2019.04.017.
3. Tran NH, Tantidhnazet S, Raocharernporn S, Kiattavornchareon S, Pairuchvej V, Wongsirichat N. Accuracy of three-dimensional planning in surgery-first orthognathic surgery: planning versus outcome. J Clin Med Res. 2018;10(5):429–36. https://doi.org/10.14740/jocmr3372w.
4. Keim RG. The evolution of Invisalign. J Clin Orthod. 2017;51(2):69–70.
5. Weir T. Clear aligners in orthodontic treatment. Aust Dent J. 2017;62(Suppl 1):58–62. https://doi.org/10.1111/adj.12480.
6. Rosvall MD, Fields HW, Ziuchkovski J, Rosenstiel SF, Johnston WM. Attractiveness, acceptability, and value of orthodontic appliances. Am J Orthod Dentofac Orthop. 2009;135(3):276.e1–12; discussion -7. https://doi.org/10.1016/j.ajodo.2008.09.020.
7. Rossini G, Parrini S, Castroflorio T, Deregibus A, Debernardi CL. Efficacy of clear aligners in controlling orthodontic tooth movement: a systematic review. Angle Orthod. 2015;85(5):881–9. https://doi.org/10.2319/061614-436.1.
8. Taub DI, Palermo V. Orthognathic surgery for the Invisalign patient. Semin Orthod. 2017;23:99–102.
9. Caminiti M, Lou T. Clear aligner orthognathic splints. J Oral Maxillofac Surg. 2019;77(5):1071.e1–8. https://doi.org/10.1016/j.joms.2018.12.012.
10. Guarda-Nardini L, Manfredini D, Ferronato G. Temporomandibular joint total replacement prosthesis: current knowledge and considerations for the future. Int J Oral Maxillofac Surg. 2008;37(2):103–10. https://doi.org/10.1016/j.ijom.2007.09.175.
11. Rollman GB, Gillespie JM. The role of psychosocial factors in temporomandibular disorders. Curr Rev Pain. 2000;4(1):71–81.
12. Dworkin SF, Turner JA, Wilson L, Massoth D, Whitney C, Huggins KH, et al. Brief group cognitive-behavioral intervention for temporomandibular disorders. Pain. 1994;59(2):175–87. https://doi.org/10.1016/0304-3959(94)90070-1.
13. Dao TT, Lavigne GJ. Oral splints: the crutches for temporomandibular disorders and bruxism? Crit Rev Oral Biol Med. 1998;9(3):345–61.
14. Dimitroulis G. The role of surgery in the management of disorders of the temporomandibular joint: a critical review of the literature. Part 1. Int J Oral Maxillofac Surg. 2005;34(2):107–13. https://doi.org/10.1016/j.ijom.2004.06.011.
15. Choi DS, Garagiola U, Kim SG. Current status of the surgery-first approach (part I): concepts and orthodontic protocols. Maxillofac Plast Reconstr Surg. 2019;41(1):10. https://doi.org/10.1186/s40902-019-0194-4.
16. Kwon TG, Han MD. Current status of surgery first approach (part II): precautions and complications. Maxillofac Plast Reconstr Surg. 2019;41(1):23. https://doi.org/10.1186/s40902-019-0206-4.
17. Janakiraman N, Feinberg M, Vishwanath M, Nalaka Jayaratne YS, Steinbacher DM, Nanda R, et al. Integration of 3-dimensional surgical and orthodontic technologies with orthognathic "surgery-first" approach in the management of unilateral condylar hyperplasia. Am J Orthod Dentofac Orthop. 2015;148(6):1054–66. https://doi.org/10.1016/j.ajodo.2015.08.012.
18. Hernández-Alfaro F, Guijarro-Martínez R, Molina-Coral A, Badía-Escriche C. "Surgery first" in bimaxillary orthognathic

surgery. J Oral Maxillofac Surg. 2011;69(6):e201–e7. https://doi.org/10.1016/j.joms.2011.01.010.
19. Liou EJW, Chen PH, Wang YC, Yu CC, Huang CS, Chen YR. Surgery-first accelerated orthognathic surgery: postoperative rapid orthodontic tooth movement. J Oral Maxillofac Surg. 2011;69(3):781–5. https://doi.org/10.1016/j.joms.2010.10.035.
20. Liou EJW, Chen PH, Wang YC, Yu CC, Huang CS, Chen YR. Surgery-first accelerated orthognathic surgery: orthodontic guidelines and setup for model surgery. J Oral Maxillofac Surg. 2011;69(3):771–80. https://doi.org/10.1016/j.joms.2010.11.011.
21. Mitsimponas K, Mehmet S, Kennedy R, Shakib K. Idiopathic condylar resorption. Br J Oral Maxillofac Surg. 2018;56(4):249–55. https://doi.org/10.1016/j.bjoms.2018.02.016.
22. Alsabban L, Amarista FJ, Mercuri LG, Perez D. Idiopathic condylar resorption: a survey and review of the literature. J Oral Maxillofac Surg. 2018;76(11):2316.e1–13. https://doi.org/10.1016/j.joms.2018.07.008.
23. He Y, Lin H, Lin Q, Lu L, Li M, Li Q, et al. Morphologic changes in idiopathic condylar resorption with different degrees of bone loss. Oral Surg Oral Med Oral Pathol Oral Radiol. 2019;128(3):332–40. https://doi.org/10.1016/j.oooo.2019.05.013.
24. Park JH, Park JJ, Papademetriou M, Suri S. Anterior open bite due to idiopathic condylar resorption during orthodontic retention of a Class II Division 1 malocclusion. Am J Orthod Dentofac Orthop. 2019;156(4):555–65. https://doi.org/10.1016/j.ajodo.2019.05.010.
25. Chigurupati R, Mehra P. Surgical management of idiopathic condylar resorption: orthognathic surgery versus temporomandibular total joint replacement. Oral Maxillofac Surg Clin North Am. 2018;30(3):355–67. https://doi.org/10.1016/j.coms.2018.05.004.
26. Raouf SR, Attia MM, Wright EF. Splint therapy is the most conservative treatment for idiopathic condylar resorption (UT CAT #2986). Tex Dent J. 2016;133(3):182.
27. Kau CH, Bejemir MP. Application of virtual three-dimensional surgery planning in management of open bite with idiopathic condylar resorption. Ann Maxillofac Surg. 2015;5(2):249–54. https://doi.org/10.4103/2231-0746.175760.

3D Prosthodontic Treatment Planning for Orthodontic Patients: Interdisciplinary Approach

13

Walaa Magdy Ahmed, Bassam Alalola, Mohammed Alsaloum, Tyler Verhaeghe, James Andrew, and Mohamed-Nur Abdallah

13.1 3D Treatment Planning Consideration for Orthodontic-Prosthodontic Patients

13.1.1 Esthetic Consideration

The idiom of beauty being in the eye of the beholder was first written over 140 years ago [1]. Esthetic dentistry, over the same time period, has not been immune to the subjectivity of beauty and has continued to evolve due to advancements in dental materials and the development of new techniques and innovative technologies [2]. Previous studies have shown that the general perception of an esthetic smile may not be as varied between dental professionals and laypeople as might be expected [3–6]. The creation of a beautiful smile, through the collective blending of artistic and scientific principles, is a process known as smile design [7]. While there is no single correct approach to this process, given its multifaceted nature, a methodical approach is recommended, often by way of a form or a checklist [7–9]. An esthetic analysis should similarly progress systematically from macro to micro, addressing five levels of esthetics: facial, oral-facial, oral, dentogingival, and dental [10]. Facial esthetics includes facial form and symmetry, and oral-facial esthetics examines the maxillomandibular and dental midline relationships to the face, while oral esthetics involves the relationship of the lips to both arches, including the teeth and gingiva. Dentogingival esthetics relates the teeth and gingiva collectively and independently, and finally, dental esthetics includes tooth shape, size, and shade within the dental arches (Figs. 13.1 and 13.2) [10]. Such a progression requires a multidisciplinary approach, particularly between the orthodontist and the prosthodontist, as shown in the cases presented in this chapter.

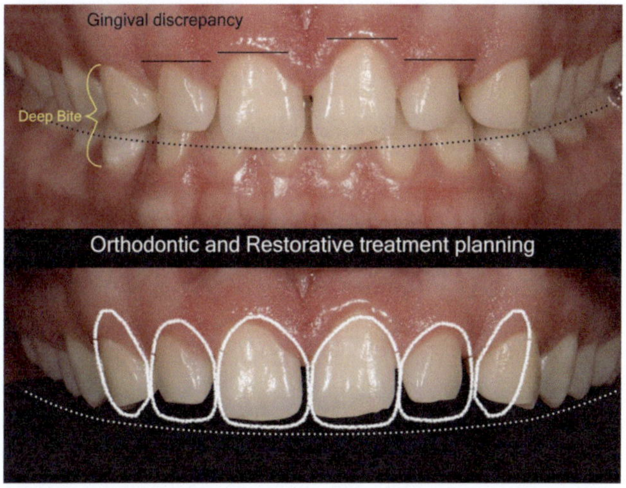

Fig. 13.1 Dentogingival esthetic considerations for orthodontic and restorative treatment planning. The gingival margins have to be symmetrical between the right and the left sides. Central incisors and canines should have the same gingival marginal level, which is slightly apical to the gingival margin of the lateral incisors

W. M. Ahmed (✉)
Department of Restorative Dentistry, Faculty of Dentistry, King Abdulaziz University, Jeddah, Saudi Arabia

Faculty of Dentistry, University of British Columbia, Vancouver, BC, Canada
e-mail: wmahmed@kau.edu.sa

B. Alalola · M. Alsaloum
College of Dentistry, King Saud bin Abdulaziz University for Health Sciences, Riyadh, Saudi Arabia

King Abdullah International Medical Research Center, Riyadh, Saudi Arabia

T. Verhaeghe · J. Andrew
Faculty of Dentistry, University of British Columbia, Vancouver, BC, Canada
e-mail: tyler.verhaeghe@alumni.ubc.ca

M.-N. Abdallah
Department of Orthodontics, School of Dentistry, University of Detroit Mercy, Detroit, MI, USA
e-mail: mohamednur.abdallah@mail.utoronto.ca

J.-M. Retrouvey, M.-N. Abdallah (eds.), *3D Diagnosis and Treatment Planning in Orthodontics*,
https://doi.org/10.1007/978-3-030-57223-5_13

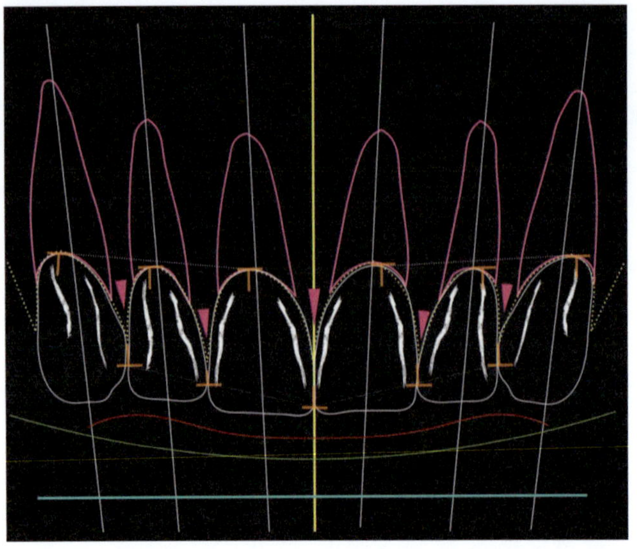

Fig. 13.2 Dental micro-esthetic considerations for orthodontic and restorative treatment planning, including height–width proportions, ideal tooth width proportions, connectors and embrasures, and gingival zenith

Generally, the maxillary anterior teeth receive the main focus when considering the smile esthetic, with the central incisors receiving significant attention, and the canines and laterals sequentially receive less visual attention as they are further from the midline (Fig. 13.1) [11]. Visual deviation in the maxillary incisal plane from an otherwise parallel to interpupillary line and posterior occlusal plane, particularly where contralateral incisor lengths are uneven, is indicative of oblique wear and requires a concerted effort between the orthodontist and prosthodontist [12]. Another esthetic example requiring the collaboration between orthodontist and prosthodontist is the excessive gingival display "gummy smile" with supraerupted, short, abraided incisors due to protrusive bruxism [12]. Whether the prosthodontist is replacing or restoring the maxillary central incisors or the entire anterior segment, the orthodontist defines the available space through the positioning of the adjacent and antagonist teeth [13]. The extent of this space is envisioned and established through mutual communication throughout treatment planning and active treatment. Further, it is essential to identify the final restorative materials at the outset of treatment planning and during orthodontic treatment prior to the definitive prosthodontic restoration [13].

Historically, esthetic analysis relied mainly on static images. However, a recent study evaluating the use of static images and video clips for analyzing posed and dynamic smiles revealed that spontaneous smiles tend to show more maxillary teeth, mandibular teeth, and gingival display when compared to posed smiles [14]. Therefore, these findings highlight the importance of considering adjunctive use of dynamic video images. Another possible paradigm shift from the traditional esthetic analysis is the facial flow concept. This concept shifts away from smiles designed using symmetry and is rather guided by mathematics and geometry in order to establish harmony with the notion that faces are often asymmetrical in nature [15] and are appreciated as such [11]. With the advent of 3D face scanners and virtual and augmented reality which can be incorporated into smartphone applications, the evolution of esthetic dentistry may, in fact, be at the precipice of a *revolution*, where perhaps, in time, machine learning and artificial intelligence will automate the esthetic analysis [2]. Nevertheless, even if beauty evolves to being in the microprocessor of a computing device, esthetics are only one of the considerations during treatment planning orthodontic-prosthodontic patients and the skilled clinician must remain cognizant of biology, occlusion, and other prosthodontic principles.

13.1.2 Biological Consideration

Ideally, dental implants should be placed after completion of facial growth to avoid the risk of infraocclusion of the implant restoration, which compromises the masticatory function and esthetic appearance [16]. Traditionally, hand-wrist radiographs and cervical vertebral maturation were used to assess the completion of facial growth. However, such methods proved to have low reliability in determining the completion of facial growth [17]. The more accurate technique is to superimpose serial lateral cephalometric radiographs every 6 months to 1 year [18]. It should be noted that even after completion of growth in adolescents, the dental implant might become infra-occluded due to continuous eruption of the teeth [19].

Five indices are usually used to assess the periodontal soft tissue status: plaque index (PI), papilla index (PpI), bleeding index (BI), probing depth (PD), and gingival index (GI) [16, 20–22]. Periodontal stability is an important factor to consider during both orthodontic and prosthodontic treatment planning. For instance, identifying the best therapeutic approach to manage maxillary lateral incisor agenesis (MLIA) has always been controversial due to the variability encountered in each clinical case. The two major alternatives being orthodontic space closure and substitution with the canines or space opening for prosthetic replacements. Clinicians that support opening the space and restoring the missing lateral incisor claim that obtaining canine guidance occlusal scheme is better for stability of occlusion and argue that it is difficult to obtain a satisfactory esthetic outcome from canine substitution due to the differences between canine and lateral incisors in terms of color, shape, and gingival level [23, 24]. On the other hand, clinicians that are inclined to close spaces and reshape the canines argue that this option is superior in terms of periodontal health and patient satisfaction as well as avoids long-term restorative work and decreases the financial burden [22, 25].

Nordquist et al. compared the two management approaches of MLIA in terms of periodontal and occlusal evaluation [21]. This study showed that the greatest plaque accumulation was observed next to the maxillary lateral incisor pontic in the case of fixed dental prosthesis (FDPs) and on the lingual surfaces of the removable partial denture in the cases that the maxillary canine substituted the maxillary lateral incisor. However, cases using dental implants to replace the missing maxillary lateral incisor after opening the space were not included in this study. Black triangles were observed in the canine substituted cases more often than cases that restored the maxillary lateral with dental implant cases after opening the space [16]. This could be attributed to the fact that the geometry of the maxillary canine is different buccolingually and mesiodistally when compared to the maxillary lateral incisor as well as the difficulty to recontour the maxillary canine to mimic the maxillary lateral incisor in the cervical region.

13.1.3 Occlusal Consideration

Skeletal and dental discrepancies could complicate the development of ideal occlusal characteristics. For example, the dental compensation that occurs in certain cases of transverse skeletal discrepancies make it more difficult to obtain ideal axial loading on the posterior teeth. Vertical discrepancies can also affect the lateral occlusal guidance scheme. Patients with increased lower anterior facial heights and vertical excess tend to demonstrate a group function occlusal scheme, whereas the occlusal scheme of patients with short lower anterior facial heights and vertical deficiency tends to be a canine guidance occlusal Scheme [26]. Studies have found no significant difference between the number of premature centric and excursive contacts, as well as the signs and symptoms of temporomandibular disorders (TMDs) between the cases were treated by canine substitution and those treated by opening the space for prosthodontic replacement when managing MLIA [21, 22].

13.2 The Orthodontic-Prosthodontic Cases

This section presents clinical cases that required a combined orthodontic and prosthodontic treatment approach with an emphasis on the digital planning steps.

13.2.1 Tooth Size Discrepancy

Tooth size discrepancy exists when the maxillary and mandibular teeth are not in proportion with each other. Tooth size discrepancy provides an additional challenge to the orthodontic treatment plan. For example, in peg-shaped maxillary lateral incisors, if no restorative plan is considered, performing inter proximal reduction (IPR) of the opposing mandibular incisors or compromising the ideal overjet and overbite is necessary to achieve an adequate occlusion. On the other hand, if considering restorative options, orthodontic treatment can prepare the space(s), either mesial or distal to the undersized teeth for placement of direct or indirect restorations. Utilizing digital tool aids in visualization, planning the final position of the teeth, and determining the restorative work are needed to achieve optimum esthetic and function outcomes.

Figure 13.3 shows a 23-year-old patient with a class II subdivision right malocclusion associated with 5 mm of crowding in the mandibular arch and mild spacing distal to left maxillary canine. The patient had a retained left mandibular primary second molar and a congenitally missing left mandibular second premolar. The retained primary molar and the undersized maxillary lateral incisors resulted in a tooth size discrepancy (maxillary deficiency/mandibular excess) [27].

The interdisciplinary treatment plan of this case involved maintaining the primary molar with the possibility of future restorative work, accepting the mandibular dental midline discrepancy, and restoring the ideal proportion of the undersized maxillary lateral incisors by opening the space distal to the maxillary lateral incisors. Prosthodontic digital diagnostic planning was performed near the end of the finishing stage of orthodontic treatment and before the removal of the fixed orthodontic appliance (Fig. 13.4). Two digital diagnostic setups were considered to address the tooth discrepancy on the right side: building up the lateral incisor (Fig. 13.4c) or building up both the lateral incisor and the canine (Fig. 13.4e, f). The decision was made to build up the distal surface of right maxillary lateral incisor and mesial surface of right maxillary canine. On the other hand, the digital diagnostic setup showed that it was sufficient to build up the dis-

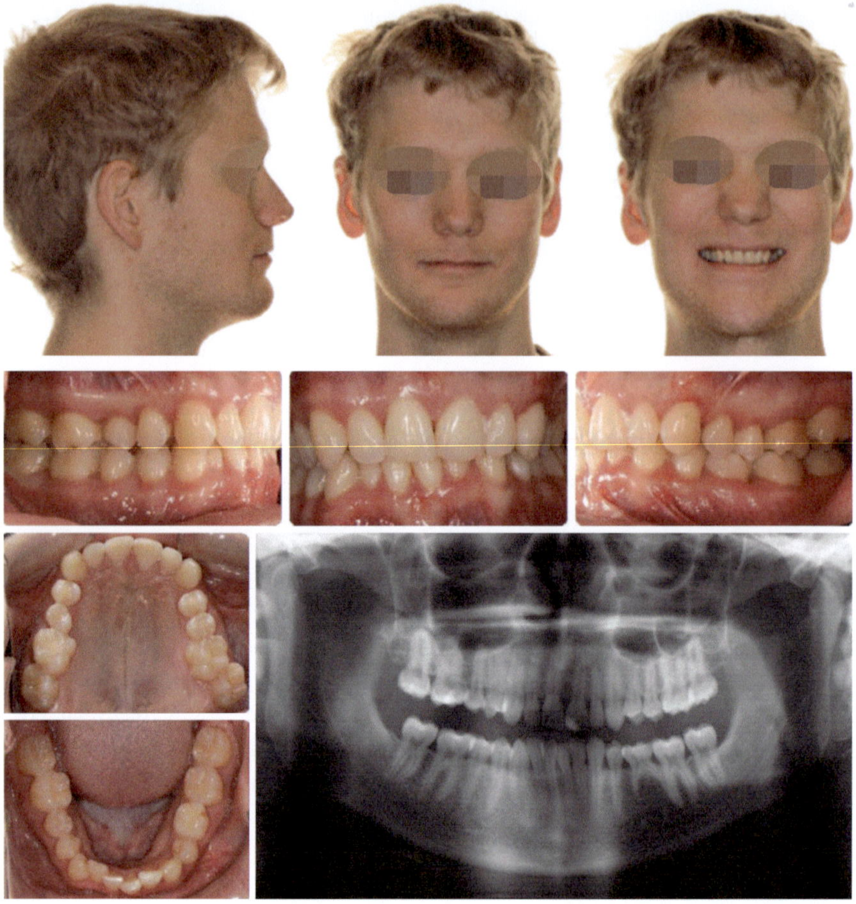

Fig. 13.3 Initial treatment records showing the mild spacing in the anterior maxillary arch distal to maxillary left canine and crowding in the anterior mandibular arch. (Courtesy of Dr. Hadeel Alohali)

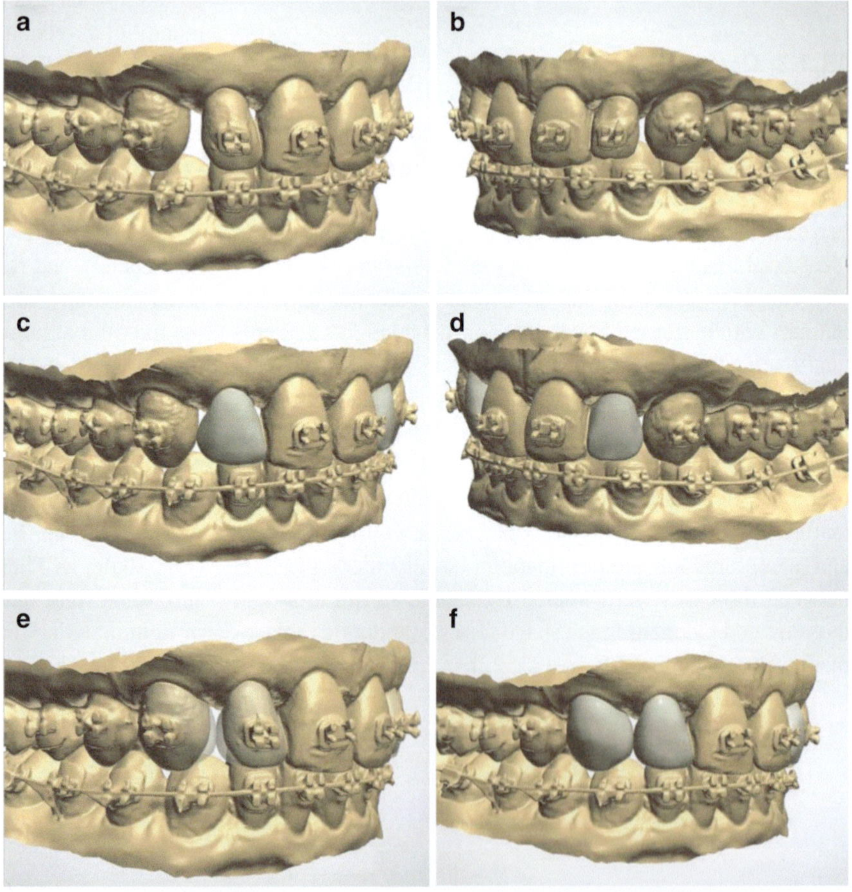

Fig. 13.4 Digital diagnostic planning for addressing the tooth size discrepancy in the anterior maxillary dentition. (**a–b**) Initial digital scans of the dentition was taken using Trios 3Shape scanner (TRIOS 3; 3Shape Inc, Copenhagen, Denmark). (**c–f**) Digital diagnostic setups including the anticipated final outcomes after performing different scenarios of tooth digital build ups. 3Shape Trios Design Studio software (3Shape Inc, Copenhagen, Denmark) was used to perform the diagnostic setups

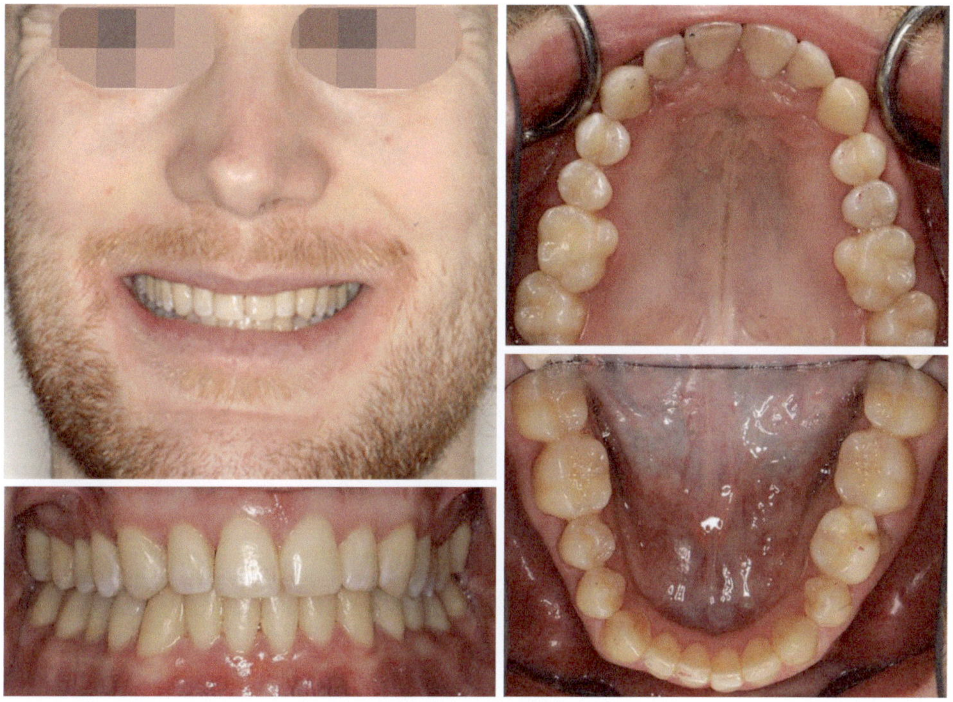

Fig. 13.5 Final treatment records after opening the spaces distal to the maxillary lateral incisors and performing composite resin build ups for the maxillary lateral incisors and the right maxillary canine

tal surface of maxillary left lateral incisor with a composite restoration to address the tooth-size discrepancy on the left side (Fig. 13.4d).

Figure 13.5 shows the final treatment outcomes after the restorative work. Certain deviations from ideal orthodontic finishing were accepted including dental midlines discrepancies, particularly the mandibular dental midline and mild class II relationship on the right side. Furthermore, the patient was advised to attend regular follow-ups to monitor the resin composite restorations in case there is a need for reparative work or additional polishing.

Figure 13.6 illustrates a 13-year-old female patient who presented to the orthodontic clinic with concerns about tooth crowding. Upon intraoral and radiographic examination, the left maxillary lateral incisor had a malformed crown shape (cylindrical) and a type-1 dens invaginatus according to Oehlers classification [28]. Such dental anomalies require additional considerations, and an interdisciplinary approach was needed to achieve ideal final results as feasible as possible (Fig. 13.6a).

The cylindrical-shaped crown of the left maxillary lateral incisor created certain functional occlusal interferences during the detailing and finishing stage of the orthodontic treatment (Fig. 13.6b). There were heavy contacts on the left maxillary lateral incisor, most probably because of its increased bucco-lingual shape, thus risking a traumatic occlusion. Due to the presence of type-1 dens invaginatus, a cone beam computed tomography (CBCT) was obtained to evaluate the thickness of enamel and dentin (Fig. 13.6c). Gradual enameloplasty was performed on the palatal surface of the lateral incisor over a 3-month period to minimize pulpal irritation as well as to create adequate and equal contacts on the maxillary anterior teeth.

The second challenge of the presence of a cylindrical-shaped crown was restoring the ideal esthetics, so a digital diagnostic setup was conducted on to facilitate accurate space assessment and possible final outcomes using a design software (3Shape Trios Design Studio software, 3Shape Inc., Copenhagen, Denmark) (Fig. 13.6d–f). The shape of the contralateral lateral incisor was copied digitally and transferred to the left maxillary lateral incisor, then the digital mock-up was modified according to the desired final form and occlusion. Two treatment options were discussed with the patient: a direct resin composite restoration and an indirect ceramic crown to reshape the left maxillary lateral incisor and consolidate the space between the left maxillary lateral incisor and canine. After assessing the dentition and occlusion, it was concluded that a 1.5 mm space between the left maxillary lateral and canine (at the narrowest point) was sufficient to allow for the fabrication of a direct resin composite restoration or a ceramic crown. A resin composite restoration was used in this case to reshape the left maxillary

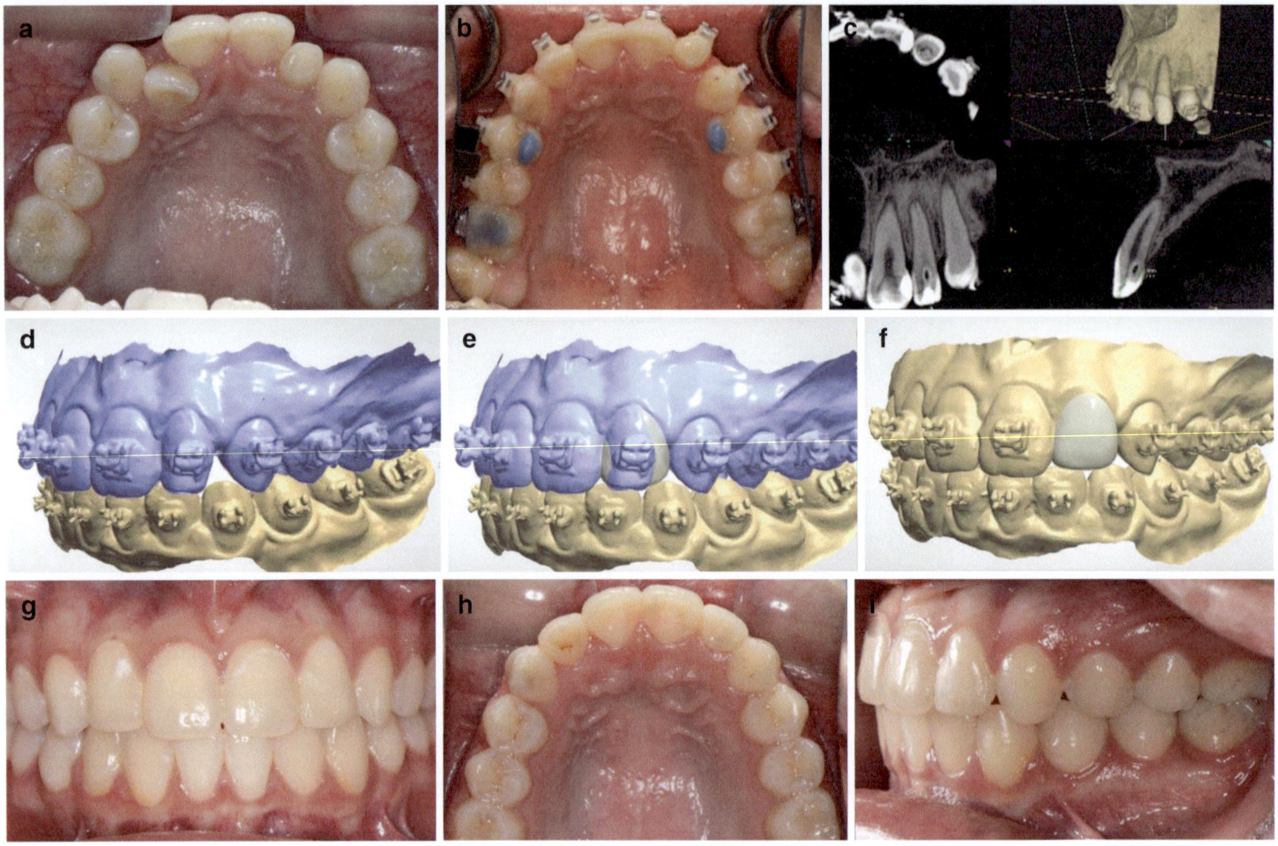

Fig. 13.6 (**a**) Initial pretreatment occlusal view of the maxillary dentition. (**b**) Progress record showing the occlusal view of the maxillary dentition. (**c**) CBCT scan illustrating the dens invaginatus in the left maxillary lateral incisor. (**d–f**) Digital diagnostic setup. (**g–i**) Intraoral photographs of the final treatment outcomes

lateral incisor and consolidate the space between left maxillary lateral incisor and canine as conservatively as possible (Fig. 13.6g–i). Restoration with a ceramic crown would also have a feasible treatment option, but it is a less conservative restorative approach and carries the risk of pulpal sensitivity and/or exposure during tooth preparation. The patient was informed of the need for annual follow-up for the possibility of repairing or re-polishing of the resin composite restoration.

When evaluating the micro esthetics results, the gingival levels on the upper canines and lateral and central incisors were not ideal because the gingival margins of the lateral incisors were more apically positioned compared to the central incisors and canines (Fig. 13.6g). That was not a major concern to the patient due to the low smile line with no gingival display on smiling.

13.2.2 Management of Congenitally Missing Maxillary Lateral Incisors

Tooth agenesis is one of the most common dental anomalies and can be defined as the congenital absence of one or more primary or permanent teeth. Tooth agenesis of permanent dentition is commonly observed in the third molar and followed by the mandibular premolars and the maxillary lateral incisors [29]. Usually undesirable compensatory movement of the neighboring and/or opposing teeth accompanies maxillary lateral incisor agenesis. Treatment planning options for congenitally missing lateral incisor(s) are either orthodontic space closure by canines substituting for the lateral incisors and reshaping the canine to mimic lateral incisor form, shape, and color or by prosthodontics involvement approaches with or without orthodontic space openings, but most commonly with orthodontic space opening [30].

Although managing missing maxillary lateral incisor(s), either unilaterally or bilaterally, might initially seem straightforward, the reality is that it requires a great deal of careful planning and consideration before deciding which management approach should be considered to achieve a predictable esthetic and functional outcomes. Several authors considered evaluating various factors before selecting the suitable therapeutic option, such as patient's age, type of malocclusion, presence or absence of crowding, facial profile, canine size, shape and color, tooth-size proportion, and smile level (Fig. 13.7) [17, 31, 32]. Specific patient criteria for canine

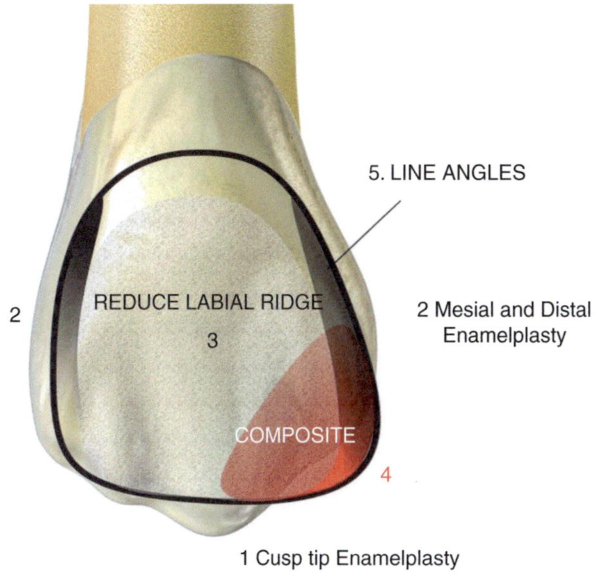

Fig. 13.7 Illustrative image demonstrating the transitional line angles and considerations when adjusting the maxillary canine to substitute for the maxillary lateral incisor

substitution should be considered in order to obtain an optimum outcome. Generally, patients with a straight to slightly convex facial profile with class II malocclusions with no crowding in the mandibular anterior teeth region or class I malocclusions with mandibular anterior crowding that necessitates tooth extractions are the types of malocclusions that present better final outcomes with the canine substitution approach.

13.2.2.1 Space Closure and Canine Substitution

The major advantage of canine substitution approach in adolescent patients is the possibility of completing the treatment at an early stage without the need of provisional restorative or prosthodontic treatment until the completion of facial growth, as is the case for the space-opening approach and implant replacement. Additionally, studies have shown that combining esthetic dentistry with the canine substitution approach yields a satisfactory long-term treatment outcome [33, 34]. Furthermore, the gingival health and dental papilla will change in synchrony with the patient's own teeth over time. However, esthetic matching of the functional occlusion may become compromised, especially with unilateral cases [22, 25].

The patient presented in Fig. 13.8 was a 13-year-old female with maxillary missing lateral incisors and complained of spacing between her anterior teeth. She presented with a class I malocclusion associated with retroclined mandibular incisors, normally inclined maxillary incisors and protrusive lips. She also had a retained primary left mandibular second molar.

It was decided after discussion with the patient and her parents to manage the malocclusion by following space closure approaches for the missing lateral incisors and mandibular second premolar to avoid the future need of prosthetic interventions and/or implant surgeries. Near the completion of orthodontic treatment, prosthodontics consultation was requested to consider reshaping the maxillary anterior teeth (Fig. 13.9).

Initial scans were obtained after removing the orthodontic archwires, but without removing the orthodontic brackets, using an intraoral scanner (TRIOS 3; 3Shape Inc., Copenhagen, Denmark). The intraoral scan file was incorporated into a design software (3Shape Trios Design Studio software, 3Shape Inc., Copenhagen, Denmark), and several digital diagnostic setups were planned. Three digital setups with their corresponding digital smile designs presented to the patient to determine the most esthetic outcome and decide whether only reshaping the maxillary canines is sufficient or the maxillary centrals and premolars should also be reshaped (Fig. 13.10).

After discussing the different possible scenarios with the patient, it was decided to reshape both maxillary centrals and maxillary canines by using resin-composite restorations. The mockup cast of reshaping maxillary central incisors and canines was printed by a 3D printer (Max X, ASIGA) using a resin material (DentaMODEL, ASIGA) and a vacuum-forming machine was used to fabricate a plastic template in order to be used as guide for reshaping the four anterior teeth (Fig. 13.10). A maxillary orthodontic retainer was modified according to the newly restored maxillary teeth, and the patient was instructed to wear it on a full-time basis to avoid creating diastema between the two maxillary central incisors.

13.2.2.2 Space Opening and Prosthodontic Replacement

Orthodontic space opening prosthodontic replacement of missing lateral incisor presents different prosthodontic treatment options including a dental implant-supported crown or a tooth-supported prosthesis. The tooth-supported prosthesis can be a resin-bonded fixed dental prothesis (FDP), a cantilever FDP, or a conventional FDP.

One of the essential considerations before deciding the most appropriate prosthodontic option is the conservation of tooth structure. From a restorative prospective, two major principles are generally followed when managing congenitally missing teeth. The first principle is to establish appropriate horizontal and vertical spaces for the missing teeth that correspond to the size of the natural teeth to be replaced. The second principle is to optimize the position of the existing teeth within the dental arches and to position the anterior teeth in an ideal overjet and overbite with proper inclination

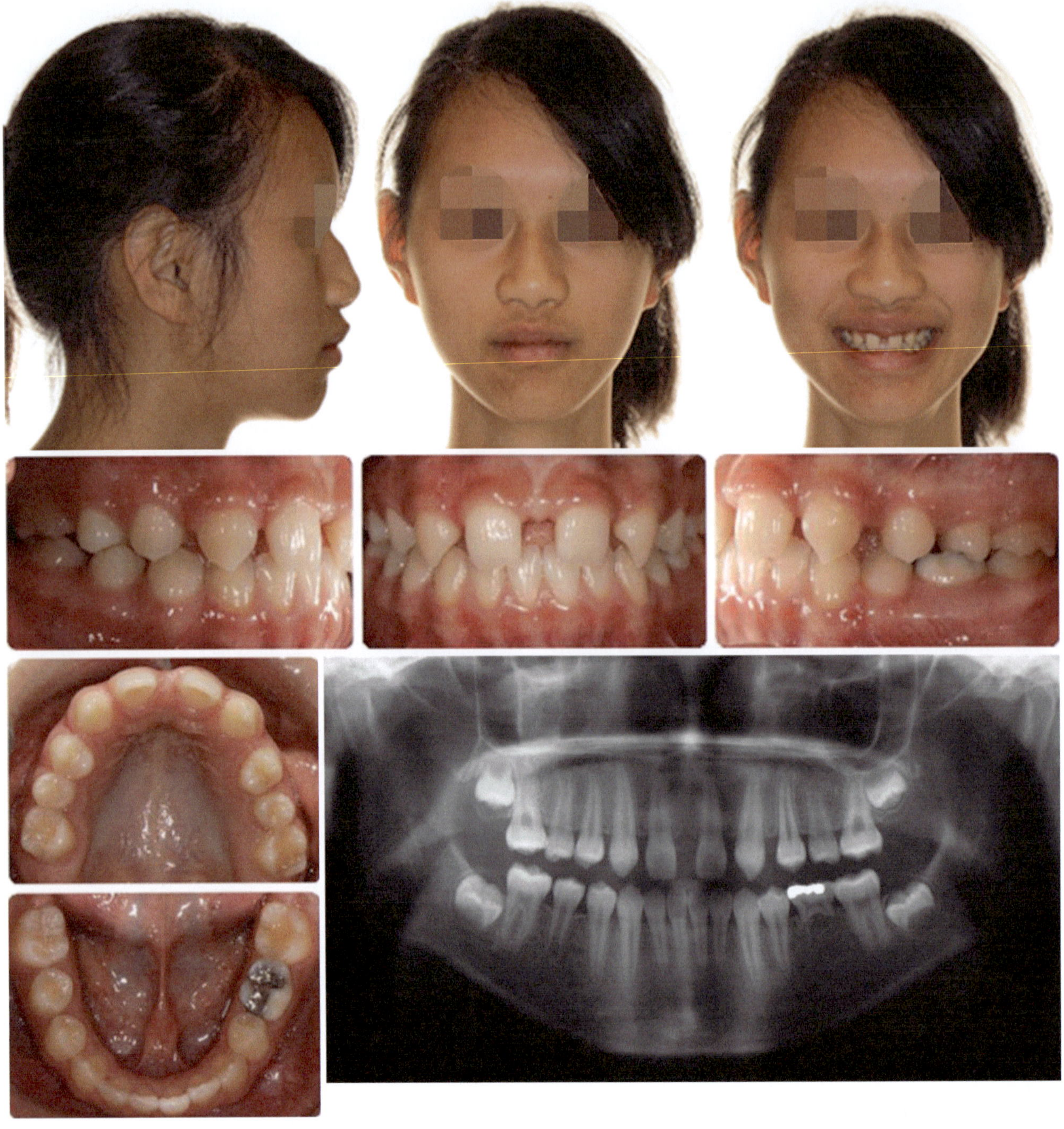

Fig. 13.8 Initial pre-orthodontic patient records. Note the congenitally missing maxillary lateral incisors. (Courtesy of Dr. Hajer Alsabban)

as much as clinically feasible without compromising the hard and soft tissues. This concept will often provide appropriate anterior guidance during excursion movements. In some circumstances, teeth can be moved into a deficient edentulous ridge to encourage the formation of alveolar bone in order to eliminate or reduce the need for bone augmentation prior to implant placement. For instance, it was proposed by Dr. Kokich that facilitating the eruption of the permanent canine mesially into the space of the missing lateral incisor can establish a more favorable implant site development. The permanent canine can then be distalized to develop the implant site with adequate bucco-lingual alveolar bone dimensions that can house an implant without the need of a bone graft [18].

Resin-Bonded Fixed Dental Prosthesis (Resin-Bonded FDP)

A resin-bonded FDP is commonly used as an interim solution to restore a single tooth space in growing children and young adults until a definitive long-term solution can be

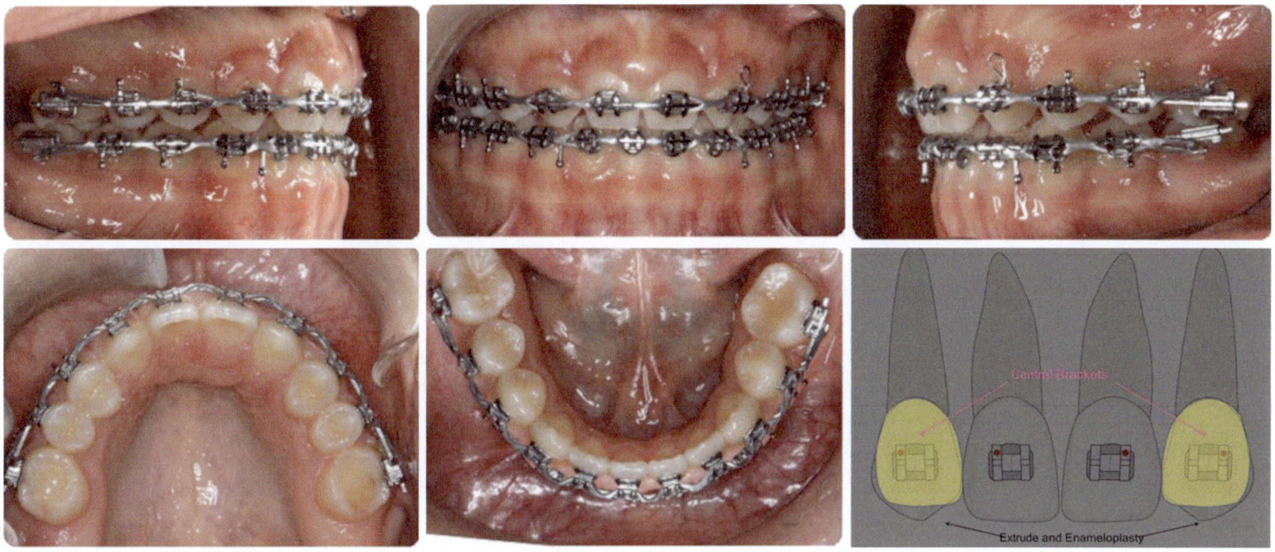

Fig. 13.9 Intraoral photographs after orthodontic space closure and before the prosthodontic consultation. (Courtesy of Dr. Hajer Alsabban)

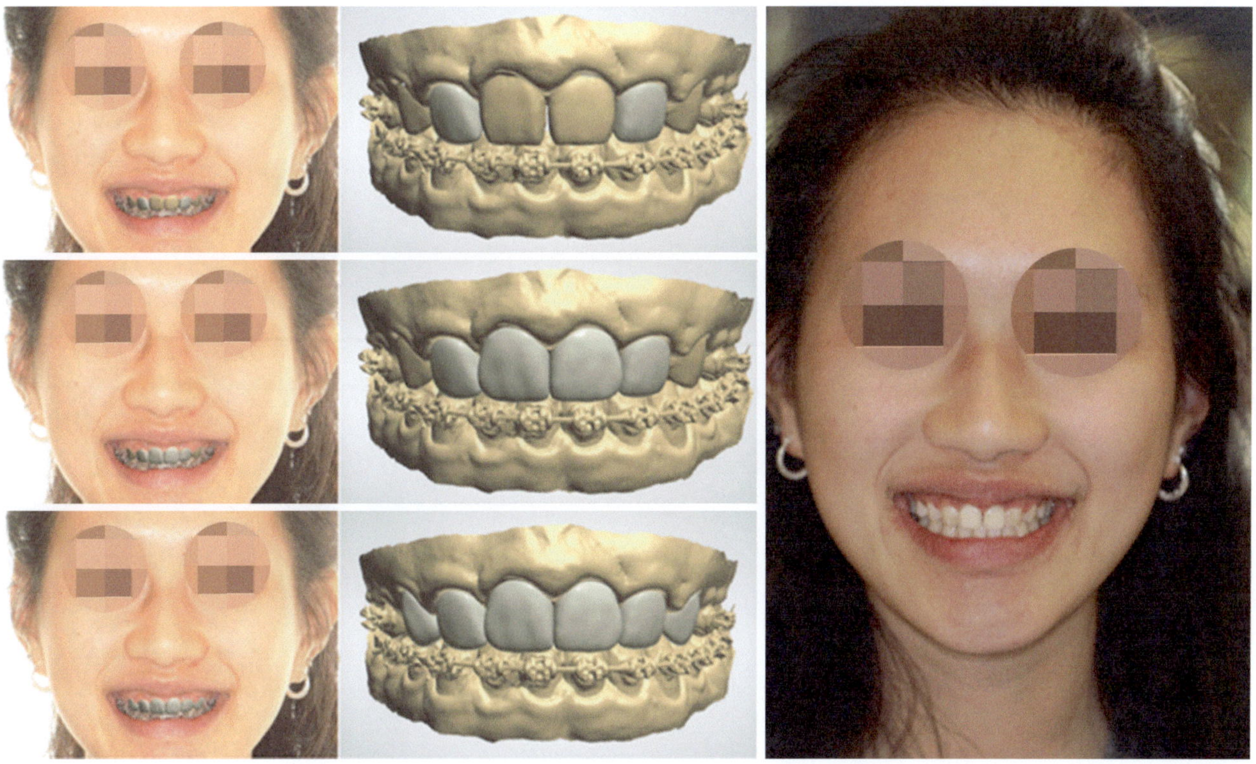

Fig. 13.10 Left column: Different digital smile designs. Middle column: Digital diagnostic setups. Right column: Post-restorative photograph after completion of the orthodontic treatment and restorative buildup of the maxillary anterior teeth with composite resin

employed. The advantage of resin-bonded FDP is that it requires minimal preparation of the adjacent teeth and is considered the most conservative tooth-supported fixed option. In addition, the fabrication time is short, and it costs less compared to a conventional FDP [35]. Although the success rate is significantly lower than that of the conventional FDP due to high debonding rate [36], it remains a viable short-term solution, until patients complete their facial growth and are more clinically suitable to receive an implant-supported prosthesis.

Resin-bonded FDP still demonstrates a high risk of debonding (15–20%) despite the advancement of dental materials and techniques of bonding agents [36]. This option is restricted to patient with certain clinical criteria that include a shallow to normal overbite, normally proclined maxillary central incisors and the absence of heavy occlusal contact on the maxillary anterior teeth. Cases of deep overbites, mobile teeth, and increased proclination of maxillary incisors showed a higher rate of failure, particularly, in patients with parafunctional habits [17].

Figure 13.11 shows an 11-year-old female patient who initially presented to the orthodontic clinic to manage spacing between the maxillary teeth due to congenitally missing maxillary lateral incisors. After consultation with the patient and her parents, it was decided to open spaces for the placement of dental implants to replace the maxillary lateral incisors when facial growth is complete.

After completion of orthodontic treatment at age 14 years, the patient received an orthodontic retainer with provisional acrylic teeth to replace the maxillary lateral incisors; however, the patient was not satisfied with the esthetic properties of the acrylic teeth. Upon prosthodontic consultation, the patient was presented with the option of restoring the missing maxillary lateral incisors with resin-bonded FDP using high translucent lithium disilicate ceramic materials until she completes her facial growth (Fig. 13.12).

After removing the maxillary fixed retainer, maxillary central incisors required a minimum finish line preparation for the fabrication of the resin-bonded FDP. However, there was no need to reduce that palatal surfaces of the incisors due to the deep concavities of the palatal surfaces. An intraoral scan was obtained using an intraoral dental scanner (TRIOS 3; 3Shape Inc., Copenhagen, Denmark). The margin of the preparation was defined digitally to facilitate the communication with the laboratory technician (Fig. 13.13).

The scan Standard Tessellation Language file (STL file) was transferred to the laboratory technician to design the prosthesis digitally (Fig. 13.14). The resin-bonded FDP was designed with sufficient thickness that can serve as a fixed retainer to avoid diastema formation.

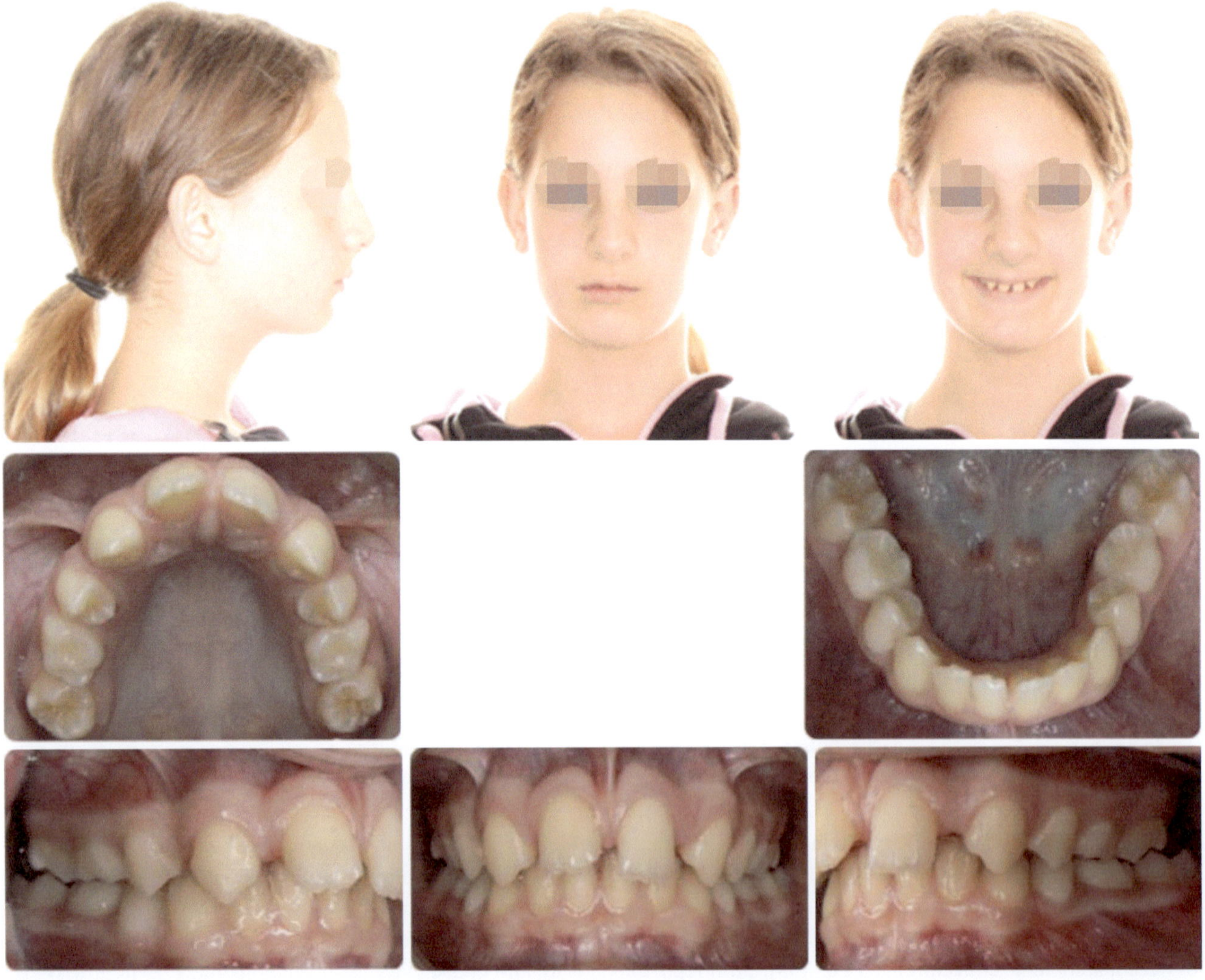

Fig. 13.11 Pre-orthodontic treatment records of a patient with congenitally missing maxillary lateral incisors. (Courtesy of Dr. Kathleen Martin)

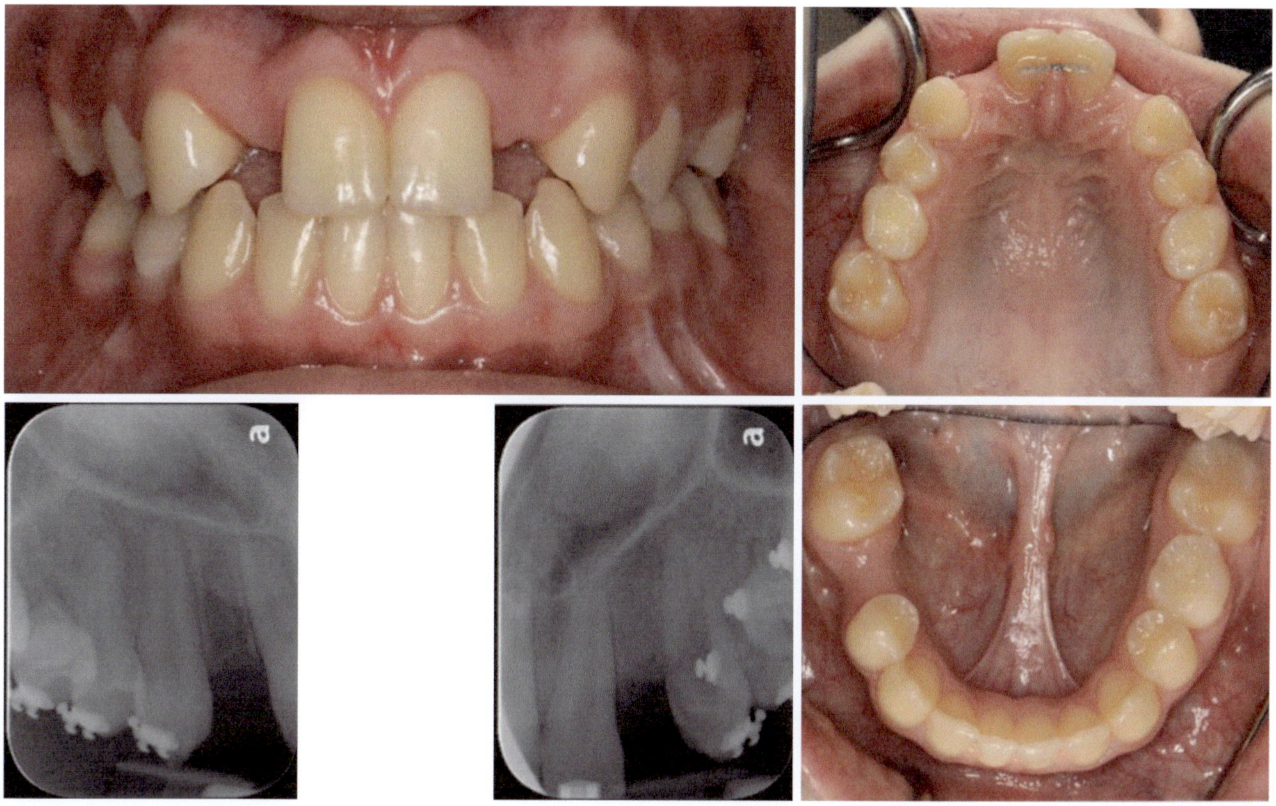

Fig. 13.12 Post-orthodontic treatment records after opening the space to replace the missing maxillary lateral incisors. (Courtesy of Dr. Kathleen Martin)

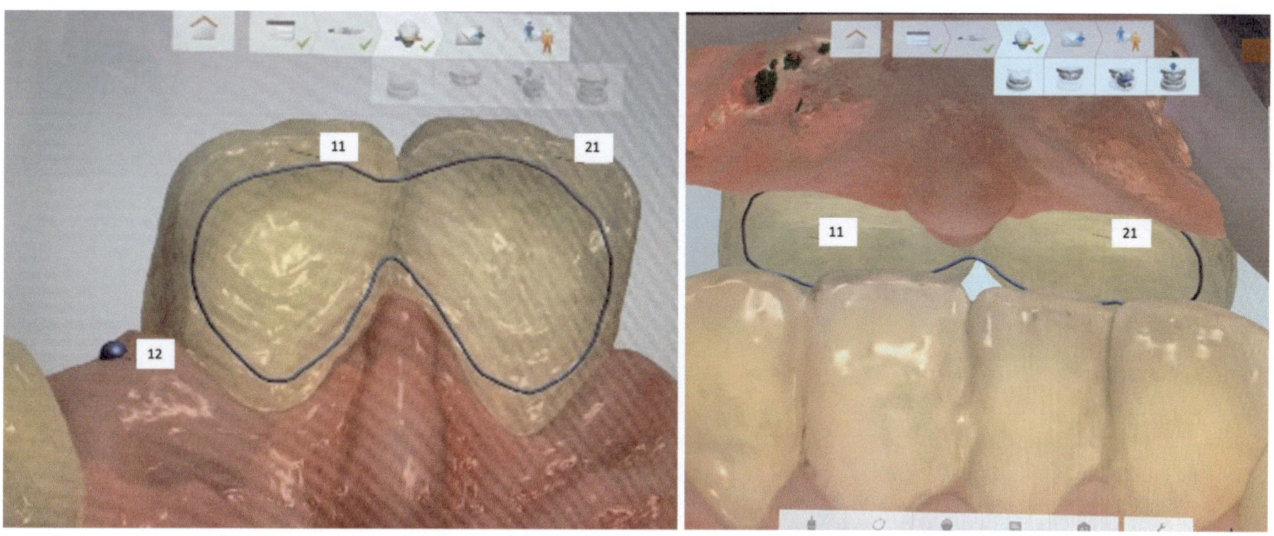

Fig. 13.13 Digital intraoral scan showing the design of the planned preparation margins. This facilitates the communication with the laboratory technician and allows proper visualization of the palatal surface of the maxillary incisors

The prosthesis was milled using lithium disilicate blocks (IPS e.max CAD, Ivoclar Vivadent, Liechtenstein). After clinical try-in was confirmed, the standard protocol of bonding lithium disilicate to tooth structure was performed to bond the prosthesis to the tooth structure using resin cement (RelyX™ unicem, 3M) (Fig. 13.15).

Cantilevered Fixed Dental Prosthesis

Another option to replace MLIA is the cantilevered FDP. This option is valid because the geometry of the maxillary canine (root length and diameter) can effectively serve as an ideal abutment for the cantilevered FDP option. This option can be successful if the occlusion of the pontic can be managed with

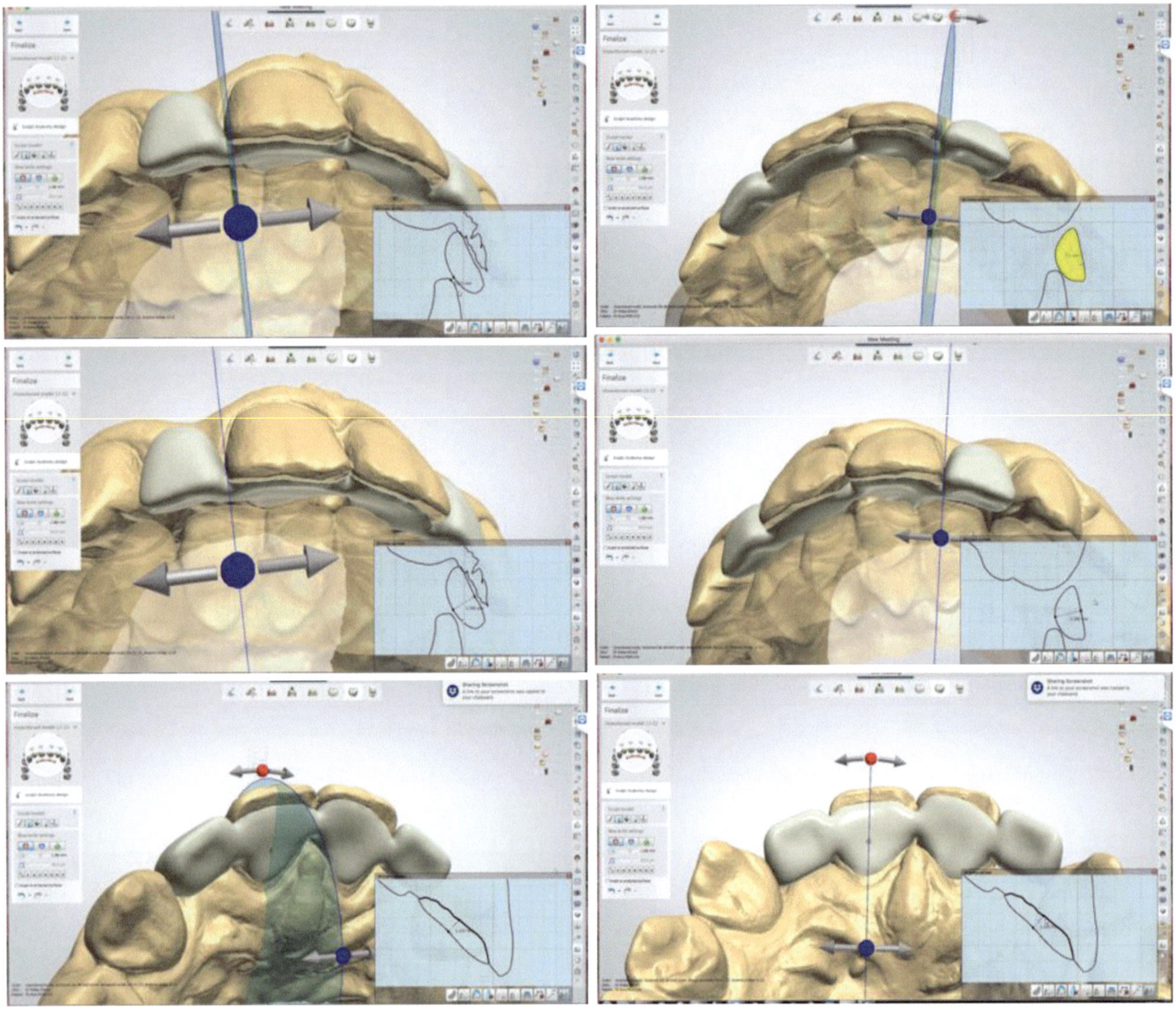

Fig. 13.14 Digital designing of splinted resin-bonded fixed dental prosthesis. The digital designing ensured adequate thickness and size (yellow) of the prosthesis especially at the connectors. Designing the prothesis digitally enhanced the visualization and optimization of the occlusion. (Courtesy of Mr. Jae Won Sim B.I.D at Paul Ro Dental Laboratory, Vancouver, Canada)

minimal eccentric contact. A partial coverage retainer can be used on the canine if there is no need to alter the shape of the canine facially; otherwise, the full coverage retainer should be considered to retain the cantilevered lateral incisor pontic. Excessive eccentric contact of the pontic showed higher risk of fracture of the restoration, loosening of the restoration, or migration of the abutment [37].

Conventional Fixed Dental Prosthesis

Conventional fixed dental prosthesis (CFDP) is considered the least conservative option to replace missing teeth. It is often indicated when the adjacent teeth have significant caries or fractures or in cases where a previous FDP needs to be replaced or if the implant-supported prosthesis option is contraindicated for the patient. Furthermore, it can be considered an option in cases that necessitate a significant alteration in the facial morphology of the teeth adjacent to the maxillary lateral incisor. The advantage of having CFDP is that it allows better control of the final occlusal outcomes. However, an important concern that should be addressed for the CFDP option is the alignment and parallelism between the long axis of maxillary central incisor(s) and the facial surface of canine(s) along the common pathway to avoid over-preparing the teeth and to achieve a parallel path of insertion. This also provides sufficient space accommodate the CFDP connector. Over-preparing the teeth, especially in the young patients, can lead to pulp exposure and necessitate the need for root canal treatment and, possibly, shorten the longevity of the teeth.

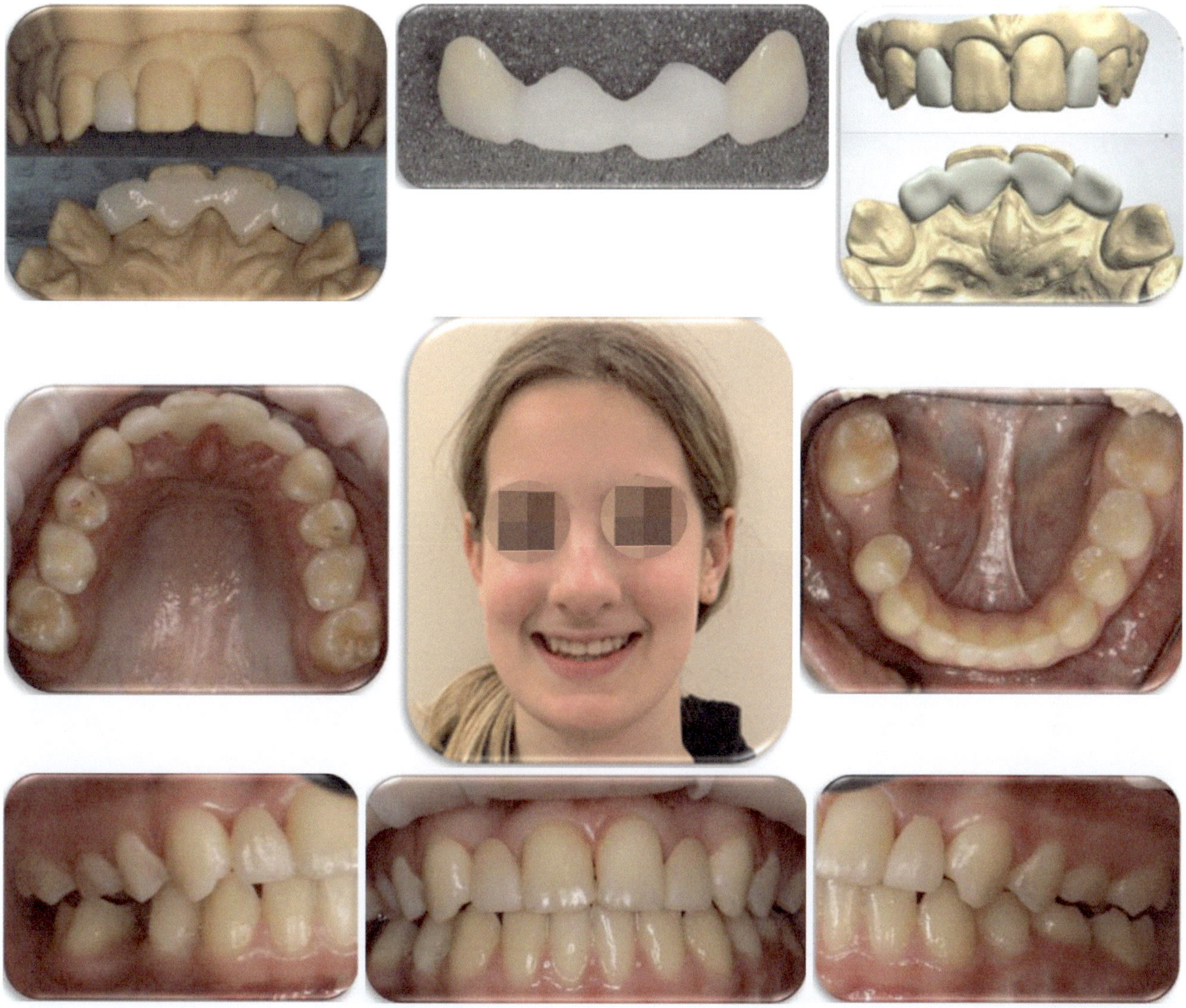

Fig. 13.15 Final records after the orthodontic and prosthodontic treatment of missing maxillary lateral incisors with lithium disilicate resin-bonded fixed dental prosthesis

13.2.3 Management of a Unilateral Impacted Canine

Figures 13.16 and 13.17 illustrate an impacted right maxillary canine in a 13-year-old female patient. The patient presented with a convex profile, competent lips, and mild hyperdivergent skeletal class II. Dentally, she had a class I molar relationship and a class II canine relationship on the left side with moderate curve of Spee and severe crowding in both the maxillary and the mandibular arches. The overjet and overbite were 1 mm and 5%, respectively, and the maxillary and mandibular incisors were proclined and protrusive. Maxillary and mandibular dental midlines were shifted to the right by 2 mm. The right maxillary canine and right mandibular second premolar were impacted.

The orthodontic treatment plan involved a fixed edgewise appliances after the extraction of the right maxillary canine, left maxillary first molar, left mandibular first premolar, and right mandibular second premolar. Premolar–canine substitution was planned in the maxillary right quadrant, and an interdisciplinary approach was followed to achieve optimum restoration of esthetics and function. The prosthodontist was consulted near the end of finishing stage of orthodontic treatment to confirm the desired final location of the right maxillary first and second premolars (Figs. 13.18 and 13.19).

Digital diagnostic setup was performed after digitally coping the shape of the contralateral canine and superimposing over the right maxillary first premolar (Fig. 13.20a, b). The setup was then finalized according to the optimum esthetic and function requirements (Fig. 13.20c–e). The patient was presented with two conservative options, resin-

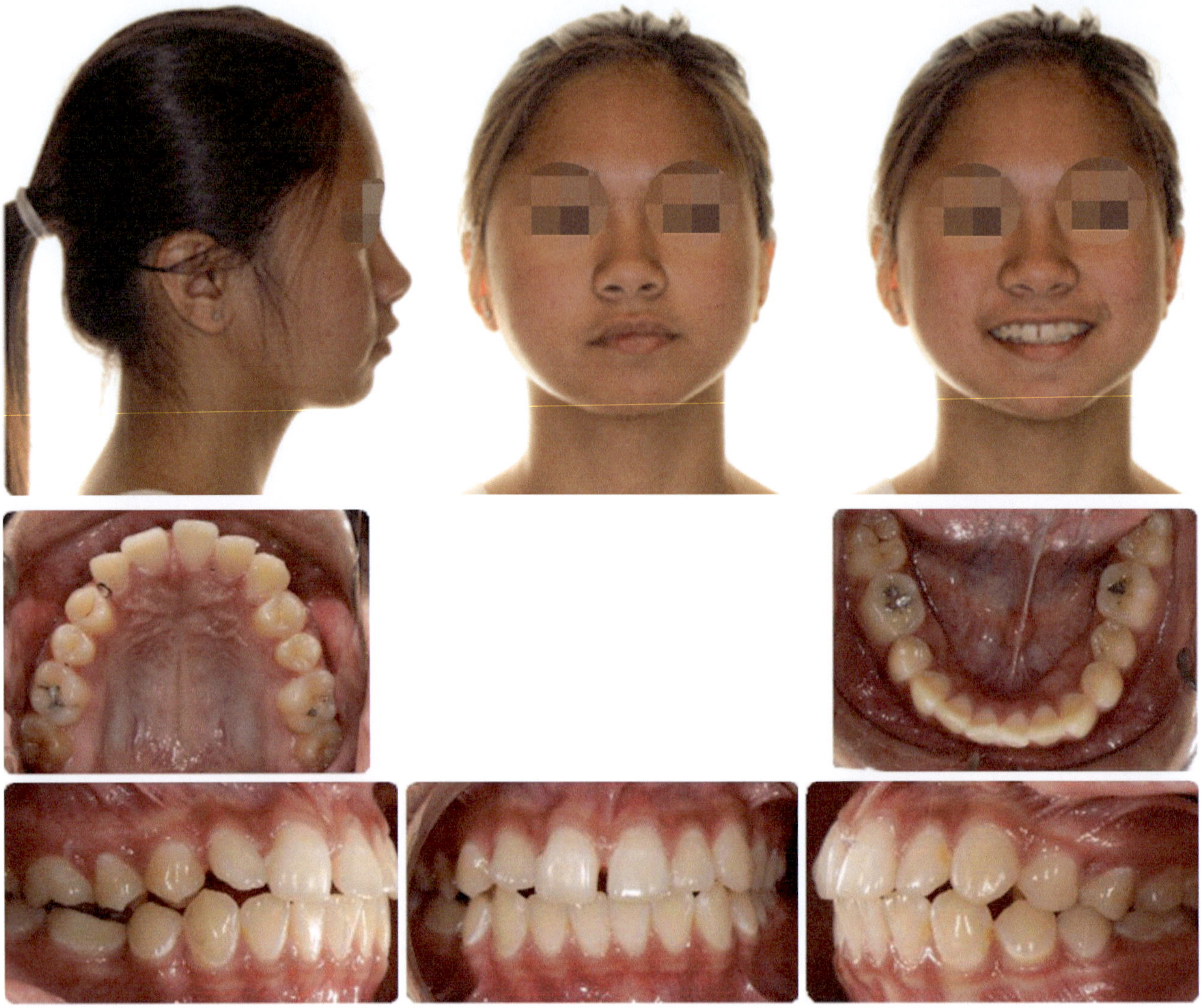

Fig. 13.16 Initial pre-orthodontic treatment records of a patient with impacted right maxillary canine and right mandibular second premolar. (Courtesy of Dr. Hajer Alsabban)

bond composite build up or porcelain veneers; however, she preferred the resin-composite option. A vacuum forming machine was used to fabricate a plastic template according to the digital diagnostic setup in order to build up the right maxillary first and second premolars with resin-composite restoration (Fig. 13.21).

13.2.4 Management of a Deep Bite Case

The patient in Fig. 13.22 is a 52-year-old female who presented to the clinic asking for veneers to improve her smile. She presented with a deep bite and associated with uneven wear of the occlusal surface of the anterior teeth. She also had an uneven gingival architecture.

The treatment plan was to improve alignment and achieve a functional occlusion to minimize the amount of tooth preparation needed combined with having a mutually protected occlusion. The patient had some periodontal and oral maxillofacial surgery prior to orthodontic treatment. Orthodontic treatment spanned over 18 months to correct bite and achieve an optimal occlusion and gingival architecture. This also minimizes the amount of tooth structure removal during the veneer preparation.

After the completion of the orthodontic treatment, the dentition was scanned digitally using an intraoral scanner, and a 2D virtual smile design was performed to involve the patient in the design and decision process. The 2D smile design was communicated to the laboratory technician on the exact size and shape of veneer design in mind. After that

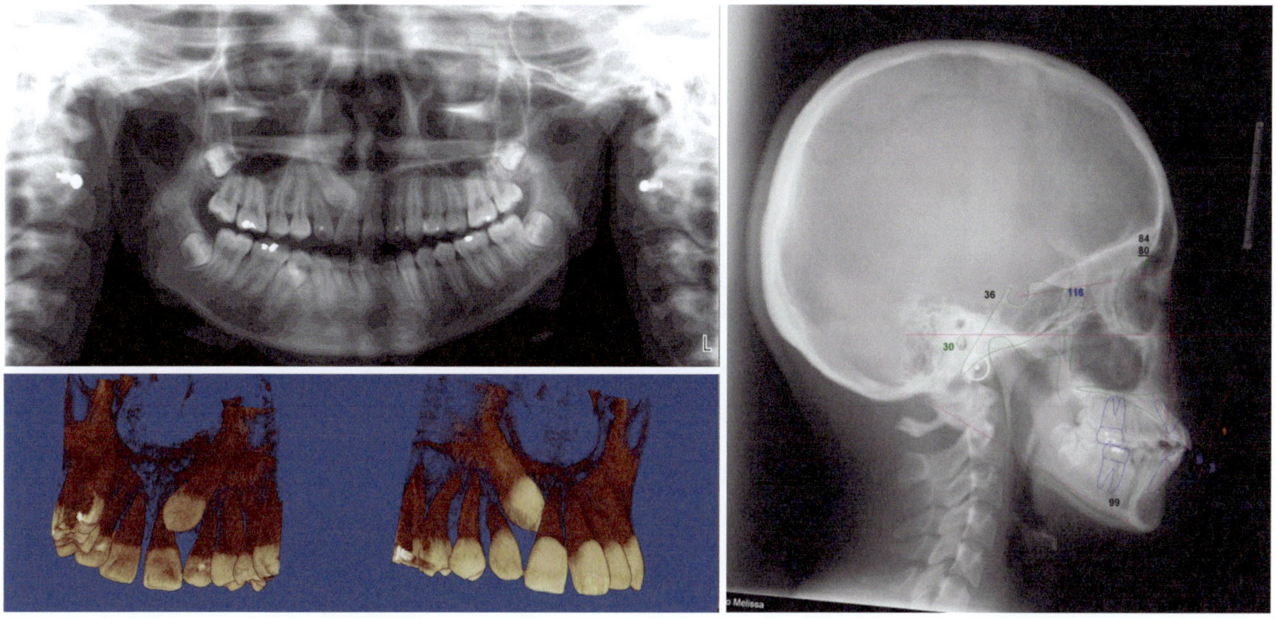

Fig. 13.17 Pre-orthodontic treatment records, top left; panoramic radiograph, bottom left; cone bean computerized tomography (CBCT) to locate impacted maxillary right canine, right; Cephalometric radiograph

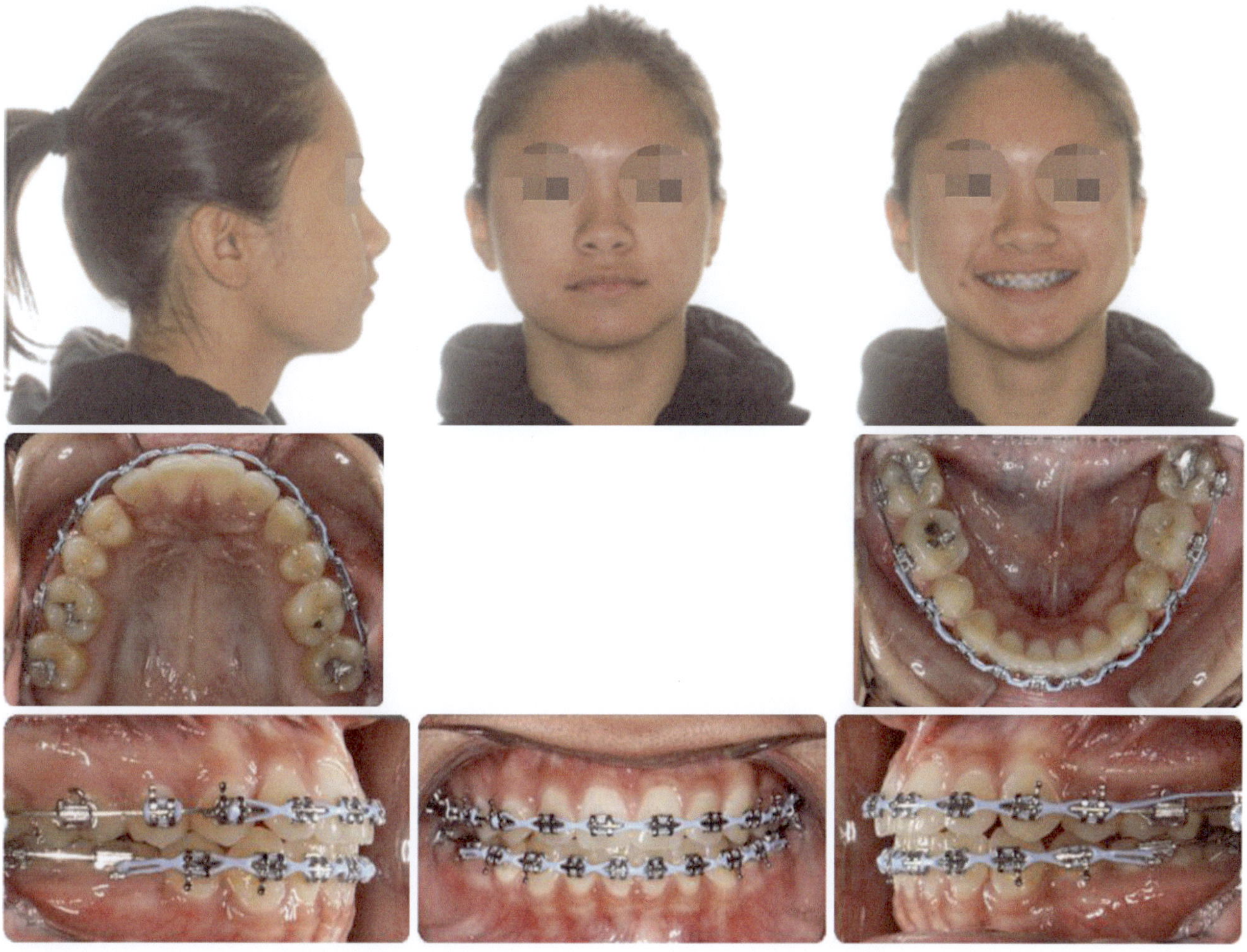

Fig. 13.18 Progress records during orthodontic treatment and after extracting impacted right maxillary canine and right mandibular second premolar. (Courtesy of Dr. Hajer Alsabban)

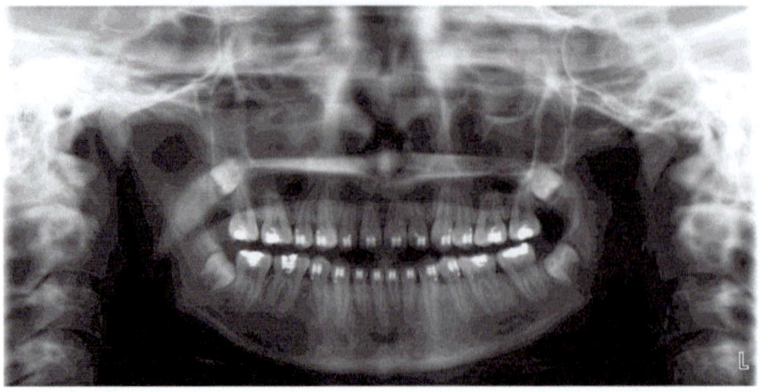

Fig. 13.19 Progress panoramic radiograph at the finishing stage of orthodontic treatment

step, a 3D digital smile design was performed, and its STL file was obtained (Fig. 13.23). A model was printed using a 3D printer and a vacuum forming machine was used to fabricate a plastic template in order to be used for clinical esthetic try-in. An esthetic mock-up was satisfactory after trying it on in the laboratory with chemically cured acrylic resin.

The template was also used as a preparation guide for veneers. Feldspathic porcelain was the material choice selected for the fabrication of the veneers due to the high esthetic demand of the patient. Preparations were performed and provisionals were placed, then in the following appointments veneers were fitted and cemented (Fig. 13.24).

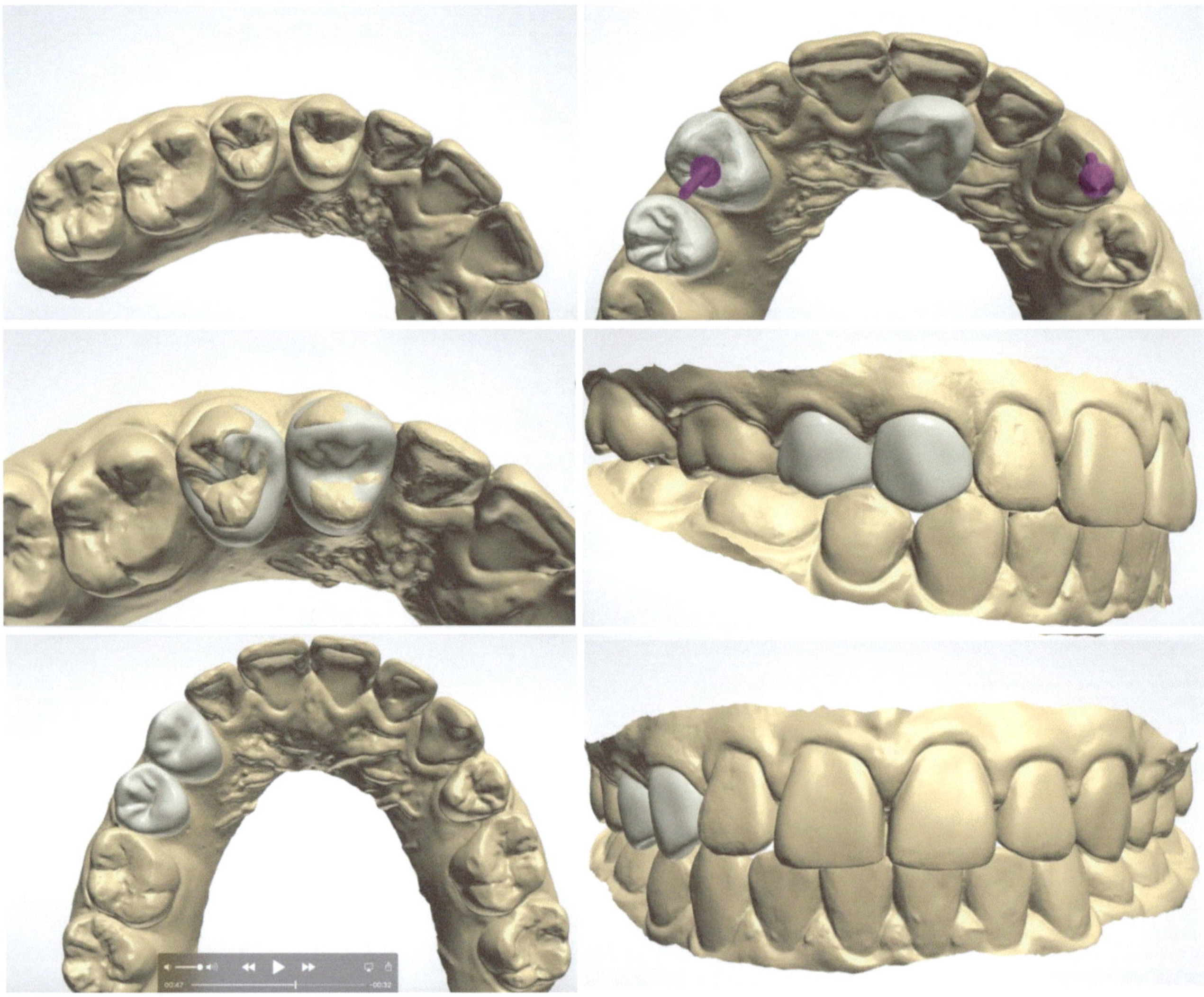

Fig. 13.20 (**a**) Digital simulation of the obtained intraoral scan. (**b**) Diagnostic mock-up of right maxillary first and second premolars was designed using 3Shape Trios Design Studio software. The black arrow points at a digital copy of the left maxillary canine which was flipped to help with designing the buildup for the left maxillary first premolars. It should be noted that the lingual cusp of the right maxillary first premolar was maintained. (**c–f**) The digital mock-up was finalized according to the esthetic and functional requirements

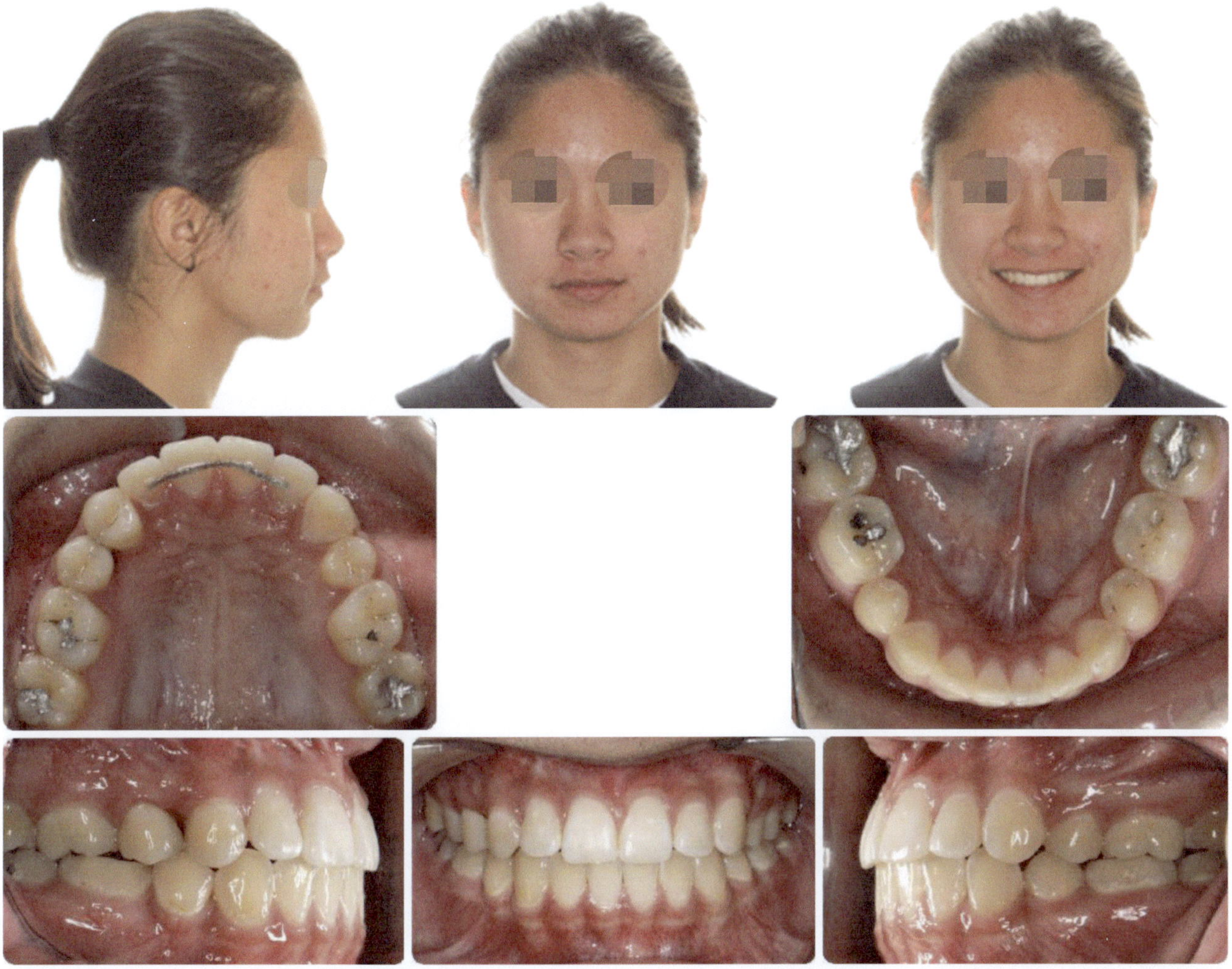

Fig. 13.21 Final records after the prosthodontic management of the reshaping right maxillary first and second premolars

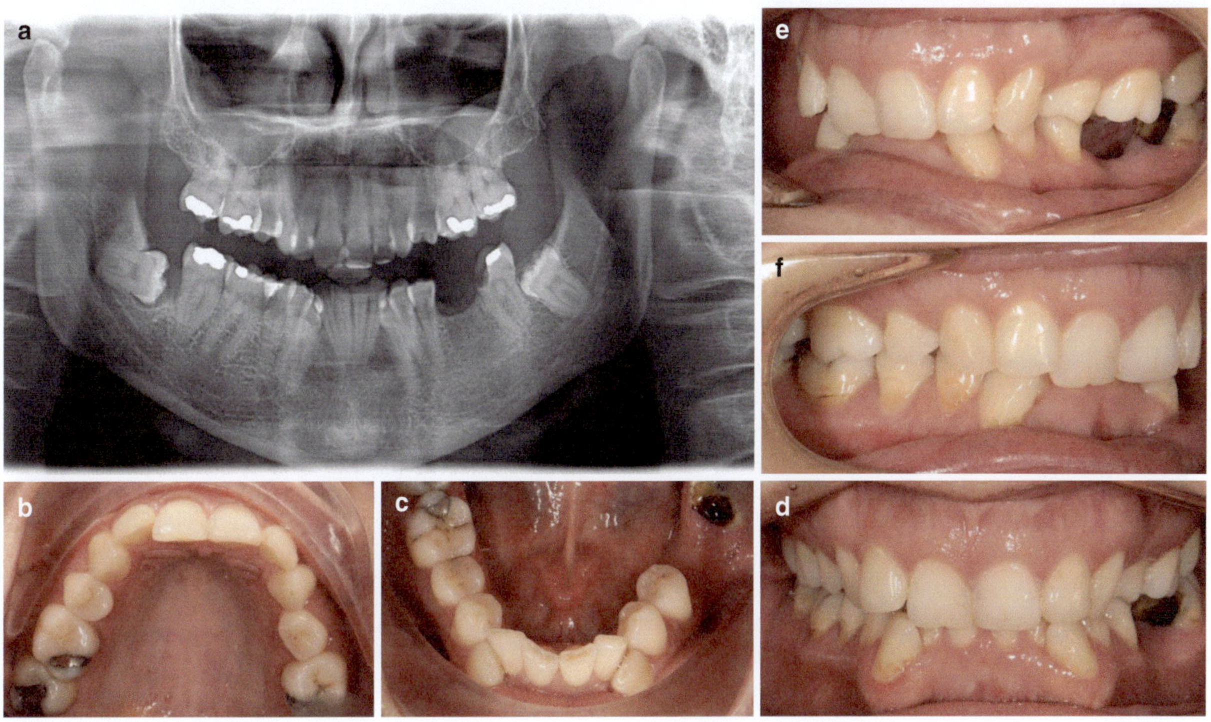

Fig. 13.22 Initial preoperative treatment records. (**a**) Panoramic radiograph. (**b–f**) Intraoral photographs

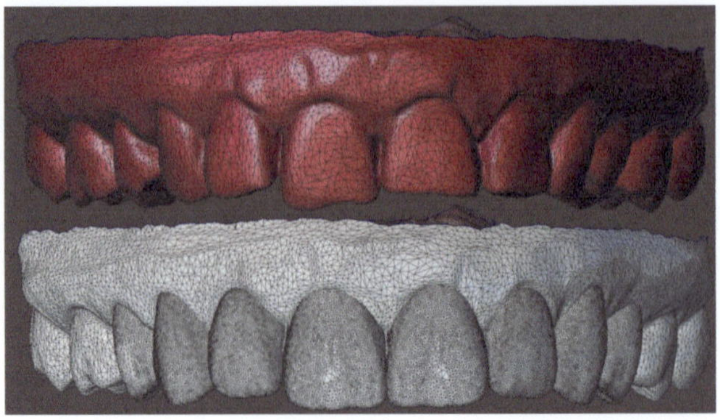

Fig. 13.23 The red digital cast is the STL file of the preliminarily intraoral scan, and the gray digital cast is the STL file after digital setups of the complete maxillary arch

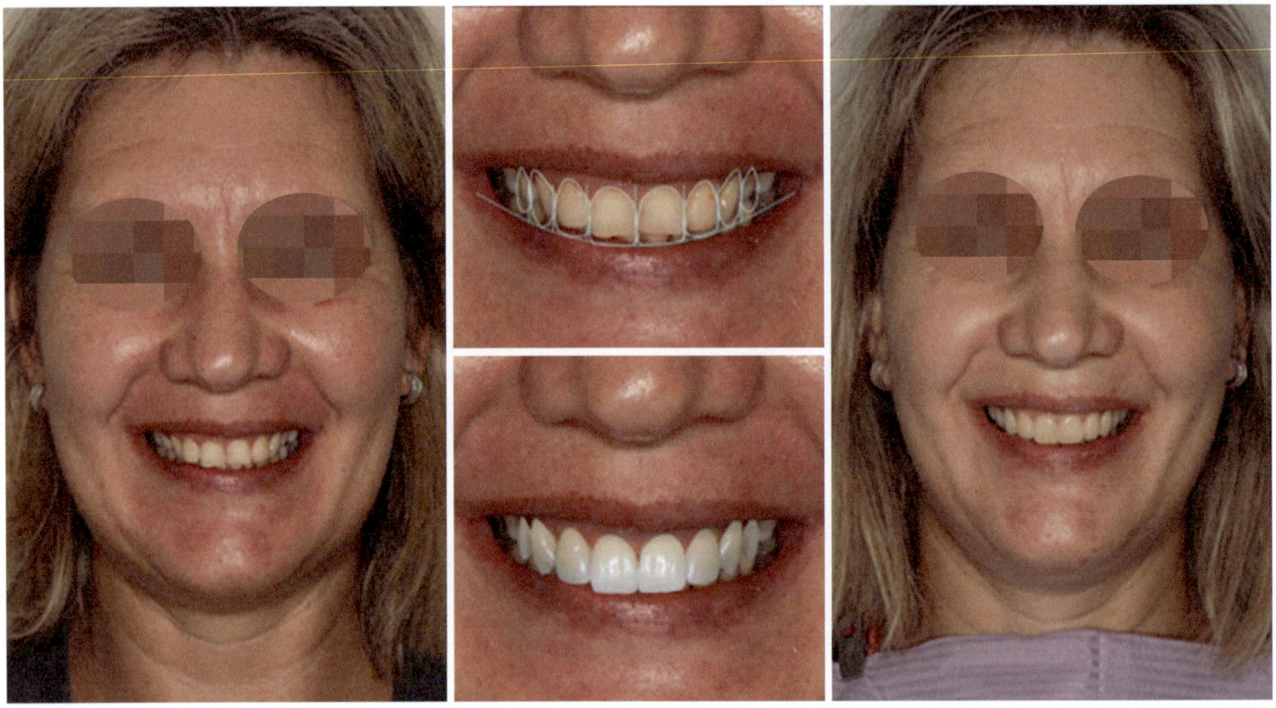

Fig. 13.24 Left and top middle photos are the initial pretreatment records, and the lower middle is the digital setups for the complete maxillary teeth; to the right is the posttreatment photograph

13.3 Summary

Digital workflow provides an efficient route for the interdisciplinary orthodontic-prosthodontic treatment planning process. It serves as a tool for 3D visualization and facilitates communication during treatment planning and execution. This chapter presented several orthodontic-prosthodontic cases that incorporated digital diagnostic setups in their treatment progress and planning. Intraoral digital scans provide high-quality simulations and images for diagnosis and the fabrication of final prostheses. Incorporating the digital diagnostic setups in your treatment planning phase helps with identifying the final orthodontic position of the teeth according to the restorative plan and consequently allows the fabrication of predictable restorative work.

Acknowledgments The authors would like to thank Mr. Jae Won Sim B.I.D at Paul Ro Dental Laboratory, Vancouver, Canada for performing the dental laboratory work. The authors would like to acknowledge and thank Professor Tarek El-Bialy at the University of Alberta, Canada for reviewing the chapter.

References

1. Molly Bawn. 1st ed. London: Smith, Elder and Company; 1878.
2. Blatz MB, Chiche G, Bahat O, Roblee R, Coachman C, Heymann HO. Evolution of aesthetic dentistry. J Dent Res. 2019;98(12):1294–304.
3. Henson ST, Lindauer SJ, Gardner WG, Shroff B, Tufekci E, Best AM. Influence of dental esthetics on social perceptions of adolescents judged by peers. Am J Orthod Dentofac Orthop. 2011;140(3):389–95.

4. Kokich VO Jr, Kiyak HA, Shapiro PA. Comparing the perception of dentists and lay people to altered dental esthetics. J Esthet Dent. 1999;11(6):311–24.
5. Machado AW, Moon W, Gandini LG Jr. Influence of maxillary incisor edge asymmetries on the perception of smile esthetics among orthodontists and laypersons. Am J Orthod Dentofac Orthop. 2013;143(5):658–64.
6. Passia N, Blatz M, Strub JR. Is the smile line a valid parameter for esthetic evaluation? A systematic literature review. Eur J Esthet Dent. 2011;6(3):314–27.
7. Davis NC. Smile design. Dent Clin North Am. 2007;51(2):299–318, vii.
8. Calamia JR, Levine JB, Lipp M, Cisneros G, Wolff MS. Smile design and treatment planning with the help of a comprehensive esthetic evaluation form. Dent Clin North Am. 2011;55(2):187–209, vii.
9. Belser UC, editor. Esthetics checklist for the fixed prosthesis. Part II: biscuit-bake try-in. Chicago: Quintessence Publishing Co; 1982.
10. McLaren EA, Garber DA, Figueira J. The photoshop smile design technique (part 1): digital dental photography. Compend Contin Educ Dent. 2013;34(10):772, 4, 6 passim.
11. Magne P, Salem P, Magne M. Influence of symmetry and balance on visual perception of a white female smile. J Prosthet Dent. 2018;120(4):573–82.
12. Kokich V. Esthetics and anterior tooth position: an orthodontic perspective. Part II: vertical position. J Esthet Dent. 1993;5(4):174–8.
13. Magne P, Magne M, Belser U. Natural and restorative oral esthetics. Part I: rationale and basic strategies for successful esthetic rehabilitations. J Esthet Dent. 1993;5(4):161–73.
14. Mahn E, Sampaio CS, Pereira da Silva B, Stanley K, Valdes AM, Gutierrez J, et al. Comparing the use of static versus dynamic images to evaluate a smile. J Prosthet Dent. 2020;123(5):739–46.
15. Silva BP, Mahn E, Stanley K, Coachman C. The facial flow concept: an organic orofacial analysis—the vertical component. J Prosthet Dent. 2019;121(2):189–94.
16. Jamilian A, Perillo L, Rosa M. Missing upper incisors: a retrospective study of orthodontic space closure versus implant. Prog Orthod. 2015;16:2.
17. Kinzer GA, Kokich VO Jr. Managing congenitally missing lateral incisors. Part III: single-tooth implants. J Esthet Restor Dent. 2005;17(4):202–10.
18. Kokich VG. Maxillary lateral incisor implants: planning with the aid of orthodontics. J Oral Maxillofac Surg. 2004;62(9 Suppl 2):48–56.
19. Bernard JP, Schatz JP, Christou P, Belser U, Kiliaridis S. Long-term vertical changes of the anterior maxillary teeth adjacent to single implants in young and mature adults. A retrospective study. J Clin Periodontol. 2004;31(11):1024–8.
20. De-Marchi LM, Pini NI, Ramos AL, Pascotto RC. Smile attractiveness of patients treated for congenitally missing maxillary lateral incisors as rated by dentists, laypersons, and the patients themselves. J Prosthet Dent. 2014;112(3):540–6.
21. Nordquist GG, McNeill RW. Orthodontic vs. restorative treatment of the congenitally absent lateral incisor—long term periodontal and occlusal evaluation. J Periodontol. 1975;46(3):139–43.
22. Robertsson S, Mohlin B. The congenitally missing upper lateral incisor. A retrospective study of orthodontic space closure versus restorative treatment. Eur J Orthod. 2000;22(6):697–710.
23. Kokich VO Jr, Kinzer GA, Janakievski J. Congenitally missing maxillary lateral incisors: restorative replacement. Counterpoint. Am J Orthod Dentofac Orthop. 2011;139(4):435, 7, 9 passim.
24. McNeill RW, Joondeph DR. Congenitally absent maxillary lateral incisors: treatment planning considerations. Angle Orthod. 1973;43(1):24–9.
25. Zachrisson BU, Rosa M, Toreskog S. Congenitally missing maxillary lateral incisors: canine substitution. Point. Am J Orthod Dentofac Orthop. 2011;139(4):434, 6, 8 passim.
26. DiPietro GJ, Moergeli JR. Significance of the Frankfort-mandibular plane angle to prosthodontics. J Prosthet Dent. 1976;36(6):624–35.
27. Bolton W. The clinical application of a tooth size analysis. Am J Orthod. 1962;48(7):504–29.
28. Oehlers FA. Dens invaginatus (dilated composite odontome). I. Variations of the invagination process and associated anterior crown forms. Oral Surg Oral Med Oral Pathol. 1957;10(11):1204–18 contd.
29. Dermaut LR, Goeffers KR, De Smit AA. Prevalence of tooth agenesis correlated with jaw relationship and dental crowding. Am J Orthod Dentofac Orthop. 1986;90(3):204–10.
30. Silveira GS, de Almeida NV, Pereira DM, Mattos CT, Mucha JN. Prosthetic replacement vs space closure for maxillary lateral incisor agenesis: a systematic review. Am J Orthod Dentofac Orthop. 2016;150(2):228–37.
31. Kinzer GA, Kokich VO Jr. Managing congenitally missing lateral incisors. Part II: tooth-supported restorations. J Esthet Restor Dent. 2005;17(2):76–84.
32. Kokich VO Jr, Kinzer GA. Managing congenitally missing lateral incisors. Part I: canine substitution. J Esthet Restor Dent. 2005;17(1):5–10.
33. Armbruster PC, Gardiner DM, Whitley JB Jr, Flerra J. The congenitally missing maxillary lateral incisor. Part 2: assessing dentists' preferences for treatment. World J Orthod. 2005;6(4):376–81.
34. Armbruster PC, Gardiner DM, Whitley JB Jr, Flerra J. The congenitally missing maxillary lateral incisor. Part 1: esthetic judgment of treatment options. World J Orthod. 2005;6(4):369–75.
35. Antonarakis GS, Prevezanos P, Gavric J, Christou P. Agenesis of maxillary lateral incisor and tooth replacement: cost-effectiveness of different treatment alternatives. Int J Prosthodont. 2014;27(3):257–63.
36. Mourshed B, Samran A, Alfagih A, Samran A, Abdulrab S, Kern M. Anterior cantilever resin-bonded fixed dental prostheses: a review of the literature. J Prosthodont. 2018;27(3):266–75.
37. Hochman N, Ginio I, Ehrlich J. The cantilever fixed partial denture: a 10-year follow-up. J Prosthet Dent. 1987;58(5):542–5.

Index

J.-M. Retrouvey, M.-N. Abdallah (eds.), *3D Diagnosis and Treatment Planning in Orthodontics*,
https://doi.org/10.1007/978-3-030-57223-5

MIX
Papier aus verantwortungsvollen Quellen
Paper from responsible sources
FSC® C105338

If you have any concerns about our products,
you can contact us on
ProductSafety@springernature.com

In case Publisher is established outside the EU,
the EU authorized representative is:
Springer Nature Customer Service Center GmbH
Europaplatz 3, 69115 Heidelberg, Germany

Printed by Libri Plureos GmbH
in Hamburg, Germany